Cirrhosis

A practical guide to management

Cirrhosis

A practical guide to management

EDITED BY

Samuel S. Lee, MD, FRCPC

Professor of Medicine
University of Calgary Cumming School of Medicine
Calgary, Canada

Richard Moreau, MD

Deputy Director
INSERM, U114, Centre de Recherche sur l'Inflammation (CRI), Paris, France;
UMRS 1149, Université Paris Diderot-Paris 7, Paris, France;
Département Hospitalo-Universitaire UNITY, Service d'Hépatologie, Hôpital Beaujon, APHP, Clichy, France

FIRST EDITION

FOREWORD BY SAMUEL S. LEE AND RICHARD MOREAU

WILEY Blackwell

Registered office: John Wiley & Sons, Ltd, The Atrium, Southern Gate, Chichester, West Sussex, PO19 8SQ, UK

Editorial offices: 9600 Garsington Road, Oxford, OX4 2DQ, UK
The Atrium, Southern Gate, Chichester, West Sussex, PO19 8SQ, UK
111 River Street, Hoboken, NJ 07030-5774, USA

For details of our global editorial offices, for customer services and for information about how to apply for permission to reuse the copyright material in this book please see our website at www.wiley.com/wiley-blackwell

Library of Congress Cataloging-in-Publication Data

Cirrhosis (Lee)
Cirrhosis : a practical guide to management / edited by Samuel S. Lee, Richard Moreau.
p. ; cm.
Includes index.
ISBN 978-1-118-27482-8 (cloth)
I. Lee, Samuel S., 1954- , editor. II. Moreau, Richard, 1951- , editor. III. Title.
[DNLM: 1. Liver Cirrhosis–diagnosis. 2. Liver Cirrhosis–therapy. 3. Liver Diseases–complications. WI 725]
RC848.C5
616.3'624–dc23

2014032682

A catalogue record for this book is available from the British Library.

Wiley also publishes its books in a variety of electronic formats. Some content that appears in print may not be available in electronic books.

Set in 8.5/12 MeridienLTStd-Roman by Thomson Digital, Noida, India

1 2015

Contents

List of contributors

Ayman A. Abdo, MD, FRCPC
Professor, Division of Gastroenterology, Department of Medicine, College of Medicine, King Saud University;
King Saud University Liver Disease Research Center, Riyadh, Saudi Arabia

Danielle Adebayo, BSc, MBBS, MRCP
Hepatology Research Fellow, Liver Failure Group,
UCL Institute for Liver and Digestive Health,
UCL Medical School, Royal Free Hospital, London, UK

Fernando Alvarez, MD
Professor of Pediatrics, Department of Pediatrics, CHU- Sainte Justine, University of Montreal, Quebec, Canada

Piero Amodio, MD
Professor of Internal Medicine, Department of Medicine (DIMED), University of Padova, Padova, Italy

Paolo Angeli, MD, PhD
Professor of Medicine, Department of Medicine (DIMED),
Unit of Hepatic Emergencies and Liver Transplantation,
University of Padova, Padova, Italy

Yasuhiro Asahina, MD, PhD
Professor, Department of Hepatitis Investigation, Tokyo Medical and Dental University, Tokyo, Japan

Sumeet K. Asrani, MD, MSc
Hepatology Fellow, Baylor University Medical Center, Dallas, Texas, USA

Soon Koo Baik, MD, PhD
Professor of Internal Medicine, Department of Internal Medicine, Yonsei University Wonju College of Medicine, Wonju, Republic of Korea

Nora V. Bergasa, MD
Chief, Department of Medicine, Metropolitan Hospital Center, New York, NY, USA;
Professor of Medicine, New York Medical College, Valhalla, New York, NY, USA

Vijay Bodh, MD
Fellow in DM (Heptology), Department of Hepatology,
Post Graduate Institute of Medical Education and Research (PGIMER), Chandigarh, India

A.K. Burroughs, MD (deceased)
The Royal Free Sheila Sherlock Liver Centre and University Department of Surgery, Department of Intensive Care, Royal Free Hospital, London, UK

Hai-Xia Cao, PhD, MD
Department of Gastroenterology, Shanghai Key Laboratory of Pediatric Gastroenterology and Nutrition,
Xinhua Hospital Affiliated to Shanghai Jiaotong University School of Medicine, Shanghai, China

Andrés Cárdenas, MD, MMSc, AGAF
Faculty Member, Senior Specialist, GI Unit, Hospital Clínic and University of Barcelona, Institut d'Investigacions Biomèdiques August Pi-Sunyer (IDIBAPS), Ciber de Enfermedades Hepaticas y Digestivas (CIBERHED)

Rodrigo Cartin-Ceba, MD
Assistant Professor of Medicine, Division of Pulmonary and Critical Care Medicine, Mayo Clinic, Rochester, MN, USA

Laurent Castera, MD, PhD
Senior Consultant in Hepatology, Department of Hepatology, Hopital Beaujon, Assistance Publique-Hôpitaux de Paris, INSERM U773, Clichy, France

Y.K. Chawla, MD, DM (Gastroenterology), FAMS
Professor, Department of Hepatology, Post Graduate Institute of Medical Education and Research (PGIMER), Chandigarh, India

Isabelle Colle, MD, PhD
Full Professor, Ghent University, Belgium;
Department of Hepatology and Gastroenterology, Algemeen Stedelijk Ziekenhuis (ASZ), Aalst, Belgium and Ghent University

Jane Collier, MD, MBChB, FRCP
Consultant in Hepatology, John Radcliffe Hospital, Oxford, UK

Alejandro Costaguta, MD
Jefe, Servicio de Gastroenterología, Hepatología y Nutrición, Sanatorio de Niños, Rosario, Santa Fe, Argentina

Emily Dannhorn, MBBS, MRCP
Specialist Registrar in Hepatology, Sheila Sherlock Liver Centre, Royal Free Hospital, London, UK

Maissa El Raziky, MD
Professor of Endemic Medicine and Hepatology, Director of the Hepatic Schistosomiasis Research Unit, Faculty of Medicine, Cairo University, Cairo, Egypt

Gamal Esmat, MD
Vice President for Graduate Studies and Research Cairo University, Professor of Endemic Medicine and Hepatology, Faculty of Medicine, Cairo University, Cairo, Egypt

Michael B. Fallon, MD
Professor of Medicine, Division of Gastroenterology, Hepatology and Nutrition, Department of Internal Medicine, The University of Texas, Health Science Center at Houston, Houston, TX, USA

Jian-Gao Fan, PhD, MD
Professor and Director, Department of Gastroenterology, Shanghai Key Laboratory of Pediatric, Gastroenterology and Nutrition, Xinhua Hospital Affiliated to Shanghai Jiaotong University School of Medicine, Shanghai, China

Adrián Gadano, MD, PhD
Associate Professor and Chief, Department of Medicine and Liver Unit, Hospital Italiano, Buenos Aires, Argentina

Anja Geerts, MD, PhD
Professor, Ghent University, Belgium;
Department of Hepatology and Gastroenterology, Ghent University Hospital, Ghent, Belgium

Pere Ginès, MD, PhD
Chairman – Liver Unit, Professor of Medicine, Liver Unit, Hospital Clínic and University of Barcelona; Institut d'Investigacions Biomèdiques August Pi-Sunyer (IDIBAPS); Ciber de Enfermedades Hepaticas y Digestivas (CIBERHED); Instituto Reina Sofía de Investigación Nefrológica (IRSIN), Barcelona, Spain

Isabel Graupera, MD
Liver Unit, Hospital Clínic and University of Barcelona; Institut d'Investigacions Biomèdiques August Pi-Sunyer (IDIBAPS), Ciber de Enfermedades Hepaticas y Digestivas (CIBERHED), Instituto Reina Sofía de Investigación Nefrológica (IRSIN), Barcelona, Spain

Thierry Gustot, MD, PhD
Associate Professor, Department of Gastroenterology and Hepato-Pancreatology, Erasme Hospital, Brussels, Belgium
Laboratory of Experimental Gastroenterology, Université Libre de Bruxelles, Brussels, Belgium;
INSERM, U773, Centre de Recherche Biomédicale Bichat-Beaujon CRB3, Paris, France

Kwang-Hyub Han, MD
Professor and Chairman, Department of Internal Medicine, Yonsei University College of Medicine, Seoul, Korea

Namiki Izumi, MD, PhD
Chief, Vice President, Department of Gastroenterology and Hepatology, Musashino Red Cross Hospital, Tokyo, Japan

Rajiv Jalan, MBBS, MD, PhD, FRCPE, FRCP
Professor of Hepatology, Liver Failure Group, UCL Institute for Liver and Digestive Health, UCL Medical School, Royal Free Hospital, London, UK

Woo Kyoung Jeong, MD, PhD
Assistant Professor of Radiology, Department of Radiology and Center for Imaging Science, Samsung Medical Center, Sungkyunkwan University School of Medicine, Seoul, Republic of Korea

Patrick S. Kamath, MD
Professor of Medicine, Division of Gastroenterology and Hepatology, Mayo Clinic College of Medicine, Rochester, MN, USA

Do Young Kim, MD, PhD
Associate Professor, Department of Internal Medicine, Yonsei University College of Medicine, Seoul, Korea

Moon Young Kim, MD, PhD
Associate Professor of Internal Medicine, Yonsei University Wonju College of Medicine, Wonju, Republic of Korea

Michael J. Krowka, MD
Professor of Medicine, Division of Pulmonary and Critical Care Medicine, Mayo Clinic, Rochester, MN, USA

Masayuki Kurosaki, MD, PhD
Director, Department of Gastroenterology and Hepatology, Musashino Red Cross Hospital, Tokyo, Japan

Samuel S. Lee, MD, FRCPC
Professor of Medicine, University of Calgary Cumming School of Medicine, Calgary, Canada

Han-Chieh Lin, MD, FAGG
Professor and Chief, Department of Gastroenterology and Hepatology, Taipei Veterans General Hospital and National Yang-Ming University School of Medicine, Taipei, Taiwan

Hongqun Liu, MD, PhD
Research Assistant Professor, University of Calgary Cumming School of Medicine, Calgary, Canada

Sebastián Marciano, MD
Assistant Professor, Liver Unit, Hospital Italiano, Buenos Aires, Argentina

Vincenzo Morabito, MBBS
Clinical Research Fellow, Liver Failure Group,
UCL Institute for Liver and Digestive Health,
UCL Medical School Royal Free Hospital, London, UK

Filippo Morando, MD
Hepatology Fellow, Department of Medicine (DIMED), University of Padova, Padova, Italy

Richard Moreau, MD
INSERM, U1149, Centre de Recherche sur l'Inflammation (CRI); UMR S 1149, Université Paris Diderot-Paris 7, Faculté de Médecine Bichat;
Département Hospitalo-Universitaire (DHU) UNITY, Service d'Hépatologie, Hôpital Beaujon, Assistance Publique-Hôpitaux de Paris, Clichy, France

James O'Beirne, MBBS (Hons), MD, FRCP, EDIC
Consultant Hepatologist, Sheila Sherlock Liver Centre, Royal Free Hospital, London, UK

Valérie Paradis, MD, PhD
Professor, Pathology Department, Beaujon Hospital, INSERM URM 1149, Paris, France

Salvatore Piano, MD
Hepatology Fellow, Department of Medicine (DIMED), University of Padova, Padova, Italy

Moises Ilan Nevah Rubin, MD
Assistant Professor of Medicine, Division of Gastroenterology, Hepatology and Nutrition, Department of Internal Medicine, The University of Texas Health Science Center at Houston, Houston, TX, USA

Faisal M. Sanai, MD, ABIM, SBG
Consultant Transplant Hepatologist, Department of Hepatobiliary Science and Liver Transplantation, King Abdul Aziz Medical City;
King Saud University Liver Disease Research Center, Riyadh, Saudi Arabia

Marco Senzolo, MD
Multivisceral Transplant Unit, Gastroenterology, Department of Surgical and Gastroenterological Sciences, University Hospital of Padova, Padova, Italy

Felix Stickel, MD
Associate Professor of Hepatology, Department of Gastroenterology and Hepatology, University Hospital Zürich, Switzerland

Nobuharu Tamaki, MD
Department of Gastroenterology and Hepatology, Musashino Red Cross Hospital, Tokyo, Japan

Xavier Verhelst, MD
Resident Hepatology, Department of Hepatology and Gastroenterology, Ghent University Hospital, Ghent, Belgium

Hans Van Vlierberghe, MD, PhD
Full Professor, Ghent University, Belgium;
Department of Hepatology and Gastroenterology,
Ghent University Hospital, Ghent, Belgium

Florence Wong, MBBS, MD, FRACP, FRCPC
Professor, Division of Gastroenterology, Department of Medicine, Toronto General Hospital, University of Toronto, Toronto, Ontario, Canada

Ying-Ying Yang, MD, PhD
Professor and Chief, Department of Medical Education, Taipei Veterans General Hospital and National Yang-Ming University School of Medicine, Taipei, Taiwan

Foreword

"Cirrhosis" is derived from the Greek word *kirrós* meaning orange or tawny. Millennia ago, ancient people including the Greeks must have been impressed by the scarred, tawny appearance of the cirrhotic liver. They recognized that such a diseased liver was associated with many complications including ascites. Indeed, throughout history, until relatively recently, the liver was judged to be the most important organ in the body by almost all civilizations. It was felt to be the seat of most emotions including courage, anger, and love. In 1628, William Harvey discovered that the heart pumped the entire blood circulation and that arteries and veins were connected by capillaries. Until then, the arterial and venous circulations were thought to be entirely separate, and the liver made and pumped venous blood. Thus, this discovery started the process of the heart supplanting the liver as the primary organ in laypeople's understanding of the body.

Cirrhosis is the end-stage process of virtually all chronic insults to the liver. Although it was originally defined as purely a histopathologic condition characterized by extensive fibrosis with architectural disorganization and nodular regeneration, physicians have known for thousands of years that many other parts of the body are affected by cirrhosis.

Any physician caring for patients with cirrhosis is familiar with the presentation of end-stage liver failure: the emaciated, malnourished, confused patient with ascites, prone to bleeding, infections, renal failure, and liver cancer. Almost all the major organ systems in the body including the brain, heart, lungs, kidneys, gut, adrenals, bones, muscles, blood and endocrine systems show evidence of dysfunction in the presence of cirrhosis. Caring for patients with these myriad complications of cirrhosis continues to challenge physicians in the twenty-first century as it did thousands of years ago. Fortunately, we now have many more ways to diagnose and treat such complications. But, with the explosion of knowledge about pathophysiology and molecular mechanisms of disease, as well as major advances in medical and surgical therapies, such "information overload" may be a problem.

To try to address that problem, 57 distinguished authorities from 15 countries provide their expert practical guidance on the management of the many facets of cirrhosis. The operative word is "practical." Authors provide concise but practical advice, often with algorithms and illustrations, to help the busy clinician care for the patient with cirrhosis and its complications.

The first part comprises eight chapters that expertly summarize the ways to diagnose cirrhosis, and its pathophysiology and prognosis. The second part consists of 20 chapters that cover all aspects of the management of each complication, from the specific conditions associated with cirrhosis that affect organs such as the brain (hepatic encephalopathy), heart (cirrhotic cardiomyopathy), lungs (hepatopulmonary syndrome), and kidneys (ascites, acute kidney injury, hyponatremia). Symptoms and major causes of mortality and morbidity such as bleeding, coagulopathy, infections, osteopenia, and pruritus are explained in concise but practical detail. Chapters on special considerations in children with cirrhosis, and drug therapy and potential hepatotoxicity complete this book.

We were privileged to work with such expert hepatologists on this text, and hope that clinicians who care for patients with cirrhosis will find it useful.

Samuel S. Lee
Richard Moreau

List of abbreviations

AAA	aromatic amino acid
AaPO2	alveolar–arterial oxygen gradient
AASLD	American Association for the Study of Liver Diseases
ACG	American College of Gastroenterology
ACLF	acute-on-chronic liver failure
ACTH	adrenocorticotropic hormone
ADC	apparent diffusion coefficient
AFP	alpha-fetoprotein
AI	adrenal insufficiency
AICF	accelerated intravascular coagulation and fibrinolysis
AIH	autoimmune hepatitis
AJCC	American Joint Committee on Cancer
AKI	acute kidney injury
AKIN	Acute Kidney Injury Network
ALD	alcoholic liver disease
ARD	ammonia reducing drug
ALK-P	alkaline phosphatase
ALT	alanine aminotransferase
AMA	anti-mitochondrial antibody
ANP	atrial natriuretic peptide
APC	argon plasma coagulation
APRI	aspartate aminotransferase: platelet ratio index
ARDS	acute respiratory distress syndrome
ARFI	acoustic radiation force impulse
ASA	American Society of Anesthesiologists
ASQ	Acoustic Structure Quantification
AST	aspartate aminotransferase
ATN	acute tubular necrosis
AUROC	area under the receiver operating characteristic curve
AVP	vasopressin
BCAA	branched chain amino acid
BCLC	Barcelona Clinic Liver Cancer
BCS	Budd–Chiari syndrome
BDT	block design test
BIA	bioelectrical impedance analysis
BMD	bone mineral density
BMI	body mass index
BMIc	body mass index corrected for fluid retention
BNP	brain natriuretic peptide
BRTO	balloon-occluded retrograde transvenous obliteration
BSP	bromsulphalein
cAMP	cyclic adenosine monophosphate
CAP	community-acquired pneumonia
CBDL	common bile duct ligation
CBG	cortisol binding globulin
CC	cholangiocarcinoma
CDS	cirrhosis discriminate score
CEUS	contrast-enhanced ultrasonography
CFTR	cystic fibrosis transmembrane regulator
CHB	chronic hepatitis B
CHE	covert hepatic encephalopathy
CHF	chronic heart failure
CI	95% confidence interval
CIOMS	Council for International Organizations of Medical Sciences
CIRCI	critical illness-related corticosteroid insufficiency
CKD	chronic kidney disease
CLD	chronic liver disease
CLDQ	Chronic Liver Disease Questionnaire
CLIF	Chronic Liver Failure (score)
CLKT	combined liver kidney transplant
CNS	central nervous system
CO	cardiac output
CPA	collagen proportionate area
CPK	creatine phosphokinase
CRH	corticotropin-releasing hormone
CRP	C-reactive protein
c-statistic	concordance statistic
CT	computed tomography
CTGF	connective tissue growth factor
CTP	Child–Turcotte–Pugh (score)
CXR	chest X-ray
DCD	donation after cardiac death
DDLT	deceased donor liver transplantation
DEXA	dual-energy X-ray absorptiometry
DIC	disseminated intravascular coagulation
DILI	drug-induced liver injury
DLCO	diffusing capacity for carbon monoxide
DN	dysplastic nodule
DST	digit symbol test
DWI	diffusion-weighted imaging
EASL	European Association for the Study of the Liver
EBL	endoscopic band ligation
ECM	extracellular matrix
EHPVO	extrahepatic portal vein obstruction
ESBL	extended-spectrum β-lactamase
ESLD	end-stage liver disease

ESPEN	European Society for Parenteral and Enteral Nutrition
ET	endothelin
FAGA	functional adrenal gland atrophy
FDA	US Food and Drug Administration
FDG-PET	fludeoxyglucose positron emission tomography
FGF	fibroblast growth factor
FRF	functional renal failure
FSC	fat-storing cell
GAVE	gastric antral vascular ectasia
GCS	Glasgow Coma Scale
Gd-EOB-DTPA	gadoliniumethoxybenzyldiethylenetriamine-pentaacetic acid
GFR	glomerular filtration rate
GGT	gamma-glutamyl transpeptidase
Gla	gamma-carboxyglutamic acid
GNB	Gram-negative bacteria
GOV	gastroesophageal varices
GPC	Gram-positive cocci
GRPR	gastrin-releasing peptide receptor
GSD	glycogen storage disease
HAART	highly active antiretroviral therapy
HAIC	hepatic arterial infusional chemotherapy
HBIG	hepatitis B immunoglobulin
HBV	hepatitis B virus
HCC	hepatocellular carcinoma
HCV	hepatitis C virus
HDL	high-density lipoprotein
HE	hepatic encephalopathy
HFSR	hand–foot skin reaction
HPA	hypothalamic–pituitary–adrenal axis
HPS	hepatopulmonary syndrome
HR	hazard ratio
HRS	hepatorenal syndrome
HRT	hormone replacement therapy
HSC	hepatic stellate cells
HTLV	human T-cell lymphotropic virus
HVPG	hepatic venous pressure gradient
ICG	indocyanine green
ICU	intensive care unit
IFN	interferon
IGV	isolated gastric varices
IL	interleukin
IM	immunoglobulin
INR	international normalized ratio
IPAH	idiopathic pulmonary artery hypertension
IQR	interquartile range
IV	intravenous
LAT	local ablative therapy
LCC	large cell change
LDH	lactic dehydrogenase
LDL	low-density lipoprotein
LDLT	living donor liver transplantation
LOLA	L-ornithine-L-aspartate
LPA	lipophosphatidic acid
LPS	lipopolysaccharide
LR	likelihood ratio
LSM	liver stiffness measure
LSPS	LSM-Spleen diameter to Platelet ratio Score
LT	liver transplantation
LVEF	left ventricular ejection fraction
MAC	mid-arm circumference
MAMC	mid-arm muscle circumference
MAO	monoamine oxidase
MAP	mean arterial pressure
MDCT	multi-detector computed tomography
MELD	model for end-stage liver disease
MHE	minimal hepatic encephalopathy
MPAP	mean pulmonary arterial pressure
MR	magnetic resonance
MRI	magnetic resonance imaging
MS	metabolic syndrome
NAFLD	nonalcoholic fatty liver disease
NAPQI	*N*-acetyl-*p*-benzoquinone imine
NASH	nonalcoholic steatohepatitis
NCPF	noncirrhotic portal fibrosis
NCT	Number Connection Test
NNRTI	non-nucleoside reverse transcriptase inhibitor
NO	nitric oxide
NRTI	nucleoside reverse transcriptase inhibitor
NSAID	nonsteroidal anti-inflammatory drug
NSBB	nonselective beta-blocker
NUNS	Non-ureic nitrogen scavenger
OR	odds ratio
PAH	pulmonary arterial hypertension
PAI	plasminogen activator inhibitor
P-ANCA	perinuclear antineutrophil cytoplasmic antibody
PAWP	pulmonary artery wedge pressure
PBC	primary biliary cirrhosis
PDE	phosphodiesterase
PDGF	platelet derived growth factor
PEG-IFN	pegylated interferon
PEI	percutaneous ethanol injection
PFIC	progressive familial intrahepatic cholestasis
PFT	pulmonary function test
PHC	portal hypertensive colopathy
PHES	Portal-Hepatic Psychometric Score
PHG	portal hypertensive gastropathy
PIVKA	proteins induced by vitamin K absence
PMX-DHP	polymyxin B-immobilized direct fiber hemoperfusion
PNALD	parenteral nutrition-associated liver disease
PPAR	peroxisomal proliferator activated receptor
PPH	portopulmonary hypertension
PPI	proton pump inhibitor
PROM	patient-reported outcome measure

PSC primary sclerosing cholangitis
PSE portosystemic encephalopathy
PT prothrombin time
PTFE polytetrafluoroethylene
PTT partial thromboplastin time
PTX pentoxifylline
PV portal vein
PVR pulmonary vascular resistance
PXR pregnane X receptor
QoL quality of life
RAI relative adrenal insufficiency
RCT randomized controlled trial
RFA radiofrequency ablation
RHC right heart catheterization
RVSP right ventricle systolic pressure
SBE spontaneous bacterial empyema
SBP spontaneous bacterial peritonitis
SCC small cell change
SF-36 Short Form (36) Health Survey
SGA subjective global assessment
SHG second harmonic generation
SIADH syndrome of inappropriate antidiuretic hormone
SIP Sickness Impact Profile
SIRS systemic inflammatory response syndrome
SLK simulaneous liver–kidney
SNP single nucleotide polymorphism
SOFA Sequential Organ Failure Assessment
SPIO superparamagnetic iron oxide
SSRI selective serotonin reuptake inhibitor
SST short Synacthen test
SSTI skin and soft tissue infections
SSWE supersonic shear-wave elastography
SVR sustained virologic response
SVR systemic vascular resistance
TACE transarterial chemoembolization
TAFI thrombin-activable fibrinolysis inhibitor
TDF tenofovir disoproxil fumarate
TE transient elastography
TGF transforming growth factor
TIPS transjugular intrahepatic portosystemic shunt
TLR toll-like receptor
TNF tumor necrosis factor
TNM tumor–node–metastasis
tPA tissue plasminogen activator
TPN total parenteral nutrition
TPO thrombopoietin
TR tricuspid regurgitant peak velocity
TST triceps skinfold thickness
TT thromboplastin time
TTE transthoracic echocardiography
UDCA ursodeoxycolic acid
UGT uridine-diphosphoglucuronate glucuronosyltransferase
US ultrasonography
UTI urinary tract infection
VEGF vascular endothelial growth factor
VLDL very low-density lipoprotein
VTTQ Virtual Touch Tissue Quantification
vWf von Willebrand factor

PART 1
Diagnosis and pathophysiology

CHAPTER 1

Clinical clues to the diagnosis of cirrhosis

Y.K. Chawla and Vijay Bodh

Department of Hepatology, Post Graduate Institute of Medical Education and Research (PGIMER), Chandigarh, India

Introduction

Cirrhosis is a diffuse process characterized by replacement of normal liver tissue by fibrosis and regenerative nodule formation [1]. The development of cirrhosis is usually an irreversible process. However, the reversal of fibrosis has been shown in certain conditions like hepatitis C, biliary obstruction, iron overload, and non-alcoholic steatohepatitis. Thus, cirrhosis is considered as a dynamic process involving pro- and anti-fibrogenic mechanisms, the former being more marked than the latter. The term cirrhosis is a histologic diagnosis and has its own unique constellation of clinical manifestations such that a clinical diagnosis of cirrhosis can be made with confidence most of the time.

The diagnosis of cirrhosis in clinical practice is based on risk factors, history and clinical findings, biochemical tests, imaging, endoscopic and histologic findings. The diagnosis of cirrhosis is not based on a single clinical parameter but a combination of above parameters and the identification and interpretation of these findings. This chapter focuses on the clinical clues that aid in the diagnosis of cirrhosis.

Clinical presentation

Cirrhosis occurs clinically as compensated cirrhosis or decompensated cirrhosis.

Compensated cirrhosis is usually diagnosed incidentally during a routine examination or biochemical test, during surgery for some other reason, or sometimes with non-specific symptoms like fatigue, anorexia, dyspepsia, weight loss, or right upper abdominal discomfort. Up to 30–40% of patients with compensated cirrhosis remain without clinical signs [2]. These patients decompensate at the rate of 10% per year and have a 50% 10-year survival rate [3].

Decompensated cirrhosis is cirrhosis complicated by one or more of the following: jaundice, ascites (with or without hepatorenal syndrome, hyponatremia, spontaneous bacterial peritonitis), hepatic encephalopathy, or variceal bleeding. The presence of these features of decompensation have a high specificity but low sensitivity for the diagnosis of cirrhosis. Decompensated cirrhosis has a 50% survival rate at 18 months [3]. These clinical manifestations are discussed subsequently.

Patient history

Abdominal distension (ascites)

Cirrhosis is the most common cause of ascites (85%) and ascites is the most common complication of cirrhosis. Up to 60% of patients with compensated cirrhosis develop ascites within 10 years [3]. Clinically, patients present with gradually progressive abdominal distension with or without pedal edema, history of weight gain, increase in waist size of clothing, sometimes with a decrease in urine output, or the development of abdominal hernias as a result of increased intra-abdominal pressure. The ascites in cirrhosis resulting from portal hypertension is usually responsive to diuretic therapy, hence such a history must be sought in any patient presenting with ascites. History of cardiac failure, renal disease, malignancy, and tuberculosis must be ruled out. A history of ascitic tap is a

Cirrhosis: A practical guide to management, First Edition. Edited by Samuel S. Lee and Richard Moreau.

strong clue to the presence of ascites, hence the nature of fluid tapped may add further valuable information to the diagnosis.

Jaundice

Jaundice as a clinical manifestation may be seen in cirrhosis depending on the degree of decompensation. Jaundice (icterus) is a clinical manifestation of hyperbilirubinemia and presents as yellow discoloration of the skin and mucous membranes. It is the most obvious sign of liver disease and is best seen in the conjunctivae. It is usually detectable when the serum level of bilirubin exceeds 2 mg/dL (34 mmol/L). Elevation of both unconjugated and conjugated bilirubin occurs in patients with hepatocellular disease resulting from impaired canalicular excretion or biliary obstruction. Unconjugated hyperbilirubinemia in cirrhosis is caused by either associated hemolysis or decreased conjugating enzyme in the endoplasmic reticulum of hepatocytes, namely bilirubin uridine-diphosphoglucuronate glucuronosyltransferase (UGT) or associated Gilbert's syndrome. Serum bilirubin levels are usually below 5 mg/dL; however, values above this may also be seen in certain patients who are in a decompensated state. A serum bilirubin level >5 mg/dL is one of the clinical defining criteria for acute on chronic liver failure [4]. The clinical significance of jaundice in cirrhosis lies in assessing the decompensated state of cirrhosis as jaundice is not specific to cirrhosis alone as it is seen in many other liver disorders and even in nonhepatic disorders.

Upper gastrointestinal bleeding

Gastroesophageal varices are present in approximately 50% of patients with cirrhosis. Up to 40% of patients with Child A cirrhosis have varices which increases to 85% in Child C cirrhosis [5]. Variceal bleeding occurs at a rate of 5–15% per year [6]. Variceal bleeding presenting as hematemesis with or without melena is one of the most common complications of cirrhosis with portal hypertension. The presentation is usually a painless, effortless bleed and may be precipitated by drugs like nonsteroidal anti-inflammatory drugs (NSAIDs). There may be associated melena which is passage of black tarry stools, which are offensive, semi-solid, and difficult to flush down the toilet. Patients may have postural hypotensive symptoms such as light-headedness and fainting episodes in cases of a significant bleed. Once a patient has a variceal bleed, the portal pressure (i.e., hepatic venous pressure gradient; HVPG) is usually >12 mmHg [7], because the development of varices occurs with HVPG >10 mmHg. However, variceal bleed alone is not a feature of cirrhosis; it may well be seen in noncirrhotic portal hypertensive conditions such as extrahepatic portal vein obstruction (EHPVO) or noncirrhotic portal fibrosis (NCPF).

Hepatic encephalopathy

Hepatic encephalopathy is a neuropsychiatric syndrome with multiple variable manifestations. It may be covert (which includes minimal hepatic encephalopathy; MHE) and stage I encephalopathy) or an overt (stage II–IV) encephalopathy. Patients with MHE may present only with cognitive dysfunction in cirrhosis. The prevalence of MHE is 30–84% [8] and that of overt hepatic encephalopathy is 30–50% in cirrhotic patients [9,10]. The presentation of hepatic encephalopathy has marked variability among patients. Drowsiness, disorientation with reference to time, place, or person, delirium, and confusion can occur. Disturbance in sleep develops early with hypersomnia and altered sleep rhythm. There is further development of apathy, somnolence, tremors, apathy, and slowness of response. As further worsening occurs, the patient may become aroused on noxious stimuli or may become deeply unresponsive and comatose. Seizures may occur, especially in deeper grades of encephalopathy. Personality disturbance is another mode of presentation in the form of irritability, euphoria, and features of social disinhibition. Patients often present with loss of bladder and bowel control. Intellectual deterioration, memory impairment, and cognitive dysfunction also frequently occur. Constructional apraxia, micrographia, slow slurred monotonous speech, dysphasia, and perseveration can all occur.

A clinician must always look for a history of precipitating factors for encephalopathy: gastrointestinal bleed, use of diuretics, infections, hyponatremia, surgery, constipation, renal failure, anemia, hypoglycemia, and, in the absence of any precipitating event, a thorough search should be made for the presence of spontaneous portosystemic shunts [11]. Any patient with hepatic encephalopathy must have any neurologic cause like meningitis, stroke, intracranial bleed, chronic subdural hematoma (especially in alcoholics) ruled out. There are various criteria for staging of hepatic encephalopathy. One of the most commonly used is the West Haven criteria as shown in Table 1.1 [12].

Table 1.1 West Haven criteria for staging of hepatic encephalopathy.

Stage	Intellectual impairment	Neuromuscular impairment
Stage 0	Normal	Normal
Minimal hepatic encephalopathy	Normal examination findings, subtle changes in work or driving	Minor abnormalities of visual perception or on psychometric or number tests
Stage 1	Personality changes, attention deficits, irritability, depressed state	Tremor and incoordination
Stage 2	Changes in sleep–wake cycle, lethargy, mood and behavioural changes, cognitive dysfunction	Asterixis, ataxic gait, speech abnormalities (slow and slurred)
Stage 3	Somnolence, confusion, disorientation, amnesia	Muscular rigidity, nystagmus, clonus, Babinski's sign, hyporeflexia
Stage 4	Stupor and coma	Oculocephalic reflex, unresponsive to noxious stimuli

Source: Ferenci et al. 2002 [12]. Reproduced with permission of John Wiley & Sons.

Etiologic history taking

Alcohol intake: how much is significant

Fatty liver develops in up to 90% of patients who drink more alcohol than 60 g/day [13]. Fibrosis progression and development of cirrhosis may occur in up to 5–15% of patients despite abstinence. Continued alcohol use increases the risk of progression to cirrhosis in 30% of patients [14]. The risk of developing cirrhosis increases with the ingestion of >60–80 g/day of alcohol for 10 years or longer in men, and >20 g/day in women. Yet, even drinking at these levels, only 6–41% develop cirrhosis [15–17]. Hence, there are several other risk factors involved in the development of alcoholic liver disease: sex (female), drinking patterns (early age of drinking, daily heavy drinking, episodic binge drinking), obesity, dietary factors, non-sex-linked genetic factors, cigarette smoking, other chronic liver disorders (hepatitis B or C, hemochromatosis, nonalcoholic fatty liver disease; NAFLD).

In a population-based cohort study of almost 7000 subjects in two northern Italian communities, even among patients with very high daily alcohol intake (>120 g/day), only 13.5% developed alcoholic liver disease (ALD). Homemade brew has variable amounts of alcohol and associated trace metals which may cause the development of liver disease with fewer years of consumption.

The history of alcohol consumption should be obtained both from the patient and family members, enquiring about alcohol-associated illnesses like pancreatitis and peripheral neuropathy, driving under the influence of alcohol, and history of any withdrawal symptoms. The amount of alcohol for reference purposes is 30 mL whisky, 360 mL beer, 120 mL wine – all equivalent to 10–11 g alcohol, and each of them is considered as one unit. The CAGE questionnaire is frequently used to assess the degree of alcohol-related problems and alcohol dependence [18].

History of other risk factors

A history including blood transfusion, surgery, needle-stick injuries, sexual contact, tattooing, skin piercing, dialysis, sharing of razors or toothbrushes must be taken to assess the risk of exposure to hepatitis B and C viruses. Metabolic risk factors include diabetes mellitus, hypertension, obesity, and dyslipidemia which must be asked about in view of nonalcoholic steatohepatitis-related cirrhosis. A family history of chronic liver disease may be relevant in certain situations like Wilson's disease, autoimmune disorders, and even hepatitis B and C-related cirrhosis. A history of abnormal involuntary movements like choreoathetosis should arouse the suspicion of Wilson's disease. Autoimmune disorders like vitiligo, diabetes mellitus, thyroid disorder, pernicious anemia, and inflammatory bowel disease are associated with autoimmune hepatitis. A past history of biliary obstruction and biliary surgery could give a clue to the diagnosis of secondary biliary cirrhosis as pruritus and fatigue may be seen in primary biliary cirrhosis. A personal history of sexual dysfunction like loss of libido, loss of secondary sexual characteristics, breast enlargement in males and amenorrhea or infertility in females are clues to hypogonadism, often seen in cirrhosis. A history of smoking is also important as it has been shown to have a role in progression of chronic liver disease: hepatitis C and alcoholic cirrhosis [19].

Examination

General examination

A patient with cirrhosis appears malnourished, with shrunken eyes, temporal hollowing, parched lips, muddy complexion of the face, dried skin (xerosis), and hyperpigmentation, with features of various nutritional deficiencies. Patients have a hyperkinetic circulation. They may also have petechiae, purpura, or ecchymotic patches suggestive of underlying coagulopathy and thrombocytopenia. Fetor hepaticus is a sign of hepatocellular failure characterized by a sweetish, slightly faecal smell of the breath similar to freshly opened corpses of mice.

Pallor indicates anemia, which may be multifactorial in cirrhosis as a result of anemia of chronic disease, hypersplenism, acute or chronic blood loss, a nutritional cause, bone marrow suppression, or an autoimmune process. Scleral icterus is usually present in patients with decompensated cirrhosis. However, all patients who are decompensated do not have scleral icterus, especially those who present with upper gastrointestinal bleed or ascites. Patients with compensated cirrhosis are usually anicteric. Scratch marks may be present in cholestatic liver disorders. Xanthelasmas and pruritic scratch marks are a clue to biliary cirrhosis. Xanthelasma often develops as a painless, yellowish, soft plaque with well-defined borders, which may enlarge over the course of weeks. Clubbing is seen in patients with cirrhosis, especially in the setting of biliary cirrhosis, hepatopulmonary syndrome, or cystic fibrosis. Cyanosis may be seen in severe degrees of hepatopulmonary syndrome. Presence of a Kayser–Fleischer ring or sunflower cataract should arouse suspicion for underlying Wilson's disease as the etiology.

Nutritional status

Malnutrition is a common complication of cirrhosis with a prevalence of 65–90% [20]. There is severe reduction of body fat and overall muscle mass [21]. These patients also have various micro and macronutrient deficiencies often manifesting clinically. Nutritional status should be assessed in all patients. Nutritional assessment by body mass index in cirrhotic patients with ascites is difficult as it overestimates the true body weight in these patients. Hence, in patients with ascites, weight correction should be carried out by reducing 14 kg in massive ascites, 6 kg in moderate ascites, and 2.2 kg in minimal ascites from the observed weight [22].

Cutaneous clues

Spider angioma

A spider angioma consists of a central arteriole with numerous small radiating vessels from it resembling a spider's legs. These spider angiomas may range from a pinhead to 0.5 cm in diameter. They are mostly seen along the vascular territory of the superior vena cava, "V" of the neck, chest, face, arms, hands, and back. They are reckoned to be distributed in relation to a gradient of skin vascular reactivity and temperature [23]. These skin lesions blanch on pressure and if large enough can be seen or felt to be pulsating [24]. A study showed the prevalence of spider angiomas was 50% in patients with alcoholic cirrhosis compared with 27% in patients with nonalcoholic cirrhosis. Overall, up to 33% of patients with cirrhosis have spider angiomas [25].

The number and size of vascular spider angiomas have been found to correlate with the severity of liver dysfunction. They may disappear with improvement in liver function or may increase in number with progression of liver dysfunction. Sometimes they may bleed profusely. They are mostly seen in association with alcoholic cirrhosis. Patients with spider angiomas have a higher frequency of variceal bleeding (36%) than patients without spider angiomas (11%). Spider angioma profile also predicts the risk of variceal bleeding, which is greater when there are >20 spider angiomas (50%) or multiple atypically located spider angiomas (66%). Large spider angiomas (>15 mm) correlate with large varices and higher risk of bleeding [26]. Other causes of spider angiomas include viral hepatitis and under normal conditions in children and adults (including pregnancy). They are mainly caused by an increase in ratio of serum estradiol to free testosterone in male patients [27]. Young age, elevated plasma vascular endothelial growth factor, and basic fibroblast growth factor have been attributed as significant independent predictors of spider nevi in cirrhotic patients [28]. For cosmetic reasons, spider angiomas can be treated with laser therapy [29]. Differential diagnosis for vascular spider angiomas include cherry hemangiomas, insect bites, Rendu–Osler–Weber syndrome, angioma serpiginosum, ataxia telangiectasia, senile angioma, disseminated essential telangiectasia, and angiokeratomas.

Palmar erythema

Palmar erythema manifests as bright red discoloration of the palms, mostly on hypothenar, thenar eminences, and pulps of the fingers. Also known as liver palms, it is a less frequent finding than vascular spider angiomas. Of patients with cirrhosis, 23% manifest palmar erythema [30]. The soles of feet may also be affected. The mottling blanches on pressure. Other causes also include familial inheritance, thyrotoxicosis, pregnancy, rheumatoid arthritis, diabetes mellitus, gestational syphilis, human T-cell lymphotropic virus type 1 (HTLV-1) associated myelopathy, leukemia, chronic febrile illnesses, and drugs (amiodarone, gemfibrozil, cholestyramine, topiramate, and albuterol or salbutamol). Similar to vascular spider angiomas, the pathogenesis of liver palms lies in the hyperestrogenic state and regional differences in the peripheral circulation of patients with cirrhosis [31].

Dupuytren's contracture

Dupuytren's contracture is a flexion contracture of the ring and little fingers brought about by thickening of the palmar fascia of the hands. It is thought to be caused by fibroblastic proliferation and disorderly collagen deposition. Normally, the palmar fascia consists of type I collagen but in Dupuytren's contracture this is replaced by type III collagen which is significantly thicker than type I. According to Wolfe et al. [32], Dupuytren's contracture was present in 66% of male alcoholic patients with cirrhosis. In Nazari's series a similar association was found in 55% of patients with alcoholic (Laënnec's) cirrhosis [33].

The exact pathogenesis and causal association in cirrhosis is not clear. It is also seen in other conditions like diabetes mellitus, alcoholism, repeated trauma, and phenytoin therapy. Male gender, age more than 40 years, people of northern Europe and Scandinavian descent, and a positive family history are risk factors for Dupuytren's contracture. The contractures are divided into three grades (based on the joint with the greatest degree of flexion contracture): grade I contractures of 5–30 degrees, grade II contractures of 30–60 degrees, and grade III contractures of 60–90+ degrees [34].

Leukonychia

Leukonychia means white nails (Terry nails) and was first described in 1954. Terry nails is a physical finding in which fingernails and/or toenails appear white with a characteristic ground glass appearance with a dark band (pink or brown) at the distal tip and the absence of a lunula. This is mainly caused by hypoalbuminemia, and can also be seen in those with chronic kidney disease, type 2 diabetes mellitus, congestive heart failure, or advanced age. The pathogenesis of these nail changes is unclear but is thought to be caused by a decrease in vascularity and an increase in connective tissue within the nail bed. Holzberg postulated that the vascular changes (dilated vasculature in the dermis of the distal band) were related to the premature aging of the nail bed, which resulted in the abnormal appearance of the nail [35–38].

Muehrcke's nails

Muehrcke's nails are paired horizontal white bands separated by normal color. The exact pathogenesis is not known but it is believed to be caused by hypoalbuminemia, hence may be seen in other conditions such as nephrotic syndrome.

Bier spots

Bier spots are small, irregularly shaped, hypopigmented patches on the arms and legs caused by venous stasis associated with functional damage to the small vessels of the skin. Bier spots disappear when pressure is applied. Raising the affected limb from a dependent position also causes Bier spots to disappear, which is not the case in true pigmentation disorders [39].

Paper-money skin

Paper-money skin (or "dollar-paper" markings) describes the condition in which the upper trunk is covered with many randomly scattered, needle-thin superficial capillaries. It often occurs in association with spider angiomas. The name comes from the resemblance to the finely chopped silk threads in American dollar bills. The condition is commonly seen in patients with alcoholic cirrhosis and may improve with hemodialysis [40].

Hypogonadism and gynecomastia

Diminished libido and potency, loss of secondary sexual hair, decreased frequency of shaving, gynecomastia, and testicular atrophy are the usual features of hypogonadism in cirrhosis. Gynecomastia is the enlargement of the male breast, defined as glandular breast tissue that is >4 cm in diameter and is often tender [41]. It is mostly seen in those with alcoholic liver disease, although spironolactone use is also a common cause for this in cirrhotic patients. It is present in up to two-thirds of patients with cirrhosis. The prevalence of gynecomastia in cirrhotic patients in one study was reported to be 44% [42]. Female patients with cirrhosis may present with infertility or amenorrhea. In cirrhosis there is a decrease in the hepatic androgen receptors and an increase in the hepatic estrogen receptors, resulting in increased estrogen: androgen ratio [43]. Hypothalamic pituitary dysfunction is also one of the mechanisms for these features. The conjugation of steroid hormones occurs in the liver and any failure of hormonal metabolism may result in steroid hormonal imbalance. Testicular atrophy is ideally measured by orchidometer; however, in the absence of the same, small volume testes, with loss of testicular sensation, is also an adequate clue for atrophy.

Parotidomegaly

Parotidomegaly is usually seen in those with alcoholic cirrhosis. It is usually caused by glandular hypertrophy as a result of adipose infiltration or acinar hypertrophy. Some authors also suggest a role for glandular dysfunction [44]. In sialosis of alcoholic origin, 60% of patients with alcoholic cirrhosis present with parotidomegaly [45], the glandular enlargement being observed already in the pre-cirrhotic phase in 12% of cases [46,47].

Other manifestations

Muscle cramps occur frequently in those with cirrhosis and are characterized by severe pain, occurring in the calf muscles, mostly during sleep or at rest, lasting for few minutes and occurring several times a week [48]. They occur in more than 70% of patients after diagnosis of cirrhosis and are related to the duration of recognized cirrhosis and the degree of liver dysfunction. The mechanism proposed includes reduced effective plasma volume and correlates with the presence of ascites, low mean arterial pressure, and plasma renin activity [49]. Neurogenic, muscular origin, deficiency of calcium, magnesium, and zinc have also been proposed as mechanisms. Lid lag and lid retraction also occur more frequently in cirrhotic patients than healthy individuals with no evidence of any thyroid dysfunction. Other oral and cutaneous manifestations include onycholysis, gingivitis, and candidiasis.

Abdominal examination

Abdominal veins

Portal hypertension caused by cirrhosis may result in dilatation of periumbilical collateral veins. Blood from the portal venous system may be shunted through the periumbilical veins and ultimately to the anterior abdominal wall veins, manifesting as caput medusa. It involves a prominent vein, the thoracoepigastric vein, which interconnects the superficial epigastric vein with the lateral thoracic vein, which is a tributary of the axillary vein. It therefore connects the superior vena cava (axillary vein) with the inferior vena cava (superficial epigastric, which drains into the femoral vein). The dilated veins appear to radiate from the umbilicus and the flow of veins when examined is away from the umbilicus. The presence of visible veins alone does not indicate portal hypertension; the distension of these veins is more important. In cases of suspected Budd–Chiari syndrome (with inferior vena caval involvement), the infra-umbilical vein flow is directed upwards and there is opening up of back veins as well.

Cruveilhier–Baumgarten murmur

A venous hum is heard in the epigastric region on auscultation because of collateral connections between the portal system and the periumbilical veins in portal hypertension, seen rarely in cirrhotic patients. Congenital patency of the umbilical vein may also cause this venous hum. These patients are associated with an increase in spontaneous hepatic encephalopathy [50].

Examination of the liver

Liver examination should focus on the size, surface, margin, consistency, and presence of any bruit. The liver span is usually 10–12 cm in men and 8–11 cm in women. A reduced liver span is a clue to the diagnosis of liver cirrhosis. A shrunken liver is usually a feature of post-necrotic cirrhosis while an enlarged liver indicates an alcohol etiology, autoimmune liver disease, hemochromatosis, or Budd–Chiari syndrome. The cirrhotic liver usually has a firm consistency, irregular or nodular surface, and irregular margins. Presence of an arterial bruit may denote the development of hepatocellular carcinoma, although it may also be seen in alcoholic hepatitis or other vascular lesions of liver. A firm liver has a sensitivity and specificity of 73% and 81%, respectively, for the diagnosis of cirrhosis [51]. The left lobe is often enlarged in cirrhosis and is a useful sign, with a sensitivity and specificity of 86% and 67% [52].

Examination of the spleen

Splenomegaly indicates portal hypertension and is a valuable sign in a suspected case of cirrhosis, especially if there are other features suggestive of cirrhosis; however, it may be enlarged in other conditions. The spleen is usually mild to moderately enlarged in cirrhosis. An unduly massive spleen should make the physician suspect coexisting portal or splenic vein thrombosis or noncirrhotic portal hypertension. Presence of splenomegaly has a very high specificity (90%) but low sensitivity (34%) [51].

There are three methods of percussion of the spleen: Nixon's method, Castell's method, and percussion of the Traube's space. Percussion of Traube's space has a sensitivity and specificity of 67% and 75%, respectively, for detecting splenomegaly [53]. Patients presenting with upper gastrointestinal bleed and splenomegaly usually indicates a diagnosis of portal hypertension and evidence of one of the features of cirrhosis may form a clue to cirrhosis. Splenomegaly is almost universal in NCPF and the average spleen is about 8 cm. In comparison to EHPVO, the spleen is usually >7 cm below costal margin in NCPF and <7 cm in EHPVO [54]. The splenomegaly in EHPVO is mild (5 cm) in 42% of patients, moderate (6–10 cm) in 40%, and massive in only 18% [55].

Examination for ascites

Jugular venous pressure can help in differentiating between cardiac ascites and hepatic ascites as it is commonly raised in cardiac but not in liver disease. Lack of rise in jugular venous pressure (negative hepatojugular reflux) can be a useful clue in cases of Budd–Chiari syndrome [56]. The hepatojugular reflux has a reported sensitivity of 24–72% and a specificity of 93–96% as a marker of right heart dysfunction [57]. The clinical finding of ascites by means of shifting dullness has a sensitivity of 83% and a specificity of 56% [58]. In cases where the shifting dullness is absent, the patient has a <10% chance of having ascites. The amount of ascites required for detection by various methods includes 30 mL for ultrasonography, 1500–2000 mL for shifting dullness. However, in the setting of a tense ascites, shifting dullness may not be apparent. A puddle sign detects up to 120 mL of free fluid [58]. Development of ascites also correlates with the degree of portal pressures such that with an HVPG of >8 mmHg, patients start developing ascites.

Neurologic examination

Asterixis, or flapping tremors, is the most characteristic neurologic abnormality detected on clinical examination in patients with overt hepatic encephalopathy. The patient's arms are outstretched, with forearms fixed and hyperextension at the wrist joint. The physician observes a rapid flexion–extension movement at the metacarpophalangeal joint, and wrist joint. Sometimes, arms, neck, jaw, protruded tongue, retracted mouth, and tightly closed eyelids are involved and the gait is ataxic. Absent at rest, less marked on movement, and maximum on sustained posture, the tremor is usually bilateral. Alternatively, asterixis can be evaluated having the patient grip the evaluator's fingers in steady fashion and is present if the patient's grip tension oscillates. Asterixis can be graded: grade 0 (no flapping motions), grade I (rare flapping motions, 1–2 per 30 seconds), grade II (occasional, irregular flaps, 3–4 per 30 seconds), grade III (frequent flaps, 5–30 per 30 seconds), and grade IV (almost continuous flapping motions) [59]. It may be seen in certain other conditions such as cardiac failure, respiratory failure, and uremia. There is no ideal test for the diagnosis of MHE. However, the Working Party recommends that the diagnosis of MHE requires a normal mental status examination and impairment in the performance of at least two of the following tests: Number Connection Test, Part A (NCT-A), Number Connection Test, Part B (NCT-B), block design test (BDT), and digit symbol test (DST) [11]. There are various neuropsychologic, neurophysiologic, and computerized tests that can be used for making the diagnosis of MHE.

The patient may have hypertonia in the initial stages and hypotonia as coma supervenes, exaggerated deep tendon reflexes or areflexia (in deep coma), flexor or extensor plantar response. In cases of hypertonia, ankle clonus must be checked. The gait is often ataxic. Patients with Wilson's disease may have extrapyramidal features like chorea, athetosis, dystonia, rigidity, dysphonia, dysarthria, and dysphagia.

A recent study analyzed the diagnostic accuracy of overall clinical impression and combination indices and models for detection of cirrhosis. The sensitivity and specificity of the overall clinical impression for the diagnosis of cirrhosis are 54% and 89%, respectively [51].

Thus, cirrhosis can be diagnosed by a combination of history and clinical examination. This diagnosis has to be confirmed by imaging or endoscopy. Its presence indicates a close observation on follow-up for development of hepatocellular carcinoma.

References

1 Anthony PP, Ishak KG, Nayak NC, Poulsen HE, Scheuer PJ, Sobin LH. The morphology of cirrhosis: definition, nomenclature and classification. Bull World Health Org 1977;55:521–40.

2 Conn HO, Atterbury CE. Cirrhosis. In: Schiff L, Schiff ER (eds) Diseases of the Liver, 6th edn. Philadelphia: JB Lippincott; 1987. pp. 725–864.

3 Gines P, Quintero E, Arroyo V, et al. Compensated cirrhosis: natural history and prognostic factors. Hepatology 1987;7:122–8.

4 Sarin SK, Kumar A, Almeida JA, et al. Acute on chronic liver failure: consensus recommendations of the Asian Pacific association for the study of the liver (APASL). Hepatol Int 2009;3:269–82.

5 Pagliaro L, D'Amico G, Pasta L, et al. Portal hypertension in cirrhosis: Natural history. In: Bosch J, Groszmann RJ (eds) Portal Hypertension: Pathophysiology and Treatment. Oxford, UK: Blackwell Scientific; 1994. pp. 72–92.

6 North Italian Endoscopic Club for the Study and Treatment of Esophageal Varices. Prediction of the first variceal hemorrhage in patients with cirrhosis of the liver and esophageal varices: a prospective multicenter study. N Engl J Med 1988;319:983–9.

7 Maruyama H, Sanyal AJ. Portal hypertension: non-surgical and surgical management. In: Schiff ER (ed.) Schiff's Diseases of the Liver, 11th edn. Blackwell Publishing: Oxford, 2012. pp. 326–61.

8 Das A, Dhiman RK, Saraswat VA, Naik SR. Prevalence and natural history of subclinical hepatic encephalopathy in cirrhosis. J Gastroenterol Hepatol 2001;16:531–5.

9 Amodio P, Del Piccolo F, Petteno E, et al. Prevalence and prognostic value of quantified electroencephalogram (EEG) alterations in cirrhotic patients. J Hepatol 2001;35:37–45.

10 Quero JC, Schalm SW. Subclinical hepatic encephalopathy. Semin Liver Dis 1996;16:321–8.

11 Watanabe A. Portal-systemic encephalopathy in non-cirrhotic patients: classification of clinical types, diagnosis and treatment. J Gastroenterol Hepatol 2000;15:969–79.

12 Ferenci P, Lockwood A, Mullen K, Tarter R, Weissenborn K, Blei AT. Hepatic encephalopathy – definition, nomenclature, diagnosis, and quantification: final report of the working party at the 11th World Congresses of Gastroenterology, Vienna, 1998. Hepatology 2002;35:716–21.

13 Crabb DW. Pathogenesis of alcoholic liver disease: newer mechanisms of injury. Keio J Med 1999;48:184–8.

14 Leevy CM. Fatty liver: a study of 270 patients with biopsy proven fatty liver and review of the literature. Medicine (Baltimore) 1962;41:249–76.

15 Mandayam S, Jamal MM, Morgan TR. Epidemiology of alcoholic liver disease. Semin Liver Dis 2004;24:217–32.

16 Bellentani S, Saccoccio G, Costa G, et al. Drinking habits as cofactors of risk for alcohol induced liver damage. The Dionysos Study Group. Gut 1997;41:845–50.

17 Day CP. Who gets alcoholic liver disease: nature or nurture? J R Coll Physicians Lond 2000;34:557–62.

18 Ewing JA. Detecting alcoholism: the CAGE questionnaire. JAMA 1984;252:1905–7.

19 Klatsky AL, Armstrong MA. Alcohol, smoking, coffee, and cirrhosis. Am J Epidemiol 1992;136:1248–57.

20 O'Brien A, Williams R. Nutrition in end-stage liver disease: principles and practice. Gastroenterology 2008;134:1729–40.

21 Periyalwar P, Dasarathy S. Malnutrition in cirrhosis: contribution and consequences of sarcopenia on metabolic and clinical responses. Clin Liver Dis 2012;16:95–131.

22 Mendenhall CI. Protein calorie malnutrition in alcoholic liver disease. In: Watson RR, Watzl B (eds) Nutrition and Alcohol. Boca Raton: CRC Press; 1992. pp. 403–28.

23 Reuben A. Along came a spider. Hepatology 2002;35:735–6.

24 Requena L, Sangueza OP. Cutaneous vascular anomalies Part I, hamartomas, malformation and dilation of pre existing vessels. J Am Acad Dermatol 1997;37:523–49.

25 Khasnis A, Gokula RM. Spider nevus. J Postgrad Med 2002;48:307–9.

26 Foutch PG, Sullivan JA, Gaines JA, Sanowski RA. Cutaneous vascular spiders in cirrhotic patients: correlation with hemorrhage from esophageal varices. Am J Gastroenterol 1988;83:723–6.

27 Li CP, Lee FY, Hwang SJ, et al. Spider angiomas in patients with liver cirrhosis: role of alcoholism and impaired liver function. Scand J Gastroenterol 1999;34:520–3.

28 Li CP, Lee FY, Hwang SJ, et al. Spider angiomas in patients with liver cirrhosis: role of vascular endothelial growth factor and basic fibroblast growth factor. World J Gastroenterol 2003;9:2832–5.

29 Scheepers JH, Quaba AA. Treatment of nevi aranei with the pulsed tunable dye laser at 585 nm. J Pediatr Surg 1995;30:101–4.

30 Serrao R, Zirwas M, English JC. Palmar erythema. Am J Clin Dermatol 2007;8:347–56.

31 Okumura H, Aramaki T, Katsuta Y, et al. Regional differences in peripheral circulation between upper and lower extremity in patients with cirrhosis. Scand J Gastroenterol 1990;25:883–9.

32 Wolfe SJ. Summerskill WHJ, Davidson CS. Thickening and contraction of the palmar fascia (Dupuytren's contracture) associated with alcoholism and hepatic cirrhosis. N Engl J Med 1956;255:559–63.

33 Nazari B. Dupuytren's contracture associated with liver disease. J Mount Sinai Hosp NY 1966;33:69–72.

34 Luck JV. Dupuytren's contracture: a new concept of the pathogenesis correlated with surgical management. J Bone Joint Surg Am 1959;41:635–64.
35 Terry R. White nails in hepatic cirrhosis. Lancet 1954;266:757–9.
36 Holzberg M, Walker HK. Terry's nails: revised definition and new correlations. Lancet 1984;1:896–9.
37 Nabai H. Nail changes before and after heart transplantation: personal observation by a physician. Cutis 1998;61:31–2.
38 Jemec GB, Kollerup G, Jensen LB, Mogensen S. Nail abnormalities in nondermatologic patients: prevalence and possible role as diagnostic aids. J Am Acad Dermatol 1995;32:977–81.
39 Peyrot I, Boulinguez S, Sparsa A, Le Meur Y, Bonnetblanc JM, Bedane C. Bier's white spots associated with scleroderma renal crisis. Clin Exp Dermatol 2007;32:165–7.
40 Satoh T, Yokozeki H, Nishioka K. Vascular spiders and paper money skin improved by hemodialysis. Dermatology 2002;205:73–4.
41 Bhasin S, Jameson JL. Disorders of the testes and male reproductive system. In: Fauci AS (ed.) Harrison's Principles of Internal Medicine, 17th edn. McGraw Hill: New York, 2008: pp. 2310–23.
42 Cavanaugh J, Niewoehner CB, Nuttall FQ. Gynecomastia and cirrhosis of the liver. Arch Intern Med 1990;150:563–5.
43 Braunstein GD. Gynecomastia. N Engl J Med 1993;328:490–5.
44 Carda C, Gomez DE, Ferraris ME, Arriaga A, Carranza M, Peydró A. alcoholic parotid sialosis: a structural and ultrastructural study. Med Oral 2004;9:24–32.
45 Borsanyi SJ. Chronic asymptomatic enlargement of the parotid glands. Ann Otol (St. Luis) 1962;71:857–67.
46 Tirapelli LF, Tirapelli DPC, Schimming BC. Ultrastructural alterations of the parotid glands of rats (Rattus norvegicus) submitted to experimental chronic alcoholism. Rev Chil Anat 2001;19:175–82.
47 Wolfe SJ, Summerskill WHJ, Davidson C. Parotid swelling, alcoholism and cirrhosis. N Engl J Med 1957;256:491–9.
48 Konikoff F, Theodor E. Painful muscle cramps: a symptom of liver cirrhosis? J Clin Gastroenterol 1986;8:669–72.
49 Angeli P, Albino G, Carraro P, et al. Cirrhosis and muscle cramps: evidence of a causal relationship. Hepatology 1996;23:264–73.
50 Lam KC, Juttner HU, Reynolds TB. Spontaneous portosystemic shunt: relationship to spontaneous encephalopathy and gastrointestinal hemorrhage. Dig Dis Sci 1981;26: 346–52.
51 Udell JA, Wang CS, Tinmouth J, et al. Does this patient with liver disease have cirrhosis? JAMA 2012;307:832–42.
52 McCormick PA, Nolan N. Palpable epigastric liver as a physical sign of cirrhosis: a prospective study. Eur J Gastroenterol Hepatol 2004;16:1331–4.
53 Dubey S, Swaroop A, Jain R, Verma K, Garg P, Agarwal S. Percussion of Traube's space: a useful index of splenic enlargement. J Assoc Physicians India 2000;48:326–8.
54 Dilawari JB, Ganguly S, Chawla Y. Noncirrhotic portal fibrosis. Indian J Gastroenterol 1992;11:31–6.
55 Dilawari JB, Chawla YK. Extrahepatic portal venous obstruction. Gut 1988;29:554–5.
56 Menon KVN, Shah V, Kamath PS. The Budd Chiari syndrome. N Engl J Med 2004;350:578–85.
57 Ewy G. The abdominojugular test: technique and hemodynamic correlates. Ann Intern Med 1988;109:456–60.
58 Cattau EL Jr, Benjamin SB, Knuff TE, Castell DO. The accuracy of the physical exam in the diagnosis of suspected ascites. JAMA 1982;247:1164–6.
59 Conn HO. Quantifying the severity of hepatic encephalopathy. In: Conn H, Bircher J (eds) Hepatic Encephalopathy: Syndromes and Treatment. Bloomington: Medi-Ed Press; 1994. pp. 13–26.

CHAPTER 2

Diagnostic laboratory tests

Ying-Ying Yang and Han-Chieh Lin
Department of Medical Education, Taipei Veterans General Hospital and National Yang-Ming University School of Medicine, Taipei, Taiwan

Introduction

There is no single biomarker for liver cirrhosis, but its existence can be suggested by some laboratory abnormalities. We would initiate a series of biochemical investigations for patients in whom clinical symptoms of chronic liver disease are noted or the characteristics of liver cirrhosis are identified by physical examination. Liver function tests commonly includes tests to detect hepatic injury (aminotransferases, alkaline phosphatase, and gamma-glutamyl transpeptidase), tests assessing hepatic metabolism (serum bilirubin and ammonia), and tests assessing hepatic biosynthetic function (albumin and prothrombin time). In addition, the magnitude of the abnormalities in blood cell counts, serum biochemistries, and other tests may suggest the severity and etiology of liver cirrhosis.

Tests that detects hepatic injury (Table 2.1)

Serum aminotransferases

Alanine aminotransferase (ALT) and aspartate aminotransferase (AST) are hepatic enzymes that are involved in amino acid metabolism. However, high levels of AST are also found in the myocardium, kidneys, pancreas, skeletal muscle, red blood cells, and other tissues. In these circumstances, ALT is considered to be a specific and cost-effective screening test for hepatic injury but this test has limits when predicting the degree of hepatic inflammation and the severity of liver fibrosis [1,2]. ALT mainly exists in the cytosol of hepatocytes, whereas AST is mainly found in the mitochondria. Both of them are released into the bloodstream when hepatocytes are injured or die. However, normal aminotransferase levels do not preclude a diagnosis of liver cirrhosis [3].

Several studies have investigated AST : ALT ratios to correlate these with the severity of hepatic fibrosis. The ratio is about 0.8 in a healthy subject. In patients with alcoholic hepatitis, the AST : ALT ratio is often greater than 2 [4], whereas patients with most forms of nonalcoholic hepatitis have a ratio of less than 1. However, as the chronic hepatitis progresses to cirrhosis, the ratio of AST : ALT may reverse, with a ratio greater than 1 having a specificity of more than 80% for liver cirrhosis and a sensitivity that varies from 32% to 83% [5–8]. This suggests that we need to check for the presence of cirrhosis in patients with nonalcoholic liver disease when the AST : ALT ratio rises above 1. Bonacini et al. [9] concluded that the modified three-parameter cirrhosis discriminate score (CDS), which is derived from three laboratory parameters –platelet count, AST : ALT ratio, and prothrombin time (PT) – has a high likelihood of detecting liver cirrhosis, with a sensitivity of 46% and a specificity of 98% when the value is 8 or above (possible total score 0~11) [6,10]. Nevertheless, two other studies have failed to confirm the predictive value of the AST : ALT ratio for liver cirrhosis [11,12]. Therefore, the clinical utility of this ratio needs further investigation and its usefulness still remains uncertain for the diagnosis of liver cirrhosis.

Serum biliary enzymes

Alkaline phosphatase (ALK-P) is present in the bile canaliculi membrane of hepatocytes. It is often mildly elevated, but less than the two or three times the upper normal limit seen in liver cirrhosis. In patients with

Cirrhosis: A practical guide to management, First Edition. Edited by Samuel S. Lee and Richard Moreau.

Table 2.1 Normal range of parameters that detect hepatic injury and metabolism.

Hepatic injury			Hepatic metabolism		
Parameter	Normal range		Parameter	Normal range	
	SI units	Usual units		SI units	Usual units
Serum ALT	Female: 0.15–0.75 μkat/L Male: 0.15–1.1 μkat/L	3–55 U/L	Serum bilirubin	1.7–17 μmol/L	0.1–1 mg/dL
Serum AST	Female: 0.25–0.6 μkat/L Male: 0.25–0.75 μkat/L	12–48 U/L	Serum amonia	17–60 μg/dL	10–35 μmol/L
Serum ALK-P	0.6–1.8 μkat/L	80–280 U/L	ICG test	Retention at 15 min <8% (3.5–10.6%)	
Serum GGT	Female: 0–0.63 μkat/L Male: 0–0.92 μkat/L	Female: <55 U/L Male: <90 U/L	BSP test	Retention at 45 min <3.5%	

ALK-P, alkaline phosphate; ALT, alanine aminotransferase; AST, aspartate aminotransferase; BSP, bromsulphalein; GGT, gamma-glutamyl transferpeptidase; ICG, indocyanine green.

primary biliary cirrhosis (PBC) and primary sclerosing cholangitis (PSC), the serum level of ALK-P is higher than patients with other etiologies of liver cirrhosis. However, ALK-P is not only present in the hepatobiliary system, but also in the intestine, bone, kidneys, and placenta. Thus, ALK-P is likely to be less specific for liver disease. Although gamma-glutamyl transpeptidase (GGT) is also present in many other tissues, such as pancreas, kidneys, heart, and lung, it is considered to be more closely correlated to liver disease [13]. In patients with alcoholic hepatitis or alcoholic liver cirrhosis, the serum level of GGT will be much higher than those having liver cirrhosis due to other etiologies.

Tests of hepatic metabolism (Table 2.1)

Serum bilirubin

Serum bilirubin levels may be normal in patients with well-compensated liver cirrhosis. It becomes raised later than ALK-P and GGT as the severity of liver cirrhosis progresses. The hyperbilirubinemia in decompensated liver cirrhosis is related to persist cholestasis, hepatocellular dysfunction, and decreased renal excretory function. As one of the parameters in Child–Pugh–Turcotte score, the serum total bilirubin level is also an important predictor of survival in cirrhotic patients. In particular, in patients with PBC, an elevated serum bilirubin level suggests a poor prognosis [14].

Serum ammonia

Ammonia is produced by enterocytes from glutamine and by colonic bacterial catabolism of nitrogenous sources, such as ingested protein and secreted urea. The intact liver will convert nearly all ammonia to urea or glutamine via the urea cycle. Elevation of blood ammonia is a common feature in patients with liver cirrhosis. Hepatic dysfunction, shunting of blood around the liver, and muscle wasting, is a common characteristic of these patients and decreases the extrahepatic removal of ammonia. Patients with hepatic encephalopathy often have hyperammonemia. Treatments that lower plasma ammonia will improve the clinical status of encephalopathy. However, cerebral ammonia metabolism is not the only causal factor that is related to the development of hepatic encephalopathy [15]. Blood ammonia is not required to make a diagnosis of hepatic encephalopathy and neither does it indicate during long-term follow-up. Furthermore, there are many nonhepatic conditions, such as infection or intestinal bleeding, that can elevate a patient's blood ammonia level. It is important to be aware of these possible precipitating factors when treating hepatic encephalopathy in cirrhotic patients.

Indocyanine green and bromsulphalein tests

These two dye tests have been used to quantify the excretory capacity of the liver. They assess reserved hepatic function during advanced liver disease, particularly among patients who will undergo resection of the liver. The bromsulphalein (BSP) test is seldom performed now because of the possibility of an anaphylactic reaction. The indocyanine green (ICG) test is able to provide a good prediction of hepatic blood flow in healthy adults, but gives low readings in patients with liver cirrhosis, who show a marked decrease in extraction of ICG [16].

Tests of hepatic biosynthetic function (Table 2.2)

Serum albumin

Albumin is exclusively synthesized in the liver with approximately 15 g produced per day (200 mg/kg of body weight per day). Hypoalbuminemia that is a consequence of decreased production often reflects severe liver damage, such as liver cirrhosis [17]. Thus, a lower serum albumin level is indicative of more severe liver cirrhosis. As one of the parameters in the Child–Pugh score, just like bilirubin, the serum albumin level also suggests the survival probability in patients with liver cirrhosis. However, cirrhotic patients with massive ascites may have hypoalbuminemia but still have adequate hepatic synthetic function because of hypervolemic dilution via a remarkable increase in plasma volume [18]. On the other hand, hypoalbuminemia is not specific for liver disease; it could be caused by nephrotic syndrome, protein losing enteropathy, malnutrition, congestive heart failure, severe sepsis, and various other diseases. Therefore it is necessary to exclude these nonhepatic etiologies before evaluating the severity or prognosis of liver cirrhosis using the patient's serum albumin level.

Prothrombin time and international normalized ratio

Liver synthesizes most of the blood coagulating proteins. These include eight coagulating factors, factor I (fibrinogen), factor II (prothrombin), factor V, factor VII, factor IX, factor X, factor XII, and factor XIII, as well as three anti-thrombotic agents, anti-thrombin III, protein C, and protein S. Among them, synthesis of factors II, VII, IX, and X is dependent on the presence of vitamin K. The reduced ability of a cirrhotic liver to synthesize these coagulating factors will result in a longer PT. However, a prolonged PT is not specific for liver disease only. It also may be caused by increased consumption of coagulating factors (such as disseminated intravascular coagulation, severe sepsis, or severe bleeding), congenital or acquired coagulopathy, and side effects of certain drugs (e.g., flomoxef, cefmetazole). After excluding these conditions, there are two common causes of prolonged PT: vitamin K deficiency and severe liver dysfunction such as liver cirrhosis. The vitamin K deficiency-related PT prolongation is caused by malnutrition, prolonged obstructive jaundice, and so on, and can be normalized within 24 hours after a single parenteral administration of vitamin K. This typically good response of vitamin K deficiency-related PT prolongation could help us differentiate that from severe hepatic dysfunction-related PT prolongation. Severe hepatic dysfunction-related PT prolongation arises from poor utility of vitamin K and cannot be corrected by exogenous vitamin K administration.

The PT can help to predict survival probability in patients with liver cirrhosis when used as a parameter of Child–Pugh score and model for end-stage liver disease (MELD) score. In patients with fulminant hepatic failure,

Table 2.2 Normal range of parameters that detect hepatic biosynthetic function, coagulating factors, cell counts and others.

Hepatic biosynthetic function		Cell counts and others	
Parameter	**Normal range in SI units**	**Parameter**	**Normal range in SI units**
Serum albumin	3.5–5.0 g/dL (usual units: 540–740 μmol/L)	Serum platelet count	$15–45 \times 10^{10}$/L
Serum PT	8.3–10.8 seconds, INR: 0.9–1.2	Serum WBC count	$4500–11\,000 \times 10^{6}$/L
Serum factor VIII	50–200% of normal (control sample) activity	Serum hemoglobin	Male: 2.02–2.79 mmol/L Female: 1.86–2.48 mmol/L
Serum factor V	70–130% of normal (control sample) activity	Serum globulin levels	23–35 g/L
Serum factor VII	60–140% of normal (control sample) activity	Serum sodium concentration	135–145 mmol/L

INR, international normalized ratio; PT, prothrombin time; WBC, white blood cells.

a PT of more than 100 seconds indicates high priority for a liver transplantation [19]. Croquet et al. [19] have found that the PT is well correlated with histologic liver fibrosis score and has a high diagnostic accuracy for severe fibrosis or cirrhosis, especially in alcoholic liver cirrhosis.

Nevertheless, the PT cannot completely represent the whole picture of the coagulating status of the patient with liver cirrhosis [21]. The occurrence of bleeding will be inferred by the decreased levels of protein C, protein S, and anti-thrombin III, which favors thrombosis and a possibly superimposed infection or other conditions [22].

The international normalized ratio (INR) is adopted in the MELD score, which is used to prioritize patients in the waiting list for liver transplant [23]. Utilization of INR in patients with liver disease has the shortcoming that it will vary wildly because of the different types of thromboplastin used in this test [24,25]. Subsequently, it will influence the MELD score. As a result, several studies have tried to develop a standard form, such as "INR liver" to avoid this kind of variation [24]. However, it is still uncertain whether the widely implementation of the INR liver for the calculation of the MELD score is essential for all cirrhotic patients [25].

Individual serum coagulating factor levels

Factor VIII

Factor VIII is an endothelium-derived pro-coagulant factor that is increased in liver cirrhosis [26]. In cirrhotic patients, serum levels of factor VIII may help to distinguish whether disease is superimposed with disseminated intravascular coagulation (DIC). The serum level of factor VIII is increased in cirrhotic patients without DIC. By contrast, serum levels of factor VIII are significantly decreased in cirrhotic patients with DIC.

Factors V and VII

Synthesis of coagulation factors II, VII, IX, and X in liver is dependent on the availability of hepatic vitamin K. In patients with cirrhosis, a simultaneous decrease in factors V and VII is a consequence of liver dysfunction. A greater decrease in serum factor VII level than serum factor V level indicates deficiency of hepatic vitamin K.

Cell counts and other biochemistry (Table 2.2)

Thrombocytopenia

Reduction in the circulating platelet count is commonly found in patients with liver cirrhosis. The mechanisms of thrombocytopenia in cirrhosis include a reduced formation of thrombopoietin (TPO) [27], sequestration by the portal hypertension-related enlarged and congestive spleen, bone marrow suppression, and autoantibody-induced destruction of platelets [28]. Among these, splenic sequestration may be the main reason that an enlarged spleen could temporarily hold up to 90% of the circulating platelets. However, unless superimposed with other conditions, such as DIC, splenic sequestration seldom leads to severe thrombocytopenia (platelet count ≤50 000/mL) [13].

Furthermore, the platelet count will also influence thrombin generation in patients with liver cirrhosis, which will affect coagulation [29]. A platelet count of more than 50 000/mm^3 is related to adequate thrombin production, while a count of 100 000/mm^3 is associated with optimal thrombin production [29]. A platelet transfusion should be given to cirrhotic patients with thrombocytopenia if they are bleeding or before undergoing an invasive procedure or surgery.

Neutropenia

Neutropenia is often noted in patients with liver cirrhosis. It is usually related to splenic margination caused by hypersplenism.

Anemia

The anemia in liver cirrhosis might result from multiple causes. Microcytic anemia may be due to iron deficiency related to gastrointestinal bleeding (e.g., via gastric antral vascular ectasia). Normocytic anemia may be associated with anemia of chronic inflammation, and macrocytic anemia may arise from alcoholic toxicity that suppresses the bone marrow.

Globulins

Remarkably elevated serum IgG may suggest the association with autoimmune hepatitis. In cirrhotic patients, increased serum IgM levels may be present in more than 90% of patients with PBC [30]. Triger and Wright [31] suggested that shunting of intestinal bacterial antigens in the portal venous blood to lymphoid tissues would induce the plasma cells leading to increased serum globulins.

Hyponatremia

Hyponatremia in liver cirrhosis mainly arises from more water retention than sodium via the kidneys due to increased activity of antidiuretic hormone [32]. The severity of hyponatremia is positively correlated with the severity of liver cirrhosis [33]. Relatively poor prognosis is noted in cirrhotic patients with serum sodium concentrations of less than 130 mEq/L [32]. Furthermore, values of less than 125 mEq/L usually suggest the impending occurrence of hepatorenal syndrome. Hyponatremia is also an important predictor for the mortality of cirrhotic patients. Ruf et al. [34,35] reported that the addition of serum sodium levels into the MELD score predicts waiting list mortality better than MELD alone.

Accuracy of routine laboratory investigations (Table 2.3)

The presence of thrombocytopenia was the single most useful laboratory investigation and performed similarly to the presence of ascites for identifying cirrhosis. A platelet count threshold of less than $160 \times 10^3/\mu L$ had the highest diagnostic accuracy, with narrow confidence intervals despite statistical heterogeneity (positive likelihood ratio (LR), 6.3; 95% confidence interval (CI) 4.3–8.3; negative LR 0.29; 95% CI 0.20–0.39). A prolonged PT or INR (LR 5.0; 95% CI 3.2–6.9), or a serum albumin less than 3.5 g/dL (LR 4.4; 95% CI 1.5–7.3) were the other findings evaluated in several studies with a summary positive LR of more than 4.0 (Table 2.3). An increased ALT or bilirubin was not useful because their confidence intervals included unity. No other single laboratory finding had a negative LR that was substantially lower (range of negative LR 0.28–1.3) than the platelet count at a threshold of $160 \times 10^3/\mu L$.

Combination indices or models for detecting cirrhosis (Table 2.4)

The AST : ALT ratio and the AST : platelet ratio index (APRI; Table 2.4) have been the most extensively studied indices and are the easiest to calculate. An AST : ALT ratio higher than 1 increases the likelihood of cirrhosis (LR 4.6; 95% CI 2.6–6.5) as does an APRI higher than 29 (LR 4.6; 95% CI 3.2–6.0).

The Bonacini cirrhosis discriminant score (CDS) combines the ALT : AST ratio with the platelet count and INR into a discriminant function with possible total values between 0 and 11; higher values increase the likelihood of cirrhosis. A Bonacini CDS higher than 7 was the most frequently studied threshold (LR 9.4; 95% CI 2.6–37). A Bonacini CDS of less than 3 makes cirrhosis less likely (negative LR 0.30; 95% CI 0.18–0.50).

Table 2.3 Diagnostic accuracy of various diagnostic laboratory tests for cirrhosis.

Parameter	Sensitivity	Specificity	Positive LR (95% CI)	*P* value	Negative LR (95% CI)	*P* value
Plalelet count × $10^3/\mu L$ <160	0.74	0.88	6.3 (4.3–8.3)	<0.001	0.29 (0.2–0.39)	<0.001
Prolonged PT/INR	0.48	0.9	5 (3.2–6.9)	<0.001	0.59 (0.39–0.75)	<0.001
Albumin <3.5 g/dL	0.45	0.9	4.4 (1.5–7.3)	<0.02	0.61 (0.41–0.81)	<0.001
AST >ULN	0.78	0.62	2.1 (1.2–3.6)	<0.001	0.38 (0.21–0.67)	<0.02
GGT >300 U/L	0.49	0.82	2.8 (1.4–5.5)		0.62 (0.46–0.38)	
ACT >ULN	0.88	0.23	1.1 (0.99–1.3)	0.08	0.54 (0.17–0.91)	0.1
Bilirubin >1.2 mg/dL	0.43	0.84	2.7 (0.85–7.9)	<0.001	0.09 (0.35–1.1)	<0.001
WBC <4 × $10^3/\mu L$	0.25	0.9	2.5 (0.72–8.7)	0.18	0.9 (0.83–0.98)	0.8
Hemoglobulin <13 g/dL	0.45	0.8	1.9 (1.3–2.7)	0.58	0.8 (0.62–1)	0.15

Data from Nicastro et al. 2010 [48].

SI conversion factor: to convert bilirubin from mg/dL to μmol/L, multiply by 17.104.

ALT, alanine aminotransferase; AST, aspartate aminotransferase; CI, confidence interval; GGT: gamma-glutamyl transpeptidase; INR, international normalized ratio; LR, likelihood ratio; PT, prothrombin time; ULN, upper limit of normal; WBC, white blood cell.

Table 2.4 Definitions of the aspartate aminotransferase: platelet ratio index, Bonacini cirrhosis discriminant score, and Lok index.

Index/Score	Correlation with cirrhosis
AST: platelet ratio index (APRI) = (AST/upper limit of normal AST) × (100/platelet count [$\times 10^3/\mu L$])	Higher values of the APRI increase the likelihood of cirrhosis and lower values decrease the likelihood of cirrhosis
Bonacini cirrhosis discriminant score (CDS) = Platelet score + ALT : AST ratio score + INR score	Higher scores identify patients with higher likelihood of cirrhosis and lower scores identify patients with lower likelihood of cirrhosis

Score	Platelets ($\times 10^3/\mu L$)	ALT:AST ratio	INR
	>340	>1.7	<1.1
1	280–340	1.2–1.7	1.1–1.4
2	220–279	0.6–1.19	>1.4
3	160–219	<0.6	
4	100–159		
5	40–99		
6	<40		

The modified Bonacini CDS has a range of possible values from 0 to 11.

Index/Score	Correlation with cirrhosis
Lok index = exp (log odds)/[1 + exp (log odds)] Log odds = −5.56 − (0.0089 × platelet count [$\times 10^3/\mu L$]) + (1.26 × AST : ALT ratio) + (5.27 × INR) The Lok index is an odds ratio normalized to possible values between 0 and 1	A higher fraction (i.e., probability) increases the likelihood of cirrhosis, while a lower fraction reduces the likelihood of cirrhosis (see also http://www.haltctrial.org/cirrhosis.html)

Data from Nicastro et al. 2010 [48].
AST, aspartate transaminase; ALT, alanine aminotransferease; INR, international normalized ratio.

The Lok index, originally derived from the Hepatitis C Antiviral Long-term Treatment against Cirrhosis (HALT-C) trial cohort, is an odds ratio normalized to probabilities between 0 and 1 which uses the same factors as the Bonacini CDS but estimates the probability of cirrhosis through a logistic model (Table 2.4). An index of less than 0.2 (which represents a probability of <20) indicates a reduced likelihood of cirrhosis (LR 0.09; 95% CI 0.03–0.31).

Specific tests for determining the etiology of liver cirrhosis

Tests for viral hepatitis

Hepatitis A and E are usually self-limited and rarely result in liver cirrhosis. Therefore we investigate for hepatitis C, hepatitis B, and possibly superimposed hepatitis D in patients with liver cirrhosis.

Tests for alcoholic liver disease

The AST : ALT ratio in patients with alcoholic liver disease is often greater than 2. A significant elevation of serum GGT is often noted in alcoholic cirrhotic patients. Nevertheless, the most important criterion in the diagnosis of alcoholic liver disease is a history of chronic alcoholism.

Tests for primary biliary cirrhosis

- Serum ALK-P concentration is always elevated in PBC in parallel with GGT, while the serum ALT and AST levels might be normal or slightly elevated. Elevation of serum bilirubin level indicates a poor prognosis [14].
- Anti-mitochondrial antibody (AMA) is the most important serologic test of PBC; it is positive in about 95% of patients [36,37]. Antinuclear antibody and

anti-smooth muscle antibody are also positive in nearly half of patients with PBC [36]. According to the good sensitivity (95%) and specificity (98%) of the above serologic markers for PBC [38], liver biopsy is not necessary for the diagnosis of PBC if the patient is positive for serum AMA [36].

- Hypereosinophilia, which is involved in its pathogenesis, can be found in the early stages of PBC [39].
- Hypercholesterolemia is a special characteristic of PBC; the total serum cholesterol concentration may exceed 1000 mg/dL in PBC patients with xanthomas [40]. In the early stage, serum levels of low-density lipoprotein (LDL) and very low-density lipoprotein (VLDL) will be mildly elevated. To compensate, the serum levels of high-density lipoprotein (HDL) will be elevated. This may be responsible for the not greatly increased risk for atherosclerosis in PBC patients with hypercholesterolemia [41].

Tests for primary sclerosing cholangitis

- The serum biochemistry shows a cholestatic pattern, while the serum levels of AST and ALT are typically less than 300 IU/L.
- Perinuclear antineutrophil cytoplasmic antibodies (P-ANCA) will be positive in 30–80% of patients with PSC, but without good specificity. Additionally, increased serum immunoglobulin M (IgM) levels are also noted in 40–50% of patients with PSC [42,43].

Tests for hereditary hemochromatosis

Transferrin saturation

Increased transferrin saturation above 60% in men and 50% in women has a good predictive ability of over 90% for patients with homozygous hereditary hemochromatosis [44]. In both genders, decreasing the cutoff value of transferrin saturation to 45% increases the sensitivity for homozygous hereditary hemochromatosis but may also increase the false positive rate.

Plasma ferritin level

Elevated plasma ferritin concentrations above 300 ng/mL in men and 200 ng/mL in women suggests iron overload. However, serum ferritin levels are less specific for iron overload than transferrin saturation because its characteristic of also as an acute phase protein that will be elevated in many other circumstances, such as inflammation and stress. Moreover, plasma ferritin concentration is less sensitive than transferrin saturation in screening for hereditary hemochromatosis because a greater degree of iron overload is required to elevate the ferritin concentration [45].

The American Association for the Study of Liver Disease (AASLD) screening guidelines in 2011 considered transferrin saturations above 45% and serum ferritin levels greater than 200 ng/mL in men and 150 ng/mL in women to be the cutoff levels for screening of patients with iron overload [46].

Tests for Wilson's disease

Serum ceruloplasmin

Serum levels of ceruloplasmin, which is synthesized by hepatocytes as the major carrier of copper in the blood, are decreased in patients with Wilson's disease. About 85–90% of patients have serum concentrations below 20 mg/dL [47]. However, the serum ceruloplasmin level alone cannot establish the diagnosis of Wilson's disease. Low serum ceruloplasmin concentrations of less than 20 mg/dL, accompanied by Kayser–Fleischer rings due to copper deposits in Descemet's membrane of patients' eyes are thought to be diagnostic.

Serum copper

Non-ceruloplasmin-bound serum copper levels are increased (often above 25 μg/dL) in patients with Wilson's disease (normal <15 μg/dL). However, the sensitivity and specificity of this test have not been well established.

Urine copper excretion

The 24-hour urinary copper excretion in patients with Wilson's disease is typically greater than 100 μg (>1.6 μmol), whereas a value of more than 40 μg/day (or more than 600 nmol/day) warrants further investigation [48]. Penicillamine challenge will greatly increase urine copper excretion and will increase the specificity for Wilson's disease. This challenge test might be performed in children who have symptoms of Wilson's disease but who have urine copper excretions of less than 100 μg in 24 hours [49]. However, the predictive value of this test in adults is unknown [50,51].

Tests for alpha-1 antitrypsin deficiency

Lower levels of serum alpha-1 antitrypsin, less than 11 μmol/L, combined with a severely deficient genotype make the diagnosis of severe alpha-1 antitrypsin deficiency [52,53]. In cirrhotic patients with the features of emphysema, young age, nonsmoker or minimal smoker, predominantly basilar changes on the chest radiograph, positive family history, and history of panniculitis or unexplained chronic liver disease, the diagnosis of alpha-1 antitrypsin deficiency should be considered [52,53].

Conclusions

There is no single biomarker for liver cirrhosis; routine laboratory tests are usually not diagnostic. However, the abnormalities found in the laboratory data may provide clues for the etiology, severity, and possible prognosis of liver cirrhosis.

The conventional liver function tests mainly include tests for hepatic injury, hepatic metabolism, and biosynthetic function. With these data and the routine blood cell count and other biochemistries, it should be possible to diagnose and evaluate the severity of liver cirrhosis.

It is important to determine the etiology of liver cirrhosis for the purposes of further treatment and to predict prognosis. The common serologic screening tests include tests for hepatitis B and C, autoimmune hepatitis, PBC, and PSC, hemochromatosis, Wilson's disease, and alpha-1 antitrypsin deficiency.

References

1 Dufour DR, Lott JA, Nolte FS, Gretch DR, Koff RS, Seeff LB. Diagnosis and monitoring of hepatic injury. II. Recommendations for use of laboratory tests in screening, diagnosis, and monitoring. Clin Chem 2000;46:2050–68.

2 Heidelbaugh J, Bruderly M. Cirrhosis and chronic liver failure: part 1. Diagnosis and evaluation. Am Fam Physician 2006;74:756–62.

3 Ellis G, Goldberg DM, Spooner RJ, Ward AM. Serum enzyme tests in diseases of the liver and biliary tree. Am J Clin Pathol 1978;70:248–58.

4 Cohen J, Kaplan M. The SGOT/SGPT ratio: an indicator of alcoholic liver disease. Dig Dis Sci 1979;24:835–8.

5 Nanji AA, French SW, Mendenhall CL. Serum aspartate aminotransferase to alanine aminotransferase ratio in human and experimental alcoholic liver disease. Enzyme 1989;41:112–5.

6 Williams A, Hoofnagle J. Relationship of serum aspartate to alanine aminotransferase in chronic hepatitis: relationship to cirrhosis. Gastroenterology 1988;95:734–9.

7 Pradat P, Alberti A, Poynard T, et al. Predictive value of ALT levels for histologic findings in chronic hepatitis C. Hepatology 2002;36:973–7.

8 Lok AS, Ghany MG, Goodman ZD, et al. Predicting cirrhosis in patients with hepatitis C based on standard laboratory tests. Hepatology 2005;42:282–92.

9 Bonacini M, Hadi G, Govindarajan S, et al. Utility of a discriminant score for diagnosing advanced fibrosis or cirrhosis in patients with chronic hepatitis C virus infection. Am J Gastroenterol 1997;92:1302–4.

10 Udell JA, Wang CS, Tinmouth J, et al. Does this patient with liver disease have cirrhosis? JAMA 2012;307:832–42.

11 Imperiale T, Said A, Cummings O, Born LJ. Need for validation of clinical decision aids: use of the AST/ALT ratio in predicting cirrhosis in chronic hepatitis C. Am J Gastroenterol 2000;95:2328–32.

12 Reedy D, Loo A, Levine R. AST/ALT ratio R1 is not diagnostic of cirrhosis in patients with chronic hepatitis C. Dig Dis Sci 1998;43:2156–9.

13 Pratt D, Kaplan M. Evaluation of the liver A: laboratory tests. In Schiff E, Sorrel M, Maddrey W (eds) Schiff's Diseases of the Liver, 8th edn. Philadelphia; Lippincott Williams & Wilkens: 1999. p. 205.

14 Krzeski P, Zych W, Kraszewska E, Milewski B, Butruk E, Habior A. Is serum bilirubin concentration the only valid prognostic marker in primary biliary cirrhosis? Hepatology 1999;30:865–9.

15 Weissenborn K, Ahl B, Fischer-Wasels D, et al. Correlations between magnetic resonance spectroscopy alterations and cerebral ammonia and glucose metabolism in cirrhotic patients with and without hepatic encephalopathy. Gut 2007;56:1736–42.

16 Wynne HA, Goudevenos J, Rawlins MD, James OF, Adams PC, Woodhouse KW. Hepatic drug clearance: the effect of age using indocyanine green as a model compound. Br J Clin Pharmacol 1990;30:634–7.

17 Rothschild MA, Oratz M, Zimmon D, Schreiber SS, Weiner I, Van Caneghem A. Albumin synthesis in cirrhotic subjects with ascites studied with carbonate-14C. J Clin Invest 1969;48:344–50.

18 Lieberman FL, Reynolds TB. Plasma volume in cirrhosis of the liver: its relation of portal hypertension, ascites and renal failure. J Clin Invest 1967;46:1297–308.

19 O'Grady JG, Alexander GJ, Hayllar KM, Williams R. Early indicators of prognosis in fulminant hepatic failure. Gastroenterology 1989;97:439–45.

20 Croquet V, Vuillemin E, Ternisien C, et al. Prothrombin index is an indirect marker of severe liver fibrosis. Eur J Gastroenterol Hepatol 2002;14:1133–41.

21 Tripodi A, Salerno F, Chantarangkul V, et al. Evidence of normal thrombin generation in cirrhosis despite abnormal conventional coagulation tests. Hepatology 2005;41:553–8.

22 Koliscak L, Maynor L. Pharmacologic prophylaxis against venous thromboembolism in hospitalized patients with

cirrhosis and associated coagulopathies. Am J Health Syst Pharm 2012;69:658–63.
23 Wiesner R, Edwards E, Freeman R, et al. Model for end-stage liver disease (MELD) and allocation of donor livers. Gastroenterology 2003;124:91–6.
24 Tripodi A, Chantarangkul V, Primignani M, et al. The international normalized ratio calibrated for liver cirrhosis (INR (liver) normalizes prothrombin time results for model for end-stage liver disease calculation. Hepatology 2007;46: 520–7.
25 Tripodi A, Chantarangkul V, Primignani M, et al. Point-of-care coagulation monitors calibrated for the international normalized ratio for cirrhosis (INR liver) can help to implement the INR liver for the calculation of the MELD score. J Hepatol 2009;51:288–95.
26 Tripodi A, Primignani M, Chantarangkul V, et al. An imbalance of pro- vs. anti-coagulation factors in plasma from patients with cirrhosis. Gastroenterology 2009;137: 2105–11.
27 Goulis J, Chau TN, Jordan S, et al. Thrombopoietin concentrations are low in patients with cirrhosis and thrombocytopenia and are restored after orthotropic liver transplantation. Gut 1999;44:754–8.
28 Kajihara M, Okazaki Y, Kato S, et al. Evaluation of platelet kinetics in patients with liver cirrhosis: similarity to idiopathic thrombocytopenia purpura. J Gastroenterol Hepatol 2007; 22:112–8.
29 Tripodi A, Primignani M, Chantarangkul V, et al. Thrombin generation in patients with cirrhosis: the role of platelets. Hepatology 2006;44:440–5.
30 Lindor KD, Gershwin ME, Poupon R, Kaplan M, Bergasa NV, Heathcote EJ; American Association for Study of Liver Diseases. Primary biliary cirrhosis. Hepatology 2009;50: 291–308.
31 Triger DR, Wright R. Hyperglobulinaemia in liver disease. Lancet 1973;301:1494–6.
32 Papadakis MA, Fraser CL, Arieff AL. Hyponatremia in patients with cirrhosis. Q J Med 1990;76:675–88.
33 Ginees P, Guevara M. Hyponatremia in cirrhosis: pathogenesis, clinical significance, and management. Hepatology 2008;48:1002–10.
34 Ruf AE, Kremers WK, Chavez LL, Descalzi VI, Podesta LG, Villami FG. Addition of serum sodium into the MELD score predicts waiting list mortality better than MELD alone. Liver Transpl 2005;11:336–43.
35 Sersté T, Gustot T, Rautou PE, et al. Severe hyponatremia is a better predictor of mortality than MELDNa in patients with cirrhosis and refractory ascites. J Hepatol 2012;57:274–80.
36 Kaplan MM, Gershwin ME. Primary biliary cirrhosis. N Engl J Med 2005;353:1261–73.
37 Poupon R. Primary biliary cirrhosis. J Hepatol 2010;52: 745–58.
38 Muratori L, Granito A, Muratori P, Pappas G, Bianchi FB. Antimitochondrial antibodies and other antibodies in primary biliary cirrhosis: diagnostic and prognostic value. Clin Liver Dis 2008;12:261–76.
39 Yamazaki K, Nakadate I, Suzuki K, Sato S, Masuda T. Eosinophilia in primary biliary cirrhosis. Am J Gastroenterol 1996;91:516–22.
40 Sorokin A, Brown JL, Thompson PD. Primary biliary cirrhosis, hyperlipidemia, and atherosclerotic risk: a systematic review. Atherosclerosis 2007;194:293–9.
41 Jahn CE, Schaefer EJ, Taam LA, et al. Lipoprotein abnormalities in primary biliary cirrhosis: association with hepatic lipase inhibition as well as altered cholesterol esterification. Gastroenterology 1985;89:1266–78.
42 Lee YM, Kaplan MM. Primary sclerosing cholangitis. N Engl J Med 1995;332:924–33.
43 Chapman R, Fevery J, Kalloo A, et al. Diagnosis and management of primary sclersing cholangitis. Hepatology 2010; 51:660–78.
44 Pippard MJ. Detection of iron overload. Lancet 1997;349: 73–4.
45 Edwards CQ, Kushner JP. Screening for hemochromatosis. N Engl J Med 1993;328:1616–20.
46 Bacon BR, Adams PC, Kowdley KV, Powell LW, Tavill AS. Diagnosis and management of hemochromatosis: 2011 practice guideline by the American Association for the Study of Liver Diseases. Hepatology 2011;54:328–43.
47 Stremmel W, Meyerrose KW, Niederau C, Hefter H. Kreuzpainter G, Strohmeyer G. Wilson disease: clinical presentation, treatment, and survival. Ann Intern Med 1991; 115:720–6.
48 Nicastro E, Ranucci G, Vajro P, Vegnente A, Iorio R. Re-evaluation of the diagnostic criteria for Wilson disease in children with mild liver disease. Hepatology 2010;52: 1948–56.
49 Müller T, Koppikar S, Taylor RM, et al. Re-evaluation of the penicillamine challenge test in the diagnosis of Wilson's disease in children. J Hepatol 2007;47:270–6.
50 Roberts EA, Schilsky ML. American Association for Study of Liver Diseases (AASLD). Diagnosis and treatment of Wilson disease: an update. Hepatology 2008;47:2089–11.
51 European Association for the Study of the Liver. EASL clinical practice guideline Wilson disease. J Hepatol 2012;56:671–85.
52 Stoller JK, Aboussouan LS. Alpha1-antitrypsin deficiency. Lancet 2005;365:2225–36.
53 Fairbanks KD, Tavill AS. Liver disease in alpha-1 antitrypsin deficiency: a review. Am J Gastroenterol 2008;103:2136–41.

CHAPTER 3

Diagnostic imaging modalities

Soon Koo Baik,[1] Moon Young Kim,[1] and Woo Kyoung Jeong[2]

[1]*Department of Internal Medicine, Yonsei University Wonju College of Medicine, Wonju, Republic of Korea*

[2]*Department of Radiology and Center for Imaging Science, Samsung Medical Center, Sungkyunkwan University School of Medicine, Seoul, Republic of Korea*

In chronic liver disease, diagnostic imaging has a significant role for patient management: diagnosis of hepatocellular carcinoma and progression to cirrhosis. As an antiviral treatment for viral hepatitis has been developed recently, the diagnosis of cirrhosis becomes more important for effective treatment. Basic diagnostic imaging modalities consist of ultrasonography (US), computed tomography (CT), and magnetic resonance imaging (MRI), and the many specific techniques derived from basic methods are developing for a convenient, noninvasive, and accurate diagnosis.

Ultrasonography-based approaches

Regardless of the underlying etiology, fibrosis is the main component of chronic liver damage that is directly related to disease severity and prognosis. Accurate estimation of the severity of fibrosis is essential for evaluating the disease state and prognosis, and is the first step toward the optimization of treatment and estimation of its response [1,2].

Liver biopsy is the gold standard for assessing fibrosis. However, standard clinical liver biopsy procedures have several limitations, including sampling errors, inter- and intraobserver variability, and invasiveness [3]. The ideal noninvasive test for diagnosing fibrosis would be simple and reproducible, readily available, less expensive than biopsy, and able to predict the full spectrum of fibrosis and to reflect any changes induced by therapy [4]. Many trials have been conducted with a view to finding this ideal test; however, no test has yet satisfied all of the aforementioned requirements. Moreover, recent advances in knowledge and treatment have led to proposals for more detailed histologic diagnosis of fibrosis, and these have made it even more difficult to find an ideal noninvasive substitute for liver biopsy sampling [5,6].

Various imaging modalities have been tried as methods for assessing liver fibrosis in chronic liver damage, including US, CT), and magnetic resonance (MR) based methods.

This chapter reviews the role of various US tests used in the diagnosis and assessment of hepatic fibrosis, including grayscale US, Doppler US, contrast-enhanced US (CEUS), and elastography.

Grayscale and Doppler US

Grayscale and Doppler US are noninvasive and relatively simple and inexpensive tests that are used to study and follow-up patients with chronic liver disease and cirrhosis. Various factors including the liver size, the bluntness of the liver edge, the coarseness of the liver parenchyma, the nodularity of the liver surface, portal vein (PV) velocity, and spleen size have been suggested as useful parameters for the US-based evaluation of chronic liver disease [7–14].

A previous study obtained a diagnostic accuracy ranging from 73% (Metavir score of ≥F2) to 84% (Metavir score of ≥F3) when using multiple grayscale US indices for fibrosis (i.e., liver length, liver surface nodularity, spleen length, and splenic vein respiratory variation) and one Doppler US index (i.e., PV velocity) [9]. Another study introduced a US scoring system using the surface pattern and the appearance of the internal echogenic bands, which relate to the irregularity of the liver texture, and demonstrated a significant correlation between US stages and the histologic staging of fibrosis [13]. Another study using the bluntness of the liver edge,

Cirrhosis: A practical guide to management, First Edition. Edited by Samuel S. Lee and Richard Moreau.

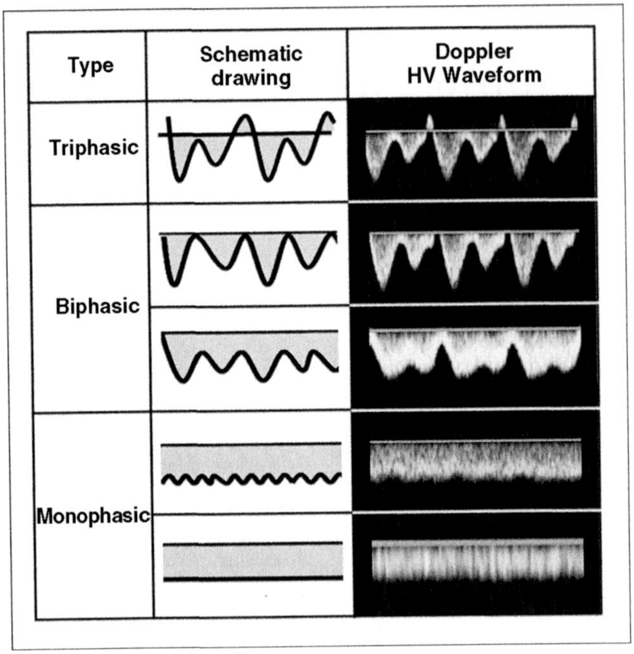

Figure 3.1 Schematic drawings and US Doppler waveforms shows classification of hepatic vein Doppler waveforms.

the irregularity of liver surface, and the coarseness of the parenchymal texture as indicators confirmed the usefulness of the US staging system [15]. However, although US can provide a qualitative assessment of the hepatic parenchyma composition, it is both subjective and operator dependent. Liver fibrosis and steatosis can have similar appearances on US and can be present at the same time in a "fatty-fibrotic pattern" [16–18]. In addition, some studies have shown that the sensitivity and specificity of US in demonstrating hepatic fibrosis are unacceptably low and that there is no correlation between US findings and the histologic stage of fibrosis on liver biopsy [19,20].

Regional hepatic and systemic hemodynamic changes are essential findings in liver fibrosis [21]. Therefore, Doppler US has been used to detect the hemodynamic changes that are known to be present from the precirrhotic stages of hepatic fibrogenesis. Doppler US indices include the PV blood volume, mean or maximum PV velocity, portal blood flow, the congestion index of the PV, effective portal liver perfusion, and resistance indices of arteries in the liver and spleen [9,21–26]. Furthermore, pulsed wave Doppler can be applied to determine the changes in waveforms of the proper hepatic arteries, PV, and hepatic vein. While the normal flow pattern in the right hepatic vein is triphasic, patients with a biphasic or monophasic flow pattern more often have advanced fibrosis (Figure 3.1) [24,27–29].

However, Doppler measurement is influenced by many patient-related factors such as respiration and timing of meals as well as observer variability and equipment differences. Furthermore, collateral pathways, hepatic steatosis, and inflammation further contribute to the measurement variability [30–32].

Taken together, grayscale and Doppler US are safe, inexpensive, and simple to use at the bedside or for outpatients, and combining multiple US indices can improve the diagnostic accuracy of cirrhosis in some conditions.

Contrast-enhanced ultrasonography

CEUS imaging represents a new US modality for the assessment of chronic liver disease. CEUS involves the intravenous administration of minute, gas-filled microbubbles that strongly enhance the intensity of signals from the intravascular flow. The various commercially available contrast agents differ in their designs and kinetics, and can therefore yield different results; they cannot be used interchangeably [33–36]. Bolus injections of microbubble agents can be used for first-pass kinetics studies, and can be used to assess transit times. It has been shown that hepatic vein transit times shorten when the liver disease worsens [33,37,38]. In theory, shorter hepatic vein transit times in patients with diffuse liver disease occur mainly secondary to arteriovenous shunting and arterializations of capillary beds in the liver and, to a lesser degree, shunting in the pulmonary and gastrointestinal capillaries. In addition, the time–intensity curve differs significantly between the normal liver parenchyma and the cirrhotic liver, with the level of decrease being related to the degree of liver damage present [39]. Comparison of the signal intensity of a region of interest within the liver parenchyma has also revealed that the accumulation of microbubbles in the liver parenchyma is decreased in nonalcoholic steatohepatitis, but not in nonalcoholic fatty liver disease or chronic viral hepatitis [40].

In conclusion, CEUS could be a simple and noninvasive test for reliably screening cirrhosis based on contrast-agent transit or the parenchymal enhancement pattern. However, this method also has some limitations in that it requires the injection of a contrast agent, considerable operator skill, and access to the relevant technology. More intensive studies and validation are needed.

Measurement of liver stiffness: transient elastography, acoustic radiation force impulse, supersonic shear-wave elastography, and real-time elastography

The increase in liver stiffness associated with chronic liver disease is primarily because of the presence of fibrosis [41]. Tissue elastography, which was introduced in 1992, is used to visualize differences in the mechanical properties between tissues [42]. The most attractive advantage of tissue elastography is the ability to quantify the viscoelasticity of the tissue, which means that it can be used for measuring hepatic fibrosis in the liver. To date, two US elastography techniques have been used to measure liver stiffness: shear-wave-based elastography and real-time elastography. Shear-wave-based elastography includes transient elastography (TE), which is the most widely used, acoustic radiation force impulse (ARFI) imaging, and supersonic shear-wave elastography (SSWE). Shear-wave-based elastography involves using an ultrasonic beam to measure the propagation velocity of a shear wave through the soft tissue under investigation, with liver stiffness being displayed in kilopascals or centimeters per second.

TE is the first commercialized elastography protocol developed to assess noninvasively the stiffness of deep soft tissues such as the liver. A mechanical vibrator generates a low-frequency elastic wave at 50 Hz to produce a shear stress in the target tissue at a distance of 4 cm, and then, as mentioned above, the velocity of the shear wave is measured using an ultrasound signal. TE has been validated extensively by numerous investigations targeted at patients with chronic liver disease and cirrhosis, and it is generally accepted that TE findings are strongly correlated with the stage of liver fibrosis. However, it does not provide a B-mode image (which is very helpful for targeting), only the right liver can be measured, and it has a higher measurement failure rate (5.5–6%), mainly because of limiting factors such as obesity and ascites [43]. ARFI imaging and SSWE use focused high-intensity, short-duration acoustic pulses instead of the mechanical vibration used in TE to produce a shear wave in the target tissue [44]. Like TE, the shear-wave velocity is observed by aiming repeated ultrasound beam pulses across the region of interest. SSWE is a new type of the shear-wave-based US elastography technique and uses multiple acoustic radiation force impulses [45]. It exhibits the remarkable feature of the viscoelastic properties in all areas within the region of interest being demonstrated on a color-coded look-up table. ARFI imaging and SSWE are expected to overcome the limitations of TE, such as measurement failures due to severe obesity, thick subcutaneous fat, and ascites. Moreover, they are able to display a grayscale US image on the background of the elastography, and so are more reliable and familiar to physicians who use conventional US. However, a high level of clinical experience and evidence are needed in order to apply either ARFI imaging or SSWE for the diagnosis of liver fibrosis.

Real-time elastography is a method derived from the static elastography technique used for the measurement of breast tissue elasticity [46,47]. It differs technically from TE in that the echo signals obtained by conventional ultrasound probes before and when under slight compression are compared and analyzed. Tissue elasticity cannot be measured directly from reflected ultrasound echoes, and so the relative tissue elasticity is calculated and displayed as a color overlay on the conventional B-mode image. It is difficult to apply pressure to the liver using an ultrasound probe, so liver stiffness is calculated from the displacement of the tissue that results automatically from pressure applied by the heartbeat. Reflected

US echoes are then used to compute the displacement and, thus, the strain distribution in the tissue.

Many clinical studies have been conducted to test the effectiveness of TE for the diagnosis of hepatic fibrosis [48,49]. TE is useful as a screening test for cirrhosis, but is not recommended for diagnosing stages other than cirrhosis because the optimal cutoffs of liver stiffness have not been validated for individual stages of fibrosis. Relatively few clinical studies have been conducted on ARFI imaging and SSWE for comparison with TE, although some studies have shown that the performance and reliability of ARFI imaging and SSWE are comparable to those of TE [44,45,50].

Measurement of liver stiffness also has a major role in estimating the severity of portal hypertension in patients with cirrhosis. Increased portal pressure is the main factor determining the clinical course of cirrhosis: variceal formation, variceal bleeding, portal hypertensive enteropathy, ascites, spontaneous bacterial peritonitis, hepatorenal syndrome, and hepatic encephalopathy are representative manifestations of decompensated cirrhosis. Measurement of the hepatic venous pressure gradient (HVPG) following hepatic venous catheterization is a surrogate marker of portal hypertension estimation, but this technique is somewhat invasive. Recent testing of the feasibility of liver stiffness measurement for detecting severe portal hypertension revealed a strong correlation with both HVPG and the presence of complications related to portal hypertension [51,52].

In conclusion, the development of various promising techniques for measuring liver stiffness have helped to overcome the limitations of conventional US, not only for evaluating hepatic fibrosis, but also for predicting the development of fatal complications related to chronic liver disease or portal hypertension, as well as the patient's prognosis.

CT- and MRI-based approaches

As mentioned above regarding US, cross-sectional imaging studies such as CT and MRI are useful imaging modalities for the diagnosis of cirrhosis (Figure 3.2). These modalities are considered as standard methods for the diagnosis of hepatocellular carcinoma (HCC) on the background of chronic liver disease, including cirrhosis [53,54]. The radiologic features of advanced cirrhosis are normally obvious: surface nodularity, prominent fibrous septa, shrinkage of liver volume, and an enlarged portal venous system including varices and splenomegaly due to portal hypertension. However, it is difficult to diagnose the early stage of cirrhosis, and so various functional techniques using CT and MRI have been developed recently and described in many hepatology and radiology journals. This chapter describes the morphologic features of cirrhosis with various etiologies and the hemodynamic and functional imaging techniques for the early diagnosis of cirrhosis and its complications.

Morphologic changes

In the advanced stages of cirrhosis, the morphologic changes in the liver can be clearly demonstrated by both CT and MRI. Although the imaging features are highly specific for cirrhosis, the sensitivity is very low for early cirrhosis. The observed nodularity of the liver surface is caused by the presence of numerous regenerative nodules and fibrotic scars.

Regenerative nodules are seldom evident on CT, but MRI reveals subtle changes such as regenerative nodules and strands of fibrosis. Regenerative nodules are composed of hepatocytes that regenerate in the fibrous scars following lobular hepatitis, and confluent necrosis of the hepatocytes [55]. Due to stepwise carcinogenesis from a regenerative nodule to a dysplastic nodule and then to HCC, cirrhotic nodules including regenerative and dysplastic nodules should be differentiated from HCC by using various MRI sequences and dynamic contrast enhancement. These cirrhotic nodules generally manifest as isoattenuating on CT, hypointense on T2-weighted MRI, and with no enhancement on arterial-phase CT and MRI, and are considered benign lesions [56]. Conversely, HCC appears with high signal intensity on T2-weighted MRI, as an early enhancement on arterial-phase CT and MRI because of its change of vascularity, and with high signal intensity on diffusion-weighted imaging (DWI) due to its high degree of cellularity [56,57].

Fibrotic scars are barely visible on conventional CT and MRI but, in patients with advanced cirrhosis, unenhanced MRI may reveal fibrotic septa as hypo- and hyperintense reticulations on T1- and T2-weighted MRI, respectively [58]. The use of either a gadolinium-based contrast agent or superparamagnetic iron oxide (SPIO) agent will result in hepatic fibrosis appearing as very clear contrast enhancement on MRI. Gadolinium-based contrast agents, except hepatocyte-specific agents

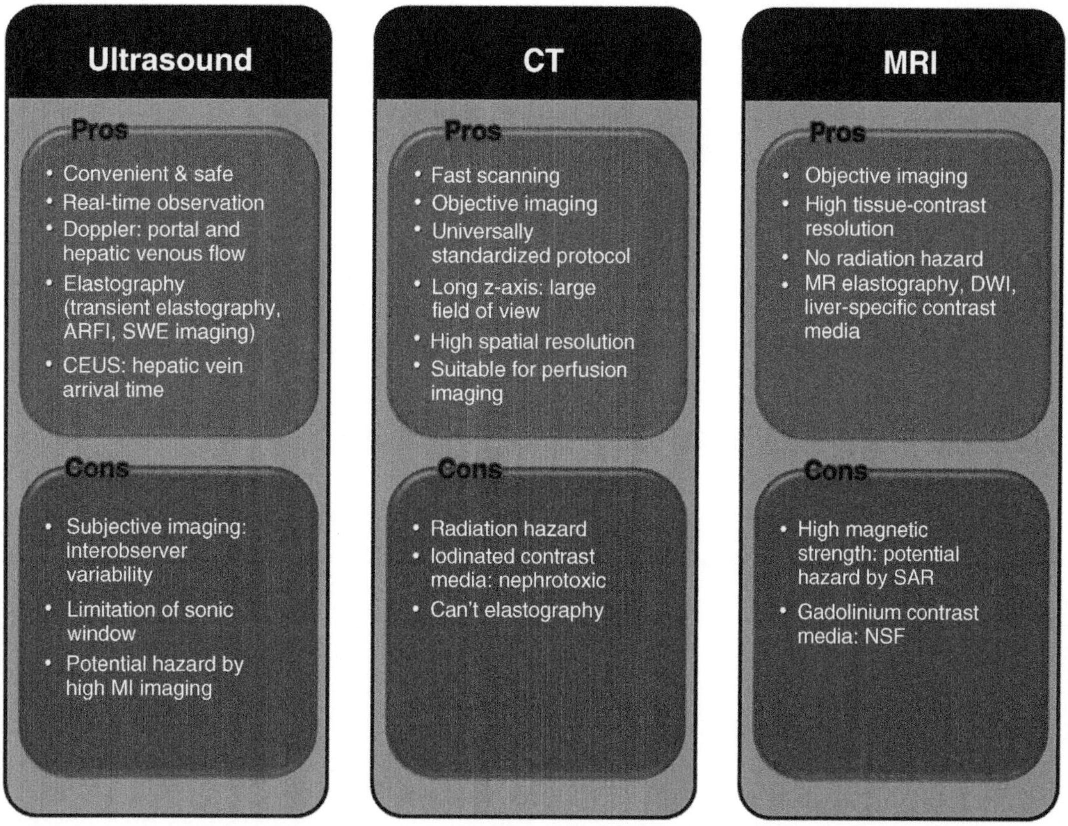

Figure 3.2 Pros and cons of imaging modalities for diagnosis of cirrhosis. ARFI, acoustic radiation force impulse; CEUS, contrast-enhanced ultrasonography; CT, computed tomography; DWI, diffusion-weighted imaging; MR, magnetic resonance; MRI, magnetic resonance imaging; NSF, nephrogenic systemic fibrosis; SAR, specific absorption rate; SWE, shear-wave elastography.

such as gadoxetate disodium or gadobenate dimeglumine, equilibrate with the extracellular matrix of the liver in the delayed phase and accumulate in fibrotic liver tissue [59]. On the other hand, the SPIO agent is not taken up into fibrous septa, but rather into Kupffer cells in the hepatic sinusoid. As the signal intensity of the SPIO agent in the Kupffer cell is decreased on T2*-weighted gradient-recalled-echo sequence imaging, the fibrous septa are brighter than the regenerative nodules in which Kupffer cells are present [60]. A hybrid enhancement technique using sequentially both SPIO and gadolinium-based agents was also introduced to synergistically improve the diagnosis of hepatic fibrosis [61,62].

Cross-sectional imaging can be used for the diagnosis of cirrhosis; thus, several imaging signs related to morphologic changes of the liver have been investigated. A modified caudate : right-lobe ratio is one of these morphologic CT signs [63], defined by using the bifurcation of the right PV as a landmark, which is considered as a lateral boundary for the caudate lobe and a medial boundary for the right lobe. According to that study, the sensitivity and accuracy for diagnosing cirrhosis was about 72% and 74%, respectively, when using a modified caudate: right-lobe ratio cutoff of greater than 0.90. The expanded gallbladder fossa sign and the right posterior hepatic notch sign are other morphologic features visible on cross-sectional imaging in cirrhosis [64]. In the normal liver, the gallbladder fits into a fossa in the plane of the major interlobar fissure. In patients with cirrhosis, the fossa is widened because of atrophy of the right liver, and filled with fat tissue. The right posterior hepatic notch is a sharp pit on the right medial posterior surface of the liver that is usually noted in patients with cirrhosis. The use of these signs produces a very high specificity and

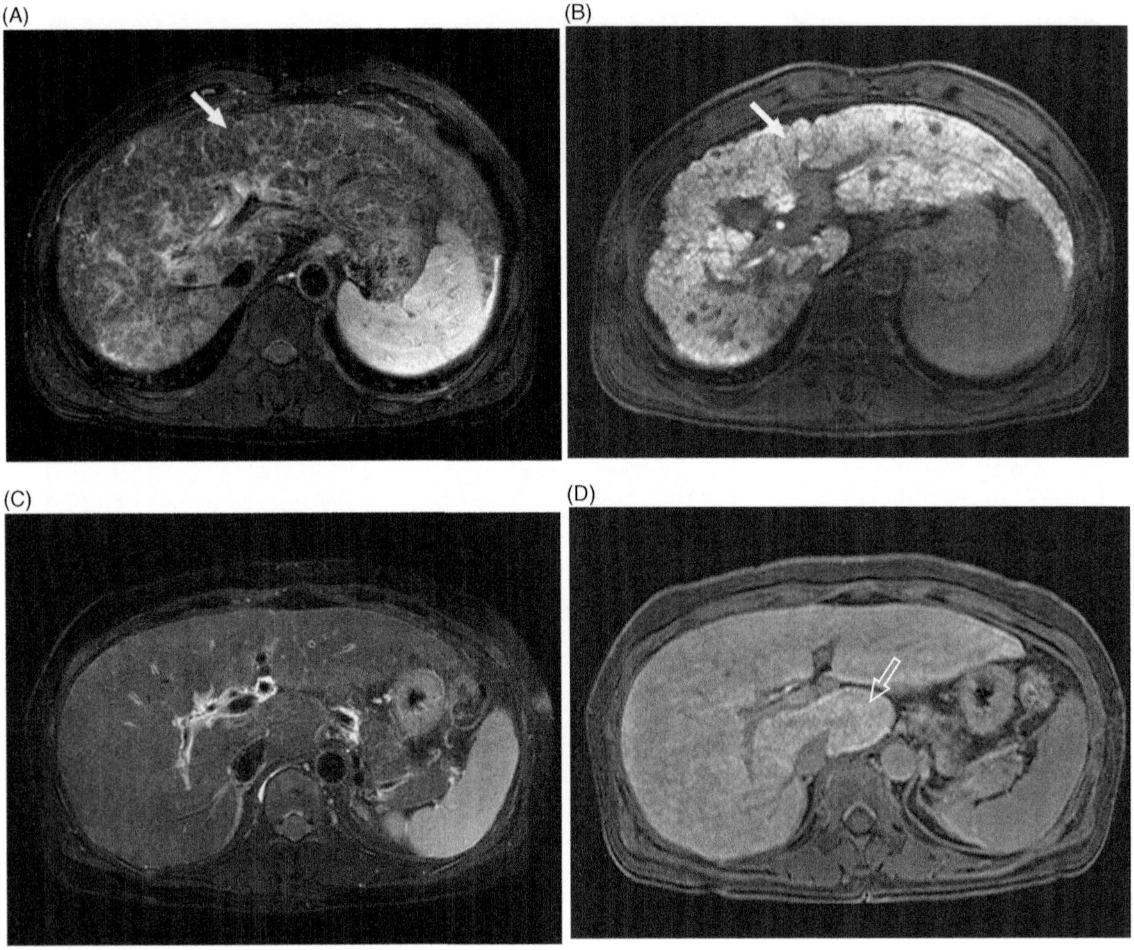

Figure 3.3 Magnetic resonance images (MRI) of cirrhosis caused by hepatitis B infection and chronic alcohol ingestion. (A and B) In a patient with hepatitis B virus-related cirrhosis, various sizes and shapes of regenerative nodules (solid arrow) and fibrotic scars are shown on T2-weighted (A) and hepatobiliary phase MRI (B). (C and D) On the contrary, regenerative nodules in alcoholic cirrhosis are very small and fibrotic scarring is not obvious on T2-weighted MRI (C). Compared with viral cirrhosis, caudate lobe (open arrow) and left liver is relatively more enlarged and right liver is less hypotrophic (D).

positive predictive value for diagnosing cirrhosis, but usually a low sensitivity. In other words, the morphologic changes associated with cirrhosis that are visible on CT and MRI are usually observed in advanced cases only; CT and MRI are thus not suitable for the early diagnosis of cirrhosis.

The progression to advanced disease will make atrophy of the right hepatic lobe and the left medial segment with hypertrophy of the left lateral segment and the caudate lobe more prominent, features that are easily demonstrated on conventional cross-section imaging modalities such as CT and MRI. These morphologic changes were previously explained by alterations of blood flow associated with the progress of cirrhosis. However, the morphologic changes differ depending upon the underlying etiology of the cirrhosis, although they overlap as the disease advances (Figure 3.3). The aforementioned findings are typical features of viral-induced cirrhosis. On the contrary, the characteristics of cirrhotic patients with a history of chronic heavy alcoholic consumption are marked hypertrophy of the caudate lobe, a higher frequency of visualization of the right posterior hepatic notch, and smaller regenerative nodules [65,66]. Primary biliary cirrhosis (PBC), a chronic and usually progressive cholestatic disease that is characterized by asymmetric destruction of bile ductules within the portal triads as a result of an autoimmune inflammatory process [67], has a morphology that is similar to other forms of cirrhosis on CT and MRI, with a small heterogeneously attenuating liver, varices, and splenomegaly [68]. A typical MR finding on T2-weighted images in end-stage PBC is the periportal halo sign [69]; DWI can aid estimation of the fibrosis grade in patients with PBC. Primary sclerosing cholangitis, another entity of chronic cholestatic disorder that is characterized by fibrosing inflammatory destruction of the bile ducts and multifocal biliary strictures [70], is also characterized by pseudotumoral enlargement of the caudate lobe along with atrophy of the peripheral hepatic segments, resulting in a lobulated contour [71]. Multiple irregular strictures of the bile ducts are also observed on MR cholangiopancreatography [72].

Hemodynamic changes

Hemodynamically, the cirrhotic liver is highly resistant to portal inflow, and the systemic response that improves the splanchnic circulation aggravates the situation, creating a vicious cycle that may result in the development of portal hypertension and its complications [73]. Basically, since CT and MRI are not functional imaging modalities, they are not appropriate for evaluating the hemodynamic changes in the liver. However, they are useful for observing the secondary changes of portal hypertension in a patient with cirrhosis, such as portosystemic collateral formation, splenomegaly, portal hypertensive gastropathy (PHG), portal hypertensive colopathy (PHC), and ascites.

The arterioportal shunt is a communication between the hepatic arterial and portal venous systems that allows arterial blood to flow into a region of the portal venous territory [74]. In patients with cirrhosis, the arterioportal shunt is usually found on the arterial phase of a CT scan. The mechanism underlying such an arterioportal shunt is not clear, but it is thought that distortion and capillarization of the hepatic sinusoid disturbs hepatic venular flow and increases intrahepatic vascular resistance, resulting in the arterial blood flow regurgitating to the PV via the arterioportal shunt [75]. Although the arterioportal shunt has minimal clinical significance, it can be mistaken for a small HCC on the arterial phase of a CT scan. Therefore, it should be differentiated from HCC by using dynamic enhanced CT and MRI; a liver-specific MR contrast agent can also be used for the diagnosis.

Esophageal and paraesophageal varices are common complications of cirrhosis, and arise from the impaired venous drainage of the esophageal vein due to increased portal venous pressure. A gastric varix is less common than an esophageal varix, occurring in about 20% in patients with portal hypertension [76]. The gastric varix can be subdivided into gastroesophageal and isolated gastric types according to its location and relationship with esophageal varices [77]. Short and posterior gastric veins are the main communicating veins of the fundal gastric varix. These circulatory collaterals are located around the esophagus and stomach, especially the esophageal and submucosal gastric varices [77]; bleeding from theses varices into the gastrointestinal tract is serious and life-threatening. Physicians generally estimate the risk of variceal bleeding using endoscopic findings such as the size, color, and location of varices [78]. However, in the era of the multi-detector CT, which enables CT scanning at a submillimeter thickness, CT can be used not only to obtain information about the cirrhotic liver itself, but also about the portal hypertension caused by cirrhosis. Various portosystemic collateral veins can also be depicted in the CT scan (Figure 3.4), and physicians can plan a strategy for the treatment of varices, including the insertion of a transjugular intrahepatic portosystemic shunt (TIPS) and balloon-occluded retrograde transvenous obliteration (BRTO). Moreover, as with endoscopy, it is now possible to demonstrate the presence of esophageal and gastric varices using CT [79–81]. The sensitivity and specificity of CT for detecting esophageal varices were found to be 96% and 55%, respectively, and 93% and 80%, respectively, for high-risk esophageal varices [80]. Use of the 1- to 3-mm multiplanar reformat or surface-shaded display can increase the specificity of CT for the risk stratification of esophageal varices [82,83]. With regard to gastric varices, the sensitivity and specificity were 83–89% and 75–79%, respectively [79]. These results are not bad, but the accuracy for small varices remains low.

Splenomegaly is another CT feature of cirrhosis, and its underlying mechanism is explained simply as congestion resulting from portal hypertension. Although the size and shape of the spleen varies among individuals, its average dimensionsin adults are <11 cm long, <7 cm

(A) (B)

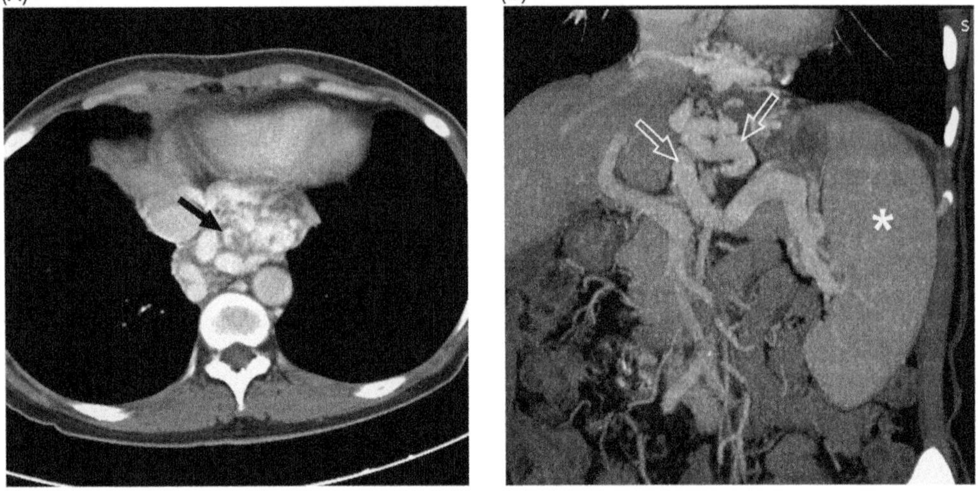

Figure 3.4 CT features of prominent esophageal and paraesophageal varices. (A) On axial scan, engorged paraesophageal collateral veins surround the esophagus with a varix (solid arrow). (B) On oblique coronal view of maximum intensity projection, a tortuous and engorged left gastric vein (open arrows) is shown, and it is connected with esophageal and paraesophageal varices. Marked splenomegaly is also noted (asterisk).

wide, and <5 cm thick. Splenomegaly is highly sensitive for the diagnosis of PH, and is weakly correlated with portal vascular resistance [84]. It is more frequently observed in patients with viral cirrhosis and PBC than in patients with alcoholic cirrhosis. The usefulness of splenic stiffness measurements obtained using MR elastography for detecting significant portal hypertension has recently been tested [85]. Along with splenomegaly, Gamna–Gandy bodies are usually found in the spleen of cirrhotic patients on gradient-echo MRI. They are caused by the deposition of hemosiderin as a result of a focal organized hemorrhagic infarct, and are seen in 9–12% of patients with portal hypertension [86].

PHG and PHC are caused by chronic venous congestion resulting from portal hypertension, which results in mucosal hyperemia and capillary ectasia in the gastric and colonic walls [87,88]. PHG is important clinically because it may be associated with acute gastric bleeding; it is responsible for up to 30% of all cases of upper gastrointestinal bleeding in patients with cirrhosis [89]. PHG is generally diagnosed by endoscopy, but CT can also show edematous gastric-wall thickening and persistent enhancement on the inner layer of the gastric wall, with or without transient segmental hypoperfusion in the gastric fundus or body on arterial-phase scanning [90,91].

MR elastography

MR elastographyis an emerging technology that is used for quantitatively assessing the elasticity of the liver [92]. Like palpation, elastography is a diagnostic modality that reveals differences in one of the mechanical properties of tissues, the elastic modulus of tissues, and this can improve the contrast between different tissues in the body as compared with other imaging modalities such as ultrasound, CT, and conventional MRI. There are three basic steps involved in performing elasticity imaging: application of excitation, measurement of the tissue response, and estimation of the mechanical parameters [93]. Excitation is applied using a pneumatic-based, pressure-activated driver composed of active and passive drivers, whereby the active driver generates a pneumatic pressure wave that is transmitted through a plastic tube to the passive driver placed over the wall of the right anterior body [94]. After generating a shear wave at a low frequency (50–500 Hz), the response in the liver tissue can be measured using phase-contrast MRI with a motion-encoding gradient that oscillates at the same frequency as the motion of the activated liver tissue [95]. A quantitative value of the mechanical shear modulus can then be calculated from the acquired MR images (Figure 3.5). The shear modulus can be calculated from the velocity of the shear wave (corresponding to the

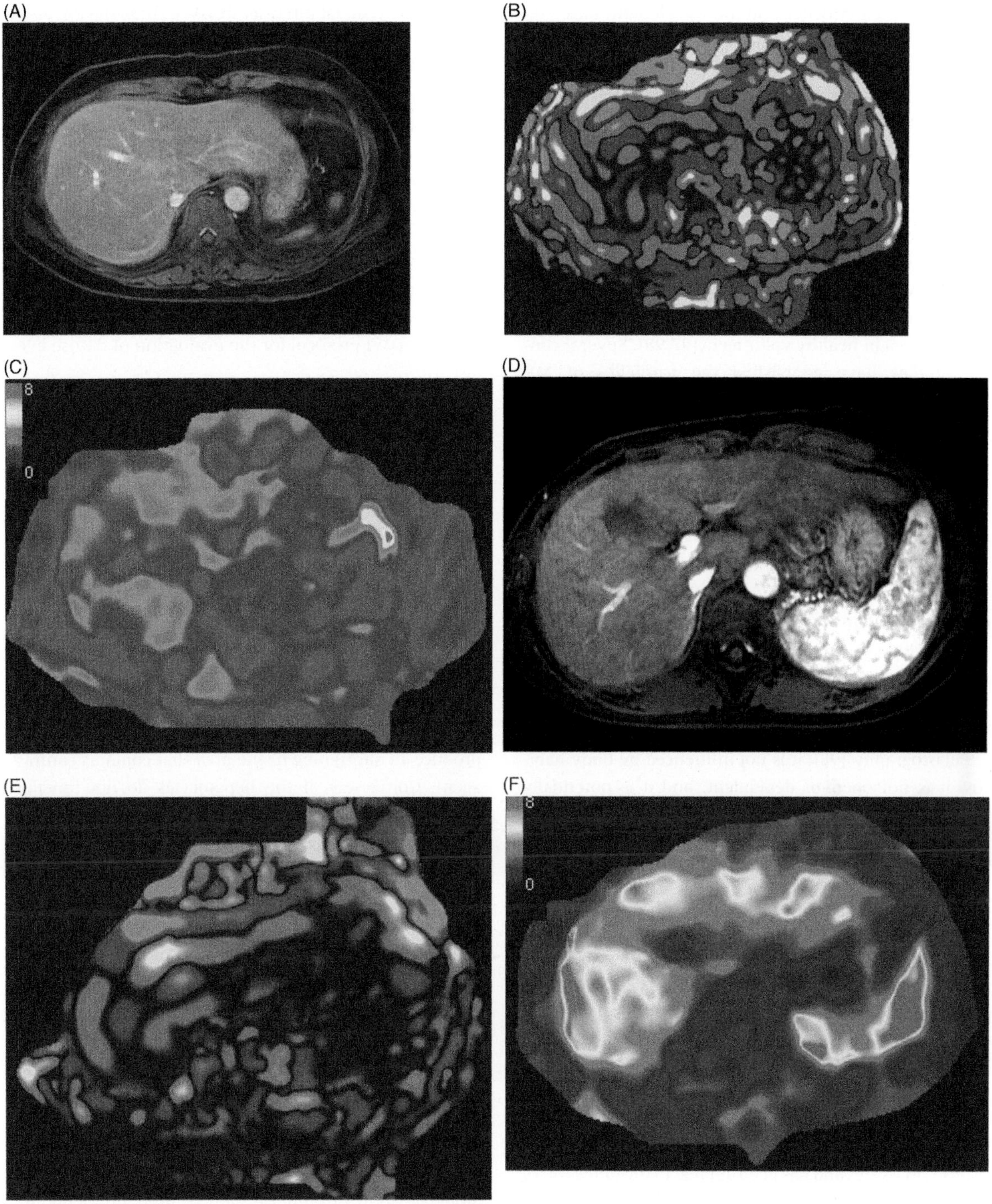

Figure 3.5 MR elastography of the normal liver (A–C) and cirrhotic liver (D–F). In the normal liver (B), shear wave passing through the liver propagates slowly compared with the cirrhotic liver (E). The elastograms show a higher mean stiffness of the cirrhotic liver (4.9 kPa; F) compared with the normal liver (1.7 kPa; C). (Courtesy of Dr. Jeong Min Lee, Department of Radiology, Seoul National University Hospital, Korea.) (See colour plate section.)

product of the frequency and the wavelength) based on the assumption that the density of the tissue is around 1000 kg/m^3. In addition, because the liver tissue moves in more than one direction, a specific reconstruction technique using the direct local inversion of the differential equation of motion is applied to estimate the complex stiffness tensor in the multidimensional displacement dataset [96].

MR elastography has been used in clinical practice for the assessment of hepatic fibrosis since 2006 [94,97]. Hepatic MR elastography is usually performed with a 60-Hz pressure wave. The shear modulus is approximately 2 kPa in healthy volunteers [97,98]. Several clinical studies have established the feasibility of MR elastography for evaluating hepatic fibrosis. In a study of 141 patients with chronic liver disease [99], the mean MR elasticity increased gradually according to the severity of hepatic fibrosis, as for liver stiffness using TE, and the diagnostic performance of MR elastography was comparable or higher than that for TE or blood testing (aspartate aminotransferase: platelet ratio index test; APRI index). Moreover, the failure rate was significantly lower for MR elastography than for TE; the causes of MR elastography failure were claustrophobia, low hepatic signal intensity related to hemochromatosis, and severe obesity (i.e., the patient did not to fit into the magnet bore).

There are several advantages of MR elastography over US elastography [92]: it is not influenced by body habitus, it is not operator dependent, and it is potentially possible to assess the entire liver. Nevertheless, although great strides have been made with MR elastography technology, several challenges remain: improving the spatial resolution, developing a high-speed imaging technique such as echo planar imaging or parallel imaging, and overcoming some of the complex mathematical problems associated with solving for mechanical anisotropy, nonlinearity, and viscoelastic behavior [93].

Other imaging techniques

Several imaging techniques have been investigated for the noninvasive diagnosis of hepatic fibrosis. DWI is a technique that assesses the freedom of diffusion of water protons in tissues and has been applied to the detection of malignant hepatic lesions such as metastasis or HCC in abdominal imaging. The diffusion of water protons may be restricted in livers with hepatic fibrosis because collagen does not contain many free unbound water protons. However, it is inappropriate to quantify the diffusivity based on the signal intensity in DWI; thus, the apparent diffusion coefficient (ADC) is calculated from two or more DWIs, representing the slope of the logarithm of intensity versus the *b* value [100]. According to several preliminary studies [101,102], a decreased ADC is correlated with increased hepatic fibrosis or stage of chronic liver disease. Challenges remain, however [103], such as: (i) the presence of potential confounders of the ADC such as perfusion, hepatic steatosis, hepatic iron deposition, and inflammation; and (ii) the ADC varying with imaging parameters such as the field strength, repetition time, echo time, and *b* value. Thus, it is necessary to develop a standard DWI protocol for the evaluation of diffuse liver disease.

Liver-specific MR contrast agents were developed to improve the conspicuity of malignant focal hepatic lesions such as HCC and metastasis [104,105]. There are two commercially available gadolinium-based contrast agents: gadobenatedimeglumin and gadoliniumethoxybenzyldiethylenetriaminepentaacetic acid (Gd-EOB-DTPA); these function as combined extracellular hepatobiliary agents. The basic mechanism underlying liver-specific enhancement is that a considerable portion of the contrast agent added to the bloodstream is taken into hepatocytes and excreted into the bile duct after some time. If the hepatocytes in a portion of the liver function normally, the contrast agent will be taken into the hepatocytes and produce T1 shortening in the area that contains contrast agent. Conversely, if the hepatocytes do not function normally or they are replaced by other cells such as metastatic tumor cells, the contrast agent will not be taken up and the signal intensity of the area will be lower than that of the normal liver. Therefore, the enhancement by liver-specific contrast agent depends on the underlying liver function: liver perfusion, vascular permeability, extracellular diffusion, and hepatocyte transporter expression. Thus, peak enhancement of the cirrhotic liver may be diminished and delayed [104,106].

Estimation of liver function by measuring the enhancement of the liver or ratio of hepatic enhancement to splenic enhancement with Gd-EOB-DTPA MRI may be an alternative to indocyanine green clearance in the work-up before major hepatic resection [107]. Hepatobiliary contrast agent can only be used for the preliminary staging of hepatic fibrosis, but a study has demonstrated that Gd-EOB-DTPA MRI is more reliable than DWI for staging hepatic fibrosis [108]. Nevertheless, pharmacokinetics analyses of Gd-EOB-DTPA MRI enhancement have several issues [104], including the lack of linearity between the signal intensity and the concentration of contrast agent. This issue also applies to MR perfusion studies. As for DWI, there are several confounders that influence Gd-EOB-DTPA enhancement that need to be addressed to enable a precise quantification of liver function: blood flow, transmembrane barriers preventing movement of the contrast agent, interaction between drugs, and individual variability of transporter expression in hepatocytes.

The use of CT and MRI in perfusion studies involves the observation of hemodynamic changes in tissues using vascular contrast media. These tools can be applied not only for assessing the response to anticancer treatment, but also for the staging of liver fibrosis and evaluation of HCC [109]. As mentioned above, the intrahepatic vessels are gradually obliterated as hepatic fibrosis advances. This results in decreases in portal blood flow and volume in the liver, but hepatic arterial flow increases by compensation, causing the development of numerous intrahepatic shunts. Therefore, most of the perfusion studies carried out to evaluate the liver have applied a dual-input kinetics model. The most important merit of CT perfusion studies is the linearity between the attenuation value (measured in Hounsfield units) and the concentration of contrast agent, meaning that the formula for obtaining the perfusion parameters is much simpler than for MRI. Moreover, the ability to perform CT scanning very rapidly improves the temporal resolution. On the other hand, repeated CT scanning is a radiation hazard, which is a very important issue that remains a major obstacle to its clinical application.

References

1 Schalm SW. The diagnosis of cirrhosis: clinical relevance and methodology. J Hepatol 1997;27:1118–9.

2 Friedman SL, Bansal MB. Reversal of hepatic fibrosis: fact or fantasy? Hepatology 2006;43:S82–8.

3 Bravo AA, Sheth SG, Chopra S. Liver biopsy. N Engl J Med 2001;344:495–500.

4 Bonekamp S, Kamel I, Solga S, Clark J. Can imaging modalities diagnose and stage hepatic fibrosis and cirrhosis accurately? J Hepatol 2009;50:17–35.

5 Ishak K, Baptista A, Bianchi L, et al. Histological grading and staging of chronic hepatitis. J Hepatol 1995;22:696–9.

6 Kim MY, Cho MY, Baik SK, et al. Histological subclassification of cirrhosis using the Laennec fibrosis scoring system correlates with clinical stage and grade of portal hypertension. J Hepatol 2011;55:1004–9.

7 Colli A, Fraquelli M, Andreoletti M, Marino B, Zucoli E, Conte D. Severe liver fibrosis or cirrhosis: accuracy of US for detection: analysis of 300 cases. Radiology 2003;227:89–94.

8 Oberti F, Valsesia E, Pilette C, et al. Noninvasive diagnosis of hepatic fibrosis or cirrhosis. Gastroenterology 1997;113: 1609–16.

9 Aubé C, Oberti F, Korali N, et al. Ultrasonographic diagnosis of hepatic fibrosis or cirrhosis. J Hepatol 1999;30:472–8.

10 Shen L, Li JQ, Zeng MD, Lu LG, Fan ST, Bao H. Correlation between ultrasonographic and pathologic diagnosis of liver fibrosis due to chronic virus hepatitis. World J Gastroenterol 2006;12:1292–5.

11 Celle G, Savarino V, Picciotto A, Magnolia MR, Scalabrini P, Dodero M. Is hepatic ultrasonography a valid alternative tool to liver biopsy? Report on 507 cases studied with both techniques. Dig Dis Sci 1988;33:467–71.

12 Gaiani S, Gramantieri L, Venturoli N, et al. What is the criterion for differentiating chronic hepatitis from compensated cirrhosis? A prospective study comparing ultrasonography and percutaneous liver biopsy. J Hepatol 1997; 27:979–85.

13 Khan KN, Yamasaki M, Yamasaki K, et al. Proposed abdominal sonographic staging to predict severity of liver diseases: analysis with peritoneoscopy and histology. Dig Dis Sci 2000;45:554–64.

14 Nicolau C, Bianchi L, Vilana R. Gray-scale ultrasound in hepatic cirrhosis and chronic hepatitis: diagnosis, screening, and intervention. Semin Ultrasound CT MR 2002; 23:3–18.

15 Nishiura T, Watanabe H, Ito M, et al. Ultrasound evaluation of the fibrosis stage in chronic liver disease by the simultaneous use of low and high frequency probes. Br J Radiol 2005;78:189–97.

16 Needleman L, Kurtz AB, Rifkin MD, Cooper HS, Pasto ME, Goldberg BB. Sonography of diffuse benign liver disease: accuracy of pattern recognition and grading. AJR Am J Roentgenol 1986;146:1011–5.

17 Saverymuttu SH, Joseph AE, Maxwell JD. Ultrasound scanning in the detection of hepatic fibrosis and steatosis. Br Med J (Clin Res Ed) 1986;292:13–5.

18 Tchelepi H, Ralls PW, Radin R, Grant E. Sonography of diffuse liver disease. J Ultrasound Med 2002;21:1023–32; quiz 1033–4.

19 Chen CH, Lin ST, Yang CC, Yeh YH, Kuo CL, Nien CK. The accuracy of sonography in predicting steatosis and fibrosis in chronic hepatitis C. Dig Dis Sci 2008;53:1699–706.

20 Kutcher R, Smith GS, Sen F, et al. Comparison of sonograms and liver histologic findings in patients with chronic hepatitis C virus infection. J Ultrasound Med 1998;17:321–5.

21 Baik SK. Haemodynamic evaluation by Doppler ultrasonography in patients with portal hypertension: a review. Liver Int 2010;30:1403–13.

22 Bolognesi M, Sacerdoti D, Mescoli C, et al. Different hemodynamic patterns of alcoholic and viral endstage cirrhosis: analysis of explanted liver weight, degree of fibrosis and splanchnic Doppler parameters. Scand J Gastroenterol 2007;42:256–62.
23 Iliopoulos P, Vlychou M, Margaritis V, et al. Gray and color Doppler ultrasonography in differentiation between chronic viral hepatitis and compensated early stage cirrhosis. J Gastrointestin Liver Dis 2007;16:279–86.
24 Haktanir A, Cihan BS, Celenk C, Cihan S. Value of Doppler sonography in assessing the progression of chronic viral hepatitis and in the diagnosis and grading of cirrhosis. J Ultrasound Med 2005;24:311–21.
25 Iwao T, Toyonaga A, Oho K, et al. Value of Doppler ultrasound parameters of portal vein and hepatic artery in the diagnosis of cirrhosis and portal hypertension. Am J Gastroenterol 1997;92:1012–7.
26 Liu CH, Lin JW, Tsai FC, et al. Noninvasive tests for the prediction of significant hepatic fibrosis in hepatitis C virus carriers with persistently normal alanine aminotransferases. Liver Int 2006;26:1087–94.
27 Arda K, Ofelli M, Calikoglu U, Olçer T, Cumhur T. Hepatic vein Doppler waveform changes in early stage (Child–Pugh A) chronic parenchymal liver disease. J Clin Ultrasound 1997;25:15–9.
28 Baik SK, Kim JW, Kim HS, et al. Recent variceal bleeding: Doppler US hepatic vein waveform in assessment of severity of portal hypertension and vasoactive drug response. Radiology 2006;240:574–80.
29 Kim MY, Baik SK, Park DH, et al. Damping index of Doppler hepatic vein waveform to assess the severity of portal hypertension and response to propranolol in liver cirrhosis: a prospective nonrandomized study. Liver Int 2007; 27:1103–10.
30 Bernatik T, Strobel D, Hahn EG, Becker D. Doppler measurements: a surrogate marker of liver fibrosis? Eur J Gastroenterol Hepatol 2002;14:383–7.
31 Lim AK, Patel N, Eckersley RJ, et al. Can Doppler sonography grade the severity of hepatitis C-related liver disease? AJR Am J Roentgenol 2005;184:1848–53.
32 Colli A, Cocciolo M, Mumoli N, Cattalini N, Fraquelli M, Conte D. Hepatic artery resistance in alcoholic liver disease. Hepatology 1998;28:1182–6.
33 Blomley MJ, Lim AK, Harvey CJ, et al. Liver microbubble transit time compared with histology and Child–Pugh score in diffuse liver disease: a cross sectional study. Gut 2003;52:1188–93.
34 Lim AK, Taylor-Robinson SD, Patel N, et al. Hepatic vein transit times using a microbubble agent can predict disease severity non-invasively in patients with hepatitis C. Gut 2005;54:128–33.
35 Lim AK, Patel N, Eckersley RJ, et al. Hepatic vein transit time of SonoVue: a comparative study with Levovist. Radiology 2006;240:130–5.
36 Klibanov AL. Ultrasound molecular imaging with targeted microbubble contrast agents. J Nucl Cardiol 2007;14: 876–84.
37 Albrecht T, Blomley MJ, Cosgrove DO, et al. Non-invasive diagnosis of hepatic cirrhosis by transit-time analysis of an ultrasound contrast agent. Lancet 1999;353:1579–83.
38 Kim MY, Suk KT, Baik SK, et al. Hepatic vein arrival time as assessed by contrast-enhanced ultrasonography is useful for the assessment of portal hypertension in compensated cirrhosis. Hepatology 2012;56:1053–62.
39 Kaneko T, Teshigawara O, Sugimoto H, et al. Signal intensity of the liver parenchyma in microbubble contrast agent in the late liver phase reflects advanced fibrosis of the liver. Liver Int 2005;25:288–93.
40 Iijima H, Moriyasu F, Tsuchiya K, et al. Decrease in accumulation of ultrasound contrast microbubbles in non-alcoholic steatohepatitis. Hepatol Res 2007;37:722–30.
41 Talwalkar JA. Elastography for detecting hepatic fibrosis: options and considerations. Gastroenterology 2008;135: 299–302.
42 Ophir J, Céspedes I, Ponnekanti H, Yazdi Y, Li X. Elastography: a quantitative method for imaging the elasticity of biological tissues. Ultrason Imaging 1991;13:111–34.
43 Foucher J, Castéra L, Bernard PH, et al. Prevalence and factors associated with failure of liver stiffness measurement using FibroScan in a prospective study of 2114 examinations. Eur J Gastroenterol Hepatol 2006;18:411–2.
44 Friedrich-Rust M, Wunder K, Kriener S, et al. Liver fibrosis in viral hepatitis: noninvasive assessment with acoustic radiation force impulse imaging versus transient elastography. Radiology 2009;252:595–604.
45 Bavu E, Gennisson JL, Couade M, et al. Noninvasive in vivo liver fibrosis evaluation using supersonic shear imaging: a clinical study on 113 hepatitis C virus patients. Ultrasound Med Biol 2011;37:1361–73.
46 Koizumi Y, Hirooka M, Kisaka Y, et al. Liver fibrosis in patients with chronic hepatitis C: noninvasive diagnosis by means of real-time tissue elastography – establishment of the method for measurement. Radiology 2011;258:610–7.
47 Friedrich-Rust M, Ong MF, Herrmann E, et al. Real-time elastography for noninvasive assessment of liver fibrosis in chronic viral hepatitis. AJR Am J Roentgenol 2007; 188:758–64.
48 Stebbing J, Farouk L, Panos G, et al. A meta-analysis of transient elastography for the detection of hepatic fibrosis. J Clin Gastroenterol 2010;44:214–9.
49 Tsochatzis EA, Gurusamy KS, Ntaoula S, Cholongitas E, Davidson BR, Burroughs AK. Elastography for the diagnosis of severity of fibrosis in chronic liver disease: a meta-analysis of diagnostic accuracy. J Hepatol 2011;54:650–9.
50 Boursier J, Isselin G, Fouchard-Hubert I, et al. Acoustic radiation force impulse: a new ultrasonographic technology for the widespread noninvasive diagnosis of liver fibrosis. Eur J Gastroenterol Hepatol 2010;22:1074–84.

51 Robic MA, Procopet B, Métivier S, et al. Liver stiffness accurately predicts portal hypertension related complications in patients with chronic liver disease: a prospective study. J Hepatol 2011;55:1017–24.
52 Vizzutti F, Arena U, Romanelli RG, et al. Liver stiffness measurement predicts severe portal hypertension in patients with HCV-related cirrhosis. Hepatology 2007;45:1290–7.
53 EASL-EORTC clinical practice guidelines: management of hepatocellular carcinoma. J Hepatol 2012;56:908–43.
54 Bruix J, Sherman M. Management of hepatocellular carcinoma: an update. Hepatology 2011;53:1020–2.
55 Theise ND, Bodenheimer HC Jr, Ferrell LD. Acute and chronic viral hepatitis. In Burt AD, Portman BC, Ferrell LD (eds) MacSween's Pathology of the Liver, 5th edn. Philadelphia: Elsevier; 2007. pp. 410–14.
56 Hussain SM, Zondervan PE, IJermans JN, Schalm SW, de Man RA, Krestin GP. Benign versus malignant hepatic nodules: MR imaging findings with pathologic correlation. Radiographics 2002;22:1023–36; discussion 1037–9.
57 Parikh T, Drew SJ, Lee VS, et al. Focal liver lesion detection and characterization with diffusion-weighted MR imaging: comparison with standard breath-hold T2-weighted imaging. Radiology 2008;246:812–22.
58 Kita K, Kita M, Sato M, Ooshima A, Yamada R. MR imaging of liver cirrhosis. Acta Radiol 1996;37:198–203.
59 Semelka RC, Chung JJ, Hussain SM, Marcos HB, Woosley JT. Chronic hepatitis: correlation of early patchy and late linear enhancement patterns on gadolinium-enhanced MR images with histopathology initial experience. J Magn Reson Imaging 2001;13:385–91.
60 Lucidarme O, Baleston F, Cadi M, et al. Non-invasive detection of liver fibrosis: Is superparamagnetic iron oxide particle-enhanced MR imaging a contributive technique? Eur Radiol 2003;13:467–74.
61 Yu JS, Shim JH, Chung JJ, Kim JH, Kim KW. Double contrast-enhanced MRI of viral hepatitis-induced cirrhosis: correlation of gross morphological signs with hepatic fibrosis. Br J Radiol 2010;83:212–7.
62 Aguirre DA, Behling CA, Alpert E, Hassanein TI, Sirlin CB. Liver fibrosis: noninvasive diagnosis with double contrast material-enhanced MR imaging. Radiology 2006;239: 425–37.
63 Awaya H, Mitchell DG, Kamishima T, Holland G, Ito K, Matsumoto T. Cirrhosis: modified caudate-right lobe ratio. Radiology 2002;224:769–74.
64 Ito K, Mitchell DG. Imaging diagnosis of cirrhosis and chronic hepatitis. Intervirology 2004;47:134–43.
65 Kim I, Jang YJ, Ryeom H, et al. Variation in hepatic segmental volume distribution according to different causes of liver cirrhosis: CT volumetric evaluation. J Comput Assist Tomogr 2012;36:220–5.
66 Okazaki H, Ito K, Fujita T, Koike S, Takano K, Matsunaga N. Discrimination of alcoholic from virus-induced cirrhosis on MR imaging. AJR Am J Roentgenol 2000;175:1677–81.
67 Kaplan MM, Gershwin ME. Primary biliary cirrhosis. N Engl J Med 2005;353:1261–73.
68 Blachar A, Federle MP, Brancatelli G. Primary biliary cirrhosis: clinical, pathologic, and helical CT findings in 53 patients. Radiology 2001;220:329–36.
69 Wenzel JS, Donohoe A, Ford KL 3rd, Glastad K, Watkins D, Molmenti E. Primary biliary cirrhosis: MR imaging findings and description of MR imaging periportal halo sign. AJR Am J Roentgenol 2001;176:885–9.
70 Silveira MG, Lindor KD. Primary sclerosing cholangitis. Can J Gastroenterol 2008;22:689–98.
71 Brancatelli G, Federle MP, Ambrosini R, et al. Cirrhosis: CT and MR imaging evaluation. Eur J Radiol 2007;61:57–69.
72 Fulcher AS, Turner MA, Franklin KJ, et al. Primary sclerosing cholangitis: evaluation with MR cholangiography: a case–control study. Radiology 2000;215:71–80.
73 Kim MY, Baik SK, Lee SS. Hemodynamic alterations in cirrhosis and portal hypertension. Korean J Hepatol 2010;16:347–52.
74 Choi BI, Lee KH, Han JK, Lee JM. Hepatic arterioportal shunts: dynamic CT and MR features. Korean J Radiol 2002;3:1–15.
75 Ahn JH, Yu JS, Hwang SH, Chung JJ, Kim JH, Kim KW. Nontumorous arterioportal shunts in the liver: CT and MRI findings considering mechanisms and fate. Eur Radiol 2010;20:385–94.
76 Sarin SK, Lahoti D, Saxena SP, Murthy NS, Makwana UK. Prevalence, classification and natural history of gastric varices: a long-term follow-up study in 568 portal hypertension patients. Hepatology 1992;16:1343–9.
77 Ryan BM, Stockbrugger RW, Ryan JM. A pathophysiologic, gastroenterologic, and radiologic approach to the management of gastric varices. Gastroenterology 2004;126: 1175–89.
78 Dell'era A, Bosch J. Review article: the relevance of portal pressure and other risk factors in acute gastro-oesophageal variceal bleeding. Aliment Pharmacol Ther 2004; 20 (Suppl 3): 8–15; discussion 16–7.
79 Zhu K, Meng X, Pang P, et al. Gastric varices in patients with portal hypertension: evaluation with multidetector row CT. J Clin Gastroenterol 2010;44:e108–15.
80 Kim H, Choi D, Gwak GY, et al. Evaluation of esophageal varices on liver computed tomography: receiver operating characteristic analyses of the performance of radiologists and endoscopists. J Gastroenterol Hepatol 2009;24:1534–40.
81 Kim SH, Lee JM, Choi JY, et al. Changes of portosystemic collaterals and splenic volume on CT after liver transplantation and factors influencing those changes. AJR Am J Roentgenol 2008;191:W8–W16.
82 Yu NC, Margolis D, Hsu M, Raman SS, Lu DS. Detection and grading of esophageal varices on liver CT: comparison of standard and thin-section multiplanar reconstructions in diagnostic accuracy. AJR Am J Roentgenol 2011; 197:643–9.

83 Kim SH, Kim YJ, Lee JM, et al. Esophageal varices in patients with cirrhosis: multidetector CT esophagography – comparison with endoscopy. Radiology 2007;242:759–68.

84 Bolognesi M, Merkel C, Sacerdoti D, Nava V, Gatta A. Role of spleen enlargement in cirrhosis with portal hypertension. Dig Liver Dis 2002;34:144–50.

85 Nedredal GI, Yin M, McKenzie T, et al. Portal hypertension correlates with splenic stiffness as measured with MR elastography. J Magn Reson Imaging 2011;34:79–87.

86 Elsayes KM, Narra VR, Mukundan G, Lewis JS Jr, Menias CO, Heiken JP. MR imaging of the spleen: spectrum of abnormalities. Radiographics 2005;25:967–82.

87 Viggiano TR, Gostout CJ. Portal hypertensive intestinal vasculopathy: a review of the clinical, endoscopic, and histopathologic features. Am J Gastroenterol 1992;87: 944–54.

88 Panés J, Bordas JM, Piqué JM, et al. Increased gastric mucosal perfusion in cirrhotic patients with portal hypertensive gastropathy. Gastroenterology 1992;103:1875–82.

89 Balan KK, Grime JS, Sutton R, Critchley M, Jenkins SA. Do alterations in the rate of gastric emptying after injection sclerotherapy for oesophageal varices play any role in the development of portal hypertensive gastropathy? HPB Surg 1999;11:141–8; discussion 148–50.

90 Kim TU, Kim S, Woo SK, et al. Dynamic CT of portal hypertensive gastropathy: significance of transient gastric perfusion defect sign. Clin Radiol 2008;63:783–90.

91 Ishihara K, Ishida R, Saito T, Teramoto K, Hosomura Y, Shibuya H. Computed tomography features of portal hypertensive gastropathy. J Comput Assist Tomogr 2004;28:832–835.

92 Talwalkar JA, Yin M, Fidler JL, Sanderson SO, Kamath PS, Ehman RL. Magnetic resonance imaging of hepatic fibrosis: emerging clinical applications. Hepatology 2008;47:332–42.

93 Mariappan YK, Glaser KJ, Ehman RL. Magnetic resonance elastography: a review. Clin Anat 2010;23:497–511.

94 Yin M, Talwalkar JA, Glaser KJ, et al. Assessment of hepatic fibrosis with magnetic resonance elastography. Clin Gastroenterol Hepatol 2007;5:1207–13.

95 Muthupillai R, Lomas DJ, Rossman PJ, Greenleaf JF, Manduca A, Ehman RL. Magnetic resonance elastography by direct visualization of propagating acoustic strain waves. Science 1995;269:1854–7.

96 Oliphant TE, Manduca A, Ehman RL, Greenleaf JF. Complex-valued stiffness reconstruction for magnetic resonance elastography by algebraic inversion of the differential equation. Magn Reson Med 2001;45:299–310.

97 Rouvière O, Yin M, Dresner MA, et al. MR elastography of the liver: preliminary results. Radiology 2006;240:440–8.

98 Hines CDG, Bley TA, Lindstrom MJ, Reeder SB. Repeatability of magnetic resonance elastography for quantification of hepatic stiffness. J Magn Reson Imaging 2010;31:725–31.

99 Huwart L, Sempoux C, Vicaut E, et al. Magnetic resonance elastography for the noninvasive staging of liver fibrosis. Gastroenterology 2008;135:32–40.

100 Koinuma M, Ohashi I, Hanafusa K, Shibuya H. Apparent diffusion coefficient measurements with diffusion-weighted magnetic resonance imaging for evaluation of hepatic fibrosis. J Magn Reson Imaging 2005;22:80–5.

101 Taouli B, Tolia AJ, Losada M, et al. Diffusion-weighted MRI for quantification of liver fibrosis: preliminary experience. AJR Am J Roentgenol 2007;189:799–806.

102 Lewin M, Poujol-Robert A, Boëlle PY, et al. Diffusion-weighted magnetic resonance imaging for the assessment of fibrosis in chronic hepatitis C. Hepatology 2007;46:658–65.

103 Faria SC, Ganesan K, Mwangi I, et al. MR imaging of liver fibrosis: current state of the art. Radiographics 2009;29: 1615–35.

104 Van Beers BE, Pastor CM, Hussain HK. Primovist, Eovist: what to expect? J Hepatol 2012;57:421–9.

105 Ringe KI, Husarik DB, Sirlin CB, Merkle EM. Gadoxetate disodium-enhanced MRI of the liver: part 1, protocol optimization and lesion appearance in the noncirrhotic liver. AJR Am J Roentgenol 2010;195:13–28.

106 Jeong WK, Byun JH, Lee SS, et al. Gadobenate dimeglumine-enhanced liver MR imaging in cirrhotic patients: quantitative and qualitative comparison of 1-hour and 3-hour delayed images. J Magn Reson Imaging 2011;33: 889–97.

107 Yamada A, Hara T, Li F, Ueda K, Kadoya M, Doi K. Quantitative evaluation of liver function with use of gadoxetate disodium-enhanced MR imaging. Radiology 2011;260: 727–33.

108 Watanabe H, Kanematsu M, Goshima S, et al. Staging hepatic fibrosis: comparison of gadoxetate disodium-enhanced and diffusion-weighted MR imaging – preliminary observations. Radiology 2011;259:142–50.

109 Haider MA, Farhadi FA, Milot L. Hepatic perfusion imaging: concepts and application. Magn Reson Imaging Clin N Am 2010;18:465–75, x.

CHAPTER 4
Histology/pathology

Valérie Paradis
Pathology Department, Beaujon Hospital, INSERM URM 1149, Paris, France

Introduction

Usually considered as the end stage of chronic liver diseases (CLD), cirrhosis is defined anatomically by the presence throughout the liver of fibrous septa that delineate parenchymal nodules of various sizes. Such parenchymal changes may favor the occurrence of clinical or pathological complications, such as liver decompensation, portal hypertension, and development of primary liver malignancies, especially hepatocellular carcinomas (HCC). Although cirrhosis has been traditionally viewed as the end stage in the evolution of CLD, increasing evidence, with the successful treatment of several risk factors, especially related to viral infections, has supported the concept of reversibility of fibrosis and cirrhosis. The cirrhotic process is rather complex, involving necro-inflammatory lesions, production and/or accumulation of extracellular matrix (ECM), and vascular reorganization. Such a morphologic picture may be appreciated best by the histologic approach which also provides, when necessary, clues for etiologic factors.

Cirrhosis: a pathologic spectrum

Cirrhosis is defined by a diffuse process characterized by fibrosis and the conversion of normal liver architecture into structurally abnormal nodules [1]. Diagnosis of cirrhosis relies on the presence of extensive fibrosis delineating parenchymal hepatocellular nodules associated with vascular abnormalities reflecting the occurrence of intrahepatic vascular shunts [2].

Fibrosis: extracellular accumulation of matrix components

Intrahepatic accumulation of ECM is observed at various sites of the parenchyma, mainly concerning the perisinusoidal space of Disse (defining the space between the vascular channel and the hepatocytes) and portal tracts. ECM deposits increase with the degree of severity of fibrosis, moving from less than 3% of the relative area in a normal liver to more than 15% in a cirrhotic liver [3–5]. In addition to such quantitative aspects, significant qualitative modifications of the ECM components are observed with prominent production of fibrillar collagens contributing to sinusoidal capillarization, a phenomenon that strongly impairs exchanges between liver cells and blood flow [6]. On liver tissue specimens, excess deposits of ECM are easily observed by specific staining (trichrome, picrosirus). Additional procedures, such as histochemistry and immunohistochemistry, are potential tools to define the main types of deposited matrix proteins (Figure 4.1). Second harmonic generation (SHG) microscopy offers the opportunity to image fibrillar collagens in unstained tissues. As liver fibrosis is mainly associated with deposition of type I and III collagens, such an approach, based on multiphoton microscopy, may be used as a collagen scoring method in CLD [7]. Interestingly, its performance has been demonstrated in a cohort study of patients with CLD related to viral hepatitis, showing further discrimination of several levels of fibrosis as assessed by semi-quantitative staging systems [8].

Production of ECM results from the activation and proliferation of fibrocompetent cells, which are able to produce and excrete the main ECM components. They

Cirrhosis: A practical guide to management, First Edition. Edited by Samuel S. Lee and Richard Moreau.

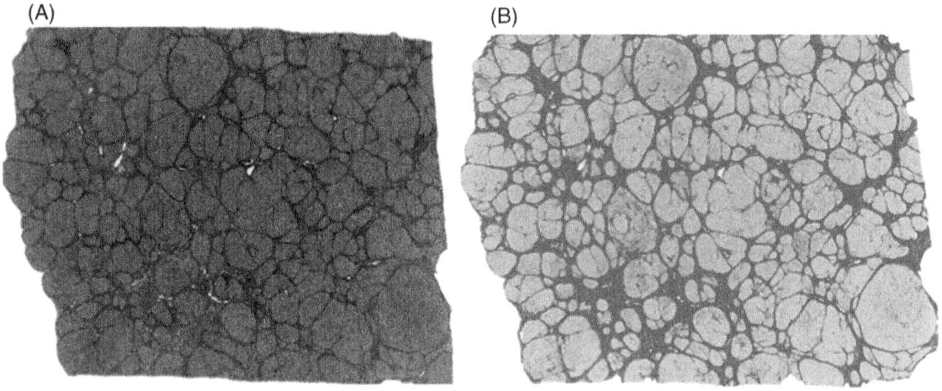

Figure 4.1 Cirrhosis at low power view. Specific stainings of fibrosis showing parenchymal nodules delineated by annular fibrous septa: (A) trichrome staining; (B) picrosirius staining. (See colour plate section.)

include hepatic stellate cells (HSC), which correspond to fat-storing cells located in the perisinusoidal space, and portal fibroblasts [9,10]. Although other cell types of the liver, such as biliary cells, are able to produce ECM components they represent a minor source of liver fibrogenesis [11]. The role of HSC has been investigated in this process where they acquire an activated phenotype of myofibroblast requiring crosstalk with mostly inflammatory cells and production of a wide range of cytokines and chemokines, such as transforming growth factor β1 (TGFβ1), connective tissue growth factor (CTGF), and so on [12,13]. Interestingly, presence of activated HSC on liver tissue sections may be identified using specific immunophenotypical markers, such as α smooth muscle actin (Figure 4.2). Such a procedure gains further insights into the dynamics of liver fibrogenesis and may be valuable in the prediction of the course of CLD, as already illustrated in the follow-up of patients transplanted for hepatitis C virus (HCV) cirrhosis [14]. The fibrous compartment is not restricted to an amorphous area of ECM components but commonly houses different cell types in addition to fibroblasts. Among these, inflammatory cells and biliary proliferation are the most prominent, even though their respective proportions may vary considerably according to the origin of the cirrhosis and its severity.

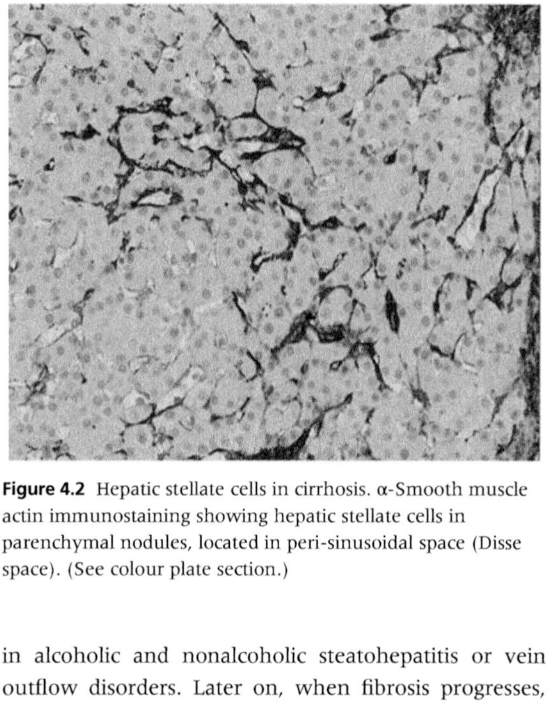

Figure 4.2 Hepatic stellate cells in cirrhosis. α-Smooth muscle actin immunostaining showing hepatic stellate cells in parenchymal nodules, located in peri-sinusoidal space (Disse space). (See colour plate section.)

Different morphologic patterns of fibrosis are recognized according to their origin and severity [15]. Thus, deposition of ECM usually starts in portal tracts and periportal areas in different contexts, including chronic viral hepatitis, autoimmune and biliary diseases, while an earlier involvement of the centrolobular zone is observed in alcoholic and nonalcoholic steatohepatitis or vein outflow disorders. Later on, when fibrosis progresses, the fibrous septa connect vascular structures to each other, leading to constitution of portal to portal, portal to central septa, or central to central septa, mainly depending on the etiologic risk factors and severity of the disease. However, at the advanced stage, all kinds of extensive septa are observed throughout the liver, hampering the recognition of the elementary anatomic structures of the liver (i.e., portal tracts and centrolobular veins). Altogether, this architectural distortion leads to a macroscopic picture of cirrhosis commonly defined by the global aspect of the liver (hypertrophic, atrophic, dysmorphic) and size of the hepatocellular nodules into macro- or micronodular according to whether the majority of the nodules are larger or smaller than 3 mm. Macronodular cirrhosis, especially observed in hepatitis B virus (HBV) infection, may be composed of nodules of several centimeters in diameter. In fact, in a significant number of cases, cirrhosis is made up of a mixture of small and large parenchymal nodules, recognized as "mixed" or "irregular" cirrhosis. Importantly, in the course of cirrhosis, the size of the nodules may evolve, with progression of micronodules to macronodules in cases of successful removal of the etiologic agent.

Vascular changes

In addition to the fibrogenic process, vascular structural changes within the intrahepatic circulation are essential to the increased vascular resistance and physiopathology of portal hypertension [16,17]. Importantly, these modifications directly correlate with the degree of fibrosis [18,19]: (i) angiogenesis, driven by hypoxia, mainly through the production of vascular endothelial growth factor (VEGF), leading to increase in vascular structures with additional shunting, and (ii) sinusoidal remodeling featured by increased density of contractile HSC around sinusoidal endothelial cells that display significant morphologic and functional changes, with the loss of their characteristic fenestra and the occurrence of a basement membrane, known as sinusoidal capillarization, resulting in sinusoidal vasoconstriction [16,17]. Such features can be seen on tissue sections showing increased number of vessels in the fibrous septa, perisinusoidal fibrosis into the nodular parenchyma, and CD34 immunostaining of the sinusoidal lining (Figure 4.3).

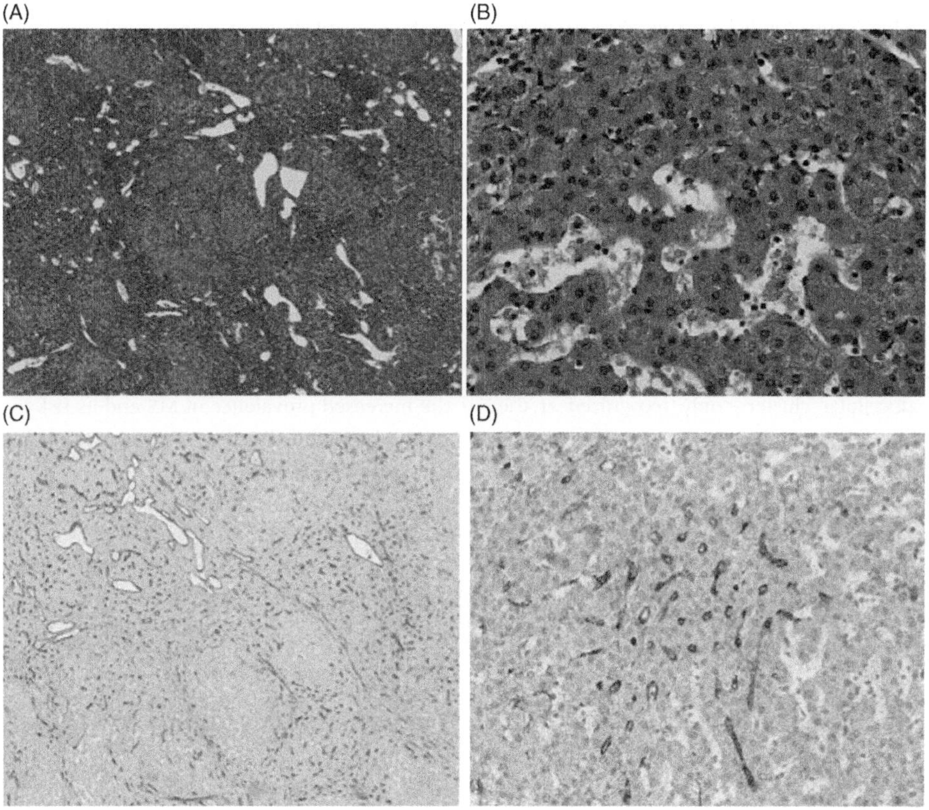

Figure 4.3 Vascular changes in cirrhosis. (A) Low magnification showing cirrhosis with vessels multiplication in fibrous septa (hematein and eosin). (B) Higher magification of cirrhotic nodule with sinusoidal dilatation. (C) CD31 immunostaining dysplaying increased vascular density. (D) Sinusoidal capillarization demonstrated by CD34 lining of endothelial cells in cirrhotic nodule. (See colour plate section.)

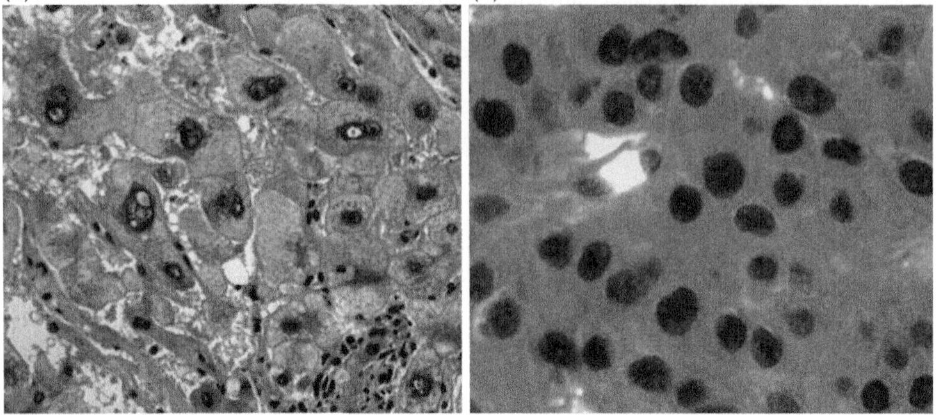

Figure 4.4 Dysplastic changes in cirrhosis. (A) Large cell change represented by large cells containing atypical nuclei of increased size. (B) Small cell change defined by foci of small hepatocytes with increased nuclear: cytoplasmic ratio (hematein and eosin). (See colour plate section.)

Parenchymal nodules: etiologic features

Besides the architectural modifications observed in cirrhosis, a wide range of elementary histologic features may be present. Among them, significant disarray of hepatocellular trabeculae is observed, with focal thickening of liver cell plates to two or three cells thick, consistent with regenerative process. Silver stainings for reticulin clearly demonstrate these changes with an irregular and focally thickened pattern. Cytologically, hepatocytes may appear regular, as eosinophilic polygonal cells, and may harbor dystrophic changes (irregularity in shape and size), or dysplastic changes. These latter modifications, now described as small or large liver cell changes, usually involve hepatocellular clusters, only recognized at the microscopic level (Figure 4.4).

Large cell change (LCC), first described in chonic hepatitis B, is defined by large cells containing atypical nuclei of increased size, sometimes multinucleated, but with a fairly normal nuclear: cytoplasmic ratio [20]. By contrast, small cell change (SCC) consists of small hepatocytes containing irregular and hyperchromatic nuclei with increased nuclear: cytoplasmic ratio [21,22]. Iron overload is commonly present in parenchymal nodules, especially in patients with advanced cirrhosis, whatever its etiology [23]. Its intensity is variable, well-demonstrated with Perls' staining, usually heterogeneous from one nodule to another, involving both macrophages and hepatocytes (Figure 4.5). Several semi-quantitative scoring systems have been developed, based on the quantity and/or the natural progression of accumulation (from periportal to centrolobular zones) [24]. In cases of hereditary hemochromatosis, a pericanalicular pattern of iron distribution is described in the hepatocytes. However, with progression of the disease and extension of fibrosis, there is loss of the characteristic gradient pattern (portal centrolobular zone) and iron overload is also seen in the biliary epithelium. Features of steatosis and steatohepatitis may also be observed in cirrhotic samples, more commonly associated with metabolic syndrome (MS) and chronic alcohol consumption [25–28]. In those settings, steatosis is prominently macrovacuolar, and, interestingly, the degree of steatosis seems to decrease with extension of fibrosis. Such an observation may explain the increased prevalence of MS and its risk factors, such as obesity and diabetes, in patients with so-called cryptogenic cirrhosis [29]. Morphologic features of steatohepatitis include clarified and ballooned hepatocytes that may contain Mallory–Denk bodies potentially associated with inflamatory cells (mostly lymphocytes in MS and neutrophil polymorphs in alcoholic diseases) (Figure 4.5).

Cirrhosis: an evolving concept

Our view of the natural history of cirrhosis has significantly changed in recent years, and cirrhosis should no longer be considered as the irreversible end stage of CLD. Rather, it is a dynamic process resulting from a fine-tuned balance between fibrogenesis and fibrolysis, and

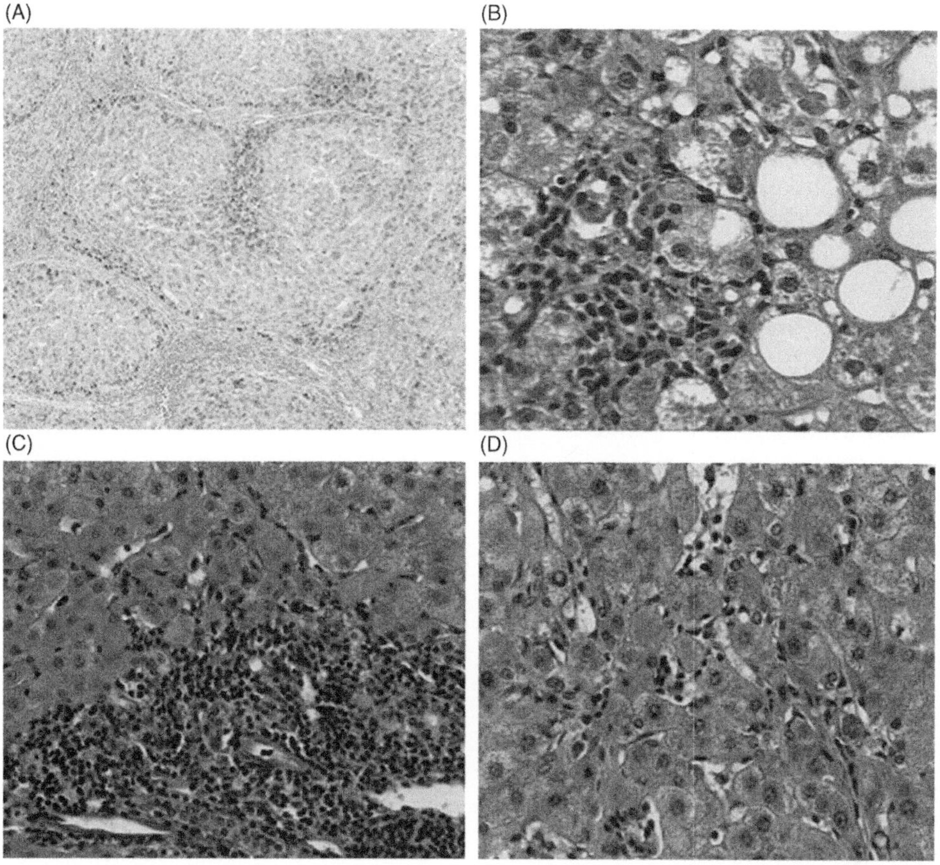

Figure 4.5 Parenchymal nodules: elementary features. (A) Iron overload in parenchymal nodules involving mainly hepatocytes with a gradient pattern (Perls' staining). (B) Steatohepatitis with ballooned hepatocytes containing Mallory–Denk bodies with inflamatory cells around (mostly lymphocytes in metabolic syndrome and neutrophil polymorphs in alcoholic diseases) (hematein and eosin). (C) Piecemeal necrosis: portal inflammation with inflammatory cells disrupting limiting plate (hematein and eosin). (D) Lobular inflammation composed of small foci of lymphocytes between hepatic cell plates (hematein and eosin). (See colour plate section.)

parenchymal extinction and regeneration. This concept has been introduced in experimental models of cirrhosis where reversibility of cirrhosis has been observed in cases where the causative agent was removed [30]. Evidence of regression of liver fibrosis and even cirrhosis has been further reported in patients with CLD of various etiologies, including viral hepatitis, autoimmune hepatitis, and alcoholic diseases [31–33]. However, the magnitude of improvement has to be qualified because, in some cases, regression may lead to a morphologic picture of "incomplete septal cirrhosis" defined by thin fibrous septa, focally incomplete, but still associated with vascular changes [34]. More recently, a study of paired pre and post-treatment liver biopsies from patients with HCV-related cirrhosis who achieved sustained viral response showed both cirrhosis regression (as evaluated by Metavir staging) and decreased collagen content (as evaluated by morphometry) in 61% and 89%, respectively, whereas no changes in sinusoidal capillarization were observed [33]. This outlines the potentially different mechanisms involved in the ECM remodeling according to localization. Importantly, metabolic zonation, assessed by glutamine synthetase and CYP2E1 expression, which is lost in cirrhotic livers, was recovered following HCV eradication, whereas normal lobular architecture was not fully recovered [33].

Altogether, the clinical and morphologic evidence points to a reconsideration of fibrosis staging, and especially

Table 4.1 Scoring systems used in chronic viral hepatitis: grading.

Grading systems	Pathologic features	Scale	Overall grade
Sheuer (1991)	Portal/periportal activity	0–4	Sum of individual
	Lobular activity	0–4	scores (0–8)
Batts and Ludwig (1995)	Piecemeal necrosis	No, minimal, mild, moderate, severe	Grade determined by severity of lesions
	Lobular activity	No, minimal, mild, moderate, severe	
Ishak (1995)	Piecemeal necrosis	0–4	Sum of individual
	Confluent necrosis	0–6	scores (0–18)
	Focal necrosis and inflammation	0–4	
	Portal inflammation	0–4	
Metavir (1996)	Piecemeal necrosis	0–3	Algorithm
	Lobular necrosis	0–2	A0–A3

staging of cirrhosis, and finally leads to the development of a more comprehensive approach to the assessment of advanced chronic liver diseases [35]. Staging of fibrosis relies on an evaluation of several histologic features including assessment of the extent of the ECM deposits, their localization within the liver lobule, and changes in lobular architecture. These features are then integrated into a semi-quantitative scoring system. Different scoring systems have been developed and several are widely used in clinical practice, especially in the field of chronic viral hepatitis for which they were initially developed [36–39]. They propose a separate grading of necro-inflammatory lesions (including piecemeal necrosis and lobular necro-inflammation) which reflects the aggressiveness of disease, and staging of the extent of fibrosis which reflects disease severity. The main features of the scoring systems are reported in Tables 4.1 and 4.2.

Staging is based on a linear numerical scale, from 0 (no fibrosis) to the highest score (4–6) for cirrhosis. It is worthy of note that, in addition to the differences in definition of the intermediate stages according to the scoring systems, the Ishak system is more discriminating for late-stage fibrosis, subdividing incomplete (stage 5) from definite cirrhosis (stage 6) [38]. Although such a level of accuracy in the Ishak system may impact reproducibility and interobserver variability, the additional information is useful because the degree of liver fibrosis, including in cirrhosis, clinically affects the prognosis of patients [40,41]. Indeed, a single-stage histologic description of cirrhosis becomes more and more challenged,

Table 4.2 Scoring systems used in chronic viral hepatitis: staging.

Staging system	Sheuer (1991)	Batts and Ludwig (1995)	METAVIR (1996)	Ishak (1995)
Stage 0	No fibrosis	No fibrosis	No fibrosis	No fibrosis
Stage 1	Enlarged PT	Portal fibrosis	Portal fibrosis without septa	Portal fibrosis of some PT with or without short septa
Stage 2	Periportal fibrosis or portal septa	Periportal fibrosis	Portal fibrosis with rare septa	Portal fibrosis of most PT with or without short septa
Stage 3	Fibrosis with architectural distorsion	Septal fibrosis with architectural distorsion	Numerous septa without cirrhosis	Portal fibrosis of most PT with occasional bridging
Stage 4	Cirrhosis (probable or definite)	Cirrhosis	Cirrhosis	Portal fibrosis of most PT with marked bridging
Stage 5	—	—	—	Incomplete cirrhosis
Stage 6	—	—	—	Cirrhosis (probable or definite)

PT, portal tract.

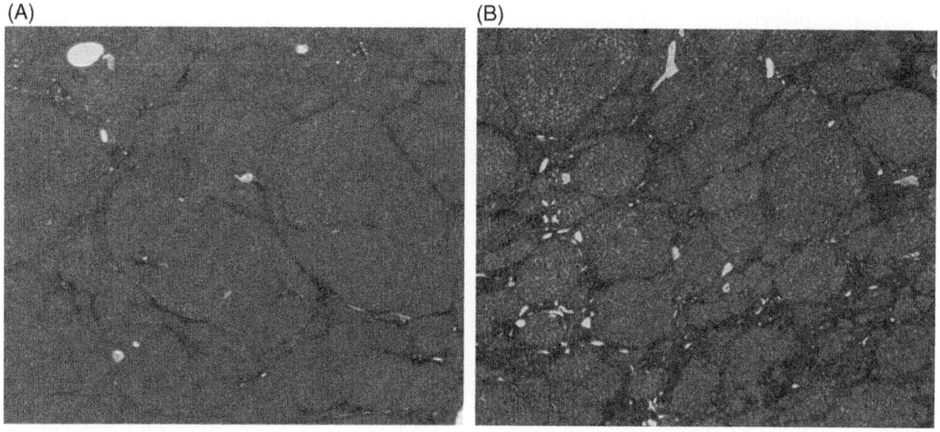

Figure 4.6 Laënnec staging. Substaging of cirrhosis is based on thickness of the fibrous septa and size of the parenchymal nodules. (A) Thin septa surrounding large sized nodules. (B) Thicker fibrous septa surrounding smaller nodules (hematein and eosin). (See colour plate section.)

given its heterogeneity and the significant beneficial impact of treatment in patients with advanced liver fibrosis [42]. Taken altogether, these data support the need to propose a more refined pathologic substaging of cirrhosis. For that purpose, the Laënnec staging system, a modification of the Metavir system, has been introduced, subdividing stage 4 (F4) into three groups (4A, 4B, and 4C) according to the thickness of the fibrous septa and the size of the nodules (Figure 4.6) [43]. Importantly, this scoring system has been further validated, showing its correlation with hepatic venous pressure gradient (HPVG), clinical severity of cirrhosis, and occurrence of liver related events, including hepatic decompensation and HCC development [44–46].

Improvements in the staging of cirrhosis are in accord with an increasing interest in quantifying fibrosis. Based on digital image analysis, morphometry allows accurate quantification of the extent of fibrosis, identified by specific staining, as a ratio of the relative area of fibrosis present on a whole-liver biopsy specimen [47–49]. Interestingly, using such approach, it has been shown that the progressive increase in the area of fibrosis observed with histologic staging systems was not linear [48]. Similarly, measurement of the collagen proportionate area (CPA) has shown good correlation with HPVG, liver stiffness, as evaluated by transient elastography, and accurately predicts further liver decompensation [50–52]. As a continuous numerical scale, morphometry is much more sensitive to minimal variations than semi-quantitative histologic scoring systems. This has been clearly demonstrated in paired pre and post-treatment liver biopsies in HCV cirrhotic patients showing that even in patients with unchanged Metavir score (F4) following a sustained viral response, a significant reduction in collagen was seen [33].

Cirrhosis: a preneoplastic condition

Although a diffuse process, cirrhosis represents a heterogeneous condition with a wide spectrum of severity associated with various complications, including malignant progression. Accordingly, approximately 80% of HCC arise on a background of advanced CLD and cirrhosis. The preneoplastic condition is supported by a description of dysplastic nodules and identification of significant molecular changes in cirrhotic parenchyma, promoting clonal expansion of hepatocytes that may subsequently become malignant. Morphologically, different kinds of preneoplastic nodules are described, including low and high grade dysplastic nodules [53]. Clinical follow-up studies demonstrated their differential rate of progression to HCC, ranging from 26% to 69% in a mean follow-up of 2.8 months [54,55]. Differential diagnosis of these nodules, and especially between high grade dysplatic and early HCC, based on architectural and cytologic features, may be difficult [53]. Molecular studies, using transcriptomics, identifying differential RNA profile expression between dysplastic nodules and HCC, provided several surrogate phenotypical diagnostic markers of HCC [56–59]. Among them, a panel composed of glypican 3, heat shock protein 70, and glutamine synthetase has demonstrated its performance in the positive diagnosis of early HCC (<2 cm), even in biopsy specimens [60,61].

Similarly to morphologic heterogeneity, cirrhotic tissue is made up of a mixture of poly- and monoclonal parenchymal nodules randomly distributed throughout the liver [62,63]. Theoretically, only monoclonal nodules would have the potential to progress to HCC. Although the diagnosis of such monoclonal nodules will certainly help to identify patients with a higher risk of malignant progression, no reliable marker has been validated so far in clinical practice. Histologically, clonal status has been shown to be associated with size, presence of iron overload, and LCC [63]. Molecularly, progressive decrease in LYVE1 mRNA expression was observed from poly- to monoclonal nodules and overt small HCC [64]. Independently of macronodules, cirrhotic parenchyma harbours an intrinsic potential to develop malignancy. Whereas LCC is associated with further development of HCC, as an independent risk factor, SCC, by sharing genetic alterations with HCC, is considered as a preneoplastic lesion. In addition, the potential involvement of hepatic progenitor cells is suggested in liver carcinogenesis given their increased occurrence along the process of CLD [65]. Interestingly, the presence of intermediate hepatobiliary cells in patients with HCV-related cirrhosis, as evaluated by cytokeratin 7 immunostaining in liver biopsy specimens, has shown to be an independent risk factor for developing HCC in multivarite analysis [66]. Finally, molecular analysis of cirrhotic tissue identified a poor prognostic signature associated with late recurrence of HCC and overall survival [67].

Replicative senescence, a physiologic process associated with progressive erosion of telomeres, is induced in several human diseases characterized by fibrosis, including in the liver [68]. Thus, in patients with chronic HCV-related hepatitis, the number of senescent cells gradually increases with fibrosis progression and is correlated with the presence of HCC, in which telomerase expression is induced [69,70]. More recently, telomere dysfunctions related to genetic mutations in some components of the telomerase complex have been isolated as risk factors for cirrhosis [71]. In the multistep pathway of liver carcinogenesis, chronic inflammation, ECM remodeling, and hepatocellular regeneration are intimately connected and may result, according to the nature of the etiologic trigger, in genetic alterations. For instance, alterations of microsatellites in genomic DNA have been reported in cirrhotic tissue, with increased frequency in cirrhosis associated with HCC [72].

Although HCC is the main primary malignancy occurring on a background of cirrhosis, cirrhosis also increases the risk for developing cholangiocarcinoma (CC). In that setting, cirrhosis is mainly observed in patients with chronic inflammatory biliary diseases, including primary sclerosing cholangitis.

Cirrhosis: a place for biopsy?

As diagnosis of cirrhosis relies on a panel of complementary features, based on clinical, biologic, and morphologic tools, and given the relative invasiveness of the biopsy, indications of biopsy are limited. Indeed, significant advances in the noninvasive diagnosis of fibrosis, provided either by physical (such as liver stiffness using transient elastography) or biochemical approaches, have challenged the place of biopsy [73]. Importantly, such techniques are more accurate in detecting advanced stages of fibrosis or cirrhosis, and, among them, transient elastography has been shown to have a higher level of perfomance than biochemical assays. Therefore, in the setting of HCV infection, an algorithm combining noninvasive methods is currently proposed.

Although liver biopsy has been considered as the reference standard for assessing fibrosis, cirrhosis heterogeneity may negatively impact on its performance, which is mainly dependent on sample size. It is admitted that a 2–3 cm length biopsy with at least 11 portal tracts is required [48,74]. However, the increased prevalence of comorbidities in patients with CLD, especially with the rising incidence of MS worldwide, may encourage the a more complete morphologic picture of liver changes to be obtained in order to offer better management to the patient. Finally, as a preneoplastic condition per se, histologic analysis of cirrhosis could potentially provide valuable information in the near future.

References

1 Anthony PP, Ishak KG, Nayack NC, Poulsen HE, Scheuer PJ, Sobin LH. The morphology of cirrhosis: definition, nomenclature and classification. Bull World Heath Organ 1977;55:521–40.

2 Crawford JM. Liver cirrhosis. In MacSween RNM, Burt AD, Portmann BC, et al (eds). Pathology of the Liver, 4th edn. London, England: Churchill Livingston; 2002. pp. 575–619.
3 Schuppan D. Structure of the extracellular matrix in normal and fibrotic liver: collagens and glycoproteins. Semin Liver Dis 1990;10:1–10.
4 Gressner AM. Hepatic fibrogenesis: the puzzle of interacting cells, fibrogenic cytokines, regulatory loops and extracellular matrix molecules. Z Gastroenterol 1992;30:5–16.
5 Rojkind M, Giambrone MA, Biempica L. Collagen types in normal and cirrhotic liver. Gastroenterology 1985;76:710–9.
6 Schaffner F, Popper H. Capillarization of the sinusoids in man. Gastroenterology 1963;44:239–42.
7 Zipfel WR, Williams RM, Webb WW. Nonlinear magic: multiphoton microscopy in the biosciences. Nat Biotechnol 2003;21:1369–77.
8 Gailhouste L, Le Grand Y, Odin C, et al. Fibrillar collagen scoring by second harmonic microscopy: a new tool in the assessment of liver fibrosis. J Hepatol 2010;52:398–406.
9 Li D, Friedman S. Liver fibrogenesis and the role of hepatic stellate cells: new insights and prospects for therapy. J Gastroenterol Hepatol 1999;14:618–33.
10 Friedman SL. Hepatic stellate cells. Prog Liver Dis 1996;14:101–30.
11 Bedossa P. The cell origin of extracellular matrix proteins. J Hepatol 1993;19:1–3.
12 Friedman S. Cytokines and fibrogenesis. Semin Liver Dis 1999;19:129–40.
13 Paradis V, Dargère D, Vidaud M, et al. Expression of connective tissue growth factor in experimental rat and human liver fibrosis. Hepatology 1999;30:968–76.
14 Russo MW, Firpi RJ, Nelson DR, Schoonhoven R, Shrestha R, Fried MW. Early hepatic stellate cell activation is associated with advanced fibrosis after liver transplantation in recipients with hepatitis C. Liver Transpl 2005;11:1235–41.
15 Pinzani M, Rombouts K. Liver fibrosis: from the bench to clinical targets. Dig Liver Dis 2004;36:231–42.
16 Fernández M, Semela D, Bruix J, Colle I, Pinzani M, Bosch J. Angiogenesis in liver disease. J Hepatol 2009;50:604–20.
17 Thabut D, Shah V. Intrahepatic angiogenesis and sinusoidal remodelling in chronic liver disease: new targets for the treatment of porta hypertension. J Hepatol 2010;53:976–80.
18 Taura K, De Minicis S, Seki E, et al. Hepatic stellate cells secrete angiopoietin 1 that induces angiogenesis in liver fibrosis. Gastroenterology 2008;135:1729–38.
19 Tugues S, Fernandez-Varo G, Munoz-Luque J, et al. Antiangiogenic treatment with sunitinib ameliorates inflammatory infiltrate, fibrosis, and portal pressure in cirrhotic rats. Hepatology 2007;46:1919–26.
20 Kim H, Oh BK, Roncalli M, et al. Large liver cell change in hepatitis-B virus-related liver cirrhosis. Hepatology 2009;50:752–62.
21 Hitiroglou P. Morphological changes of early human hepatocarcinogenesis. Semin Liver Dis 2004;24:65–75.
22 Chang O, Yano Y, Masuzawa A, Fukushima N, Teramura K, Hayashi Y. The cytological characteristics of small cell change of dysplasia in small hepatic nodules. Oncol Rep 2010;23:1229–32.
23 23- Ludwig J, Hashimoto E, Porayko MK, Moyer TP, Baldus WP. Hemosiderosis in cirrhosis: a study of 447 native livers. Gastroenterology 1997;112:882–8.
24 Turlin B, Deugnier Y. Evaluation and interpretation of iron in the liver. Semin Diagn Pathol 1998;15:237–45.
25 McSween RN, Burt AD. Histologic spectrum of alcoholic liver disease. Semin Liver Dis 1986;6:221–32.
26 26- Burt AD, Mutton A, Day CP. Diagnosis and interpretation of steatosis and steatohepatitis. Semin Diagn Pathol 1998;15:246–58.
27 Ludwig J, Viggiano TR, McGill DB, Oh BJ. Non-alcoholic steato-hepatitis: Mayo Clinic experiences with a hitherto unnamed disease. Mayo Clin Proc 1980;55:434–8.
28 Brunt EM. Non-alcoholic steatohepatitis: definition and pathology. Semin Liver Dis 2001;21:3–16.
29 Bugianesi E, Leone N, Vanni E, et al. Expanding the natural history of nonalcoholic steatohepatitis: from cryptogenic cirrhosis to hepatocellular carcinoma. Gastroenterology 2002;123:134–40.
30 Iredale JP, Benyon RC, Pickering J, et al. Mechanisms of spontaneous resolution of rat liver fibrosis: hepatic stellate cell apoptosis and reduced hepatic expression of metalloproteinase inhibitors. J Clin Invest 1998;102:538–49.
31 Poynard T, McHutchison J, Manns M, et al. Impact of pegylated interferon alfa-2b and ribavirin on liver fibrosis in patients with chronic hepatitis C. Gastroenterology 2002;122:1303–13.
32 George SL, Bacon BR, Brunt EM, Mihindukulasuriya KL, Hoffmann J, Di Bisceglie AM. Clinical, virologic, histologic, and biochemical outcomes after successful HCV therapy. Hepatology 2009;49:729–38.
33 D'Ambrosio R, Aghemo A, Rumi AG, et al. A morphometric and immunohistochemical study to assess the benefit of a sustained virological response in hepatitis C virus patients with cirrhosis. Hepatology 2012;56:532–43.
34 Wanless IR, Nakashima E, Sherman M. Regression of human cirrhosis: morphologic features and the genesis of incomplete septal cirrhosis. Arch Pathol Lab Med 2000;124:1599–607.
35 Hytiroglou P, Dale CS, Alves V, et al. Beyond "cirrhosis": a proposal from the international Liver Pathology Study Group. Am J Clin Pathol 2012;137:5–9.
36 Sheuer PJ. Classification of chronic viral hepatitis: a need for reassessment. J Hepatol 1991;13:372–4.
37 Batts KP, Ludwig J. Chronic hepatitis: an update on terminology and reporting. Am J Surg Pathol 1995;19:1409–17.
38 Ishak K, Baptista A, Bianchi L, et al. Histological grading and staging of chronic hepatitis. J Hepatol 1995;22:696–9.
39 Bedossa P, Poynard T. An algorithm for the grading of activity in chronic hepatitis C: The METAVIR Cooperative Study Group. Hepatology 1996;24:289–93.

40 D'Amico G, Garci-Tsao G, Pagliaro L. Natural history and prognostic indicators of survival in cirrhosis: a systematic review of 118 studies. J Hepatol 2006;44:217–31.

41 Nagula S, Jain D, Groszmann RJ, Garcia-Tsao G. Histological-hemodynamics correlations in cirrhosis: a histological classification of the severity of cirrhosis. J Hepatol 2006;44:111–7.

42 Garcia-Tsao G, Friedman S, Iredale J, Pinzani M. Now there are many (stages) where before there was one: in search of a pathophysiological classification of cirrhosis. Hepatology 2010;51:1445–9.

43 Kutami RGN, Girgrah N, Wanless IR, et al. The Laennec grading system for assessment of hepatic fibrosis: validation by correlation with wedged hepatic vein pressure and clinical features. Hepatology 2000;32:407A.

44 Kim MY, Cho MY, Baik SK, et al. Histological sub-classification of cirrhosis using the Laennec fibrosis scoring system correlates with clinical stage and grade of portal hypertension. J Hepatol 2011;55:1004–9.

45 Kim SU, Oh HJ, Wanless IR, Lee S, Han KH, Park YN. The Laennec staging system for histological sub-classification of cirrhosis is useful for stratification of prognosis in patients with liver cirrhosis. J Hepatol 2012;57:556–63.

46 Rastogi A, Maiwall R, Bihari C, et al. Cirrhosis histology and Laennec staging system correlate with high portal pressure. Histopathology 2013;62:731–41.

47 Pilette C, Rousselet MC, Bedossa P, et al. Histopathological evaluation of liver fibrosis: quantitative image analysis vs semi-quantitative scores. J Hepatol 1998;27:1–8.

48 Bedossa P, Dargère D, Paradis V. Sampling variability of liver fibrosis in chronic hepatitis C. Hepatology 2003;38:1449–57.

49 Caballero T, Perez-Milena A, Masseroli M, et al. Liver fibrosis assessment with semiquantitative indexes and image analysis quantification in sustained-responder and non-responder interferon-treated patients with chronic hepatitis C. J Hepatol 2001;34:740–7.

50 Calvaruso V, Burroughs AK, Dhillon AP, et al. Computer-assisted image analysis ofliver collagen: relationship to Ishak scoring and hepatic venous pressure gradient. Hepatology 2009;49:1236–44.

51 Sethasine S, Jain D, Groszmann RJ, Garcia-Tsao G. Quantitative histological-hemodynamic correlations in cirrhosis. Hepatology 2012;55:1146–53.

52 Isgro G, Garcovich M, Luong TV, et al. Collagen proportion-ate area: the most appropriate index to correlate with transient elastography. Hepatology 2010; 52(Suppl): 411A.

53 International Consensus Group for Hepatocellular Neoplasia: The International Consensus Group for Hepatocellular Neoplasia. Pathologic diagnosis of early hepatocellular carcinoma: a report of the international consensus group for hepatocellular neoplasia. Hepatology 2009;49:658–64.

54 Borzio M, Fargion S, Borzio F, et al. Impact of large regenerative, low grade and high grade dysplastic nodules in hepatocellular carcinoma development. J Hepatol 2003;39: 208–14.

55 Kobayashi M, Ikeda K, Hosaka T, et al. Dysplastic nodules frequently develop into hepatocellular carcinoma in patients with chronic viral heopatitis and cirrhosis. Cancer 2006;106:636–47.

56 Paradis V, Bièche I, Dargère D, et al. Molecular profiling of hepatocellular carcinomas (HCC) using a large-scale real-time RT-PCR approach: determination of a molecular diagnostic index. Am J Pathol 2003;163:733–41.

57 Llovet JM, Chen Y, Wurmbach E, et al. A molecular signature to discriminate dysplastic nodules from early hepatocellular carcinoma in HCV cirrhosis. Gastroenterology 2006;131:1758–67.

58 Wang XY, Degos F, Dubois S, et al. Glypican-3 expression in hepatocellular tumors: diagnostic value for preneoplastic lesions and hepatocellular carcinomas. Hum Pathol 2006;37:1435–41.

59 Libbrecht L, Severi T, Cassiman D, et al. Glypican-3 expression distinguishes small hepatocellular carcinomas from cirrhosis, dysplastic nodules, and focal nodular hyperplasia-like nodules. Am J Surg Pathol 2006;30:1405–11.

60 Di Tommaso L, Franchi G, Park YN, et al. Diagnostic value of HSP70, Glypican 3 and Glutamine synthetase i hepatocellular nodules in cirrhosis. Hepatology 2007;45:725–34.

61 Di Tommaso L, Destro A, Seok JY, et al. The application of markers (HSP70 GPC3 and GS) in liver biopsies is useful for detection of hepatocellular carcinoma. J Hepatol 2009;50:746–54.

62 Paradis V, Laurendeau I, Vidaud M, Bedossa P. Clonal analysis of macronodules in cirrhosis. Hepatology 1998;28:953–8.

63 Paradis V, Dargère D, Bonvoust F, et al. Clonal analysis of micronodules in virus C-induced liver cirrhosis using laser capture microdissection (LCM) and Humara Assay. Lab Invest 2000;80:1553–9.

64 Colombat M, Paradis V, Bièche I, et al. Quantitative RT-PCR in cirrhotic nodules reveals gene expression changes associated with liver carcinogenesis. J Pathol 2003;201:260–7.

65 Roskams T, Kojiro M. Pathology of early hepatocellular carcinoma: conventional and molecular diagnosis. Semin Liver Dis 2010;30:17–25.

66 Ziol M, Nault JC, Aout M, et al. Intermediate hepatobiliary cells predict an increased risk of hepatocarcinogenesis in patients with hepatitis C virus-related cirrhosis. Gastroenterology 2010;139:335–43.

67 Hoshida Y, Villanueva A, Kobayashi M, et al. Gene expression in fixed tissues and outcome in hepatocellular carcinoma. N Engl J Med 2008;359:1995–2004.

68 Calado RT, Young NS. Telomere diseases. N Engl J Med 2009;361:2353–65.

69 Paradis V, Youssef N, Dargère D, et al. Replicative senescence in normal liver, chronic hepatitis C, and hepatocellular carcinoma. Hum Pathol 2001;32:327–32.

70 Youssef N, Paradis V, Ferlicot S, Bedossa P. In situ detection of telomerase enzymatic activity in hepatocellular carcinoma, cirrhosis, chronic hepatitis and normal liver. J Pathol 2001;194:459–65.

71 Calado RT, Brudno J, Mehta P, et al. Constitutional telomerase mutations are genetic risk factors for cirrhosis. Hepatology 2011;53:1600–7.

72 Nagai H, Emi M, Terada Y, et al. DNA alterations during multi-step development of human hepatocellular carcinomas revealed by laser capture microdissection. Hepatol Res 2003;26:199–208.

73 Castera L. Noninvasive methods to assess liver disease in patients with hepatitis B or C. Gastroenterology 2012; 142:1293–302.

74 Colloredo G, Guido M, Sonzogni A, Leandro G. Impact of liver biopsy size on histological evaluation of chronic viral hepatitis: the smaller the sample, the milder the disease. J Hepatol 2003;39:239–44.

CHAPTER 5

Fibrosis and fibrogenesis

Namiki Izumi,[1] Nobuharu Tamaki,[1] Yasuhiro Asahina,[2] and Masayuki Kurosaki[1]

[1] *Department of Gastroenterology and Hepatology, Musashino Red Cross Hospital, Tokyo, Japan*
[2] *Department of Hepatitis Investigation, Tokyo Medical and Dental University, Tokyo, Japan*

Introduction

Cirrhosis is derived from advanced fibrosis of the liver caused by hepatitis B or C virus infection, autoimmune liver disease, alcoholic or metabolic disorders. To prevent the development of cirrhosis, it is important to be able to predict the degree of the fibrosis of the liver and prevent its progression. Recently, remarkable progress has been made in estimating the degree of hepatic fibrosis and in understanding the importance of a single-nucleotide polymorphism involved in the progression of fibrosis. Understanding the mechanism of fibrogenesis is fundamental to preventing the progression to cirrhosis.

Mechanism of liver fibrosis in hepatitis B and C

Liver fibrosis arises from a variety of factors including hepatitis B and C viruses (HBV and HCV), autoimmunity, alcohol, and metabolic abnormalities such as steatosis [1]. The degree of fibrosis is assessed by liver biopsy, and classified according to international standards [2]. The mechanism of development of fibrosis differs for HBV and HCV and a frequent problem that needs to be addressed is how to assess liver fibrosis without the need for a liver biopsy.

Fundamentally, in both HBV and HCV infections, fibrosis develops in areas of necrosis. Differences between these mechanisms of fibrosis were analyzed and when phospho-Smad 2 staining was performed, a correlation between the amount of staining and the stage of fibrosis was observed in steatosis, steatohepatitis, and hepatitis B, but no such relationship was found for hepatitis C. On the other hand, interleukin 13 (IL-13) immunostaining was correlated with the stage of fibrosis in steatosis, steatohepatitis and in hepatitis C, while there was no such relationship with hepatitis B [3]. This is believed to illustrate one of the differences in the mechanisms of fibrosis. Transforming growth factor β (TGF-β) and IL-13 signaling differs depending on the cause of the liver fibrosis: TGF-β1 predominance is associated with HBV-related liver fibrogenesis, while IL-13 predominance is detected in HCV infection. In addition, an increase in natural killer T cells was seen in a study of HBV using transgenic mice and this is considered to be the mechanism that triggers the activation of fat-storing cells (FSCs) in the liver, leading to liver fibrosis [4].

On the other hand, there are numerous reports of liver fibrosis arising from HCV infection. It has been shown that HCV produces reactive oxygen species, inducing TGF-β1 and causes liver fibrosis to occur [5]. It also has been shown by a meta-analysis that steatosis is an independent risk factor for liver fibrosis in cases of HCV infection [6]. In nonalcoholic steatohepatitis and HCV infection, hepatic insulin signaling is impaired and down-regulation of insulin-sensitive targets is observed; this has been shown to be associated with apoptosis and fibrogenesis [7]. In an Asian study, hepatic fibrosis was also found to be associated with insulin resistance based on a homeostatic model assessment of insulin resistance in infections with HCV genotypes 2 and 3 [8]. In HCV infection, 25-hydroxyvitamin D blood levels are low and cytochrome P27A1, a liver 25-hydroxylating enzyme, correlates with 25-hydroxyvitamin D serum levels, which are said to be associated with liver fibrosis [9].

Cirrhosis: A practical guide to management, First Edition. Edited by Samuel S. Lee and Richard Moreau.

Diagnosis of liver fibrosis by imaging

FibroScan, a transient elastography tool developed and produced by Echosens (Paris, France), was introduced in 2005 as a method for assessing the progression of liver fibrosis [10]. This method uses a thin cylindrical probe placed close to the liver to send a 1-period 50-Hz shear wave through the surface of the body to the liver and measure the propagation velocity [11]. Later, advances were made with the development of devices that measure liver stiffness using abdominal ultrasound. Virtual Touch Tissue Quantification (VTTQ) developed by Siemens AG (Munich, Germany), is a method for measuring tissue stiffness from a shear wave generated by an acoustic radiation force impulse (ARFI) with a 300-μs push pulse and measurement of the propagation velocity [12,13]. Acoustic Structure Quantification (ASQ) (Toshiba, Tokyo, Japan) was established from echogenicity distribution within the region of interest of the liver, a mean value was calculated, and expressed as liver stiffness. An example of measurement of liver stiffness using ASQ is shown in Figure 5.1.

Although the gold standard for the diagnosis of liver fibrosis is liver biopsy, there are associated risks of complications and it cannot be repeatedly performed. Sampling errors and diagnostic mistakes by pathologists also are problematic [14,15]. Measuring liver stiffness is one way to resolve these problems. The relationship between liver fibrosis and HCV can be shown with the FibroScan tool, which can be used to diagnose F3 and F4 advanced cases of fibrosis [16]. However, liver stiffness measurements are uninterpretable in nearly one in five cases because of obesity, increased waist circumference, or operator inexperience [17].

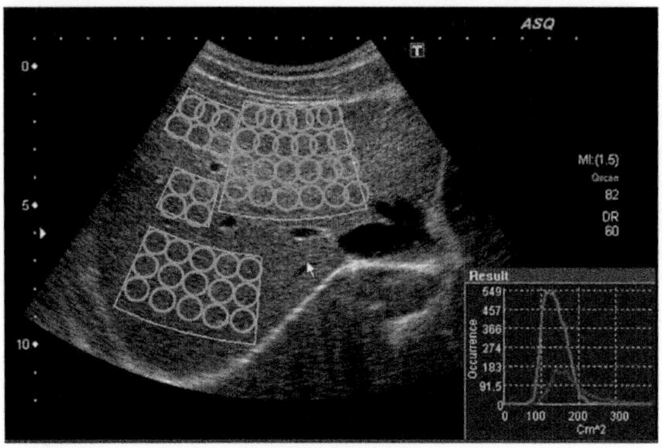

Figure 5.1 Measurement of liver stiffness using acoustic radiation force impulse. The region of interest is established by abdominal ultrasound and the stiffness of this site can be measured. (See colour plate section.)

Diagnosis of liver fibrosis by laboratory tests

Links to liver fibrosis have been reported for the results of blood tests that can be clinically measured. For example, links between the aspartate aminotransferase : alanine aminotransferase (AST : ALT) ratio [18] and AST : platelet ratio index [19,20] and liver fibrosis have been observed and are reported to be clinically useful. The FibroTest blood marker test (BioPredictive, Paris, France), a combination of basic serum markers such as α2-globulin, gammaglobulin, and apolipoprotein, has been reported to be useful for inferring liver fibrosis [21,22]. On the other hand, the FIB-4 index, which is calculated based only on age, AST, ALT, and platelet counts measured by general clinical laboratory tests, is reportedly useful for reflecting advanced F3–F4 liver fibrosis: when the FIB-4 score is less than 1.45, the negative predictive value for F3–F4 is 90% and when the FIB-4 score is greater than 3.25, the positive predictive value for F3–F4 is 80% [23,24]. It has been shown that these noninvasive markers of liver fibrosis are useful for predicting liver-related mortality [25] and the occurrence of hepatocellular carcinoma [26]. The FIB-4 index was evaluated in patients who underwent liver biopsy and a positive correlation was noted as shown in Figure 5.2. However, there is overlap among F2, F3, and F4. When we investigated the relationship between FIB-4 and the progression of liver fibrosis in patients with chronic HCV infection who had undergone two or more liver biopsies, we found a good correlation and therefore believe that this is a good index for estimating prognosis and evaluating the therapeutic effect of interferon (Figure 5.3) [27]. On the other hand, APRI score, which is calculated as (AST/ULN)/platelet (10^9/L) was shown to correlated with the fibrosis stage, but there are overlaps between F3 and F4 (Figure 5.4).

From these results, a diagnostic algorithm for fibrosis of the liver in patients with chronic HCV infection, without liver biopsy, was produced and is shown in Figure 5.4. Seventy-five per cent of patients with a FIB-4 index of 3 or greater, and ASQ score 120 or greater, are estimated

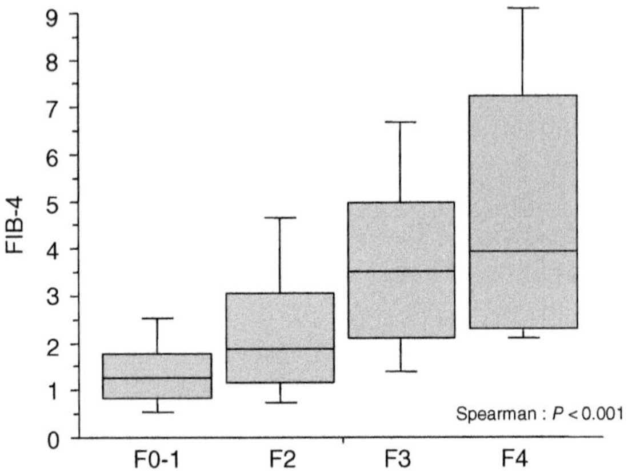

Figure 5.2 The relationship between FIB-4 index score and liver fibrosis in patients with chronic hepatitis C virus infection who had undergone two liver biopsies. (Tamaki et al. 2012 [27]. Reproduced with permission of John Wiley & Sons.)

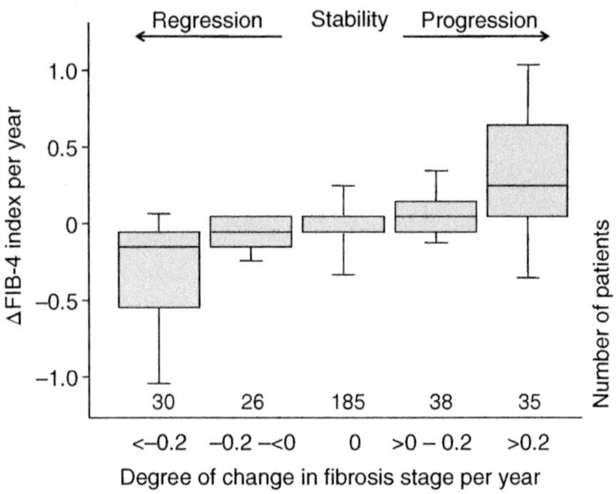

Figure 5.3 The relationship between FIB-4 and the progression of liver fibrosis in patients with chronic hepatitis C virus infection who had undergone two or more liver biopsies. There was a good correlation and FIB-4 is likely to be a good index for estimating prognosis and evaluating the therapeutic effect of interferon (Tamaki et al. 2012 [27]. Reproduced with permission of John Wiley & Sons.)

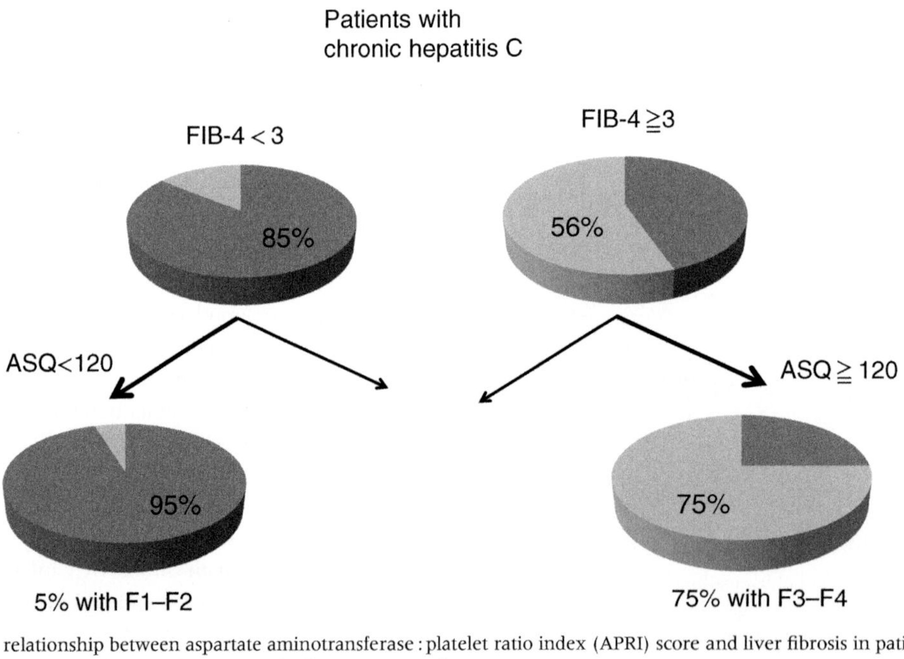

Figure 5.4 The relationship between aspartate aminotransferase : platelet ratio index (APRI) score and liver fibrosis in patients with chronic hepatitis C virus infection. There is overlap between F3 and F4.

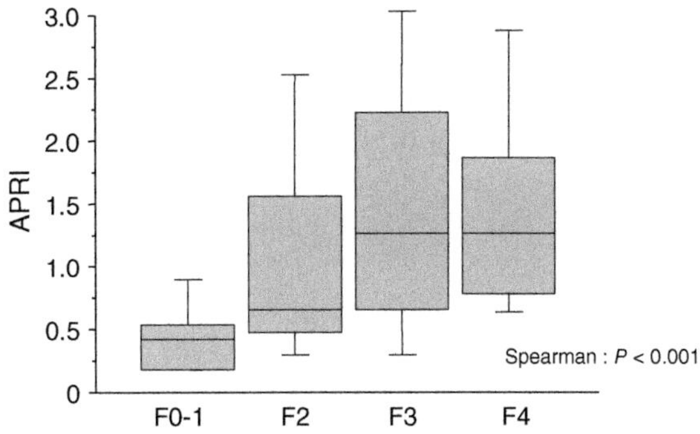

Figure 5.5 Diagnostic algorithm for advanced fibrosis with F3 and F4 by FIB-4 index and Acoustic Structure Quantification (ASQ). Seventy-five per cent of patients with a FIB-4 index of 3 or greater, and ASQ score of 120 or greater, were estimated to have the stage of F3–F4 fibrosis. Only 5% of patients with a FIB-4 index below 3 and ASQ score less than 120 were predicted to have the advanced fibrosis at stage of F3–F4. Thus, fibrosis stage was estimated with 89% accuracy in 53% of the patients with chronic hepatitis C without liver biopsy.

to have stage F3–F4 fibrosis. Only 5% of the patients with an FIB-4 index below 3, and ASQ score less than 120, are predicted to have advanced fibrosis stage of F3–F4. Thus, fibrosis stage was estimated with 89% accuracy without liver biopsy in 53% of the patients with chronic HCV infection.

Cell types involved in liver fibrosis

With long-term liver damage, hepatocyte loss and/or necrosis and regeneration repeat persistently. Cells involved in the inflammatory response aggregate in areas of necrosis, and an extracellular matrix composed primarily of type I collagen is generated and grows. If inflammation is transient, the remaining hepatocytes regenerate and proliferate, the collagen degenerates, fiber-producing cells go into apoptosis, and the tissue recovers. However, if liver damage is prolonged, the balance between hepatocellular necrosis and regeneration is disrupted and fibers are deposited and accumulate in the necrotic tissue. FSC are believed to be the cells primarily responsible for synthesizing fiber in the liver. Close interactions among activated Kupffer cells and damaged hepatocytes in the vicinity, platelets and sinusoidal endothelial cells, and bile duct epithelial cells have an important role in the activation of FSCs; monocytes circulating in the blood are also reported to be involved.

FSCs, myofibroblasts, and fibrocytes contribute to the production of collagen in the liver. It has been shown that the origin of collagen production differs in FSCs and myofibroblasts. Specifically, it has been reported that portal myofibroblasts present in the portal region react differently to specific markers and apoptosis stimulation than to FSCs [28]; it also has been shown that bile duct epithelial cells and hepatocytes are converted to myofibroblasts via epithelial–mesenchymal transition [29,30]. In addition, bone marrow-derived cells and fibrocytes in the bloodstream may adhere to the liver and differentiate into FSCs [31].

FSCs are located in the space of Disse, a gap between a sinusoid and a hepatic cord, and with the cell body in contact with sinusoidal endothelial cells. Branch-like protrusions extend from FSCs and wrap around the sinusoidal endothelial cells; the other side of the cell body being in contact with hepatocytes. FSCs function as liver-specific pericytes and regulate the sinusoidal microcirculation by contracting and relaxing in response to exposure to vasoactive mediators such as endothelin, nitric oxide, and carbon monoxide. It has been shown that FSCs produce osteopontin, an oxidative stress-induced cytokine, and that FSCs may change to a profibrogenic phenotype and enhance the production of collagen-1 [32]. Consequently, it is possible that osteopontin promotes the production of collagen-1 as a key cytokine of the extracellular matrix and contributes to liver fibrosis and scarring.

If the liver is damaged, the function and morphology of the FSCs are dramatically altered, the traits of the cells are changed to those of myofibroblasts, which have different properties, and these cells are regarded as activated FSCs [33]. Specifically, FSCs are activated through a receptor-dependent signaling cascade by TGF-β1 and platelet-derived growth factor secreted by aggregated platelets and macrophages derived from monocytes, and Kupffer cells activated by local inflammation of the liver.

In activated FSCs, stored vitamin A is lost and levels decrease, desmin (a cytoskeletal protein) and α-smooth muscle actin increase, enhancing their contractile capability and producing excessive quantities of extracellular matrix materials, mainly type I collagen. When FSCs are activated, latent TGF-β1 is generated; this is activated by plasminogen activator/plasmin, enhancing the autocrine-like production of type I collagen. In addition, tissue inhibitor matrix of metalloproteinases, which are collagenase inhibitors, are produced and inhibit the breakdown of the extracellular matrix and accumulate locally in the tissues. Tissue inhibitor matrix of metalloproteinase-1 contributes to the continuous FSC activation because it inhibits the apoptosis of FSCs [34].

However, the involvement of immunity in FSC activation also has been analyzed and it has been shown that in HCV infection, fibrosis may be induced when FSCs are activated by the phagocytosis of lymphocytes [35]. When the role of ghrelin was investigated in rats administered CCl_4 or subjected to bile duct ligation, fibrosis was inhibited by the administration of recombinant ghrelin, myofibroblast accumulation decreased, and the fibrogenic properties of FSC were reduced [36]. Based on these findings, it may be possible to use ghrelin as an antifibrotic therapy.

Genes involved in liver fibrosis

CXCL1, a ligand for CXC chemokine-receptor 2 which is expressed on FSCs, is believed to be involved in FSC activation and an analysis has been carried out to determine whether CXCL1 rs4074 polymorphism is linked to the expression of CXCL1 and the progression of liver fibrosis in chronic HCV infection. The results indicated a high frequency of the A allele in type C hepatic cirrhosis and that this is a risk factor for liver fibrosis [37]. Whether a single-nucleotide polymorphism of the antizyme inhibitor (AzI) gene is involved in slow fibrosis progression was investigated separately. A novel splice variation was found whereby a single-nucleotide polymorphism of the *AZIN1* gene regulates FSC liver fibrosis [38].

Onset and progression of liver fibrosis

Cytokines (chemokines) derived from nearby cell groups, oxidative stress, and mediators that produce FSCs themselves are involved in FSC activation as well as in the onset and progression of liver fibrosis. Injured hepatocytes are a source of lipid peroxide and excess reactive oxygen species produced by mitochondria in hepatocytes as well as proteins and cellular membranes from injured hepatocytes become FSC activating factors [39,40]. In addition, if bivalent iron (Fe^{2+}) overaccumulates in hepatocytes, it has a potent oxidative effect due to the Fenton reaction and produces OH radicals, which induce hepatocellular apoptosis and enhance fibrosis via FSC activation. TGF- β, TGF-α, insulin-like growth factor and binding proteins, hepatocyte growth factor, vascular endothelial growth factor, and IL-6 are believed to be cytokines derived from hepatocytes. However, Kupffer cells, which are hepatic macrophages, also produce various inflammatory cytokines. Kupffer cells are indigenous macrophages that adhere to sinusoidal endothelial cells on the inside of a sinusoid and phagocytose or process foreign bodies coming from the digestive track and primarily contained in the portal vein, as well as waste products produced in the body. Kupffer cells are activated by oxidative stress in a liver disorder and by endotoxins derived from enterobacteria via toll-like receptor 4 and CD14 [41]. Chemokines derived from Kupffer cells also have an important role. Activated Kupffer cells produce platelet-derived growth factor and TGF-β and these induce FSC activation.

Regulation and treatment of liver fibrosis

Liver fibrosis is initiated by the overaccumulation of extracellular matrix materials in the parenchyma, primarily type I collagen produced by activated FSCs. Consequently, inhibiting the production and promoting the breakdown of the extracellular matrix based on inhibiting or eliminating FSC activation is considered to be effective for treating liver fibrosis. Inhibiting FSC growth and activation and inhibiting collagen production have been discussed.

Interferon (IFN) inhibits the activation of FSCs *in vitro* and *in vivo*. IFN-γ alone inhibits the expression of smooth muscle α-actin and cell contraction observed using the collagen gel method. The inhibitory effect of IFN-α and IFN-β on FSC growth facilitates the induction of FSC apoptosis. It has been reported that the FSC activity that promotes collagen gene expression is inhibited by IFN-α and IFN-γ, and that the intracellular signaling factors phosphorylated Stat-1 and p300 contribute to this effect [42].

Recently, clinical tests of antifibrosis therapies have been conducted using the angiotensin II blockers candesartan and irbesartan [43,44]. There are already many angiotensin-converting enzyme inhibitors and angiotensin I receptor antagonists that are used as antihypertensive drugs. Human and rodent FSCs express components of the renin–angiotensin system [45] and it has been shown in an animal model that the use of these inhibitors regulates FCS activation and fibrosis.

The recent development of molecular target drugs for various types of malignant tumors has been remarkable. Angiogenic inhibitors (such as sorafenib), which are substances that block receptor-dependent Raf-MEK-ERK signaling to growth factors such as vascular endothelial growth factor and epidermal growth factor, inhibit the angiogenesis of cells composing the stroma that nourishes liver cancer [46]. In the fibrous septa of a fibrotic liver, not only is there growth of activated FSCs and myofibroblast-like cells, but angiogenesis also occurs along the septa. As a result, it is likely that tumor suppression itself has an antifibrotic dimension. In the future, it will be necessary to consider inhibiting liver fibrosis with molecular target drugs.

References

1 Asahina K, Tsai SY, Li P, et al. Mesenchymal organ of hepatic stellate cells, submesotheliat cells, and perivasclular mesenchymal cells during mouse liver development. Hepatology 2009;49:998–1011.

2 Desmet VJ, Gerber M, Hoofnagle JH, Manns M, Scheuer PJ. Classification of chronic hepatitis: diagnosis, grading and staging. Hepatology 1994;19:1513–20.

3 Weng HL, Liu Y, Chen JL, et al. The etiology of liver damage imparts cytokines transforming factor beta 1 or interleukin-13 as driving forces in fibrogenesis. Hepatology 2009;50:230–43.

4 Jin Z, Sun R, Wei H, Gao X, Chen Y, Tian Z. Accelerated liver fibrosis in hepatitis B virus transgenic mice: involvement of natural killer T cells. Hepatology 2011;53:219–29.

5 Lin W, Tsai WL, Shao RX, et al. Hepatitis C virus regulates transforming growth factor beta 1 production through the generation of reactive oxygen species in a nuclear factor kappa B-dependent manner. Gastroenterology 2010;138: 2509–18.

6 Leandro G, Mangia A, Hui J, et al. HCV Meta-Analysis (on) individual Patients' Data Study Group. Relationship between steatosis, inflammation, and fibrosis in chronic hepatitis C: a meta-analysis of individual patient data. Gastroenterology 2006;130:1636–42.

7 Carcia-Monzon C, Lo Iacono O, Mayoral R, et al. Hepatic insulin resistance is associated with increased apoptosis and fibrogenesis in nonalcoholic steatohepatitis and chronic hepatitis C. J Hepatol 2011;54:142–52.

8 Patel K, Thompson AJ, Chuang WL, et al. Insulin resistance is independently associated with significant fibrosisi in Asian chronic hepatitis C genotype 2 or 3 patients. J Gastroenterol Hepatol 2011;26:1182–8.

9 Petta S, Camma C, Scazzone C, et al. Low vitamin D serum level is related to severe fibrosis and low responsiveness to interferon-based therapy in genotype 1 chronic hepatitis C. Hepatology 2010;51:1158–67.

10 Castéra L, Vergniol J, Foucher J, et al. Prospective comparison of transient elastography, Fibrotest, APRI, and liver biopsy for the assessment of fibrosis in chronic hepatitis C. Gastroenterology 2005;128:343–50.

11 Ziol M, Handra-Luca A, Kettaneh A, et al. Noninvasive assessment of the liver fibrosis by measurement of stiffness in patients with chronic hepatitis C. Hepatology 2005;41: 48–54.

12 Nightingale K, McAleavey S, Trahay G. Shear-wave generation using acoustic radiation force: in vivo and ex vivo results. Ultrasound Med Biol 2003;29:1715–23.

13 Friedrich-Rust M, Wunder K, Kriener S, et al. Liver fibrosis in viral hepatitis: noninvasive assessment with acoustic radiation force impulse imaging versus transient elastography. Radiology 2009;252:595–604.

14 Regev A, Berho M, Jeffers LJ, et al. Sampling error and intraobserver varidation in liver biopsy in patients with HCV infection. Am J Gastrenterol 2002;26:2614–8.

15 Bedossa P, Dargere D, Paradis V. Sampling variability of liver fibrosis in chronic hepatitis C. Hepatology 2003;38:1449–57.

16 Lucidarme D, Foucher J, Le Bail B, et al. Factors of accuracy of transient elastography (fibroscan) for the diagnosis of liver fibrosis in chronic hepatitis C. Hepatology 2009;49:1083–9.

17 Castera L, Le Bail B, Roudot-Thoraval F, et al. Early detection in routine clinical practice of cirrhosis and oesophageal varices in chronic hepatitis C: comparison of transient elastography (FibroScan) with standard laboratory tests and non-invasive scores. J Hepatol 2009;50:59–68.

18 Williams AL, Hoofnagle JH. Ratio of serum aspirate to alanine aminotransferase in chronic hepatitis: relationship to cirrhosis. Gastroenterology 1988;95:734–9.

19 Wai CT, Greenson JK, Fontana RJ, et al. A simple non-invasive index can predict both significant fibrosis and cirrhosis in patients with chronic hepatitis C. Hepatology 2003;38:518–26.

20 Lin ZH, Xin YN, Dong QJ, et al. Performance of the aspirate aminotransferase-to-platelet ratio index for the staging of hepatitis C-related fibrosis: an update meta-analysis. Hepatology 2011;53:726–36.

21 Imbert-Bismut F, Ratziu V, Pieroni L, et al. MULTIVIRC Group. Biochemical markers of liver fibrosis in patients with hepatitis C virus infection: a prospective study. Lancet 2001;357:1069–75.

22 Sebastiani G, Vario A, Guido M, et al. Stepwise combination algorithms of non-invasive markers to diagnose significant fibrosis in chronic hepatitis C. J Hepatol 2006;44:686–93.

23 Sterling RK, Lissen E, Clumeck N, et al. Development of a simple noninvasive index to predict significant fibrosis in patients with HIV/HCV coinfection. Hepatology 2006;43: 1317–25.

24 Vallet-Pichard A, Mallet V, Nalpas B, et al. FIB-4: an inexpensive and accurate marker of fibrosis in HCV infection: comparison with liver biopsy and fibrotest. Hepatology 2007;46:32–6.
25 Nunes D, Fleming C, Offner G, et al. Noninvasive markers of liver fibrosis are highly predictive of liver-related death in a cohort of HCV-infected individuals with and without infection. Am J Gastroenterol 2010;105:1346–53.
26 Fung J, Lai CL, Seto WK, Wong DK, Yuen MF. Prognostic significance of liver stiffness for hepatocellular carcinoma and mortality in HBe-Ag negative chronic hepatitis B. J Viral Hepat 2011;18:738–44.
27 Tamaki N, Kurosaki M, Tanaka K, et al. Non-invasive estimation of fibrosis progression overtime using the FIB-4 index in chronic hepatitis C. J Viral Hepat 2013;20:72–6.
28 Battaller R, Brenner DA. Liver fibrosis. J Clin Invest 2005; 115:209–18.
29 Wynn TA. Cellular and molecular mechanisms of fibrosis. J Pathol 2008;214:199–210.
30 Zeisberg M, Yang C, Martino M, et al. Fibrosis derived from hepatocytes in liver fibrosis via epithelial to mesenchymal transition. J Biol Chem 2007;282; 23337–47.
31 Iredale JP. Models of liver fibrosis: exploring the dynamic nature of inflammation and repair in a solid organ. J Clin Invest 2007;117:539–48.
32 Urtasun R, Lopategi A, George J, et al. Osteopontin, and oxidative stress sensitive cytokine, upregulates collagen-1 via integrin $\alpha(v)\beta(3)$ engagement and PI3K/pAkt/NFκB signaling. Hepatology 2012;55:594–608.
33 Friedman SL. Molecular regulation of hepatic fibrosis, and integrated cellular response to tissue injury. J Biol Chem 2000;275:2247–50.
34 Friedman SL. Hepatic stellate cells: protein, multifunctional, and enigmatic cells of the liver. Physiol Rev 2008;88:125–72.
35 Muhanna N, Doron S, Wald O, et al. Activation of hepatic stellate cells after phagocytosis of lymphocytes: a novel pathway of fibrogenesis. Hepatology 2008;48:963–77.
36 Moreno M, Chaves JF, Sancho-Bru P, et al. Ghrelin attenuates hepatocellular injury and liver fibrogenesis in rodents and influences firrosis progression in humans. Hepatology 2010;51:974–85.
37 Nischalke HD, Berger C, Luda C, et al. The CXCL1 re 4074 allele is associated with enhanced CXCL1 responses to TLR2 ligands and predisposes to cirrhosis in HCV genotype 1-infected Caucasian patients. J Hepatol 2012;56:758–64.
38 Paris AJ, Snapir Z, Christopherson CD, et al. A polymorphism that delays fibrosis in hepatitis C promotes alternative splicing of AZIN1, reducing fibrogenesis. Hepatology 2011; 54:2198–207.
39 Kristensen DB, Kawada N, Imamura K, et al. Proteome analysis of rat hepatic stellate cells. Hepatology 2000;32: 268–77.
40 Kawada N, Kristensen DB, Asahina K, et al. Characterization of a stellate cell activation-associated protein (STAP) with peroxidase activity found in rat hepatic stellate cells. J Biol Chem 2001;276:25318–23.
41 Seki E, De Minicis S, Osterreicher CH, et al. TLR4 enhances TGF-beta signaling and hepatic fibrosis. Nat Med 2007; 13:1324–32.
42 Fischer R, Cariers A, Reinehr R, Häussinger D. Caspase 9-dependent killing of hepatic stellate cells by activated Kupffer cells. Gastroenterology 2002;123:845–61.
43 Yokohama S, Yoneda M, Haneda M, et al. Therapeutic efficacy of an angiotensin II receptor antagonist in patients with nonalcoholic steatohepatitis. Hepatology 2004;40:1222–5.
44 Hirose Am Ono M, Saibara T, Nozaki Y, et al. Angiotensin II type 1 receptor blocker inhibits fibrosis in rat nonalcoholic steatohepatitis. Hepatology 2007;45:1375–81.
45 Oakley F, Teoh V, Ching-A-Sue G, et al. Angiotensin II activates I kappa B kinase phosphorylation of RelA at Ser 536 to promote myofibroblast survival and liver fibrosis. Gastroenterology 2009;136:2334–44.
46 Llovet M, Bruix J. Molecular targeted therapies in hepatocellular carcinoma. Hepatology 2008;48:1312–27.

CHAPTER 6

Non-invasive diagnosis tests

Laurent Castera

Department of Hepatology, Hopital Beaujon, Assistance Publique-Hôpitaux de Paris, INSERM U773, Clichy, France

Introduction

Prognosis and management of chronic liver diseases greatly depend on the amount and progression of liver fibrosis. For many years, liver biopsy has been considered the "gold standard" for evaluation of hepatic fibrosis [1]. However, liver biopsy is an invasive procedure with rare but potentially life-threatening complications and prone to sampling errors. These limitations as well as the availability of powerful viral tools and new antiviral drugs have rapidly decreased the use of liver biopsy in viral hepatitis and led to the development of noninvasive methodologies for the assessment of fibrosis. Among the currently available noninvasive methods, there are two distinct approaches: (i) a "biologic" approach based on the dosage of serum biomarkers of fibrosis; (ii) a "physical" approach based on the measurement of liver stiffness using transient elastography (TE) [2]. Although complementary, these two approaches are based on differing rationale and conception: TE measures liver stiffness related to elasticity, which corresponds to a genuine and intrinsic physical property of liver parenchyma, whereas serum biomarkers are combinations of several not strictly liver-specific blood parameters optimized to mimic fibrosis stages as assessed by liver biopsy [3].

This chapter reviews the different methods that are currently available for the noninvasive evaluation of cirrhosis and also discusses their advantages and inconveniences for the management of patients with chronic liver disease.

Biologic approach: serum biomarkers of liver fibrosis

Currently available serum biomarkers

Many serum biomarkers have been evaluated for their ability to determine stage of liver fibrosis, mainly in patients with chronic hepatitis C virus infection (for review see [4,5]). Among the proposed markers, the so-called direct markers reflect the deposition or removal of extracellular matrix in the liver. These include glycoproteins such as serum hyaluronate, laminin, and YKL-40, collagens such as procollagen III N-peptide and type IV collagen, collagenases, and their inhibitors such as matrix metalloproteases and tissue inhibitory metalloprotease-1. So-called indirect markers include factors that can be measured in routine blood tests, such as the prothrombin index, platelet count, and ratio of aspartate aminotransferase to alanine aminotransferase (AST : ALT), which indicate alterations in hepatic function. Results from measurements of direct and indirect markers can be combined and used in diagnosis; the FibroTest® (BioPredictive, Paris, France) was the first algorithm that combined these data [6]. Several other scores [7–16] have been proposed – four are protected by patents and commercially available

Cirrhosis: A practical guide to management, First Edition. Edited by Samuel S. Lee and Richard Moreau.

Table 6.1 Proposed serum biomarkers for noninvasive evaluation of cirrhosis in chronic liver disease.

- FibroTest® (α2-macroglobulin, GGT, apolipoprotein A1, haptoglobin, total bilirubin, age, and gender)
- AST : platelet ratio (APRI) (AST and platelet count)
- Enhanced Liver Fibrosis score® (ELF) (age, hyaluronate, MMP-3, and TIMP-1)
- Lok index (platelet count, AST : ALT ratio, and INR)
- Goteborg University Cirrhosis Index (GUCI) (AST, INR, and platelet count)
- Hepascore® (bilirubin, γGT, hyaluronate, α2-macroglobulin, age, and gender)
- Fibrometers® (platelet count, prothrombin index, AST, α2-macroglobulin, hyaluronate, urea, and age)
- Virahep-C model (AST, platelet count, alkaline phosphatase, and age)
- FIB-4 (platelet count, ALT, and AST)
- HALT-C model (hyaluronic acid, TIMP-1, and platelet count)
- NAFLD Fibrosis Score (NFS) (age, BMI, hyperglycemia/diabetes, AST : ALT ratio, platelet count, and albumin)
- BARD score (BMI, AST : ALT ratio, and diabetes)

ALT, alanine aminotransferase; AST, aspartate aminotransferase; BMI, body mass index; GGT, gamma-glutamyl transpepsidase; INR, international normaized ratio; MMP, matrix metalloproteinase; TIMP, tissue inhibitor of metalloproteinase.

(Table 6.1). Nonproprietary methods use published models, based on routinely available laboratory tests.

Diagnostic performances of serum biomarkers

Diagnostic performances for cirrhosis of these different scores are summarized in Table 6.2. The most widely used and validated are the aspartate aminotransferase: platelet ratio index (APRI; a free nonpatented index) and the FibroTest® (a patented test that is not widely available). In a meta-analysis [17], which analyzed results from 6259 HCV patients from 33 studies, the mean area under the receiver operating characteristic curve (AUROC) values from the APRI in diagnosis of cirrhosis were 0.83.

When compared and validated externally in patients with hepatitis C virus infection [18–22], the different patented scores have similar performances for the diagnosis of cirrhosis. In the largest study to date (n = 1307 patients with viral hepatitis) comparing prospectively the most popular patented scores (FibroTest®, FibroMeter®, HepaScore®) with the nonpatented score (APRI), the AUROCs ranged from from 0.77 to 0.86 with no significant difference between the scores [22]. Although nonpatented scores such as FIB-4 and APRI may have slightly lower performance, they are cost-free, easy to calculate, and available almost everywhere. Regarding nonalcoholic fatty liver disease (NAFLD), among the limited number of serum biomarkers available, the NAFLD fibrosis score has been the most studied thus far [14,23–26].

Advantages and limitations of serum biomarkers

The practical advantages of analyzing serum biomarkers to measure fibrosis include their high applicability (>95%) and inter-laboratory reproducibility [27,28], and their potential widespread availability. However, none are liver specific – their results can be influenced by comorbid conditions and they require critical interpretation of results. For instance, FibroTest® and HepaScore® produce false positive results in patients with Gilbert's syndrome or hemolysis, because these patients have hyperbilirubinemia [29]. Similarly, acute hepatitis can produce false positive results in the APRI, Forns index, FIB-4, or FibroMeter® tests, which all measure levels of aminotransferases.

Physical approach: measurement of liver stiffness

Transient elastography

Principles and reproducibility

Liver fibrosis can be staged using TE (FibroScan®, Echosens, Paris, France) [30], which measures the velocity of a low-frequency (50 Hz) elastic shear wave propagating through the liver. This velocity is directly related to tissue stiffness, the elastic modulus (expressed as $E = 3\rho v^2$, where v is the shear velocity and ρ is the density of tissue, assumed to be constant). The stiffer the tissue, the faster the shear wave propagates. TE measures liver stiffness in a volume that approximates a cylinder that is 1 cm wide and 4 cm long, 25–65 mm below skin surface. The results are expressed in kilopascals (kPa), and range from 2.5 to 75 kPa; a normal value is around 5 kPa [31–33].

Diagnostic performances of transient elastography

The two index studies suggesting the interest of TE in the assessment of liver fibrosis have been conducted in

Table 6.2 Diagnostic performance of currently available serum biomarkers of fibrosis for cirrhosis (F4) in chronic liver disease.

Scores	Year	Etiologies	Patients (n)	F4 (%)	Cutoffs	AUROC	Sensitivity (%)	Specificity (%)	+LR	– LR
FibroTest® [6]	2001	HCV	1197	14	>0.74	0.82	63	84	4.0	0.4
APRI [7]	2003	HCV	476	17	<1.0 ≥2.0	0.89	57–89	75–93	3.6–8.1	0.1–0.5
ELF® [8]	2004	HCV	1021	NA	NA	0.89	91	69	2.9	0.4
Lok Index [9]	2005	HCV	1141	38	<0.2 ≥0.5	0.81	40–98	53–99	2.1–40.0	0.04–0.6
Hepascore® [10]	2005	HCV	211	16	>0.84	0.89	71	89	6.5	0.3
GUCI [11]	2005	HCV	179	12	>1.0	0.85	80	78	3.6	0.3
FIB-4 [13]	2007	HCV	847	17*	<1.45 >3.25	0.85	38–74	81–98	3.9–19.0	0.3–0.6
NFS [14]	2007	NAFLD	733	27*	<–1.455 >0.676	0.82	43–77	97–97	10.0–13.3	0.6–0.7
BARD score [15]	2008	NAFLD	669	30*	≥2	0.81	—	—	—	—
HALT-C model [16]	2008	HCV	512	38	<0.2 >0.5	0.81	47–88	45–92	1.6–5.9	0.3–0.6
Fibrometers® [22]	2010	HCV HBV	1204	13.6	NA	0.86	44	95	8.8	0.6

*F3–F4 patients.

AUROC, area under ROC curve; HBV, chronic hepatitis B; HCV, chronic hepatitis C; +LR, positive likelihood ratio; –LR, negative likelihood ratio; NA not availableNAFLD, non fatty alcoholic liver disease.

patients with chronic hepatitis C virus infection [34,35]. Many other groups have confirmed these results since [22,36–38], also in chronic liver diseases other than hepatitis C [39–42], including chronic hepatitis B [43–45], cholestatic liver diseases (primary biliary cirrhosis and primary sclerosing cholangitis) [46], alcoholic liver disease [47,48], and NAFLD [49–51]. As shown in Table 6.3, AUROCs range from 0.90 to 0.99 for the diagnosis of cirrhosis.

Several meta-analyses [52–55] have confirmed the high diagnostic performance of TE for cirrhosis, with mean AUROC values of 0.94 [54]. In a meta-analysis of 40 studies (32 papers and 8 abstracts), sensitivity and specificity values were 0.83 and 0.89 for patients with cirrhosis, respecively. However, only 9 studies (comprising 1364 patients) had acceptable standards for liver biopsy and TE, which limit the conclusions. It will therefore be important to perform meta-analyses of data from individual patients.

TE thus appears to be a reliable method for the diagnosis of cirrhosis, better at excluding than at predicting cirrhosis. For instance, in a population of 1007 patients with different chronic liver diseases, a cutoff value of 14.6 kPa yielded positive and negative predictive values of 74% and 96%, respectively [41]. Interestingly, proposed cutoff values for cirrhosis ranged from 11 kPa in patients with hepatitis B virus infection to 22.7 kPa in patients with alcoholic liver disease. Some researchers have proposed that cutoff values be adapted based on causes of liver disease [41]. However, differences among cutoff values could result from differences in prevalence of cirrhosis among study populations (ranging from 8% to 25%). A cutoff value for one population might not be applicable to another, which has a different prevalence of disease. Most studies used single cutoff values for patients with cirrhosis or advanced fibrosis, but more information can be obtained when values are interpreted as a continuum. For example, when liver stiffness values range from 2.5 to 7 kPa, fibrosis is likely mild or absent, whereas when values are above 13 kPa, cirrhosis is likely [56].

Table 6.3 Diagnostic performance of transient elastography for cirrhosis (F4) in chronic liver disease.

Authors	Year	Etiologies	Patients (n)	F4 (%)	Cutoffs (kPa)	AUROC	Sensitivity (%)	Specificity (%)	+LR	– LR
Castera et al. [35]	2005	HCV	183	25	12.5	0.95	87	91	9.7	0.1
Ziol et al. [34]	2005	HCV	251	19	14.6	0.87	86	96	23.1	0.1
Corpechot et al. [46]	2006	PBC-PSC	95	16	17.3	0.96	93	95	18.6	0.07
Gomez-Dominguez et al. [40]	2006	Mixed	94	17	16.0	0.94	89	96	22.25	0.11
Ganne-Carrie et al. [41]	2006	Mixed	775	15	14.6	0.95	79	95	15.8	0.11
Foucher et al. [42]	2006	Mixed	354	13	17.6	0.96	77	97	25.66	0.23
Fraquelli et al. [39]	2007	Mixed	200	12	11.9	0.90	91	89	8.27	0.1
Coco et al. [43]	2007	HCV HBV	228	20	14.0	0.96	78	98	39.0	0.22
Lupsor et al. [37]	2008	HCV	324	21	11.9	0.94	87	91	9.7	0.1
Arena et al. [36]	2008	HCV	150	19	14.8	0.98	94	92	11.3	0.1
Yoneda et al. [49]	2008	NAFLD	97	9	17.0	0.99	100	97	33.33	0
Nguyen-Khac et al. [48]	2008	ALD	103	32	19.5	0.92	86	84	5.37	0.16
Nahon et al. [47]	2008	ALD	147	54	22.7	0.87	84	83	5.24	0.19
Marcellin et al. [45]	2009	HBV	173	8	11.0	0.93	93	87	7.0	0.08
Chan et al. [44]	2009	HBV	161	25	9.0	0.93	98	75	3.92	0.02
Wong et al. [51]	2010	NAFLD	246	10	10.3	0.95	92	88	7.5	0.1
Degos et al. [22]	2010	HCV, HBV, HCV-HIV	1307	14	12.9	0.90	72	89	6.8	0.3
Zarski et al. [71]	2012	HCV	382	14	12.9	0.93	77	90	7.7	0.25

ALD, alcoholic liver disease; AUROC, area under ROC curve; HBV, chronic hepatitis B; HCV, chronic hepatitis C; +LR positive likelihood ratio; –LR negative likelihood ratio; NAFLD, non-fatty alcoholic liver disease; PBC-PSC, primary biliary cirrhosis primary sclerosing cholangitis.

Advantages and limitations of transient elastography

Advantages to TE include a short procedure time (<5 minutes), immediate results, and the ability to perform the test at the bedside or in an outpatient clinic – it is not a difficult procedure to learn. However, the interpretation of TE results should be always in the hands of an expert clinician and should be made with information regarding patient demographics, disease etiology, and essential laboratory parameters as well as manufacturer's recommendations (number of valid shots ≥10; success rate (the ratio of valid shots to the total number of shots) ≥60%; and interquartile range (IQR, reflecting the variability of measurements) less than 30% of the median liver stiffness measure (LSM) value (IQR/LSM ≤30%) [56].

Although TE analysis has excellent inter- and intraobserver agreement [39,57], its applicability (80%) is not as good as that of serum biomarkers. Failure to obtain any measurement has been reported in 3% of cases and unreliable results (not meeting manufacturer's recommendations) have been reported for 16% [58], mostly resulting from patient obesity or limited operator experience. A new probe (XL) has been proposed to overcome these limitations for overweight and obese patients [59]. Apart from obese patients, TE results can also be difficult to obtain from patients with narrow intercostal space and are impossible to obtain from patients with ascites [30]. The liver is an organ wrapped in a distensible but nonelastic envelope (Glisson's capsule), so additional space-occupying tissue abnormalities, such as edema, inflammation, extrahepatic cholestasis, or congestion, can interfere with measurements of liver stiffness, independently of fibrosis. Indeed, the extent of necroinflammatory activity has been shown to influence TE measurements in patients with viral hepatitis with a steady increase of liver stiffness values in parallel with the degree of histologic activity [36,39,44]. Consistent with these results, the risk of overestimating liver stiffness values has been reported in case of ALT flares in patients with acute viral hepatitis or chronic hepatitis B virus infection [43,60,61] as well as in cases of extra-hepatic cholestasis [62] or congestive heart failure [63]. The influence of steatosis is still a matter of debate [36,64].

Alternatives to transient elastography

Several other liver elasticity-based imaging techniques are being developed, including acoustic radiation force impulse imaging (ARFI) and magnetic resonance (MR) elastography and lately ShearWave elastography (SWE; Aixplorer®, Supersonic Imagine, Aix en Provence, France) [65].

ARFI involves mechanical excitation of tissue using short-duration (~262 μsec) acoustic pulses that propagate shear waves and generate localized, μ-scale displacements in tissue [66]. The shear-wave velocity (expressed in m/s) is measured in a smaller region than in TE (10 mm long and 6 mm wide), but can be chosen by the operator. The major advantage of ARFI is that it can be easily implemented on a modified commercial ultrasound machine (Acuson 2000 Virtual Touch™ Tissue Quantification, Siemens Healthcare, Erlangen, Germany). However, ARFI values, in contrast to TE values, have a narrow range (0.5–4.4 m/sec) limits definitions of cutoff values for patient management decisions.

MR elastography uses a modified phase-contrast method to image the propagation characteristics of the shear wave in the liver [67]. Elasticity is quantified by MR elastography (expressed in kPa) using a formula that determines the shear modulus, which is equivalent to one-third the Young's modulus used with TE [68]. The theoretical advantages of MR elastography include its ability to analyze almost the entire liver and its applicability to patients with obesity or ascites. However, MR elastography cannot be performed in livers of patients with iron overload, because of signal-to-noise limitations, and it is too costly and time-consuming to use in routine practice.

ARFI has been the most studied thus far but there are only limited data on the accuracy of MR elastography and SWE. Preliminary results indicate that the accuracy of ARFI, MR elastography, and SWE is similar to that of TE for cirrhosis. However, most studies are based on small samples of heterogeneous populations and did not always use liver biopsy as reference. Further validation is warranted.

Comparison and combination of approaches

TE appears to be best suited for cirrhosis screening, because it has a higher level of performance than biomarker assays at least in the context of viral hepatitis. In contrast to what has been shown for significant fibrosis [35], combining TE with biomarkers does not increase diagnostic accuracy for cirrhosis in patients with chronic hepatitis C virus infection [69–71]. However, the applicability of TE is lower (80% vs 95% for biomarker assays), and the performance levels of these diagnostics might not differ for intention-to-diagnose analysis [71]. Data regarding combination of TE and biomarkers in other liver diseases such as hepatitis B or NAFLD are awaited.

Monitoring of disease progression and prognosis

Noninvasive methods can be used to identify patients with cirrhosis who are at risk of disease progression. Compensated cirrhosis is classified as that without varices (stage 1) or with varices (stage 2). Compensated cirrhosis could be further subdivided, as that with no portal hypertension, portal hypertension that is not clinically-significant (hepatic venous pressure gradient, HVPG, <10 mmHg), or clinically significant portal hypertension (HVPG ≥10 mmHg) [72].

Measurements of liver stiffness might be used to assess clinical outcomes because they correlate with the severity of liver disease [42], according to a retrospective study conducted in a single center. This study provided the first "proof of concept" that liver stiffness is a prognostic factor for patients with cirrhosis. Furthermore, liver stiffness correlates with portal pressure (based on the HVPG) [73–76], which accurately predicts clinical events [77]. Interestingly, there was a high degree of correlation between liver stiffness and only HVPG values below 10–12 mmHg [74]. This indicates that beyond a certain degree of portal pressure (above 10–12 mmHg), development of portal hypertension is at least partially independent from the simple accumulation of fibrillar extracellular matrix, which is responsible for the increase in liver stiffness. Conversely, repeated measurements of liver stiffness, over time, might be made during the first year after liver transplantation, to identify patients with early stage recurrence of severe hepatitis C recurrence, and reduce the need for follow-up liver biopsies [73,78,79].

Liver stiffness values have also been correlated with the presence of esophageal varices. However, the diagnostic accuracy of TE (specificity below 60%) is too low for identification of patients with esophageal varices in clinical practice [80]. When biomarkers were compared, in a large-scale multicentre study of factors to predict which patients would develop high risk esophageal varices (large esophageal varices, those with red signs, or decompensated cirrhosis), the combination of Lok index and Forns index had the best diagnostic performance, avoiding endoscopy in around one-third of patients [81]. When compared with serum biomarkers, TE did not perform better for the detection of esophageal varices and large esophageal varices [69]. However, a strategy combining TE with spleen diameter and platelet count (referred as LSPS for LSM-Spleen diameter to Platelet ratio Score) has been shown to increase diagnostic accuracy for detecting high risk esophageal varices in patients with hepatitis B virus-related cirrhosis [82] and has been recently confirmed in patients with cirrhosis from various etiologies [83]. Interestingly, LSPS appeared as a reliable predictor of esophageal varices bleeding risk in these patients [84]. These findings are consistent with those of a study that reported that liver stiffness values can be as effective as HVPG measurements in predicting which patients with develop clinical decompensation and portal hypertension-related complications [85]. For instance, at a cutoff of 21.1 kPa, TE had a 100% negative predictive value for the occurrence of portal hypertension-related complications; if these results are confirmed, TE could be used as a prognostic tool [86]. Very recently, the measurement of spleen stiffness using either TE or ARFI has been proposed with promising results that require further validation [87–89].

In summary, TE results can identify patients most likely to develop clinically significant portal hypertension, but are not sufficient to identify patients with esophageal varices, in clinical practice, or replace endoscopy analysis of cirrhotic patients [80]. Given its likely prognostic value for patients with cirrhosis, TE could be used to discriminate rapidly among patients at different stages of progression of compensated cirrhosis, and place them in different risk categories [90].

Non-invasive methods can also be used in determining prognosis. Large, prospective cohort studies in Asia of patients with hepatitis B or C correlated liver stiffness values with hepatocellular carcinoma (HCC) occurrence [91–93]. Among 866 Japanese patients with hepatitis C virus infection, the cumulative incidence of HCC within 3 years was as high as 38.5%, among subjects with baseline liver stiffness values >25 kPa, compared with 0.4% among subjects with values ≤10 kPa [91]. Although measurements of liver stiffness could be used to identify patients at risk of developing HCC, more data are needed before they could be integrated into an HCC surveillance program.

Prognosis of patients with chronic liver disease related to viral hepatitis or other causes can be determined using TE [85,94] and assays for serum biomarkers such as FibroTest® [95–97], ELF® [98,99], APRI and FIB-4 [100], as well as for models based on standard laboratory tests [101,102]. The potential of noninvasive methods for predicting clinical outcomes seems to be greater than that of liver biopsy, probably because the non-invasive tests measure ongoing pathophysiologic processes and functions that a biopsy cannot. Additional advantages of assays for serum biomarkers and TE over histologic scoring systems are that they provide a range of continuous values, instead of a limited number of categories [103].

Conclusions

Significant progress has been made over the past decade regarding assessment of hepatic fibrosis in patients with chronic liver disease, highlighting the fact that there is no perfect method. On the one hand, there is increasing awareness that liver biopsy is an imperfect gold standard. On the other hand, an increasing number of noninvasive tests are now available for which TE, Fibrotest®, and APRI are the most extensively validated. These tests are already widely used in routine clinical practice in France, resulting in a significant decrease in the need for liver biopsy [104]. However, it is likely that noninvasive methods will reduce but not completely abolish the need for liver biopsy [105]. We believe that liver biopsy and noninvasive methods, particularly TE, should be employed as an integrated system to allow a more efficient and convenient management of patients with chronic liver disease [106].

It is important to investigate the prognostic value of noninvasive methods of fibrosis detection, particularly TE, for patients with cirrhosis; these tests could be used to classify patients with cirrhosis and assign them to different categories of risk for clinical outcomes. TE has limitations and is challenged by other technologies to measure liver stiffness, such as ARFI, MR elastography, and SWE, whose place in clinical practice remains to be defined.

References

1 Bravo AA, Sheth SG, Chopra S. Liver biopsy. N Engl J Med 2001;344:495–500.
2 Castera L, Pinzani M. Non-invasive assessment of liver fibrosis: are we ready? Lancet 2010;375:1419–20.
3 Bedossa P, Carrat F. Liver biopsy: the best, not the gold standard. J Hepatol 2009;50:1–3.
4 Pinzani M, Vizzutti F, Arena U, Marra F. Technology Insight: noninvasive assessment of liver fibrosis by biochemical scores and elastography. Nat Clin Pract Gastroenterol Hepatol 2008;5:95–106.
5 Castera L. Noninvasive methods to assess liver disease in patients with hepatitis B or C. Gastroenterology 2012;142: 1293–302, e4.
6 Imbert-Bismut F, Ratziu V, Pieroni L, Charlotte F, Benhamou Y, Poynard T. Biochemical markers of liver fibrosis in patients with hepatitis C virus infection: a prospective study. Lancet 2001;357:1069–75.
7 Wai CT, Greenson JK, Fontana RJ, et al. A simple noninvasive index can predict both significant fibrosis and cirrhosis in patients with chronic hepatitis C. Hepatology 2003;38:518–26.
8 Rosenberg WM, Voelker M, Thiel R, et al. Serum markers detect the presence of liver fibrosis: A cohort study. Gastroenterology 2004;127:1704–13.
9 Lok AS, Ghany MG, Goodman ZD, et al. Predicting cirrhosis in patients with hepatitis C based on standard laboratory tests: results of the HALT-C cohort. Hepatology 2005;42:282–92.
10 Adams LA, Bulsara M, Rossi E, et al. Hepascore: an accurate validated predictor of liver fibrosis in chronic hepatitis C infection. Clin Chem 2005;51:1867–73.
11 Islam S, Antonsson L, Westin J, Lagging M. Cirrhosis in hepatitis C virus-infected patients can be excluded using an index of standard biochemical serum markers. Scand J Gastroenterol 2005;40:867–72.
12 Cales P, Oberti F, Michalak S, et al. A novel panel of blood markers to assess the degree of liver fibrosis. Hepatology 2005;42:1373–81.
13 Vallet-Pichard A, Mallet V, Nalpas B, et al. FIB-4: an inexpensive and accurate marker of fibrosis in HCV infection. comparison with liver biopsy and fibrotest. Hepatology 2007;46:32–6.
14 Angulo P, Hui JM, Marchesini G, et al. The NAFLD fibrosis score: a noninvasive system that identifies liver fibrosis in patients with NAFLD. Hepatology 2007;45:846–54.
15 Harrison SA, Oliver D, Arnold HL, Gogia S, Neuschwander-Tetri BA. Development and validation of a simple NAFLD clinical scoring system for identifying patients without advanced disease. Gut 2008;57:1441–7.
16 Fontana RJ, Goodman ZD, Dienstag JL, et al. Relationship of serum fibrosis markers with liver fibrosis stage and collagen content in patients with advanced chronic hepatitis C. Hepatology 2008;47:789–98.
17 Lin ZH, Xin YN, Dong QJ, et al. Performance of the aspartate aminotransferase-to-platelet ratio index for the staging of hepatitis C-related fibrosis: an updated meta-analysis. Hepatology 2011;53:726–36.
18 Parkes J, Guha IN, Roderick P, Rosenberg W. Performance of serum marker panels for liver fibrosis in chronic hepatitis C. J Hepatol 2006;44:462–74.
19 Halfon P, Bacq Y, De Muret A, et al. Comparison of test performance profile for blood tests of liver fibrosis in chronic hepatitis C. J Hepatol 2007;46:395–402.
20 Leroy V, Hilleret MN, Sturm N, et al. Prospective comparison of six non-invasive scores for the diagnosis of liver fibrosis in chronic hepatitis C. J Hepatol 2007;46:775–82.
21 Cales P, de Ledinghen V, Halfon P, et al. Evaluating the accuracy and increasing the reliable diagnosis rate of blood tests for liver fibrosis in chronic hepatitis C. Liver Int 2008;28:1352–62.
22 Degos F, Perez P, Roche B, et al. Diagnostic accuracy of FibroScan and comparison to liver fibrosis biomarkers in chronic viral hepatitis: a multicenter prospective study (the FIBROSTIC study). J Hepatol 2010;53:1013–21.
23 Guha IN, Parkes J, Roderick P, et al. Noninvasive markers of fibrosis in nonalcoholic fatty liver disease: validating the European Liver Fibrosis Panel and exploring simple markers. Hepatology 2008;47:455–60.
24 Cales P, Laine F, Boursier J, et al. Comparison of blood tests for liver fibrosis specific or not to NAFLD. J Hepatol 2009;50:165–73.
25 Shah AG, Lydecker A, Murray K, Tetri BN, Contos MJ, Sanyal AJ. Comparison of noninvasive markers of fibrosis in patients with nonalcoholic fatty liver disease. Clin Gastroenterol Hepatol 2009;7:1104–12.
26 McPherson S, Stewart SF, Henderson E, Burt AD, Day CP. Simple non-invasive fibrosis scoring systems can reliably exclude advanced fibrosis in patients with non-alcoholic fatty liver disease. Gut 2010;59:1265–9.
27 Cales P, Veillon P, Konate A, et al. Reproducibility of blood tests of liver fibrosis in clinical practice. Clin Biochem 2008;41:10–8.

28 Imbert-Bismut F, Messous D, Thibaut V, et al. Intra-laboratory analytical variability of biochemical markers of fibrosis (Fibrotest) and activity (Actitest) and reference ranges in healthy blood donors. Clin Chem Lab Med 2004;42: 323–33.

29 Poynard T, Munteanu M, Imbert-Bismut F, et al. Prospective analysis of discordant results between biochemical markers and biopsy in patients with chronic hepatitis C. Clin Chem 2004;50:1344–55.

30 Sandrin L, Fourquet B, Hasquenoph JM, et al. Transient elastography: a new noninvasive method for assessment of hepatic fibrosis. Ultrasound Med Biol 2003;29:1705–13.

31 Roulot D, Czernichow S, Le Clesiau H, Costes JL, Vergnaud AC, Beaugrand M. Liver stiffness values in apparently healthy subjects: influence of gender and metabolic syndrome. J Hepatol 2008;48:606–13.

32 Kim SU, Choi GH, Han WK, et al. What are "true normal" liver stiffness values using FibroScan?: a prospective study in healthy living liver and kidney donors in South Korea. Liver Int 2010;30:268–74.

33 Colombo S, Belloli L, Zaccanelli M, et al. Normal liver stiffness and its determinants in healthy blood donors. Dig Liver Dis 2011;43:231–6.

34 Ziol M, Handra-Luca A, Kettaneh A, et al. Noninvasive assessment of liver fibrosis by measurement of stiffness in patients with chronic hepatitis C. Hepatology 2005;41: 48–54.

35 Castera L, Vergniol J, Foucher J, et al. Prospective comparison of transient elastography, Fibrotest, APRI, and liver biopsy for the assessment of fibrosis in chronic hepatitis C. Gastroenterology 2005;128:343–50.

36 Arena U, Vizzutti F, Abraldes JG, et al. Reliability of transient elastography for the diagnosis of advanced fibrosis in chronic hepatitis C. Gut 2008;57:1288–93.

37 Lupsor M, Badea R, Stefanescu H, et al. Analysis of histopathological changes that influence liver stiffness in chronic hepatitis C: results from a cohort of 324 patients. J Gastrointestin Liver Dis 2008;17:155–63.

38 Zarski JP, Sturm N, Guechot J, et al. Comparison of nine blood tests and transient elastography for liver fibrosis in chronic hepatitis C: the ANRS HCEP-23 study. J Hepatol 2012;56:55–62.

39 Fraquelli M, Rigamonti C, Casazza G, et al. Reproducibility of transient elastography in the evaluation of liver fibrosis in patients with chronic liver disease. Gut 2007;56:968–73.

40 Gomez-Dominguez E, Mendoza J, Rubio S, Moreno-Monteagudo JA, Garcia-Buey L, Moreno-Otero R. Transient elastography: a valid alternative to biopsy in patients with chronic liver disease. Aliment Pharmacol Ther 2006;24:513–8.

41 Ganne-Carrie N, Ziol M, de Ledinghen V, et al. Accuracy of liver stiffness measurement for the diagnosis of cirrhosis in patients with chronic liver diseases. Hepatology 2006;44: 1511–7.

42 Foucher J, Chanteloup E, Vergniol J, et al. Diagnosis of cirrhosis by transient elastography (FibroScan): a prospective study. Gut 2006;55:403–8.

43 Coco B, Oliveri F, Maina AM, et al. Transient elastography: a new surrogate marker of liver fibrosis influenced by major changes of transaminases. J Viral Hepat 2007;14: 360–9.

44 Chan HL, Wong GL, Choi PC, et al. Alanine aminotransferase-based algorithms of liver stiffness measurement by transient elastography (Fibroscan) for liver fibrosis in chronic hepatitis B. J Viral Hepat 2009;16:36–44.

45 Marcellin P, Ziol M, Bedossa P, et al. Non-invasive assessment of liver fibrosis by stiffness measurement in patients with chronic hepatitis B. Liver Int 2009;29:242–7.

46 Corpechot C, El Naggar A, Poujol-Robert A, et al. Assessment of biliary fibrosis by transient elastography in patients with PBC and PSC. Hepatology 2006;43:1118–24.

47 Nahon P, Kettaneh A, Tengher-Barna I, et al. Assessment of liver fibrosis using transient elastography in patients with alcoholic liver disease. J Hepatol 2008;49:1062–8.

48 Nguyen-Khac E, Chatelain D, Tramier B, et al. Assessment of asymptomatic liver fibrosis in alcoholic patients using fibroscan: prospective comparison with 7 non-invasive laboratory tests. Aliment Pharmacol Ther 2008:1188–98.

49 Yoneda M, Yoneda M, Mawatari H, et al. Noninvasive assessment of liver fibrosis by measurement of stiffness in patients with nonalcoholic fatty liver disease (NAFLD). Dig Liver Dis 2008;40:371–8.

50 Nobili V, Vizzutti F, Arena U, et al. Accuracy and reproducibility of transient elastography for the diagnosis of fibrosis in pediatric nonalcoholic steatohepatitis. Hepatology 2008;48:442–8.

51 Wong VW, Vergniol J, Wong GL, et al. Diagnosis of fibrosis and cirrhosis using liver stiffness measurement in nonalcoholic fatty liver disease. Hepatology 2010;51: 454–62.

52 Shaheen AA, Wan AF, Myers RP. FibroTest and FibroScan for the prediction of hepatitis C-related fibrosis: a systematic review of diagnostic test accuracy. Am J Gastroenterol 2007;102:2589–600.

53 Talwalkar JA, Kurtz DM, Schoenleber SJ, West CP, Montori VM. Ultrasound-based transient elastography for the detection of hepatic fibrosis: systematic review and meta-analysis. Clin Gastroenterol Hepatol 2007;5:1214–20.

54 Friedrich-Rust M, Ong MF, Martens S, et al. Performance of transient elastography for the staging of liver fibrosis: a meta-analysis. Gastroenterology 2008;134:960–74.

55 Tsochatzis EA, Gurusamy KS, Ntaoula S, Cholongitas E, Davidson BR, Burroughs AK. Elastography for the diagnosis of severity of fibrosis in chronic liver disease: a meta-analysis of diagnostic accuracy. J Hepatol 2011;54:650–9.

56 Castera L, Forns X, Alberti A. Non-invasive evaluation of liver fibrosis using transient elastography. J Hepatol 2008;48:835–47.

57 Boursier J, Konate A, Gorea G, et al. Reproducibility of liver stiffness measurement by ultrasonographic elastometry. Clin Gastroenterol Hepatol 2008;6:1263–9.
58 Castera L, Foucher J, Bernard PH, et al. Pitfalls of liver stiffness measurement: A 5-year prospective study of 13, 369 examinations. Hepatology 2010;51:828–35.
59 Myers RP, Pomier-Layrargues G, Kirsch R, et al. Feasibility and diagnostic performance of the FibroScan XL probe for liver stiffness measurement in overweight and obese patients. Hepatology 2012;55:199–208.
60 Sagir A, Erhardt A, Schmitt M, Haussinger D. Transient elastography is unreliable for detection of cirrhosis in patients with acute liver damage. Hepatology 2007;47:592–5.
61 Arena U, Vizzutti F, Corti G, et al. Acute viral hepatitis increases liver stiffness values measured by transient elastography. Hepatology 2008;47:380–4.
62 Millonig G, Reimann FM, Friedrich S, et al. Extrahepatic cholestasis increases liver stiffness (FibroScan) irrespective of fibrosis. Hepatology 2008;48:1718–23.
63 Millonig G, Friedrich S, Adolf S, et al. Liver stiffness is directly influenced by central venous pressure. J Hepatol 2010;52:206–10.
64 Fraquelli M, Rigamonti C, Casazza G, et al. Etiology-related determinants of liver stiffness values in chronic viral hepatitis B or C. J Hepatol 2011;54:621–8.
65 Berzigotti A, Castera L. Update on ultrasound imaging of liver fibrosis. J Hepatol 2013;59:180–2.
66 Nightingale K, Soo MS, Nightingale R, Trahey G. Acoustic radiation force impulse imaging: in vivo demonstration of clinical feasibility. Ultrasound Med Biol 2002;28:227–35.
67 Muthupillai R, Lomas DJ, Rossman PJ, Greenleaf JF, Manduca A, Ehman RL. Magnetic resonance elastography by direct visualization of propagating acoustic strain waves. Science 1995;269:1854–7.
68 Talwalkar JA, Yin M, Fidler JL, Sanderson SO, Kamath PS, Ehman RL. Magnetic resonance imaging of hepatic fibrosis: emerging clinical applications. Hepatology 2008;47:332–42.
69 Castera L, Le Bail B, Roudot-Thoraval F, et al. Early detection in routine clinical practice of cirrhosis and oesophageal varices in chronic hepatitis C: comparison of transient elastography (FibroScan) with standard laboratory tests and non-invasive scores. J Hepatol 2009;50:59–68.
70 Boursier J, de Ledinghen V, Zarski JP, et al. A new combination of blood test and fibroscan for accurate non-invasive diagnosis of liver fibrosis stages in chronic hepatitis C. Am J Gastroenterol 2011;106:1255–63.
71 Zarski JP, Sturm N, Guechot J, et al. Comparison of nine blood tests and transient elastography for liver fibrosis in chronic hepatitis C: the ANRS HCEP-23 study. J Hepatol 2012;56:55–62.
72 Garcia-Tsao G, Friedman S, Iredale J, Pinzani M. Now there are many (stages) where before there was one: in search of a pathophysiological classification of cirrhosis. Hepatology 2010;51:1445–9.
73 Carrion JA, Navasa M, Bosch J, Bruguera M, Gilabert R, Forns X. Transient elastography for diagnosis of advanced fibrosis and portal hypertension in patients with hepatitis C recurrence after liver transplantation. Liver Transpl 2006;12:1791–8.
74 Vizzutti F, Arena U, Romanelli RG, et al. Liver stiffness measurement predicts severe portal hypertension in patients with HCV-related cirrhosis. Hepatology 2007;45:1290–7.
75 Bureau C, Metivier S, Peron JM, et al. Transient elastography accurately predicts presence of significant portal hypertension in patients with chronic liver disease. Aliment Pharmacol Ther 2008;27:1261–8.
76 Lemoine M, Katsahian S, Ziol M, et al. Liver stiffness measurement as a predictive tool of clinically significant portal hypertension in patients with compensated hepatitis C virus or alcohol-related cirrhosis. Aliment Pharmacol Ther 2008;28:1102–10.
77 Ripoll C, Groszmann R, Garcia-Tsao G, et al. Hepatic venous pressure gradient predicts clinical decompensation in patients with compensated cirrhosis. Gastroenterology 2007;133:481–8.
78 Rigamonti C, Donato MF, Fraquelli M, et al. Transient elastography predicts fibrosis progression in patients with recurrent hepatitis c after liver transplantation. Gut 2008;57:821–7.
79 Carrion JA, Torres F, Crespo G, et al. Liver stiffness identifies two different patterns of fibrosis progression in patients with hepatitis C virus recurrence after liver transplantation. Hepatology 2010;51:23–34.
80 Castera L, Pinzani M, Bosch J. Noninvasive evaluation of portal hypertension using transient elastography. J Hepatol 2012;56:696–703.
81 Sebastiani G, Tempesta D, Fattovich G, et al. Prediction of oesophageal varices in hepatic cirrhosis by simple serum non-invasive markers: results of a multicenter, large-scale study. J Hepatol 2010;53:630–8.
82 Kim BK, Han KH, Park JY, et al. A liver stiffness measurement-based, noninvasive prediction model for high-risk esophageal varices in B-viral liver cirrhosis. Am J Gastroenterol 2010;105:1382–90.
83 Berzigotti A, Seijo S, Arena U, et al. Elastography, spleen size, and platelet count identify portal hypertension in patients with compensated cirrhosis. Gastroenterology 2013;144:102–11 e1.
84 Kim BK, Kim do Y, Han KH, et al. Risk assessment of esophageal variceal bleeding in B-viral liver cirrhosis by a liver stiffness measurement-based model. Am J Gastroenterol 2011;106: 1654-62, 730.
85 Robic MA, Procopet B, Metivier S, et al. Liver stiffness accurately predicts portal hypertension related complications in patients with chronic liver disease: a prospective study. J Hepatol 2011;55:1017–24.
86 Bosch J. Soft technique, hard end-points. J Hepatol 2011;55:955–6.

87 Castera L, Garcia-Tsao G. When the spleen gets tough, the varices get going. Gastroenterology 2013;144:19–22.
88 Colecchia A, Montrone L, Scaioli E, et al. Measurement of spleen stiffness to evaluate portal hypertension and the presence of esophageal varices in patients with HCV-related cirrhosis. Gastroenterology 2012;143:646–54.
89 Takuma Y, Nouso K, Morimoto Y, et al. Measurement of spleen stiffness by acoustic radiation force impulse imaging identifies cirrhotic patients with esophageal varices. Gastroenterology 2012;144: 92–101 e2.
90 Castera L. Liver stiffness and hepatocellular carcinoma: liaisons dangereuses? Hepatology 2009;49:1793–4.
91 Masuzaki R, Tateishi R, Yoshida H, et al. Prospective risk assessment for hepatocellular carcinoma development in patients with chronic hepatitis C by transient elastography. Hepatology 2009;49:1954–61.
92 Fung J, Lai CL, Seto WK, Wong DK, Yuen MF. Prognostic significance of liver stiffness for hepatocellular carcinoma and mortality in HBeAg-negative chronic hepatitis B. J Viral Hepat 2011;18:738–44.
93 Jung KS, Kim SU, Ahn SH, et al. Risk assessment of hepatitis B virus-related hepatocellular carcinoma development using liver stiffness measurement (FibroScan). Hepatology 2011;53:885–94.
94 Vergniol J, Foucher J, Terrebonne E, et al. Noninvasive tests for fibrosis and liver stiffness predict 5-year outcomes of patients with chronic hepatitis C. Gastroenterology 2011;140: 1970-9, 9 e1–3.
95 Ngo Y, Munteanu M, Messous D, et al. A prospective analysis of the prognostic value of biomarkers (FibroTest) in patients with chronic hepatitis C. Clin Chem 2006;52:1887–96.
96 Ngo Y, Benhamou Y, Thibault V, et al. An accurate definition of the status of inactive hepatitis B virus carrier by a combination of biomarkers (FibroTest-ActiTest) and viral load. PLoS One 2008;3:e2573.
97 Naveau S, Gaude G, Asnacios A, et al. Diagnostic and prognostic values of noninvasive biomarkers of fibrosis in patients with alcoholic liver disease. Hepatology 2009;49: 97–105.
98 Mayo MJ, Parkes J, Adams-Huet B, et al. Prediction of clinical outcomes in primary biliary cirrhosis by serum enhanced liver fibrosis assay. Hepatology 2008;48:1549–57.
99 Parkes J, Roderick P, Harris S, et al. Enhanced liver fibrosis test can predict clinical outcomes in patients with chronic liver disease. Gut 2010;59:1245–51.
100 Nunes D, Fleming C, Offner G, et al. Noninvasive markers of liver fibrosis are highly predictive of liver-related death in a cohort of HCV-infected individuals with and without HIV infection. Am J Gastroenterol 2010;105:1346–53.
101 Ghany MG, Lok AS, Everhart JE, et al. Predicting clinical and histologic outcomes based on standard laboratory tests in advanced chronic hepatitis C. Gastroenterology 2010; 138:136–46.
102 Fontana RJ, Dienstag JL, Bonkovsky HL, et al. Serum fibrosis markers are associated with liver disease progression in non-responder patients with chronic hepatitis C. Gut 2010;59:1401–9.
103 Pinzani M. Noninvasive methods for the assessment of liver fibrosis: a window open on the future? Hepatology 2011;54:1476–7.
104 Castera L, Denis J, Babany G, Roudot-Thoraval F. Evolving practices of non-invasive markers of liver fibrosis in patients with chronic hepatitis C in France: time for new guidelines? J Hepatol 2007;46:528–9.
105 Sebastiani G, Alberti A. Noninvasive fibrosis biomarkers reduce but not substitute the need for liver biopsy. World J Gastroenterol 2006;12:3682–94.
106 Castera L, Pinzani M. Biopsy and non-invasive methods for the diagnosis of liver fibrosis: does it take two to tango? Gut 2010;59:861–6.

CHAPTER 7

Evaluating prognosis[1]

Sumeet K. Asrani[1] and Patrick S. Kamath[2]

[1]*Baylor University Medical Center, Dallas, Texas, USA*

[2]*Division of Gastroenterology and Hepatology, Mayo Clinic College of Medicine, Rochester, MN, USA*

Introduction

Liver-related mortality is the eighth leading cause of death in the United States and is responsible for a significant proportion of premature mortality; among persons aged 45–64 years, it is the third leading cause of death [1]. Unfortunately, the overall prognosis of patients with cirrhosis remains poor in the recent era. Patients with cirrhosis can have compensated disease for several years or have evidence of decompensation, manifested by complications of portal hypertension. Compared to the general population, persons with compensated cirrhosis have a fivefold (hazard ratio, HR, 4.7; 95% confidence interval, CI, 4.4–5.0) and persons with decompensated cirrhosis have a 10-fold (HR 9.7; 95% CI 8.9–10.6) increased risk of death [2]. However, there is wide variability in rates of morbidity and mortality among patients with cirrhosis. Early identification of factors that portend poor outcomes is important to initiate relevant measures early on in the disease course. This chapter addresses the natural history of cirrhosis, discusses prognosis, and evaluates several models that identify cirrhotic patients at highest risk for poor outcomes.

Natural history

The natural history of cirrhosis has been well described. Mortality estimates vary based on the setting (inpatient, intensive care unit, community), stage (compensated or decompensated), and etiology of disease. A large systemic review of heterogeneous prognostic studies showed that the median survival for cirrhotic patients was 2.8 years. Median survival was approximately 12 years and 2 years for persons with compensated and decompensated cirrhosis, respectively [3]. The 1-year cumulative survival was 78% (95% for compensated cirrhosis and 61% for decompensated cirrhosis). As expected, lower survival was seen in hospital-based studies. Using data from a Danish nationwide population-based hospital registry, subjects diagnosed with cirrhosis (1995–2006) were identified. The overall 1-year survival probability was 66% after 1 year, 38% after 5 years, and 22% after 10 years [4]. The majority of the deaths were cirrhosis-related rather than due to the presence of medical comorbidities. In another population-based study, the overall survival for persons with compensated cirrhosis was 87% (versus 75%) at 1 year and 67% (versus 45%) at 5 years [2]. Most of the deaths among subjects with compensated cirrhosis occurred due to a transition to a decompensated state and subsequent consequences of the complications.

To refine prognosis of persons with cirrhosis, four stages of cirrhosis have been proposed, with stages 1 and 2 representing compensated cirrhosis [3]. Stage 1 is characterized by absence of ascites or varices. Stage 2 is characterized by the presence of nonbleeding varices but absence of ascites. Stage 3 is characterized by ascites with or without esophageal varices in a patient that has never bled. Stage 4 is characterized by variceal bleeding with or

[1] Materials appearing in this chapter prepared by individuals as part of their official duties as United States government employees are not covered by the copyright of the book, and any views expressed therein do not necessarily represent the views of the United States government. Such individuals' participation in the Work is not meant to serve as an official endorsement of any statement to the extent that such statement may conflict with any official position of the United States Government.

Cirrhosis: A practical guide to management, First Edition. Edited by Samuel S. Lee and Richard Moreau.

without ascites. Based on this initial classification, in a large systematic review the 1-year survival was 99%, 96.6%, 80%, and 43%, respectively. However, recent studies have not shown a markedly higher mortality with stage 4 than stage 3. Better management of variceal bleeding may have potentially led to improved survival in patients with variceal bleed and relatively lower survival in patients with ascites regardless of their varices status. Development of hepatic encephalopathy (HE) is an emerging negative prognostic indicator. Among alcoholics studied in the Danish National Health registry (1993–2005), the median survival in patients without complications was 48 months. The 1-year survival rate was 83% (absence of complications), 80% (variceal bleeding), 71% (ascites), 51% (ascites and variceal bleeding), and 36% (HE, alone or in combination) [5].

Infection and renal failure are common causes of mortality in patients with cirrhosis. Compared with uninfected patients, cirrhotic patients with infections have almost a fourfold increase in mortality (odds ratio, OR, 3.8; 95% CI 2.1–4.2). Infections may be spontaneous or related to complications of portal hypertension such as gastrointestinal bleeding or ascites. In a recent meta-analysis, the overall median mortality of infected patients was 38%: 30.3% at 1 month and 63% at 12 months (1-year survival 37%). In a subset of studies with spontaneous bacterial peritonitis (SBP), the median mortality was 44% (1-year survival was 34%) [6].

Renal failure is also common in patients with cirrhosis awaiting liver transplant and is often multifactorial [7,8]. When compared with patients without renal failure, cirrhotic patients with renal dysfunction have a significantly increased risk of death (OR 7.6; 95% CI 5.4–10.8) [9]. Among patients with cirrhosis, the median mortality rate for those with renal failure is 58% at 1 month and 63% at 1 year [9]. Hence, given that the median survival at 1 year is 37% with either renal dysfunction and/or infection (and refractory ascites), presence of one of these factors may represent a more advanced stage in addition to the four stages proposed above.

Given that the majority of deaths in patients with compensated cirrhosis is due to progression to a decompensated state and the development of its ensuing complications, knowledge of the risk of progression is important. The 10-year probability of risk of decompensation from a compensated state in a single-center study (1968–1980, median follow-up 63 months) was 58% [10]. Progression of cirrhosis from a compensated state (D'Amico stage 1 and 2) to a decompensated state (stage 3 and 4) has been examined in population-based studies. In an analysis of a large population-based United Kingdom General Practice Research Database (1987–2002), the age and gender adjusted rate of decompensation from compensated state was 12% per year [11]. This rate was faster during the first year after diagnosis (31%) and 5–7% in subsequent years. Other studies suggest a uniform rate of progression of 6–9% per year [3]. Yearly rates of decompensation likely vary by underlying disease with reported annual progression rates of 4% for viral hepatitis C, 6–10% for alcoholic cirrhosis with higher rates in patients with active alcohol use or development of alcoholic hepatitis, and 10% in persons with hepatitis B [12].

Besides assigning prognosis by clinical stage of disease, several models have been proposed to assist further in prognostication. This includes models to predict mortality or capture transition from a compensated to decompensated state.

Child–Pugh score

The Child's score was initially designed to predict the outcome after surgery for portal hypertension (portocaval shunting and transection of the esophagus) in cirrhotic patients (Table 7.1). Based on the variables shown in Table 7.1, cirrhotic patients are stratified into three categories: Child–Pugh grades A (5–6 points), B (7–9 points), or C (10–15 points). The factors, in addition to an evaluation of liver dysfunction, are also a gauge of organ dysfunction [13]. The median 1-year survival is 95% for Child A, 80% for Child B, and 45% for Child C cirrhosis. Correspondingly, the 2-year survival is 90%, 70%, and 38%, respectively [3,14]. Child–Pugh score is an independent predictor of mortality in compensated or decompensated liver disease (e.g., ascites, bleeding esophageal varices) and within etiologies of liver disease (e.g., chronic hepatitis C, cholestatic liver disease, or alcoholic liver disease).

Several limitations of the Child–Pugh score are noted. This includes equal weight assigned to all components with lack of statistical validity (e.g., ascites and coagulopathy get the same numerical weight), categorization

Table 7.1 Prognostic scores in assessment of patients with cirrhosis.

Child–Pugh Score			
	1 point	**2 points**	**3 points**
Total bilirubin (mg/dL)	≤2	2–3	>3
Serum albumin (g/dL)	>3.5	2.8–3.5	<2.8
INR	<1.7	1.7–2.3	>2.3
Ascites	None	Mild	Moderate to severe
Hepatic encephalopathy	None	Grade I–II	Grade III–IV
Points	**Stage**		
5–6	A		
7–9	B		
10–15	C		

MELD score [17]

MELD score = $3.8 * \log_e$ (bilirubin mg/dL) + $11.2 * \log_e$(INR) + $9.6 * \log_e$ (creatinine mg/dL) + 6.4

MELD Na [43]

MELD Na = MELD − Na − [0.025 × MELD × (140 − Na)] + 140,

where the serum sodium concentration (Na) is bound between 125 and 140 mmol/L

ReFit MELD [47]

ReFit MELD = $4.082 * \log_e$(bilirubin) + $8.485 * \log_e$(creatinine) + $10.671 * \log_e$(INR) + 7.432

where bilirubin is bilirubin bounded below by 1 mg/dL; creatinine is creatinine capped by 0.8 mg/dL below and 3 mg/dL above, and; INR is INR bounded by 1 below and 3 above. Renal replacement therapy = 3 mg/dL

of continuous variable, subjective nature of assessment for some of the variables (ascites, encephalopathy), possible redundancy (inclusion both international normalized ratio, INR, and albumin), influence of interlaboratory variability (e.g., prothrombin time, albumin), empiric cutoff values for variables, ceiling effect of variables (bilirubin 5 mg/dL and 25 mg/dL get the same points), lack of inclusion of cause of liver disease, and inability to account for reversibility of treating the underlying cause (e.g., cessation of alcohol abuse).

MELD score

The model for end-stage liver disease (MELD) score, akin to the Child–Pugh score, was devised as an objective predictor of early mortality in patients undergoing elective placement of transjugular intrahepatic portosystemic shunts (TIPS) [15]. The model contains three objective variables: serum creatinine, bilirubin, and INR (Table 7.1). The MELD score has high concordance (c-statistic 0.83) to predict risk of death within 3 months. This implies that 83 out of a 100 times, in a pair of randomly drawn patients, the model correctly predicts which patient will die first [16]. The model has been validated in several independent cohorts of patients with varying levels of liver disease severity (e.g., hospitalized and ambulatory patients), as well as patients of geographically and temporally diverse origin [17]. It is a good predictor of long-term survival (e.g., c-statistic 0.75 for 1-year survival), across several different populations (e.g., c-statistic 0.83 for alcoholic hepatitis, acute liver failure) as well as a good prognostic marker in decompensated liver disease (e.g., variceal bleeding, infections), and surgery [18–22]. The etiology of liver disease and individual complications of portal hypertension do not significantly enhance the prognostic information captured by the MELD score [16,17].

Overall, the MELD score is used a common metric of underlying disease severity [16]. The benefits of the MELD score lie in its simplicity, use of a continuous scale, and incorporation of easily available objective laboratory parameters. It has been shown to be superior to clinical judgment in identifying mortality risk [23]. Variables are ranked based on their importance and no ceiling effect is observed [24].

There are obvious limitations. The MELD score was created in a select population without acute reversible causes of decompensation (e.g., infection). Further, it does not capture prognosis in certain conditions (e.g., portopulmonary hypertension) or certain complications (e.g., hepatocellular carcinoma, HCC) [25]. The total bilirubin rather than direct bilirubin is used. However, the former is not a superior predictor than the latter (unpublished data). Serum creatinine is highly weighted in patients with liver disease. However, it is known that inclusion of serum creatinine is suboptimal among cirrhotic patients [26–28]. Measured glomerular filtration rate (GFR, e.g., by iothalamate clearance measurement) is better at assessing prognosis [26,27]. A multivariable model that incorporates calculated GFR and/or serum sodium is superior to the MELD score [28]. Serum creatinine measured is not standardized and may be overestimated in patients with high serum bilirubin [29]. Serum creatinine may underestimate the severity of renal dysfunction among women as a function of less muscle mass [30]. The prothrombin time, as a reflection of synthetic dysfunction, may be manipulated by persons who have artificially higher INR when on warfarin-based anticoagulation [31,32]. There is interlaboratory variation in assays that measure INR based on measurement techniques [33,34]. Though a liver-specific INR is more accurate, practical implementation across centers may be hard to achieve [32,35].

MELD modifications

Several models have been proposed to refine and improve the prognostic ability of the MELD score. The primary driving force has been estimating the prognosis of patients listed for liver transplantation and an assessment of their short-term mortality. This includes measurement of serial MELD scores, addition of variables (e.g., serum sodium), or reweighting components of the MELD score.

Delta MELD

A change in MELD scores, for example in patients with decompensated liver disease, may be associated with worse outcomes than other subjects with stable MELD score. However, the change in MELD (delta MELD) is not a significant predictor in multivariable analysis after adjusting for baseline MELD, which by definition is inherently higher, and repeated measurements of MELD score, which are more frequent in sicker patients [36,37].

Serum sodium and MELD-Na

Serum sodium concentration, a reflection of more advanced liver disease, is as an important prognostic factor [38–41]. Hyponatremia is associated with neurologic dysfunction, refractory ascites, hepatorenal syndrome, and death from liver disease [8,42]. Hyponatremia is an independent predictor of survival at 3 and 12 months [43,44]. Further, patients with hyponatremia are more likely to drop out while awaiting liver transplantation [45]. Hyponatremia is likely a marker for advanced renal dysfunction that is not accurately captured by creatinine-based measures. Even after adjusting for the MELD scores, a 1 mmol/L decrease in serum sodium concentration (125–140 mmol/L) is associated with a 5–10% increase in mortality [43,44]. This is particularly evident in patients with a low MELD score (Table 7.1). Serum sodium assessment is widely measured objective and easily available. Limitations of the serum sodium include potential for manipulation.

Re weighting components of MELD

Recently, attempts have been made to reweigh the components of the MELD score using a contemporary dataset [46,47] which improves the predictive ability of MELD based score to (c-statistic >0.85). Further validation is awaited (see Table 7.1)

MELD XI

As mentioned above, the role of INR in the MELD score is contentious. Heuman et al. [48] examined a model without INR (MELD-XI) for liver transplant candidates on stable oral anticoagulation. The model was still less accurate than MELD, suggesting that even in those patients, INR somehow carries prognostic information.

The INR can be elevated in patients receiving warfarin. Hence, an elevated INR may not accurately capture disease severity, especially because calibration for deriving INR is based on samples from persons on oral anticoagulation [33,34]. Less variability in INR is observed if calibration is done using samples from persons with liver disease (ISI_{liver}). Though incorporation of ISI_{liver} may improve MELD-based prediction models, it is practically cumbersome to incorporate [35]. But, despite the valid concerns, derivation of the MELD score using updated data suggests that the INR in its current form continues to be an excellent predictor of survival with a c-statistic upwards of 0.85 [47]. The incremental improvement in the predictive ability of a model that incorporates ISI_{liver} is unknown.

Child–Pugh score versus MELD score

The Child–Pugh score provides a global prognostic scale for cirrhotic patients at large, in patients with both compensated and decompensated cirrhosis. Studies show that the MELD score may be better suited for patients with decompensated liver disease. The MELD score was designed to predict short-term mortality; for longer term mortality prediction, the MELD score may not be superior to the Child–Pugh score [49–51].

Hepatic venous pressure gradient

Most deaths in persons with compensated cirrhosis occur as a result of transition to a decompensated state. Hence, prediction of development of decompensation as well as mortality specifically due to portal hypertension-related complications is important. This transition is not entirely explained by the prognostic models noted in previous sections.

By definition, portal hypertension is a pathologically abnormal portal pressure of 6 mmHg or above. The hepatic venous pressure gradient (HVPG) is an indirect reflection of the portal pressure across the liver [52]. For example, varices form only when HVPG reaches 10 mmHg with a clinically significant risk of bleeding occurring at an HVPG greater than 12 mmHg. Serum albumin, MELD score, and HVPG are independent predictors of development of decompensation from a compensated state [53,54]. An HVPG <10 mmHg has a 90% negative predictive value of development of clinical decompensation over 4 years [53].

Elevated HVPG is an independent predictor of mortality with a purported 3% increase in mortality per 1 mmHg increase in HVPG [55]. A single HVPG measurement greater than 20 mmHg is associated with worse probability of survival (1-year mortality 64% vs. 20%; $P<0.01$) and early rebleeding from varices [56,57]. Other factors that encapsulate advanced liver disease, such as serum sodium, are also important. A combination of both of hyponatremia (serum sodium <130 mmol/L) and HPVG >20 mmHg is associated with a significantly worse prognosis than either alone. However, it is unclear whether addition of HVPG to MELD of Child–Pugh stage based prediction significantly improves the predictive capabilities of a prognostic model [57].

Given that elevated HVPG is associated with poor outcomes, the benefit of a reduction in HVPG has been studied. In addition to age and serum albumin, an HVPG reduction upwards of 20% or to a gradient less than 12 mmHg is an independent predictor of reduction in risk of variceal bleeding, development of other complications of portal hypertension and is associated with improved survival [58–60]. In a large systematic review, such an HVPG reduction was associated with a 60% decrease in the odds of mortality (OR 0.39) [60]. HVPG elevation is also an independent predictor of development of HCC [61].

Measurement of HVPG, though important for prognosis, is not widely available and is invasive. Alternate noninvasive measures have been studied. Liver stiffness, as measured by transient elastography or magnetic resonance elastography is predictive of cirrhosis and presence of clinically significant portal hypertension; however, it is unclear whether the severity of portal hypertension can be accurately graded by these methods, as is possible with HVPG [62]. There are several encouraging studies. In patients with chronic liver disease, getting simultaneous measurement of HVPG and liver stiffness over a 2-year follow-up both methods were accurate to determine complications related to portal hypertension (area under the receiver operating characteristic curve, AUROC, >0.83) [63]. It is unclear whether addition of MELD or Child–Pugh scores to noninvasive measures can identify patients *at risk* for clinical decompensation. However, this technology appears promising, especially if serial measurements are obtained [64].

Variceal bleed

The natural history and prognosis of cirrhotic patients with variceal bleeding has been well studied. In patients without evidence of variceal bleeding and no history of varices, rate of development of varices was 3–5% at 1 year and 22–28% at 3 years, suggesting that overall esophageal varices develop at a rate of 7–8% per year [65,66]. As mentioned above, an HVPG greater than 10 mmHg is a predictor of development of varices. It may be possible that in patients with compensated cirrhosis, a decrease in at least 10% of HVPG from baseline may help prevent development of varices [67,68].

Progression of small varices to medium or large varices occurs at a rate of 5–12% at 1 year and 31% at 3 years [68]. Predictors of progression include higher Child–Pugh class, alcohol-related cirrhosis and high risk stigmata of bleed (e.g., red wale marks); the 1-year rate of progression is 22% (versus 2%) if any one of the above factors is present. The risk of bleeding in patient with small varices is higher than in patients without varices (12% versus 2%) [66].

The annual risk of variceal bleeding is 5–15%; the highest risk occurs within the first year (15%) in persons with large varices [69,70]. Despite significant strides in the management of varices and acute bleeding episodes, the mortality remains high at 15–20% [71,72]. Predictors of bleeding include presence of decompensated cirrhosis (Child B or C), size of varices, and presence of high risk stigmata upon endoscopy (red wale marks) [69].

The risk of further rebleeding, mortality, and complications is highest within the first 6 weeks [73]. Table 7.2 shows some of the factors associated with rebleeding or early mortality. Overall, there is a 20% failure rate in controlling the initial bleeding episode within 5 days, and up to a 60% rate of rebleeding in 1 year [74]. In prognostic studies conducted in the current era with standard of care interventions (antibiotics, vasoactive drugs, and endoscopic band ligation, EBL), the risk of early rebleeding or treatment failure was 15–21%, with the risk of early mortality being 6–24% [75]. Predictors of rebleeding or treatment failure include MELD score, Child–Pugh score, elevated HVPG ≥20 mmHg, development of infections, and endoscopic appearance (active bleeding, clot on varix, and shock) [72,75]. Recurrent variceal bleeding is lower among patients that achieve a reduction in HVPG to less than 12 mmHg or a 20% reduction in baseline HVPG values [60]. The role of HVPG guided therapy remains unclear [74]. Predictors of mortality include the above factors and HCC, worsening renal function, use of steroids, and advanced age [70,75].

Table 7.2 Selected independent prognostic factors of rebleeding and mortality within 6 weeks.

Rebleeding
Baseline liver function
Child–Pugh score and class
MELD score
Cirrhosis etiology (nonalcoholic)
Portal vein thrombosis
Hepatic venous pressure gradient ≥20 mmHg
Intensity of hemorrhage
Active bleeding
Clot at varix
Transfusion volume
Hemodynamic shock
Development of complications
Bacterial infection
Mortality
Baseline Liver Function
Child–Pugh score and class
MELD score
Albumin
Encephalopathy
Bilirubin
Hepatocellular carcinoma
Intensity of hemorrhage
Active bleeding
Hematemesis
Transfusion volume
Development of complications
Bacterial infection
Renal failure
Early rebleeding
Other
Digestive cancer
Age >60 years
Corticosteroid use
Inpatient status

Adapted from Augustin, 2011 [75].

Surgery and cirrhosis

Nonliver transplant surgery in patients with cirrhosis can be associated with significant risk of mortality. The prognosis of patients with cirrhosis undergoing surgery varies by stage of disease. Studies in the 1980s and 1990s have shown that mortality rates for patients undergoing surgery were 10% for those with Child's class A, 30% for those with Child's class B, and 76–82% for those with Child's class C cirrhosis. Predictors of perioperative complications and mortality in the pre MELD era included a elevated Child–Pugh score, advanced age, gender, type of surgery and ensuing perioperative complications, and higher American Society of Anesthesiologists (ASA) physical status rating [76]. Several studies have identified objective methods to evaluate prognosis in the last decade. In patients undergoing cardiac surgery, Child–Pugh score and MELD score were significant (P <0.01) predictors of mortality. A cutoff Child–Pugh score >7 was found to have a sensitivity and specificity of 86% and 92% for mortality, with a negative predictive value of 97% [77]. In this small study, 10% of patients in Child–Pugh class A died compared to 67% and 100% of Child B and C patients, respectively [77]. In patients undergoing non-transplant surgery (including cholecystectomies, hernia repairs, and exploratory laparotomies), the MELD score was a significant predictor or mortality. For persons undergoing intraabdominal procedures, the c-statistic for predicting 1-month mortality was 0.80 [78].

Between MELD scores of 5 and 20 there was a 1%, and for MELD scores greater than 20 there was an additional 2% increase in mortality risk with each integer increase in MELD score. Another study examined the 90-day mortality after major surgery compared with cirrhotic patients undergoing minor surgical procedures and ambulatory cirrhotic patients. In multivariable analysis, the MELD score, ASA class, and age predicted mortality at 30 and 90 days, 1 year, and long term, independently of type or year of surgery. This mortality relationship was seen through the 20-year follow-up. A linear relationship in mortality risk was observed (Table 7.3) with mortality ranging from 10% (MELD <8), 18–32% (8–15), upwards of 55% in MELD >15, and 90% in MELD >26. The c-statistic was 0.82 for 90-day mortality with the MELD score; this increased to 0.84 on addition of age and ASA class. Age above 70 added an equivalent risk of 3 additional MELD points, and ASA class IV added an equivalent risk of 5.5 additional MELD points [22].

Table 7.3 Risk of mortality among persons with cirrhosis undergoing nontransplant surgery. Percentage mortality is provided.

MELD score	7 days	30 days	90 days	1 year
0–7	1.9	5.7	9.7	19.2
8–11	3.3	10.3	17.7	28.9
12–15	7.7	25.4	32.3	45.0
16–20	14.6	44.0	55.8	70.5
21–25	23.0	53.8	66.7	84.6
≥26	30.0	90.0	90.0	100

Adapted from Teh, 2007 [22].

Intensive care for cirrhotic patients

Admission to the intensive care unit (ICU) is common in patients with decompensated cirrhosis; approximately 26 000 cirrhotic patients are admitted annually across the United States. Common indications include variceal bleeding, infection or sepsis, alcoholic hepatitis, or hepatic encephalopathy. The in-hospital mortality in these patients is greater than 50%; the majority of deaths are infection related [79]. In a single center study, survival rates in the ICU, in hospital, and at 6 months were 59%, 46%, and 38%, respectively [80]. Mortality in cirrhotic patients with severe sepsis requiring organ support was 65–90%, compared with 33–39% in those without [81]. Recent studies show that mortality may have improved [81].

Several prognostic models have been evaluated. The MELD score or Child–Pugh score may not be able to identify the subgroup of cirrhotic patients at highest risk of mortality [82]. Overall, general ICU scores seem to be superior to "liver-oriented" prognostic scores in this context. Infection, elevated bilirubin level, and requirement for mechanical ventilation or vasopressor therapy are independently associated with poor survival [83]. A recent single center analysis of liver-related admissions to the ICU showed that the Sequential Organ Failure Assessment (SOFA) and the Simplified Acute Physiology Score (SAPS II) scores were the best predictors of survival with the AUROC of 0.92 and 0.89, respectively, compared with the MELD score (0.83), and Child–Pugh score (0.79). The most common cause of infection was SBP or pneumonia. Fungal infections were universally fatal. Mortality, by number of organ failures, ranged from 2.8% (one organ) to 91% (three organs). Higher mortality with multiple organ failures is also seen in other studies [80]. Prior studies have also confirmed the good discrimination offered by the SOFA score (AUROC 0.83–0.85) [84] on day of admission or 72 hours after admission [80]. Hence, sequential measurement of SOFA as an example may be important. Serum lactate also has prognostic value [85]. Unfortunately, these scores simply reflect the severity of the patient's current medical status rather than predict development of such complications.

Acute-on-chronic liver failure

Acute-on-chronic liver failure (ACLF) describes an acute deterioration in cirrhotic patients of pre-existing chronic liver disease due to a precipitating event (most common infection), often necessitating intensive care and associated with high short-term mortality due to end organ dysfunction. An element of reversibility in nearly 50% is suggested in patients with ACLF, implying that early intervention in this group may be helpful. Precipitants include infection, acute hepatitis (alcohol, drug-induced liver injury viral hepatitis, ischemia), portal vein thrombosis, or extrahepatic insults such as trauma or surgery [86]. Common manifestations include HE, hyperbilirubinemia, coagulopathy, and potentially cardiovascular dysfunction. The notable features of ACLF include an element of reversibility with the possibility that short-term mortality may be avoided if early recognition and treatment of the precipitant is initiated. The type of precipitant matters: infection is an important negative prognostic indicator. The SOFA score helps identify patients most likely to survive the hospitalization [87]. Once again, though the SOFA score is an excellent predictor, it reflects the degree and magnitude of organ failure rather than predicts it. Factors that help identify patients at highest risk to develop multiorgan dysfunction are yet to be determined [88].

Disease-specific models

The above sections outline prediction of prognosis based on clinical stage. Several models have been proposed to predict prognosis within a disease subset (Table 7.4).

Cholestatic liver disease

The probability of survival among patients with primary biliary cirrhosis is predicted by the Mayo risk score. The

Table 7.4 Prognostic models in alcoholic hepatitis.

Maddrey discriminant factor (score ≥32 poor prognosis)

MDF = 4.6 (patient's PT – control PT) + total bilirubin (mg/dL)

where PT = prothrombin time

Model for end-stage liver disease (MELD) score (≥18 poor prognosis) [17]

$$\text{MELD score} = 3.8 * \log_e(\text{bilirubin mg/dL}) + 11.2 * \log_e(\text{INR}) + 9.6 * \log_e(\text{creatinine mg/dL}) + 6.4$$

Glasgow alcoholic hepatitis score (score >8 on day 1 or day 7 poor prognosis) [97]

	1	2	3
Age	<50	≥50	—
WCC	<15	≥15	—
Urea (mmol/L)	<5	≥5	—
PT ratio	<1.5	1.5–2.0	≥2
Bilirubin (mg/dL)	<7.3	7.3–14.6	≥14.6

PT, prothrombin time; WCC, white cell count.

Age, serum bilirubin, INR, and serum creatinine score (score >9 poor prognosis) [102]

$$\text{ABIC score}: (\text{age} \times 0.1) + (\text{serum bilirubin} \times 0.08) + (\text{serum creatinine} \times 0.3) + (\text{INR} \times 0.8)$$

Lille model (6-month survival probability of patients with a Lille model above 0.45 is about 25%) [100]

$$\text{Lille model}: 3.19 - 0.101 * (\text{age in years}) + 0.147 * (\text{albumin day 0 in g/L}) + 0.0165 * (\text{evolution in bilirubin level in mmol/L})$$
$$-0.206 * (\text{renal insufficiency 0 if absent 1 if present}) - 0.0065 * (\text{bilirubin day 0 in mmol/L}) - 0.0096 * (\text{prothrombin time in seconds})$$

score includes age, bilirubin, albumin, prothrombin time, and edema to predict probability of survival without transplantation. The risk of post-transplant mortality increases above a score of 7.8, suggesting transplant evaluation should be initiated prior to reaching the threshold [89–92]. For primary sclerosing cholangitis, the primary sclerosing cholangitis (PSC) Mayo risk score incorporates age, serum bilirubin, aspartate aminotransferase (AST), albumin, and evidence of variceal bleeding to estimate survival within the ensuing 4 years [93,94]. The models are available at http://www.mayoclinic.org/gi-rst/mayomodel2.html.

Alcoholic hepatitis

Several models have been proposed to identify the risk of short-term mortality in patients with alcoholic hepatitis (Table 7.4). These models may assist in predicting the patients most likely to benefit from corticosteroid treatment. A Maddrey sore above 32 identifies the patients most likely to benefit from corticosteroid therapy. Other models have been derived to assess short-term mortality. An early decrease in bilirubin with therapy is an important prognostic indicator. For example, the Lille model assessed early response to corticosteroid therapy within the first 7 days as reflected by a change in serum bilirubin. According to the model parameters, patients with a score above 0.45 had a 6-month mortality rate of 75%, while those with a score below 0.45 had a mortality rate of only 15%. The MELD score, MELD Na score, Glasgow alcoholic hepatitis score, Lille score, and the ABIC score have been compared. In a selected Danish population, all tests shared similar performance characteristics. The 28-day mortality was 16% with a 6-month mortality of 40%. The predictive ability of the several models were similar, with an AUROC around 0.74–0.78 for predicting 1-month mortality. The ability to predict mortality was improved by rescoring on day 7 [95–100].

Conclusions

Prognostic models are helpful to determine the risk of adverse outcomes based on clinical stage, clinical scenario, and underlying liver disease. Rather than pursuing a reactive plan of care in the treatment of patients with advanced liver disease, a proactive approach is needed to prevent the development of complications [101].

References

1 Asrani SK, Kamath PS, Pedersen R, et al. Liver related mortality in the US is underestimated. Hepatology [Meeting Abstract] 2010;52:408A–A.

2 Fleming KM, Aithal GP, Card TR, West J. All-cause mortality in people with cirrhosis compared with the general population: a population-based cohort study. Liver Int 2012;32:79–84.

3 D'Amico G, Garcia-Tsao G, Pagliaro L. Natural history and prognostic indicators of survival in cirrhosis: a systematic review of 118 studies. J Hepatol 2006;44:217–31.

4 Jepsen P, Vilstrup H, Andersen PK, Lash TL, Sørensen HT. Comorbidity and survival of Danish cirrhosis patients: a nationwide population-based cohort study. Hepatology 2008;48:214–20.

5 Jepsen P, Ott P, Andersen PK, Sorensen HT, Vilstrup H. Clinical course of alcoholic liver cirrhosis: a Danish population-based cohort study. Hepatology 2010;51:1675–82.

6 Arvaniti V, D'Amico G, Fede G, et al. Infections in patients with cirrhosis increase mortality four-fold and should be used in determining prognosis. Gastroenterology 2010;139: 1246–56, 56 e1–5.

7 Garcia-Tsao G, Parikh CR, Viola A. Acute kidney injury in cirrhosis. Hepatology 2008;48:2064–77.

8 Gines P, Schrier RW. Renal failure in cirrhosis. N Engl J Med. 2009;361:1279–90.

9 Fede G, D'Amico G, Arvaniti V, et al. Renal failure and cirrhosis: a systematic review of mortality and prognosis. J Hepatol 2012;56:810–8.

10 Gines P, Quintero E, Arroyo V, et al. Compensated cirrhosis: natural history and prognostic factors. Hepatology 1987;7: 122–8.

11 Fleming KM, Aithal GP, Card TR, West J. The rate of decompensation and clinical progression of disease in people with cirrhosis: a cohort study. Aliment Pharmacol Ther 2010;32:1343–50.

12 Schuppan D, Afdhal NH. Liver cirrhosis. Lancet 2008;371: 838–51.

13 Durand F, Valla D. Assessment of prognosis of cirrhosis. Semin Liver Dis 2008;28:110–22.

14 Infante-Rivard C, Esnaola S, Villeneuve JP. Clinical and statistical validity of conventional prognostic factors in predicting short-term survival among cirrhotics. Hepatology 1987;7:660–4.

15 Malinchoc M, Kamath PS, Gordon FD, Peine CJ, Rank J, Ter Borg PCJ. A model to predict poor survival in patients undergoing transjugular intrahepatic portosystemic shunts. Hepatology 2000;31:864–71.

16 Kamath PS, Kim WR. The model for end-stage liver disease (MELD). Hepatology 2007;45:797–805.

17 Kamath PS, Wiesner RH, Malinchoc M, et al. A model to predict survival in patients with end-stage liver disease. Hepatology 2001;33:464–70.

18 Yantorno SE, Kremers WK, Ruf AE, Trentadue JJ, Podesta LG, Villamil FG. MELD is superior to King's college and Clichy's criteria to assess prognosis in fulminant hepatic failure. Liver Transpl 2007;13:822–8.
19 Kremers WK, van IM, Kim WR, et al. MELD score as a predictor of pretransplant and posttransplant survival in OPTN/UNOS status 1 patients. Hepatology 2004;39:764–9.
20 Alessandria C, Ozdogan O, Guevara M, et al. MELD score and clinical type predict prognosis in hepatorenal syndrome: relevance to liver transplantation. Hepatology 2005;41:1282–9.
21 Northup PG, Wanamaker RC, Lee YD, Adams RB, Berg CL. Model for end-stage liver disease (MELD) predicts nontransplant surgical mortality in patients with cirrhosis. Ann Surg 2005;242:244–51.
22 Teh SH, Nagorney DM, Stevens SR, et al. Risk factors for mortality after surgery in patients with cirrhosis. Gastroenterology 2007;132:1261–9.
23 Fink MA, Angus PW, Gow PJ, et al. Liver transplant recipient selection: MELD vs. clinical judgment. Liver Transpl 2005;11:621–6.
24 Bernardi M, Gitto S, Biselli M. The MELD score in patients awaiting liver transplant: strengths and weaknesses. J Hepatol 2011;54:1297–306.
25 Wiesner R, Lake JR, Freeman RB, Gish RG. Model for end-stage liver disease (MELD) exception guidelines. Liver Transpl 2006;12 (Suppl 3): S85–7.
26 Francoz C, Glotz D, Moreau R, Durand F. The evaluation of renal function and disease in patients with cirrhosis. J Hepatol 2010;52:605–13.
27 Francoz C, Prie D, Abdelrazek W, et al. Inaccuracies of creatinine and creatinine-based equations in candidates for liver transplantation with low creatinine: impact on the model for end-stage liver disease score. Liver Transpl 2010;16:1169–77.
28 Lim YS, Larson TS, Benson JT, et al. Serum sodium, renal function, and survival of patients with end-stage liver disease. J Hepatol 2010;52:523–8.
29 Cholongitas E, Marelli L, Kerry A, et al. Different methods of creatinine measurement significantly affect MELD scores. Liver Transpl 2007;13:523–9.
30 Cholongitas E, Marelli L, Kerry A, et al. Female liver transplant recipients with the same GFR as male recipients have lower MELD scores: a systematic bias. Am J Transplant 2007;7:685–92.
31 Arjal R, Trotter JF. International normalized ratio of prothrombin time in the model for end-stage liver disease score: an unreliable measure. Clin Liver Dis 2009;13:67–71.
32 Trotter JF, Olson J, Lefkowitz J, Smith AD, Arjal R, Kenison J. Changes in international normalized ratio (INR) and model for endstage liver disease (MELD) based on selection of clinical laboratory. Am J Transplant 2007;7:1624–8.
33 Bellest L, Eschwege V, Poupon R, Chazouilleres O, Robert A. A modified international normalized ratio as an effective way of prothrombin time standardization in hepatology. Hepatology 2007;46:528–34.
34 Tripodi A, Chantarangkul V, Primignani M, et al. The international normalized ratio calibrated for cirrhosis (INR(liver)) normalizes prothrombin time results for model for end-stage liver disease calculation. Hepatology 2007;46:520–7.
35 Porte RJ, Lisman T, Tripodi A, Caldwell SH, Trotter JF. The International Normalized Ratio (INR) in the MELD score: problems and solutions. Am J Transplant 2010;10:1349–53.
36 Bambha K, Kim WR, Kremers W, et al. Predicting survival among patients listed for liver transplantation: an assessment of serial MELD measurements. Am J Transplant 2004;4:1798–804.
37 D'Amico G. Developing concepts on MELD: delta and cutoffs. J Hepatol [Comment Editorial Review] 2005;42:790–2.
38 Biggins SW, Kim WR, Terrault NA, et al. Evidence-based incorporation of serum sodium concentration into MELD. Gastroenterology 2006;130:1652–60.
39 Biggins SW, Rodriguez HJ, Bacchetti P, Bass NM, Roberts JP, Terrault NA. Serum sodium predicts mortality in patients listed for liver transplantation. Hepatology 2005;41:32–9.
40 Heuman D, Abou-assi SG, Habib A, et al. Persistent ascites and low serum sodium identify patients with cirrhosis and low MELD scores who are at high risk for early death. Hepatology 2004;40:802–10.
41 Ruf AE, Kremers W, Chavez LL, Descalzi VI, Podesta LG, Villamil FG. Addition of serum sodium into the MELD score predicts waiting list mortality better than MELD alone. Liver Transpl 2005;11:336–43.
42 Gines P, Guevara M. Hyponatremia in cirrhosis: pathogenesis, clinical significance, and management. Hepatology 2008;48:1002–10.
43 Kim WR, Biggins SW, Kremers WK, et al. Hyponatremia and mortality among patients on the liver-transplant waiting list. N Engl J Med. 2008;359:1018–26.
44 Londono MC, Cardenas A, Guevara M, et al. MELD score and serum sodium in the prediction of survival of patients with cirrhosis awaiting liver transplantation. Gut 2007;56:1283–90.
45 Biselli M, Gitto S, Gramenzi A, et al. Six score systems to evaluate candidates with advanced cirrhosis for orthotopic liver transplant: Which is the winner? Liver Transpl 2010;16:964–73.
46 Sharma P, Schaubel DE, Sima CS, Merion RM, Lok AS. Reweighting the model for end-stage liver disease score components. Gastroenterology 2008;135:1575–81.
47 Leise MD, Kim WR, Kremers WK, Larson JJ, Benson JT, Therneau TM. A revised model for end-stage liver disease optimizes prediction of mortality among patients awaiting liver transplantation. Gastroenterology 2011;140:1952–60.
48 Heuman DM, Mihas AA, Habib A, et al. MELD-XI: a rational approach to "sickest first" liver transplantation in cirrhotic

patients requiring anticoagulant therapy. Liver Transpl 2007;13:30–7.

49 Cholongitas E, Papatheodoridis GV, Vangeli M, Terreni N, Patch D, Burroughs AK. Systematic review: the model for end-stage liver disease: should it replace Child–Pugh's classification for assessing prognosis in cirrhosis? Aliment Pharmacol Ther 2005;22:1079–89.

50 Durand F, Valla D. Assessment of the prognosis of cirrhosis: Child–Pugh versus MELD. J Hepatol 2005;42 (Suppl 1): S100–7.

51 Said A, Williams J, Holden J, et al. Model for end-stage liver disease score predicts mortality across a broad spectrum of liver disease. J Hepatol 2004;40:897–903.

52 Albilllos A, Garcia-Tsao G. Classification of cirrhosis: the clinical use of HVPG measurements. Dis Markers 2011;31:121–8.

53 Ripoll C, Groszmann R, Garcia-Tsao G, et al. Hepatic venous pressure gradient predicts clinical decompensation in patients with compensated cirrhosis. Gastroenterology 2007;133:481–8.

54 Ripoll C, Lastra P, Rincon D, Catalina V, Banares R. Comparison of MELD, HVPG, and their changes to predict clinically relevant endpoints in cirrhosis. Scand J Gastroenterol 2012;47:204–11.

55 Ripoll C, Banares R, Rincon D, et al. Influence of hepatic venous pressure gradient on the prediction of survival of patients with cirrhosis in the MELD era. Hepatology 2005;42:793–801.

56 Moitinho E, Escorsell A, Bandi JC, et al. Prognostic value of early measurements of portal pressure in acute variceal bleeding. Gastroenterology 1999;117:626–31.

57 Abraldes JG, Villanueva C, Banares R, et al. Hepatic venous pressure gradient and prognosis in patients with acute variceal bleeding treated with pharmacologic and endoscopic therapy. J Hepatol 2008;48:229–36.

58 Abraldes JG, Tarantino I, Turnes J, Garcia-Pagan JC, Rodes J, Bosch J. Hemodynamic response to pharmacological treatment of portal hypertension and long-term prognosis of cirrhosis. Hepatology 2003;37:902–8.

59 Albillos A, Banares R, Gonzalez M, et al. Value of the hepatic venous pressure gradient to monitor drug therapy for portal hypertension: a meta-analysis. Am J Gastroenterol 2007;102:1116–26.

60 D'Amico G, Garcia-Pagan JC, Luca A, Bosch J. Hepatic vein pressure gradient reduction and prevention of variceal bleeding in cirrhosis: a systematic review. Gastroenterology 2006;131:1611–24.

61 Ripoll C, Groszmann RJ, Garcia-Tsao G, et al. Hepatic venous pressure gradient predicts development of hepatocellular carcinoma independently of severity of cirrhosis. J Hepatol 2009;50:923–8.

62 Berzigotti A, Ashkenazi E, Reverter E, Abraldes JG, Bosch J. Non-invasive diagnostic and prognostic evaluation of liver cirrhosis and portal hypertension. Dis Markers 2011;31: 129–38.

63 Robic MA, Procopet B, Métivier S, et al. Liver stiffness accurately predicts portal hypertension related complications in patients with chronic liver disease: a prospective study. J Hepatol 2011;55:1017–24.

64 Corpechot C, Carrat F, Poujol-Robert A, et al. Noninvasive elastography-based assessment of liver fibrosis progression and prognosis in primary biliary cirrhosis. Hepatology 2012;56:198–208.

65 Groszmann RJ, Garcia-Tsao G, Bosch Jet al. Beta-blockers to prevent gastroesophageal varices in patients with cirrhosis. N Engl J Med 2005;353:2254–61.

66 Merli M, Nicolini G, Angeloni S, et al. Incidence and natural history of small esophageal varices in cirrhotic patients. J Hepatol 2003;38:266–72.

67 Poca M, Puente A, Graupera I, Villanueva C. Prognostic markers in patients with cirrhosis and portal hypertension who have not bled. Dis Markers 2011;31:147–54.

68 Groszmann RJ, Garcia-Tsao G, Bosch J, et al. Beta-blockers to prevent gastroesophageal varices in patients with cirrhosis. N Engl J Med 2005;353:2254–61.

69 North Italian Endoscopic Club for the Study and Treatment of Esophageal Varices. Prediction of the first variceal hemorrhage in patients with cirrhosis of the liver and esophageal varices: a prospective multicenter study. N Engl J Med 1988;319:983–9.

70 de Franchis R. Revising consensus in portal hypertension: report of the Baveno V consensus workshop on methodology of diagnosis and therapy in portal hypertension. J Hepatol 2010;53:762–8.

71 Garcia-Tsao G, Bosch J. Management of varices and variceal hemorrhage in cirrhosis. N Engl J Med 2010;362:823–32.

72 Bambha K, Kim WR, Pedersen R, Bida JP, Kremers WK, Kamath PS. Predictors of early re-bleeding and mortality after acute variceal haemorrhage in patients with cirrhosis. Gut 2008;57:814–20.

73 Graham DY, Smith JL. The course of patients after variceal hemorrhage. Gastroenterology 1981;80:800–9.

74 Garcia-Tsao G, Sanyal AJ, Grace ND, Carey W. Prevention and management of gastroesophageal varices and variceal hemorrhage in cirrhosis. Hepatology 2007;46:922–38.

75 Augustin S, Genescà J. Diagnostic and prognostic markers in liver cirrhosis. Dis Markers 2011;31:119–20.

76 Ziser A, Plevak DJ, Wiesner RH, Rakela J, Offord KP, Brown DL. Morbidity and mortality in cirrhotic patients undergoing anesthesia and surgery. Anesthesiology 1999;90: 42–53.

77 Suman A, Barnes DS, Zein NN, Levinthal GN, Connor JT, Carey WD. Predicting outcome after cardiac surgery in patients with cirrhosis: a comparison of Child–Pugh and MELD scores. Clin Gastroenterol Hepatol 2004;2:719–23.

78 Northup PG, Wanamaker RC, Lee VD, Adams RB, Berg CL. Model for End-Stage Liver Disease (MELD) predicts non-transplant surgical mortality in patients with cirrhosis. Ann Surg 2005;242:244–51.

79 Olson JC, Wendon JA, Kramer DJ, et al. Intensive care of the patient with cirrhosis. Hepatology 2011;54:1864–72.
80 Das V, Boelle PY, Galbois A, et al. Cirrhotic patients in the medical intensive care unit: early prognosis and long-term survival. Crit Care Med 2010;38:2108–16.
81 O'Brien AJ, Welch CA, Singer M, Harrison DA. Prevalence and outcome of cirrhosis patients admitted to UK intensive care: a comparison against dialysis-dependent chronic renal failure patients. Intensive Care Med 2012;38:991–1000.
82 Cholongitas E, Marelli L, Shusang V, et al. A systematic review of the performance of the Model for End-Stage Liver Disease (MELD) in the setting of liver transplantation. Liver Transplant 2006;12:1049–61.
83 Levesque E, Hoti E, Azoulay D, et al. Prospective evaluation of the prognostic scores for cirrhotic patients admitted to an intensive care unit. J Hepatol 2012;56:95–102.
84 Cholongitas E, Senzolo M, Patch D, et al. Risk factors, sequential organ failure assessment and model for end-stage liver disease scores for predicting short term mortality in cirrhotic patients admitted to intensive care unit. Aliment Pharmacol Ther 2006;23:883–93.
85 Cholongitas E, Agarwal B, Antoniadis N, Burroughs AK. Patients with cirrhosis admitted to an intensive care unit. J Hepatol 2012;57:230–1.
86 Jalan R, Gines P, Olson JC, et al. Acute-on-chronic liver failure. J Hepatol 2012;57:1336–48.
87 Katoonizadeh A, Laleman W, Verslype C, et al. Early features of acute-on-chronic alcoholic liver failure: a prospective cohort study. Gut 2010;59:1561–9.
88 Olson JC, Kamath PS. Acute-on-chronic liver failure: what are the implications? Curr Gastroenterol Rep 2012;14:63–6.
89 Murtaugh PA, Dickson ER, Van Dam GM, et al. Primary biliary cirrhosis: prediction of short-term survival based on repeated patient visits. Hepatology 1994;20:126–34.
90 Dickson ER, Grambsch PM, Fleming TR, Fisher LD, Langworthy A. Prognosis in primary biliary cirrhosis: model for decision making. Hepatology 1989;10:1–7.
91 Grambsch PM, Dickson ER, Kaplan M, LeSage G, Fleming TR, Langworthy AL. Extramural cross-validation of the Mayo primary biliary cirrhosis survival model establishes its generalizability. Hepatology 1989;10:846–50.
92 Kim WR, Wiesner RH, Therneau TM, et al. Optimal timing of liver transplantation for primary biliary cirrhosis. Hepatology 1998 Jul; 28 (1): 33–8.
93 Kim WR, Therneau TM, Wiesner RH, et al. A revised natural history model for primary sclerosing cholangitis. Mayo Clin Proc 2000;75:688–94.
94 Talwalkar JA, Seaberg E, Kim WR, Wiesner RH. Predicting clinical and economic outcomes after liver transplantation using the Mayo primary sclerosing cholangitis model and Child–Pugh score. National Institutes of Diabetes and Digestive and Kidney Diseases Liver Transplantation Database Group. Liver Transpl 2000;6:753–8.
95 Sandahl TD, Jepsen P, Ott P, Vilstrup H. Validation of prognostic scores for clinical use in patients with alcoholic hepatitis. Scand J Gastroenterol 2011;46:1127–32.
96 Carithers RL Jr, Herlong HF, Diehl AM, et al. Methylprednisolone therapy in patients with severe alcoholic hepatitis: a randomized multicenter trial. Ann Intern Med 1989; 110:685–90.
97 Forrest EH, Evans CD, Stewart S, et al. Analysis of factors predictive of mortality in alcoholic hepatitis and derivation and validation of the Glasgow alcoholic hepatitis score. Gut 2005;54:1174–9.
98 Dunn W, Jamil LH, Brown LS, et al. MELD accurately predicts mortality in patients with alcoholic hepatitis. Hepatology 2005;41:353–8.
99 Mathurin P, Abdelnour M, Ramond MJ, et al. Early change in bilirubin levels is an important prognostic factor in severe alcoholic hepatitis treated with prednisolone. Hepatology 2003;38:1363–9.
100 Louvet A, Naveau S, Abdelnour M, et al. The Lille model: a new tool for therapeutic strategy in patients with severe alcoholic hepatitis treated with steroids. Hepatology 2007;45: 1348–54.
101 Tsochatzis EA, Bosch J, Burroughs AK. A new therapeutic paradigm for patients with cirrhosis. Hepatology 2012; 56:1983–92.
102 Dominguez M, Rincon D, Abraldes JG, et al. A new scoring system for prognostic stratification of patients with alcoholic hepatitis. Am J Gastroenterol 2008;103:2747–56.

CHAPTER 8

End-stage liver failure: liver transplant evaluation

Sebastián Marciano[1] and Adrián Gadano[2]
[1]*Liver Unit, Hospital Italiano, Buenos Aires, Argentina*
[2]*Department of Medicine and Liver Unit, Hospital Italiano, Buenos Aires, Argentina*

Introduction

The first attempt at human liver transplantation (LT) was performed by Thomas Starzl in 1963, but it was not until 1967 that a successful procedure was performed. As the initial immunosuppressive regimens were not potent enough, an acceptable survival was not possible. The implementation of more efficient immunosuppressive therapy, particularly cyclosporine in the 1980s, was associated with an improvement in survival. Since then other major developments in surgical techniques, newer immunosuppression regimens and preservation solutions have continued to impact favorably on the long-term postoperative course.

LT should be considered in patients with irreversible acute or chronic liver failure, in selected patients with malignant liver tumors, and in patients with genetic or metabolic disorders in which the liver is responsible for the damage to other organs. As with any other medical intervention, it is indicated when the risk of death related to the liver disease is outweighed by the benefits to be obtained from LT. Risks and benefits are not always easy to balance, but if the selection of candidates is precise, successful outcomes can be achieved. The ideal scenario to transplant a patient would be at the exact moment when the predicted life expectancy related to the liver disease is estimated to be shorter than the one that would be achieved with LT. Unfortunately, the identification of this very precise moment is challenged by at least two factors. First, organ donation is far from being plentiful enough to meet the requirements of the candidates on the waiting list. Second, mortality on the waiting list is not always accurately predicted.

Cirrhosis-related end-stage liver disease is the leading cause of LT worldwide. This chapter reviews how to select and evaluate patients with cirrhosis for LT.

Epidemiology

The etiology of cirrhosis leading to LT varies worldwide. Chronic hepatitis C is the leading cause in the United States, Europe, and Latin American countries [1–3]. In other regions such as Southeast Asia and Sub-Saharan Africa, chronic hepatitis B is the main cause of cirrhosis leading to LT [4].

A recent report from the European Liver Transplant Registry stated that cirrhosis was the indication for LT in 58% of patients, with the following distribution: viral (39%), alcoholic (33%), primary biliary cirrhosis (9%), unknown (8%), autoimmune (4%), and other (7%) [1]. No definitive cause for cirrhosis can be identified in up to 20% of patients who have end-stage liver disease (cryptogenic cirrhosis); however, many of these patients most likely have "burned-out" nonalcoholic steatohepatitis [5].

Data reported by the Organ Procurement Transplant Network (OPTN) from the United States show that the average age of adult recipients has increased steadily over the past 10 years. In 2009, approximately 75% of adult

Cirrhosis: A practical guide to management, First Edition. Edited by Samuel S. Lee and Richard Moreau.

recipients were older than 50 years and male recipients predominated, with a 2 : 1 male : female ratio [6].

Surgical aspects of liver transplantation

It is not the objective of this chapter to review surgical issues in detail. However, some strategies aimed to increase the availability of transplantable livers are discussed.

In most cases livers are procured from cadaveric donors. In an attempt to increase the availability of cadaveric donors, some countries have implemented transplantation from donors after cardiac death, known as DCD donors. This strategy is associated with a greater risk of complications after LT, especially biliary complications [7]. To minimize the risk, careful selection of these donors is mandatory.

Split LT is a strategy in which a liver from a cadaveric donor is used to transplant two patients, generally a child and an adult [8]. Domino LT is a more recent strategy that consists of transplanting the explanted livers of patients that are undergoing LT for metabolic or genetic diseases that do not compromise liver function [9]. The largest experience is with hereditary amyloidosis, which is an autosomal dominant disease characterized by the production of a mutant protein (most often transtiretin) by the liver. These patients develop progressive neuropathy and cardiomyopathy but if LT is performed in a timely manner the symptoms can stabilize or regress. As it takes two to five decades for patients to develop the symptoms, these normally functioning livers can be transplanted into patients with decompensated cirrhosis or hepatocellular carcinoma (HCC). Of course, the risk for the recipient of these livers is the development of hereditary amyloidosis so this strategy should not be used in young patients.

Living donors are also used in LT. In fact, in some countries, cadaveric donor LT is not performed because of religious or cultural issues and living donors are exclusively used [10]. The main impediment to this technique is the balance between the donor's and the recipient's risks. The remnant liver in the donor and the transplanted liver in the recipient must be sufficient to provide an adequate liver function. This balance is easily achieved in an adult donor and a pediatric recipient. In Figure 8.1 an algorithm for the evaluation of a possible living donor is shown.

Patient selection

LT in patients with cirrhosis is indicated when life expectancy related to the end-stage liver disease is considered to be significantly reduced. Less frequently, LT in patients with cirrhosis is indicated when the quality of life is compromised as a result of specific complications that are not necessarily related to a reduced life expectancy, for example, severe intractable pruritus in patients with cholestatic diseases.

The risk of death in patients with cirrhosis is mainly related to its specific complications, which determine the transition from compensated to decompensated cirrhosis. As reviewed in other chapters, survival of patients with compensated cirrhosis has been reported to average 10–12 years [11]. Performing LT in these patients would imply more risks than benefits. However, when complications such as encephalopathy and ascites arise, survival at 5 years is reduced to 20–50% [11]. As the survival rate at 5 years after LT is around 75% in large series, performing LT in these patients is justified [12].

The use of scores such as the Child–Turcotte–Pugh (CTP) and the model for end-stage liver disease (MELD) [13,14] constitutes another way of predicting survival in patients with cirrhosis (Figure 8.2).

The quality of life of patients with cirrhosis is not reflected by any of the scores and it is difficult to assess on clinical grounds. Mostly, quality of life is reduced as the complications of cirrhosis appear. When evaluating a patient with cirrhosis in terms of LT candidacy, attention has to be focused on the development of clinical complications, on the calculation of the CTP and MELD scores, and on the assessment of quality of life. Specific aspects of each of these issues are reviewed.

Complications of cirrhosis

The development of ascites, encephalopathy, hyperbilirubinemia, or variceal bleeding is considered by most authors to mark the transition from compensated to decompensated cirrhosis. Survival in these patients is reduced to less than 50% at 5 years [11] and then LT is justified. The particular case of variceal bleeding as the only complication in patients with well-preserved liver function (CTP A) must be considered separately. In this scenario, in which strategies aimed at reducing the risk of new bleeding events can offer the patient an acceptable life expectancy, LT should not be indicated.

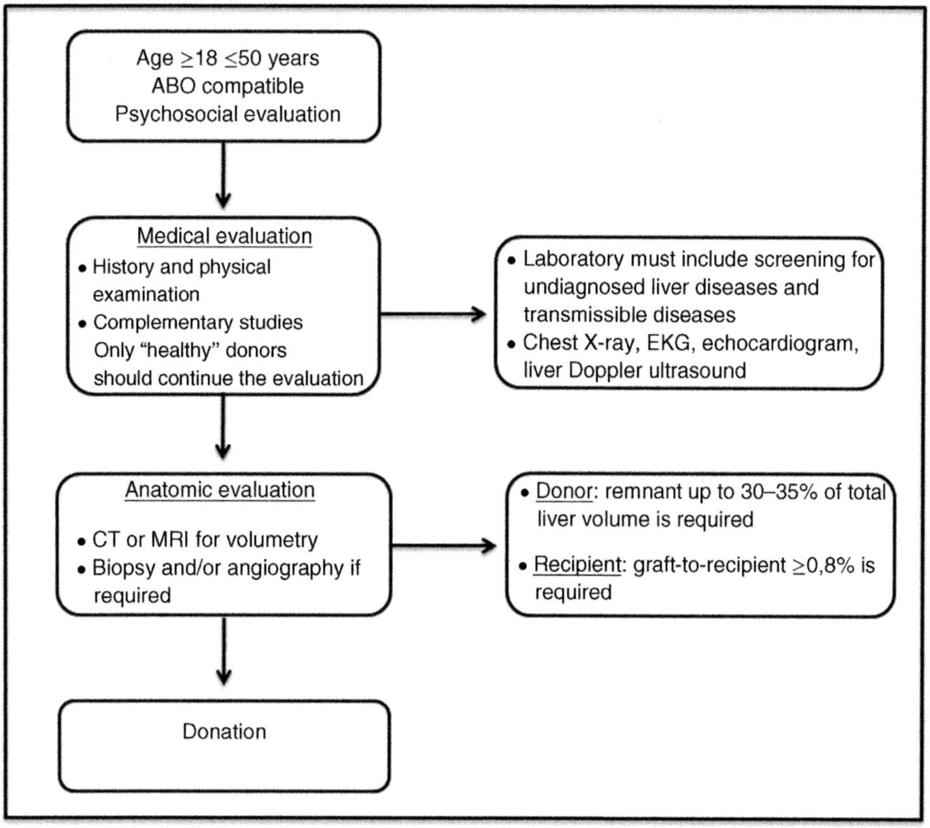

Figure 8.1 Evaluation of a potential living donor for liver transplantation.

Other complications like HCC and hepatopulmonary syndrome (HPS) are clearly associated with a reduction in survival, even though they are not recognized as causes of "decompensation" of cirrhosis by most authors. These complications share the fact that they are clear indications for LT. Nevertheless, they must fulfill specific criteria for the transplantation to be safe (see contraindications).

LT is an excellent treatment for early (stage A) HCC because it removes not only the tumor, but also the oncogenic parenchyma [15]. The downside of LT in patients with HCC is recurrence. The best results are achieved when the Milan criteria are applied: one solitary nodule <5 cm or up to three nodules <3 cm without vascular invasion or extrahepatic spread [15]. The study performed by Mazzaferro et al. [15] that was responsible for the wide application of these criteria showed a survival rate of 83% at 4 years, with a chance of recurrence of 8% in patients fulfilling these criteria. The possibility of expanding these criteria to larger nodules or more than three nodules has been evaluated with variable results. What is clear from the experience is that the risk of recurrence increases when transplanting patients with higher tumor burdens [16].

In many countries, patients with HCC fulfilling Milan criteria are prioritized on the waiting list. Once listed, if a long waiting period is anticipated (>6 months), strategies such as transarterial chemoembolization or percutaneous ablation are applied to control tumor growth [17].

In selected patients with cirrhosis, single small nodules (<2 cm), no portal hypertension, and well-preserved liver function, surgical resection or percutaneous ablation achieves great results and should be the treatment of choice as long as patients do not have other indications for LT [16].

HPS is associated with a 2-year survival rate of less than 50% [18]. As there is no other specific treatment for this condition, LT is indicated. Resolution of the hypoxemia

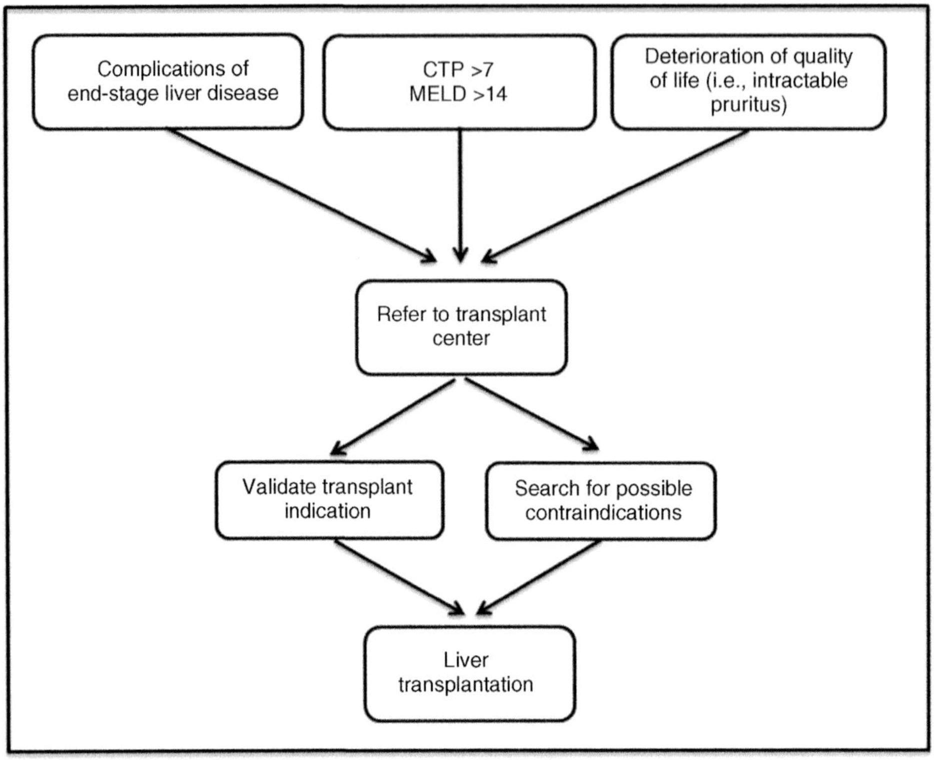

Figure 8.2 Evaluation of patients with end-stage liver disease for liver transplantation. CTP, Child–Turcotte–Pugh score; MELD, model for end-stage liver disease.

occurs in most cases in a variable time after LT. However, the severity of abnormality of gas exchange has to be evaluated with caution before LT. Patients with HPS are also prioritized on the waiting list in many countries in order to prevent progression of disease and worsening of hypoxemia [19].

In conclusion, patients with cirrhosis who develop any of the following complications in the absence of contra-indications have to be referred for LT: ascites, encephalopathy, jaundice, variceal bleeding (except CTP A), HCC, and HPS.

Scores that predict mortality: CTP and MELD

The CTP score was originally designed to predict mortality following portosystemic shunts, [13] then it was found to be a good predictor of mortality in many other settings. As three of the five variables included in the CTP score are clinical complications of cirrhosis (i.e., ascites, encephalopathy, and jaundice), patients with high CTP scores have already developed these complications and have a clear indication for LT. A CTP score of ≥7 are considered to be sufficient criteria to list a patient for LT [20].

The MELD score was originally designed to predict mortality after the placement of portosystemic shunts [14]. Like the CTP score, it was then found to be of great value in predicting mortality in other settings. In fact, the MELD score is the allocation system adopted by many countries recently because of its capacity to accurately predict 3-month mortality on the waiting list [14]. As the MELD score is calculated from creatinine, INR, and bilirubin levels, it does not always reflect the complications of cirrhosis and it is not infrequent to observe patients with decompensated cirrhosis with low MELD scores. The opposite is also possible; patients with high MELD scores who have not developed clinical complications. In general, performing LT in patients with MELD scores lower than 15 would not be justified, because it would imply more risks than benefits [20]. However, the decision to transplant a patient cannot depend on a single score and the clinical situation and quality of life should be taken into consideration.

Further refinement of MELD should improve fairness in organ allocation. Other variables such as sodium or age have been incorporated into the formula with this intention, but with discordant results [21]. For this reason, the interaction between MELD and sodium was evaluated in a large cohort of patients on the waiting list in the United States (OPTN). The authors found that compared with the MELD score, the addition of sodium (MELD Na score) provided better calibration and discrimination of the risk of death among candidates for LT.

In conclusion, the CTP and the MELD scores are very useful tools to predict mortality in patients with cirrhosis. Patients with CTP score >7 and MELD score >14 should be considered for LT. These scores do not substitute but complement the clinical evaluation of a cirrhotic patient when determining candidacy for LT.

Quality of life as an indication for LT

Most patients with decompensated cirrhosis have a poor quality of life, perhaps directly related to specific complications such as refractory ascites that requires repeated paracenteses at short intervals, and chronic encephalopathy. In these cases, the indication for LT is obvious and mainly related to the mortality implied by each of the complications. However, a minority of patients present a reduced quality of life without having the classic complications of cirrhosis or high CTP and MELD scores. This is frequently observed in patients with cholestatic diseases complicated with refractory pruritus. There is no accurate way of measuring quality of life in these cases as this aspect is not incorporated in any allocation system. Transplantation of patients with deteriorated quality of life but without a reduction in life expectancy is controversial, because it would limit the opportunities for other patients at risk of death to be transplanted.

Evaluation of candidates for liver transplantation

Once the decision to transplant a patient has been made, the next step is to perform a thorough evaluation of the candidate in order to detect possible contraindications for LT and to determine individual risks related to the surgery. In general, each transplant center designs a protocol to evaluate the candidate. The clinical history and physical examination together with specific diagnostic tests are performed with special attention to the following aspects.

Extrahepatic diseases The candidates are considered at increased high risk in the presence of any severe extrahepatic disease that might interfere with the surgery or with the postoperative course. Cardiovascular and respiratory diseases not related to the cirrhosis are the most common conditions that might contraindicate LT.

Coronary artery disease and chronic obstructive pulmonary disease are frequently detected during the evaluation of a candidate. Most centers perform cardiovascular (EKG, echocardiography) and respiratory (chest X-ray, pulmonary function tests, oxygen saturation) assessments in the pretransplant evaluation.

As dobutamine stress echocardiography seems to be an effective screening test for occult coronary disease, some guidelines recommend it in patients with risk factors [20]. However, there is no general agreement on the matter. Cardiac catheterization should be performed in patients with positive stress tests in order to confirm and to further delineate the extent of the coronary disease. It should also be performed in patients with known coronary artery disease [20].

In the evaluation of pulmonary disease, further studies (e.g., computed tomography, diffusion tests) are performed if the medical history and physical examination or the initial work-up suggest advanced disease. Any other diseases must be evaluated together with the specialist so as to estimate the specific risks.

Extrahepatic malignancies As immunosuppression might increase the risk of recurrence and de novo malignancies, patients with a history of extrahepatic malignancies must have a prudent period of control before LT. At present, there is no consensus on the optimal window of time between oncologic cure and LT. A period of at least a 5-year tumor-free interval before LT seems adequate [22] but the decision should be taken on a case-by-case basis.

Nutritional status Both obese and malnourished patients are frequently evaluated for LT. Even though there is no general agreement, morbid obesity and severe malnutrition should be considered contraindications for LT. When possible, every effort should be made to help obese patients to achieve weight loss before LT [20]. The nutritional status of malnourished patients can be improved by means of enteral or parenteral nutrition to improve post-LT outcomes [23]. However, this is difficult to achieve in patients with advanced cirrhosis.

Alcohol and substance abuse Cigarette smoking is associated with worse outcomes in terms of specific complications in the postoperative period and with higher risks of coronary artery disease and malignancies [24,25]. Even though smoking is not a major contraindication for LT, all candidates should be encouraged to try to abstain from smoking [20]. A history of heavy alcohol consumption or even active alcohol consumption is frequently observed in patients who are being evaluated for LT. Most centers require a 6-month abstinence period before LT [26]. This requirement has two main objectives. The first is related to the chance of liver function improvement, which may be achieved with abstinence in selected cases. The second objective aims to detect patients at risk of relapse after LT [27].

It is essential to rule out drug abuse (e.g., opiates, sedatives, cannabinoids). This behavior denotes a high-risk group requiring psychiatric assessment and treatment. Active drug abuse is a relative contraindication to be listed for LT [28]. Such patients tend to be poorly compliant with post-transplantation care and follow-up, and thus have worse outcomes.

Age and psychosocial issues Age is no longer considered an absolute contraindication. Physiologic age, rather than chronologic age, dictates the individual's suitability for candidacy [28]. However, older patients have lower long-term survival rates after transplantation than younger individuals, mainly because of an increased risk of death from malignancies and comorbidities [20].

Individuals should meet reasonable expectations of compliance after LT. Therefore, any significant psychiatric disorders must be under medical control. In addition, patients must have adequate support during the perioperative period. This aspect is usually evaluated by a social worker and a mental health worker in the pre-transplant evaluation.

Osteoporosis As pathologic fractures are common after LT, screening and subsequent treatment or prevention of osteoporosis are mandatory in patients with cirrhosis prior to the procedure [20].

Hepatocellular carcinoma Post-LT results in patients with HCC fulfilling Milan criteria are excellent. Most centers consider HCC exceeding Milan criteria a formal contraindication for LT. However, some strategies might be applied in order to reduce the tumor burden in patients who exceed Milan criteria. Transarterial chemoembolization or percutaneous ablation might be indicated as a strategy to downstage or downsize the HCC and make some selected candidates suitable for LT [16]. Extrahepatic disease including portal and/or hepatic vein invasion is considered a major contraindication for LT [20].

Hepatopulmonary syndrome Patients with severe hypoxemia (PO2 <30 mmHg) have increased perioperative mortality and an expected survival of less than 12 months after LT [29]. There is no agreement on what degree of hypoxemia would contraindicate LT. For some centers, a PO2 <50 mmHg is considered a contraindication. Every effort should be made in order to perform LT before this level of hypoxemia is reached. This is the reason why most countries prioritize patients on the waiting list when the PaO2 >50 mmHg [19].

Portopulmonary hypertension Severe portopulmonary hypertension (PPH), defined as a mean pulmonary arterial pressure (MPAP) of ≥45 mmHg, is an absolute contraindication for LT, because mortality in the postoperative period is almost universal [30]. Patients with moderate PPH, defined as MPAP of 35–45 mmHg, should be evaluated with caution and candidacy should be determined on a case-by-case basis. Post-LT mortality rate in these patients might be as high as 50%. Patients with mild PPH, defined as a MPAP of 25–34 mmHg, are good candidates for LT [20].

Surgical issues Careful evaluation of portal vein patency by imaging is important in order to detect portal vein thrombosis, a frequent complication of end-stage liver disease. In some cases of diffuse thrombosis of the portal and mesenteric veins, LT might be technically not feasible [20]. Even though it is not a contraindication for LT, a higher risk of bleeding and of surgical complications is observed in patients with previous abdominal surgeries [20].

Cholangiocarcinoma In patients with end-stage liver disease secondary to primary sclerosing cholangitis, cholangiocarcinoma is a feared and frequent complication.

These patients should be excluded from consideration for LT because of the high incidence of recurrence [20].

Liver transplantation in patients with cirrhosis and renal failure

Renal failure prior to LT is a strong predictor of renal failure, other complications, and death after LT [31–33]. Acute renal failure is common in patients with end-stage liver disease, with an estimated prevalence of 30% [11]. Mortality in patients who are transplanted with acute renal failure might be as high as 50% at 12 months [34]. It is important to determine the etiology of renal failure, because patients with hepatorenal syndrome are likely to recover renal function after LT [34]. However, other etiologies of renal failure might not improve or might even worsen after LT and therefore may require simultaneous liver–kidney (SLK) transplantation [34].

The decision to perform an LT or an SLK transplant in this setting is not easy. If a single LT is performed and the renal function does not improve or it worsens after the procedure, the outcome is poor. On the other hand, if an SLK transplant is performed in cases in which the renal function might have recovered after a single LT, not only the morbidity and mortality related to the transplant increase, but also a kidney is unnecessarily removed from the donors' pool. The First International Liver Transplantation Society Expert Panel Consensus Conference on Renal Insufficiency laid out criteria for qualifying patients for SLK transplantation (Table 8.1) [34].

Hyponatremia is a frequent complication of end-stage liver disease. Approximately one-third of the candidates present some degree of hyponatremia at the time of LT. These patients have an increased rate of infectious and neurologic complications after LT. Rapid correction of hyponatremia after LT is associated with neurologic complications such as seizures and central pontine myelinolysis [35–37] so it is highly recommended to try to resolve this complication before LT is performed.

Table 8.1 Criteria for simultaneous liver–kidney transplantation.

- End-stage renal disease and dialysis
- No dialysis but a glomerular filtration rate <30 mL/minute *and* proteinuria >3 g/day with a 24-hour urine protein: creatinine ratio >3
- Acute kidney injury and a requirement for dialysis at least 2 times per week for more than 6 weeks

Table 8.2 Criteria for selection of HIV-positive patients for liver transplantation.

- CD4 counts >200 cell/mL or >100 cell/mL in the presence of portal hypertension
- Absence of viremia
- Absence of AIDS-defining illness after immune reconstitution
- Therapeutic options available if HIV disease reactivates

Liver transplantation in HIV-positive patients

The improvement of antiretroviral therapy changed the history of HIV disease, which is nowadays a controllable chronic disease [38]. End-stage liver disease has evolved as a significant cause of morbidity and mortality in HIV-positive patients [39,40]. Most cases of cirrhosis in the HIV-positive population are secondary to hepatitis C virus (HCV) co-infection [40]. Chronic hepatitis B and alcohol-related cirrhosis are also frequent in HIV-positive patients [40].

Performing LT in HIV-positive patients is complex and requires a multidisciplinary approach to select the adequate candidate (Table 8.2). Interactions between antiretrovirals and immunosuppressors on one hand, and severe HCV recurrence on the other hand, are the most challenging issues. Survival after LT in HIV-positive/HCV-negative patients is similar to the survival achieved in the HIV-negative population [41]. LT in HIV- positive/HCV-positive patients is associated with lower patient and graft survival than HCV mono-infected patients. Better refinement in recipient and donor selection will probably improve the outcomes in these patients [41].

Conclusions

LT is the only curative treatment for patients with decompensated cirrhosis. Excellent results are obtained when the candidate is property selected and evaluated. As contraindications for LT undergo frequent modifications, a case-by-case approach in consultation with the transplant center is suggested in complex cases. Most countries use the MELD allocating system. This strategy is under constant revision and might be refined or replaced in the near future. Mortality on the waiting list continues to pose a large problem. Only improvement in procurement and deceased donations might reverse this situation.

References

1 European Liver Transplant Registry. http://www.eltr.org/spip.php?rubrique37/ (accessed 24 August 2014).

2 Curry MP. Hepatitis B and hepatitis C viruses in liver transplantation. Transplantation 2004;78:955–63.

3 Hepp J, Innocenti FA. Liver transplantation in Latin America: current status. Transplant Proc 2004;36:1667–8.

4 Ganem D, Prince AM. Hepatitis B virus infection: natural history and clinical consequences. N Engl J Med 2004;350: 1118–29.

5 Angulo P. Nonalcoholic fatty liver disease and liver transplantation. Liver Transpl 2006;12:523–34.

6 OPTN and SRTR Annual Data Report 2010. http://srtr.transplant.hrsa.gov/annual_reports/2010/flash/03_liver/index.html (accessed September 3, 2014).

7 Foley DP, Fernandez LA, Leverson G, et al. Donation after cardiac death. Ann Surg 2005;242:724–31.

8 Renz JF, Emond JC, Yersiz H, Ascher NL, Busuttil RW. Split-liver transplantation in the United States: outcomes of a national survey. Ann Surg 2004;239:172–81.

9 Okamoto S, Wixner J, Obayashi K, et al. Liver transplantation for familial amyloidotic polyneuropathy: impact on Swedish patients' survival. Liver Transpl 2009;15:1229–35.

10 Otte JB, Ville-de-Goyet J, Reding R, et al. Pediatric liver transplantation: from the full-size liver graft to reduced, split, and living related liver transplantation. Pediatr Surg Int 1998;13:308–18.

11 D'Amico G, Garcia-Tsao G, Pagliaro L. Natural history and prognostic indicators of survival in cirrhosis: a systematic review of 118 studies. J Hepatol 2006;44:217–31.

12 Pomfret EA, Fryer JP, Sima CS, Lake JR, Merion MR. Liver and intestine transplantation in the United States, 1996–2005. Am J Transplant 2007;7:1376–89.

13 Child CG, Turcotte JG, Surgery and portal hypertension. Major Probl Clin Surg 1964;1:1–85.

14 Kamath PS, Kim WR. The Model for End-Stage Liver Disease (MELD). Hepatology 2007;45:797–805.

15 Mazzaferro V, Regalia E, Doci R, et al. Liver transplantation for the treatment of small hepatocellular carcinomas in patients with cirrhosis. N Engl J Med 1996;334:693–9.

16 Mendizabal M, Reddy KR. Current management of hepatocellular carcinoma. Med Clin North Am 2009;93:885–900.

17 Bruix J, Sherman M. Management of hepatocellular carcinoma. Hepatology 2005;42:1208–36.

18 Swanson KL, Wiesner RH, Krowka MJ. Natural history of hepatopulmonary syndrome: Impact of liver transplantation in the United States, 1996–2005. Am J Transplant 2007;7: 1376–89.

19 Krowka MJ, Porayko MK, Plevak DJ, et al. Hepatopulmonary syndrome with progressive hypoxemia as an indication for liver transplantation: case reports and literature review. Mayo Clinic Proc 1997;72:44–53.

20 Murray KF, Carithers RL. AASLD practice guidelines: evaluation of the patient for liver transplantation. Hepatology 2005;41:1407–32.

21 Biggins SW, Kim WR, Terrault NA, et al. Evidence-based incorporation of serum sodium concentration into MELD. Gastroenterology 2006;130:1652–60.

22 Ahmed A, Keeffe EB. Current indications and contraindications for liver transplantation. Clin Liver Dis 2007;11: 227–47.

23 Plauth M, Merli M, Kondrup J, et al. ESPEN guidelines for nutrition in liver disease and transplantation. Clin Nutr 1997;14:43–5.

24 Herrero JI, Lucena JF, Quiroga J, et al. Liver transplant recipients older than 60 years have lower survival and higher incidence of malignancy. Am J Transplant 2003; 3:1407–12.

25 Pungpapong S, Manzarbeitia C, Ortiz J, et al. Cigarette smoking is associated with an increased incidence of vascular complications after liver transplantation. Liver Transpl 2002;8:582–7.

26 Everhart JE, Beresford TP. Liver transplantation for alcoholic liver disease: a survey of transplantation programs in the United States. Liver Transpl Surg 1997;3:220–6.

27 Osorio RW, Ascher NL, Avery M, Bacchetti P, Roberts JP, Lake Jr. Predicting recidivism after orthotopic liver transplantation for alcoholic liver disease. Hepatology 1994;20: 105–10.

28 Varma V, Mehta N, Kumaran V, Nundy S. Indications and contraindications for liver transplantation. Int J Hepatol 2011;2011:1–9.

29 Schenk P, Schoniger-Hekele M, Fuhrmann V, Madl C, Silberhumer G, Muller C. Prognostic significance of the hepatopulmonary syndrome in patients with cirrhosis. Gastroenterology 2003;125:1042–52.

30 Krowka MJ, Plevak DJ, Findlay JY, Rosen CB, Wiesner RH, Krom RA. Pulmonary hemodynamics and perioperative cardiopulmonary-related mortality in patients with portopulmonary hypertension undergoing liver transplantation. Liver Transpl 2000;6:443–50.

31 Lafayette RA, Pare G, Schmid CH, King AJ, Rohrer RJ, Nasraway SA. Pretransplant renal dysfunction predicts poorer outcome in liver transplantation. Clin Nephrol 1997;48:159–64.

32 Bilbao I, Charco R, Balsells J, et al. Risk factors for acute renal failure requiring dialysis after liver transplantation. Clin Transplant 1998;12:123–9.
33 Nair S, Verma S, Thuluvath PJ. Pretransplant renal function predicts survival in patients undergoing orthotopic liver transplantation. Hepatology 2002;35:1179–85.
34 Charlton MR, Wall WJ, Ojo AO, et al. Report of the first international liver transplantation society expert panel consensus conference on renal insufficiency in liver transplantation. Liver Transpl 2009;15:S1–S23.
35 Estol CJ, Faris AA, Martinez AJ, Ahdab-Barmada M. Central pontine myelinolysis after liver transplantation. Neurology 1989;39:493–8.
36 Wszolek ZK, McComb RD, Pfeiffer RF, et al. Pontine and extrapontine myelinolysis following liver transplantation: relationship to serum sodium. Transplantation 1989;48:1006–12.
37 Pujol A, Graus F, Rimola A, et al. Predictive factors of in-hospital CNS complications following liver transplantation. Neurology 1994;44:1226–30.
38 Palella FJ, Delaney KM, Moorman AC, et al. Declining morbidity and mortality among patients with advanced human immunodeficiency virus infection. HIV Outpatients Study Investigators. N Engl J Med 1998;338:853–60.
39 Soriano V, Miró JM, García-Samaniego J, et al. Consensus conference on chronic viral hepatitis and HIV infection: updated Spanish recommendations. J Viral Hepat 2004;11:2–17.
40 Roland M, Stock P. Liver transplantation in HIV-infected recipients. Semin Liver Dis 2006;26:273–84.
41 Roland ME, Barin B, Carlson L, et al. HIV-infected liver and kidney transplant recipients: 1- and 3-year outcomes. Am J Transplant 2008;8:355–65.

PART 2
Complications of cirrhosis

CHAPTER 9
Acute-on-chronic liver failure

Danielle Adebayo, Vincenzo Morabito, and Rajiv Jalan
Liver Failure Group, UCL Institute for Liver and Digestive Health, UCL Medical School, Royal Free Hospital, London, UK

Introduction and definitions

Acute-on-chronic liver failure (ACLF) is a new clinical entity defined as an acute deterioration of pre-existing chronic liver disease, usually relating to a precipitating event characterized by a marked systemic inflammatory response, organ failure, and a high mortality rate [1,2]. Three types of ACLF have recently been described based on whether there is underlying cirrhosis [3]:

- *Type A ACLF* occurs in patients with chronic liver disease but no underlying cirrhosis (e.g., hepatitis B reactivation).
- *Type B ACLF* occurs in patients with well-compensated cirrhosis who rapidly deteriorate following a major hepatic insult.
- *Type C ACLF* occurs in patients with decompensated cirrhosis.

It is important to differentiate ACLF from chronic decompensation due to progression of cirrhosis as ACLF often results from an acute insult so there is an element of reversibility. Early recognition and aggressive treatment of the syndrome may reduce the high mortality rate associated with this condition. Figure 9.1 illustrates the difference in clinical course between ACLF and decompensated liver disease [4].

Epidemiology

The results from the recently published CANONIC study involving 1343 patients [1] carried out under the umbrella of the Chronic Liver Failure-EASL consortium has allowed the hepatology community to gain a better understanding not only of the epidemiology, but also of the diagnostic criteria and prognosis of ACLF. The syndrome is relatively common and is present in 23% of patients on admission or develops in a further 11% during hospitalization [1]. ACLF is associated with a 28-day mortality that is 15 times higher than patients with no ACLF [1]. It was once thought that in patients with ACLF who recovered from the acute insult, the long-term outcome was comparable to that of the patients with compensated cirrhosis. However, it is now known that in the subgroup of ACLF patients who develop organ failure and are discharged from hospital, future development of organ failure is common and nearly all the patients die within 3 years [5], suggesting that the occurrence of organ failure truly alters the natural history of the disease.

Pathophysiology

The pathophysiology of ACLF can be explained using the PIRO concept, which was initially developed for use in the sepsis setting [6]. Using this concept in ACLF, "P" stands for *predisposition*, predisposing factors that make a cirrhotic individual more likely to develop ACLF and organ failure. "I" represents the acute *insult or precipitating event*. "R" stands for the *inflammatory/immune response*, which occurs as a consequence of the acute insult. "O" signifies *organ dysfunction*, which is the final sequela of the inflammatory response generated following the acute insult [4].

Predisposition (P)

In a large prospective study of ACLF patients conducted over 6 years [5], it was clearly highlighted that cirrhotic patients who develop organ failure following an acute insult were more likely to be of male gender, have a high Child–Pugh or MELD score. The CANONIC study has provided more robust data demonstrating that patients

Cirrhosis: A practical guide to management, First Edition. Edited by Samuel S. Lee and Richard Moreau.

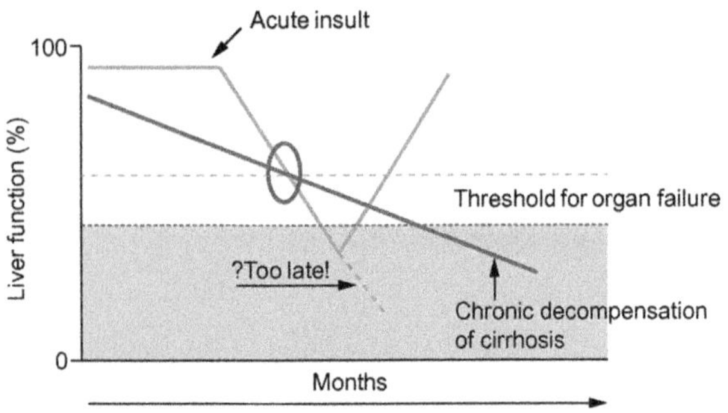

Figure 9.1 Representation of the clinical concept of acute-on-chronic liver failure (ACLF). This figure describes the clinical concept of ACLF to distinguish it from chronic decompensated cirrhosis. The black line describes the course of a patient with chronic decompensation of cirrhosis that during the evolution of their liver disease will at some point develop organ dysfunction. This is usually in association with advanced liver disease where the only option for treatment is liver transplantation and the chances of reversibility of liver disease are very limited. This is in contradistinction to the patient with ACLF (depicted by the solid gray line) who may often have a good liver reserve and can deteriorate acutely over a short period, usually in association with a precipitating illness that results in organ failure and high risk of death. The patient may also have advanced liver disease but be stable and deteriorate acutely following a precipitating event, and progress to organ failure. By contrast, this patient has the potential for reversibility and recovery to the state the patient was in prior to the acute event. Source: Jalan et al, 2012 [4]. Reproduced with permission of Elsevier.

with ACLF at enrollment are younger and are more likely to have alcoholic cirrhosis as the underlying cause for their cirrhosis but less likely to have hepatitis C virus-related cirrhosis [1,7].

Precipitating events/acute insult (I)

As patients with ACLF have previously stable disease on a background of either well-compensated or decompensated disease, and thus have a variable functional mass at the time of insult, the precipitants in ACLF are widely variable [8]. From the CANONIC study data, in 57% of patients, ACLF develops following an identifiable precipitating event. By extension, 43% of patients with ACLF did not have an identifiable precipitating event. In patients with an identifiable precipitant, bacterial infection was the most common cause and was observed in 33% of patients [1]. As well as bacterial infections such as spontaneous bacterial peritonitis and urinary tract infections, viral infections are also recognized precipitants of ACLF. For example, acute hepatitis A infection superimposed in a patient with chronic hepatitis B cirrhosis is associated with a higher risk of ACLF and thus a high mortality rate [9]. Cirrhotic patients who develop acute hepatitis B and E infections also have a high risk of developing ACLF and death [10,11]. Active alcoholism was another identified precipitant in the CANONIC study [1]. Table 9.1 summarizes precipitants of ACLF that have been described in the literature to date:

Table 9.1 Common precipitating events in acute-on-chronic liver failure (ACLF). The precipitants may directly affect the liver or may be a consequence of an extrahepatic insult.

Hepatic precipitants of ACLF	Extrahepatic precipitants of ACLF
Alcoholic hepatitis	Infection
Acute viral hepatitis (A, B, E)	Variceal hemorrhage
Drug-induced liver injury	Surgery
Portal vein thrombosis	Trauma
Ischemic hepatitis	

Inflammatory response (R)

Following the initial insult, there is an altered host response to injury resulting in an excessive systemic inflammatory response. This induces tissue damage and subsequent organ failure. In fact, the most striking difference between patients that develop ACLF and those that do not is that patients with ACLF demonstrate a more severe degree of inflammation [1]. The mechanism by which dysregulated inflammation occurs in ACLF appears to be multifactorial.

In addition to the precipitating insult (which may be infectious or non-infectious), there is abundant evidence in the literature to suggest that cirrhotic patients have increased bacterial translocation secondary to increased intestinal permeability and changes in intestinal microflora. Thus, patients with ACLF have increased levels of circulating endotoxins and are essentially exposed to two sources of insults. Indirect evidence of bacterial translocation in cirrhotic patients is derived from studies that have shown that up to 31% of non-infected cirrhotic patients are positive for bacterial DNA in serum and ascitic fluid. Furthermore, this group of patients were more likely to die over a 12-month follow-up period than patients who were bacterial DNA negative with the most common cause of death being ACLF [12].

Despite the insults, ACLF patients are unable to generate an adequate immune response because of a dysfunctional innate immune system [4,13,14]. In patients with ACLF, the Kupffer cells (resident macrophages of the liver and main effectors of innate immune system) are bypassed because of the presence of multiple intra- and extrahepatic shunts leading to failure to effectively clear endotoxins. In addition, the reduced protein synthesis that occurs in cirrhosis results in defective in complement production. This means that the opsonization capacity of the Kupffer cells is reduced and thus bacterial phagocytosis is impaired [14]. Another contributing factor to an altered host response in ACLF is a phenomenon known as "immune paralysis," akin to that seen in sepsis, and associated with a high mortality. It has been demonstrated that in ACLF patients there is reduced tumor necrosis factor α (TNF-α) production following stimulation with lipopolysaccharide. There is also a reduced expression of HLA-DR (an antigen-presenting receptor complex) on peripheral monocytes [15].

The consequence of the immune dysfunction is that the initiating insult overwhelms the host immune system leading to an exaggerated release of pro-inflammatory cytokines into the systemic circulation. This results in systemic inflammatory response syndrome (SIRS) [13,14,16]. SIRS is defined as the clinical expression of an abnormal generalized inflammatory reaction in organs distant from the initiating insult [16]. It is reported that up to 42% of ACLF patients who develop organ dysfunction have evidence of SIRS despite the absence of infection in these patients [5]. In addition, in the CANONIC study, the patients with ACLF had significantly higher plasma levels of C-reactive protein than patients without ACLF [1]. The presence of SIRS is associated with more severe encephalopathy, an increased incidence of bacterial infection, and renal failure [17]. SIRS also occurs more frequently in nonsurvivors of ACLF than in survivors [5].

Innate immune dysfunction also results in macrocirculatory dysfunction. It is known that patients with ACLF have a hyperdynamic circulation and high cardiac output. There is also peripheral vasodilatation and a low systemic vascular resistance resulting in a reduced effective arterial volume and a decrease in mean arterial blood pressure. The consequence of these circulatory changes is end-organ hypoperfusion. This, in combination with a SIRS response, may result in organ failure, multi-organ failure, and ultimately death [13].

Organ dysfunction (O)

Organ failure has a central role in the clinical course of ACLF occurring in one-third of hospitalized patients with chronic liver disease [1]. In addition to the liver, the organs commonly affected include the kidneys, brain, circulatory system, and adrenal glands. In the CANONIC study, the diagnosis of organ failure was defined as in Table 9.2.

Liver The hallmark of the liver manifestation of ACLF is hyperbilirubinemia and coagulopathy. Hyperbilirubinemia arises as a result of reduced detoxification function of the liver. In addition, the reduction in the liver's synthetic function leads to a decrease in the production of coagulation factors and, as a consequence, coagulopathy results. Hyperbilirubinemia and coagulation failure have been identified as independent predictors of mortality in

Table 9.2 The EASL-CLIF consortium diagnostic criteria for ACLF in patients with chronic liver disease following an acute decompensation.

Organ system	Variable	Value
Liver	Bilirubin (mg/dL)	>12
Kidney	Creatinine (mg/dL)	≥2 or renal replacement
Brain	Hepatic encephalopathy (HE) grade	III–IV
Coagulation	International normalized ratio (INR)	>2.5
Circulation	Vasopressor	Any use of vasopressors
Lungs	PaO/FiO_2 SpO_2/FiO_2	<200 <214

No-ACLF
- Patients with no organ failure
- Patients with single hepatic coagulation, circulation or respiratory failure, serum creatinine <1.5 mg/dL, and no HE
- Patients with cerebral failure and serum creatinine <1.5 mg/dL

ACLF-1
- Patients with single kidney failure
- Patients with other single failure with: serum creatinine ≥1.5 and <2 mg/dL; HE grade I–II

ACLF-2
- Patients with two organ failures

ACLF-3
- Patients with three or more organ failures

Data from Moreau et al., 2013 [1]. Reproduced with permission of Elsevier.

ACLF [4,5,18,19]. Histopathologically, it appears that the presence of cholestasis is associated with increased risk of infection and balloon degeneration may be associated with poorer outcome. The mechanism of cell death in this syndrome remains unclear.

Kidneys Kidney function is almost universally altered in patients with ACLF [20]. Renal failure defined using the EASL-CLIF criteria is associated with a higher mortality risk than any other organ failure [3]. The most common causes of kidney failure are pre-renal azotemia, hepatorenal syndrome, and acute tubular necrosis [21]. SIRS is present in approximately 40% of patients with functional renal failure. In addition, the presence of SIRS in patients with functional renal failure was associated with an in-hospital mortality rate of 68% [22]. Further evidence that SIRS has an important role in kidney failure associated with ACLF is derived from studies that have shown the use of anti-inflammatory agents such as pentoxifylline improves renal function or significantly decreases the risk of developing renal failure in patients with alcoholic hepatitis [23,24].

Hepatorenal syndrome (HRS) is the development of functional renal failure in patients with advanced liver disease. Type 1 HRS, which occurs in an acute setting, is a rapidly progressive decline in renal function associated with a mortality rate of 80% at 2 weeks [25]. Our current understanding is that HRS develops as a result of the hemodynamic dysregulation associated with portal hypertension. In this setting, splanchnic vasodilatation leads to decreased effective arterial volume resulting in severe renal vasoconstriction and hypoperfusion. Activation of the sympathetic nervous system through a hepatorenal reflex arc is also thought to have a role. In addition, there is altered renal blood flow autoregulation in patients with HRS. However, attempts to restore this circulatory dysfunction with the use of splanchnic vasoconstrictors (terlipressin) and volume expanders (albumin) only improves renal function in about 40–50% of patients [26]. These observations indicate that other pathophysiologic mechanisms may be responsible for the development of HRS. Indeed, recent studies have demonstrated histopathologic evidence of renal tubular cell death associated with apoptosis, increased renal tubular expression of toll-like receptor 4 (TLR4), and increased urinary markers of acute kidney injury such as nGAL and more recently urinary TLR4 providing possible novel biomarkers and approaches to therapy [27].

Brain Hepatic encephalopathy (HE) can occur either as a precipitating factor or a consequence of ACLF. It is a feature in up to 75% of patients with ACLF [28]. Brain edema is central to the development of HE in ACLF. Hyperammonemia occurs in ACLF because of a reduction in the liver's detoxifying abilities. This high level of ammonia then diffuses into the brain. Once in the brain, it combines with glutamate to form glutamine. An increase in brain glutamine levels results in astrocyte swelling. Hyponatremia, another common finding in ACLF patients, also exacerbates astrocyte swelling because of differences in osmolality between the intracellular and the extracellular compartments [29,30]. Systemic inflammation also has a role in astrocyte swelling and cerebral edema. Patients with evidence of infection or SIRS are more likely to develop severe encephalopathy [31]. It is likely that a synergy exists between hyperammonemia and inflammation. The high level of ammonia may prime the brain to the deleterious effect of superimposed inflammation, by induction of microglial cells, which have a large repertoire for cytokine production. This explains why measures that reduce the ammonia levels or levels of endotoxemia reduce the occurrence of HE [4,32–34]. Recently, it has been shown that HE occurring in the context of ACLF is associated with an extremely poor prognosis [35].

Adrenals Adrenal insufficiency occurs in 68% of patients with cirrhosis and septic shock. Although the mechanism responsible for this is not clear, it may be related to reduction in adrenal blood flow, which occurs as a consequence of circulatory changes in ALCF. In addition, high levels of pro-inflammatory cytokines seen in ACLF inhibit cortisol synthesis. Adrenal insufficiency may contribute to the development of multiorgan failure in ACLF [36].

There is emerging evidence to suggest that extrahepatic organ failure may be more important in determining prognosis in ACLF [1,37]. Figure 9.2 summarizes our current understanding of the pathophysiology of ACLF.

Management and prognosis

As ACLF is a potentially reversible condition, every effort should be made to avoid further liver injury, identify any treatable precipitating illness early, support affected organs, and treat any complications until the liver

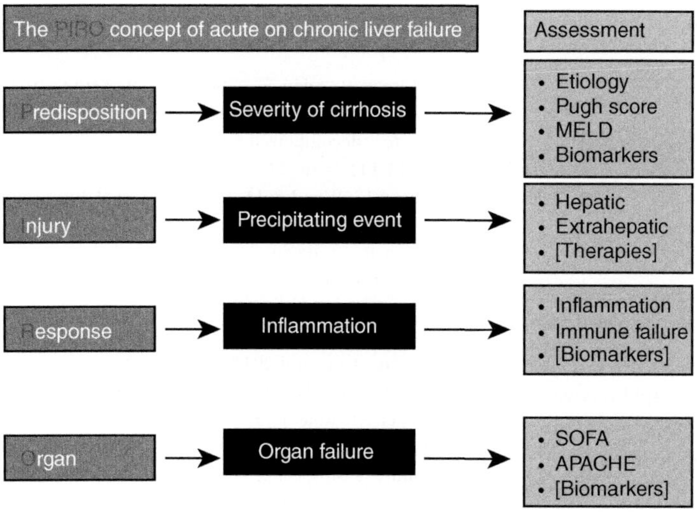

Figure 9.2 The PIRO concept of acute-on-chronic liver failure (ACLF). In patients with ACLF, it is useful to think about the PIRO concept in determining pathogenesis and prognosis. "Predisposition" is indicated by the severity of the underlying illness. "Injury" by the nature and severity of the precipitating event. "Response" by host response to injury, which determines the severity of inflammation and risk of infection. "Organs" by the extent of organ failure. Jalan et al., 2012 [4]. Reproduced with permission of Elsevier.

recovers. The main aim of management is to prevent the development of multi-organ failure, which is associated with a high mortality rate.

Patients diagnosed with ACLF should be admitted to a high dependency unit setting. General principles of management involve nutritional support, the use of intravenous antibiotics, ventilatory support, and inotropes.

Patients with renal insufficiency may require renal replacement therapy. In those with variceal hemorrhage, rapid control of the bleeding episode should be achieved either by endoscopy or insertion of a transjugular intrahepatic stent shunt. Attention should also be paid to nutritional support.

Liver support devices are intended to take over the liver's detoxification functions in patients with ACLF until liver transplantation, recovery, or futility [4]. There are two types of liver support devices available:

1 *Non-biologic systems* are the best-studied artificial liver support devices. The molecular adsorbent recirculating systems (MARS) and fractionated separation and adsorption system (Prometheus) are examples of non-biologic artificial devices that are based on the principle of albumin dialysis [38]. It is known that these devices allow the elimination of albumin-bound and water-soluble substances such as bilirubin, bile acids, and ammonia, which accumulate in liver failure [39]. The use of these devices can also encourage the elimination of inflammatory molecules, reduce nitric oxide, and improve systemic and hepatic hemodynamics [40]. A recent prospective, multicenter randomized controlled trial in ACLF patients using the MARS device failed to show a survival benefit using the device. However, MARS had an acceptable safety profile, significant dialysis effect, and nonsignificantly improved severe HE [41]. The HELIOS study is a multicenter randomized control trial that investigated the survival of ACLF patients treated with Prometheus. The use of Prometheus did not increase the probability of survival [42]. It is likely that modifications to the current devices will be necessary to improve their efficacy for use in ALCF patients as the clearance efficiency for albumin bound substances is still relatively low in all systems available today [4,38]. Recently, several anti-endotoxin strategies have been proposed as adjuvant therapy for endotoxin activity. Polymyxin B-immobilized fiber direct hemoperfusion (PMX-DHP) has been reported to be safe and effective in septic patients [43,44] and has demonstrated the ability to selectively remove endotoxin from the bloodstream, favorably impacting patient outcomes [45]. A retrospective study with ACLF patients provides interesting insight about the management of endotoxemia. PMX-DHP showed a

Table 9.3 Table showing the 28th and 90th day mortality according to ACLF grade.

Group	28-day mortality (%)	90-day mortality (%)
No-ACLF	4.7	14
ACLF-1	22.1	40.7
ACLF-2	32	52.35
ACLF-3	76.7	79.1

Data from Moreau et al., 2013 [1]. Reproduced with permission of Elsevier.

decrease of endotoxin levels, a more rapid recovery of hemodynamic stability, and reversal of the inflammatory state (TNF-α and IL-6) in the first 48 hours of treatment. In addition, a 100% survival was observed at 30-day follow-up [46].

2 *Bioartificial systems* use a bioreactor containing hepatocytes from human and animal sources coupled to a blood purification device to improve detoxification [38]. Examples of these devices are extracorporeal liver assist device (ELAD), which uses immortalized human hepatocyte cell lines, and HepatAssist, which uses porcine hepatocytes. There is a paucity of data regarding the use of these devices in ACLF patients.

Liver transplantation is the definitive treatment option in patients who fail to respond to supportive care. However, there is currently no means of high-urgency listing of these patients. Therefore, there is a high mortality in ACLF patients that do manage to make in onto the transplant list because this condition is associated with a high short-term mortality and timing is crucial. Table 9.3 shows the 28-day and 90-day mortality in the patients enrolled in the CANONIC study. In ACLF patients who are transplanted, the survival rates are similar to those in patients transplanted for other liver condition [47].

Conclusions

In summary, ACLF is a distinct clinical entity that has to be considered as a "syndrome." There are now data on the presentation and course of patients with this profile of liver failure. A better understanding of the pathogenesis of multi-organ failure in ACLF is crucial for the development of specific therapeutic approaches and further research in this area is required.

References

1 Moreau R, Jalan R, Gines P, et al. Acute-on-chronic liver failure is a distinct syndrome that develops in patients with acute decompensation of cirrhosis. Gastroenterology 2013;144:1426–37.
2 Olson JC, Wendon JA, Kramer DJ, et al. Intensive care of the patient with cirrhosis. Hepatology 2011;54:1864–72.
3 Jalan R, Yurdayin C, Bajaj JS, et al. Toward an improved definition of acute-on-chronic liver failure. Gastroenterology 2014;147:4–10.
4 Jalan R, Gines P, Olson JC, et al. Acute-on-chronic liver failure. J Hepatol 2012;57:1336–48.
5 Jalan R, Stadlbauer V, Sen S, Cheshire L, Chang YM, Mookerjee RP. Role of predisposition, injury, response and organ failure in the prognosis of patients with acute-on-chronic liver failure: a prospective cohort study. Crit Care 2012;16:R227.
6 Angus DC, Burgner D, Wunderink R, et al. The PIRO concept: P is for predisposition. Crit Care 2003;7:248–51.
7 Moreau, R. Arroyo, V. Acute on chronic liver failure: a new clinical entity. Clin Gastroenterol Hepatol 2014; in press.
8 Olson JC, Kamath PS. Acute-on-chronic liver failure: what are the implications? Curr Gastroenterol Rep 2012;14:63–6.
9 Keeffe EB. Is hepatitis A more severe in patients with chronic hepatitis B and other chronic liver diseases? Am J Gastroenterol 1995;90:201–5.
10 Garg H, Sarin SK, Kumar M, Garg V, Sharma BC, Kumar A. Tenofovir improves the outcome in patients with spontaneous reactivation of hepatitis B presenting as acute-on-chronic liver failure. Hepatology 2011;53:774–80.
11 Kumar Acharya S, Kumar Sharma P, Singh R, et al. Hepatitis E virus (HEV) infection in patients with cirrhosis is associated with rapid decompensation and death. J Hepatol 2007;46:387–94.
12 Zapater P, Francés R, González-Navajas JM, et al. Serum and ascitic fluid bacterial DNA: a new independent prognostic factor in noninfected patients with cirrhosis. Hepatology 2008;48:1924–31.
13 Laleman W, Verbeke L, Meersseman P, et al. Acute-on-chronic liver failure: current concepts on definition, pathogenesis, clinical manifestations and potential therapeutic interventions. Expert Rev Gastroenterol Hepatol 2011;5:523–37; quiz 537.
14 Verbeke L, Nevens F, Laleman W. Bench-to-beside review: acute-on-chronic liver failure – linking the gut, liver and systemic circulation. Crit Care 2011;15:233.
15 Wasmuth HE, Kunz D, Graf J, et al. Hyperglycemia at admission to the intensive care unit is associated with elevated serum concentrations of interleukin-6 and reduced ex vivo secretion of tumor necrosis factor-alpha. Crit Care Med 2004;32:1109–14.
16 Antoniades CG, Berry PA, Wendon JA, Vergani D. The importance of immune dysfunction in determining outcome in acute liver failure. J Hepatol 2008;49:845–61.

17 Leithead JA, Ferguson JW, Bates CM, et al. The systemic inflammatory response syndrome is predictive of renal dysfunction in patients with non-paracetamol-induced acute liver failure. Gut 2009;58:443–9.
18 Singh N, Gayowski T, Wagener MM, Marino IR. Outcome of patients with cirrhosis requiring intensive care unit support: prospective assessment of predictors of mortality. J Gastroenterol 1998;33:73–9.
19 Zimmerman JE, Wagner DP, Seneff MG, et al. Intensive care unit admissions with cirrhosis: risk-stratifying patient groups and predicting individual survival. Hepatology 1996;23:1393–401.
20 Cardena A, Gines P. Acute-on-chronic liver failure: the kidneys. Curr Opin Crit Care 2011;17:184–9.
21 Hartleb M, Gutkowski K. Kidneys in chronic liver diseases. World J Gastroenterol 2012;18:3035–49.
22 Thabut D, Massard J, Gangloff A, et al. Model for end-stage liver disease score and systemic inflammatory response are major prognostic factors in patients with cirrhosis and acute functional renal failure. Hepatology 2007;46:1872–82.
23 Akriviadis E, Botla R, Briggs W, Han S, Reynolds T, Shakil O. Pentoxifylline improves short-term survival in severe acute alcoholic hepatitis: a double-blind, placebo-controlled trial. Gastroenterology 2000;119:1637–48.
24 Mookerjee RP, Sen S, Davies NA, Hodges SJ, Williams R, Jalan R. Tumour necrosis factor alpha is an important mediator of portal and systemic haemodynamic derangements in alcoholic hepatitis. Gut 2003;52:1182–7.
25 Ginès A, Escorsell A, Ginès P, et al. Incidence, predictive factors, and prognosis of the hepatorenal syndrome in cirrhosis with ascites. Gastroenterology 1993;105:229–36.
26 Fabrizi F, Dixit V, Martin P. Meta-analysis: terlipressin therapy for the hepatorenal syndrome. Aliment Pharmacol Ther 2006;24:935–44.
27 Shah N, Dhar D, El Zahraa Mohammed F, et al. Prevention of acute kidney injury in a rodent model of cirrhosis following selective gut decontamination is associated with reduced renal TLR4 expression. J Hepatol 2012;56:1047–53.
28 Katoonizadeh A, Laleman W, Verslype C, et al. Early features of acute-on-chronic alcoholic liver failure: a prospective cohort study. Gut 2010;59:1561–9.
29 Cordoba J, Garcia-Martinez R, Simon-Talero M. Hyponatremic and hepatic encephalopathies: similarities, differences and coexistence. Metab Brain Dis 2010;25:73–80.
30 Garcia-Martinez R, Cordoba J. Acute-on-chronic liver failure: the brain. Curr Opin Crit Care 2011;17:177–83.
31 Shawcross DL, Sharifi Y, Canavan JB, et al. Infection and systemic inflammation, not ammonia, are associated with Grade 3/4 hepatic encephalopathy, but not mortality in cirrhosis. J Hepatol 2011;54:640–9.
32 Bass NM, Mullen KD, Sanyal A, et al. Rifaximin treatment in hepatic encephalopathy. N Engl J Med 2010;362:1071–81.
33 Wright G, Davies NA, Shawcross DL, et al. Endotoxemia produces coma and brain swelling in bile duct ligated rats. Hepatology 2007;45:1517–26.
34 Wright G, Vairappan B, Stadlbauer V, Mookerjee RP, Davies NA, Jalan R. Reduction in hyperammonaemia by ornithine phenylacetate prevents lipopolysaccharide-induced brain edema and coma in cirrhotic rats. Liver Int 2012;32: 410–9.
35 Cordoba J, Ventura-Cots M, Simón-Talero M, et al. Characteristics, risk factors, and mortality of cirrhotic patients hospitalized for hepatic encephalopathy with and without acute-on-chronic liver failure (ACLF). J Hepatol 2014;60:275–81.
36 Fernández J, Escorsell A, Zabalza M, et al. Adrenal insufficiency in patients with cirrhosis and septic shock: effect of treatment with hydrocortisone on survival. Hepatology 2006;44:1288–95.
37 Bajaj JS, O'Leary JG, Reddy KR, et al. Survival in infection-related acute-on-chronic liver failure is defined by extrahepatic organ failures. Hepatology 2014;60:250–6.
38 Krisper P, Stadlbauer V, Stauber RE. Clearing of toxic substances: are there differences between the available liver support devices? Liver Int 2011;31 (Suppl 3): 5–8.
39 Krisper P, Haditsch B, Stauber R, et al. In vivo quantification of liver dialysis: comparison of albumin dialysis and fractionated plasma separation. J Hepatol 2005;43:451–7.
40 Sen S, Davies NA, Mookerjee RP, et al. Pathophysiological effects of albumin dialysis in acute-on-chronic liver failure: a randomized controlled study. Liver Transpl 2004;10: 1109–19.
41 Bañares R, Nevens F, Larsen FS, et al. Extracorporeal albumin dialysis with the molecular adsorbent recirculating system in acute-on-chronic liver failure: the RELIEF trial. Hepatology 2013;57:1153–62.
42 Kribben A, Gerken G, Haag S, et al. Effects of fractionated plasma separation and adsorption on survival in patients with acute-on-chronic liver failure. Gastroenterology 2012;142:782–9.
43 Cruz DN, Perazella MA, Bellomo R, et al. Effectiveness of polymyxin B-immobilized fiber column in sepsis: a systematic review. Crit Care 2007;11:R47.
44 Shimizu T, Endo Y, Tsuchihashi H, Akabori H, Yamamoto H, Tani T. Endotoxin apheresis for sepsis. Transfus Apher Sci 2006;35:271–82.
45 Foreman MG, Mannino DM, Moss M. Cirrhosis as a risk factor for sepsis and death: analysis of the National Hospital Discharge Survey. Chest 2003;124:1016–20.
46 Novelli G, Morabito V, Pugliese F, et al. Management of sepsis during MARS treatment in acute on chronic liver failure. Transplant Proc 2011;43:1085–90.
47 Chan AC, Fan ST, Lo CM, et al. Liver transplantation for acute-on-chronic liver failure. Hepatol Int 2009;3:571–81.

CHAPTER 10
Hepatocellular carcinoma

Kwang-Hyub Han and Do Young Kim
Department of Internal Medicine, Yonsei University College of Medicine, Seoul, Korea

Introduction

Hepatocellular carcinoma (HCC) accounts for 70–85% of the total primary liver cancers worldwide [1]. HCC is diagnosed in more than a half million people annually and is a fatal disease, the second most frequent cause of cancer-related deaths in males [2]. The global distribution of HCC prevalence represents a difference in etiologic factors of HCC among geographic areas. The highest prevalence of HCC in Eastern Asia and sub-Saharan Africa primarily comes from chronic hepatitis B virus (HBV) infection in these areas. Hepatitis C virus (HCV) infection is also a major cause of HCC development in the United States, Japan, and central European countries [3]. Depending on the region, there are other risk factors including alcohol, obesity, and nonalcoholic steatohepatitis (NASH), α-1 antitrypsin deficiency, hemochromatosis, autoimmune hepatitis, and Wilson's disease [4]. Cirrhosis is recognized as the most important risk factor of HCC, and the annual risk of HCC development is 3–8% in HBV-associated cirrhosis and 1–7% in HCV-related cirrhosis [4,5]. In addition, the probability of HCC development is directly correlated with the stage of liver fibrosis in patients with chronic liver disease [6].

Clinical features

The symptoms caused by HCC are variable, nonspecific, and hard to differentiate from complications of cirrhosis per se. Although fatigue and loss of appetite might be the initial symptoms, patients with early stage HCC usually do not present with any symptoms. Abdominal pain is uncommon, but when present usually signifies a very large tumor extending to the surface of liver capsule or extrahepatic spread. Weight loss and unexplained fever are alarming signs that should trigger a search for HCC in cirrhotic patients. Deterioration of hepatic function in cirrhotic patients, from compensated to decompensated state, or aggravation of cirrhotic complications can be accompanied by HCC development. HCC invasion to the portal vein may decrease blood flow into the liver, which in turn leads to jaundice, ascites, edema, hepatic encephalopathy, or variceal hemorrhage. When HCC grows and metastasizes to other organs, varied symptoms of new onset can occur, such as bone pain (bony metastasis), dyspnea (lung metastasis), and neurologic symptoms (brain or spinal metastasis).

On physical examination, a palpable mass with or without tenderness on the right upper quadrant is often a finding to suggest that HCC has already progressed to an advanced stage. Jaundice is a bad prognostic sign, and implies HCC invasion into the portal vein or bile duct, or poor underlying liver function. Other signs including muscle wasting, pitting edema, ascites, and palmar erythema are not specific to HCC because they can also be observed as cirrhotic complications.

Surveillance of HCC

Screening is a one-time application of tests for detecting a disease at an early stage. For HCC, the term "surveillance," which is repeated application of screening, is more appropriate because patients with risk factors have life-long probability of developing HCC [7]. As surveillance has been found to significantly reduce HCC mortality by detecting more cancers at an early stage, it is recommended in high risk populations (i.e., cirrhotics with or without chronic HBV or HCV infections) [8]. Surveillance is usually performed using abdominal ultrasound (US) and

Cirrhosis: A practical guide to management, First Edition. Edited by Samuel S. Lee and Richard Moreau.

serum alpha-fetoprotein (AFP) measurement at regular intervals [9]. However, US is more sensitive and specific than AFP elevation for early detection of HCC [10]. The incorporation of serologic markers in surveillance program to complement US is a matter of debate. Any tumor marker including serum AFP is not recommended as a surveillance test in Western countries because of its inadequate sensitivity and specificity [10–13]. On the contrary, data from clinical practice suggest that performance of AFP might be better than US and that combination of US and AFP could improve sensitivity to 90% with minimal loss of specificity [14]. The interval for HCC surveillance in cirrhotic patients has been set at 6–12 months, based on the estimated tumor growth rate. Six-month interval seems to be superior to 12 month in terms of detection of early stage HCC, application of curative treatment, and overall survival [15].

Diagnosis and staging

Unlike other solid tumors, the diagnosis of HCC is largely made by noninvasive methods such as computed tomography (CT) scan and magnetic resonance imaging (MRI). Although liver biopsy for pathologic confirmation has several limitations of false-targeting, risk of bleeding complication, and tumor seeding, it is currently the gold standard of HCC diagnosis [16]. However, the increasing accuracy and specificity of imaging studies has largely eliminated the need for routine liver biopsy (Figure 10.3).

HCC usually takes a multi-step carcinogenesis from chronic inflammation to low or high grade dysplastic nodule (DN) and to small HCC. DN, a pre-cancerous lesion, is characterized by a distinctly nodular lesion (1 cm in size) differing from the surrounding liver parenchyma regarding size, color and texture, and bulges on the cut surface. The cellular atypia is at least moderate in high grade DN, compared with mild in low grade DN, but insufficient for HCC diagnosis. The differentiation between high grade DN and well-differentiated HCC is often difficult and identification of stromal invasion of tumor cells supports the HCC diagnosis [17].

Dynamic contrast-enhanced CT scan is an essential part of HCC diagnosis. Furthermore, the enhanced speed and flexibility of multi-detector CT (MDCT) has enabled higher spatial and temporal resolution of small lesions. Following rapid intravenous infusion of contrast, images are acquired at various time intervals corresponding to the phase of contrast enhancement. HCC derives blood flow predominantly from the hepatic artery and tends to enhance during the arterial phase or 2–40 seconds after contrast infusion. On the contrary, the surrounding hepatic parenchyma obtains 75–80% of its blood flow through the portal vein and is best demonstrated 50–90 seconds after contrast infusion during the portal phase. This "arterial enhancement" and "venous washout'" are a pattern typical of HCC on dynamic CT scan (Figure 10.1) [18]. MRI offers higher tissue contrast than CT in the evaluation of HCC. Moreover, gadoxetic acid, which behaves as an extracellular agent in the early phase and as a hepatobiliary agent in delayed phase, may allow for accurate diagnosis based on hemodynamics and hepatocyte function (Figure 10.2). MR scan using this contrast agent appears to have better performance than multi-phase CT scan in the differentiation of HCC from chronic liver disease, especially for a lesion <1 cm [19,20].

Contrast-enhanced ultrasound (CEUS) is an imaging technique that uses microbubble contrast agents that are small (3–5 μm) enough to pass thorough the pulmonary circulation. After a bolus injection, the contrast agents show strong vascular enhancement and slowly diffuse into the blood over about 5 minutes [21]. In particular, Sonazoid, a new contrast agent, can be engulfed by Kupffer cells and has a postvascular phase which begins 10 minutes after contrast injection and lasts for 60 minutes. Lack of Kupffer cells in HCC shows an enhancement defect in postvascular phase while benign lesions show sustained enhancement [22]. The advantages of CEUS over dynamic CT or MRI are no deterioration of renal function, real-time assessment of enhancement pattern, and good tolerability [21].

Clinical criteria for noninvasive diagnosis of HCC has been evolving with the increasing accuracy of dynamic studies such as CT and MRI scans. In cirrhotic patients, a nodule or mass >2 cm can be diagnosed as HCC if the imaging finding is compatible with HCC (i.e., arterial hypervascularity and portal/venous washout), in one of multi-phase CT and MRI. A nodule between 1 and 2 cm poses a diagnostic challenge even by biopsy [23–25]. It remains controversial whether one or two dynamic imaging modalities are necessary for the lesion sized 1–2 cm. For a lesion less than 1 cm, repeated US follow-up with a 3–4 month interval is recommended to see any growth, because most of the lesions are large regenerative nodules

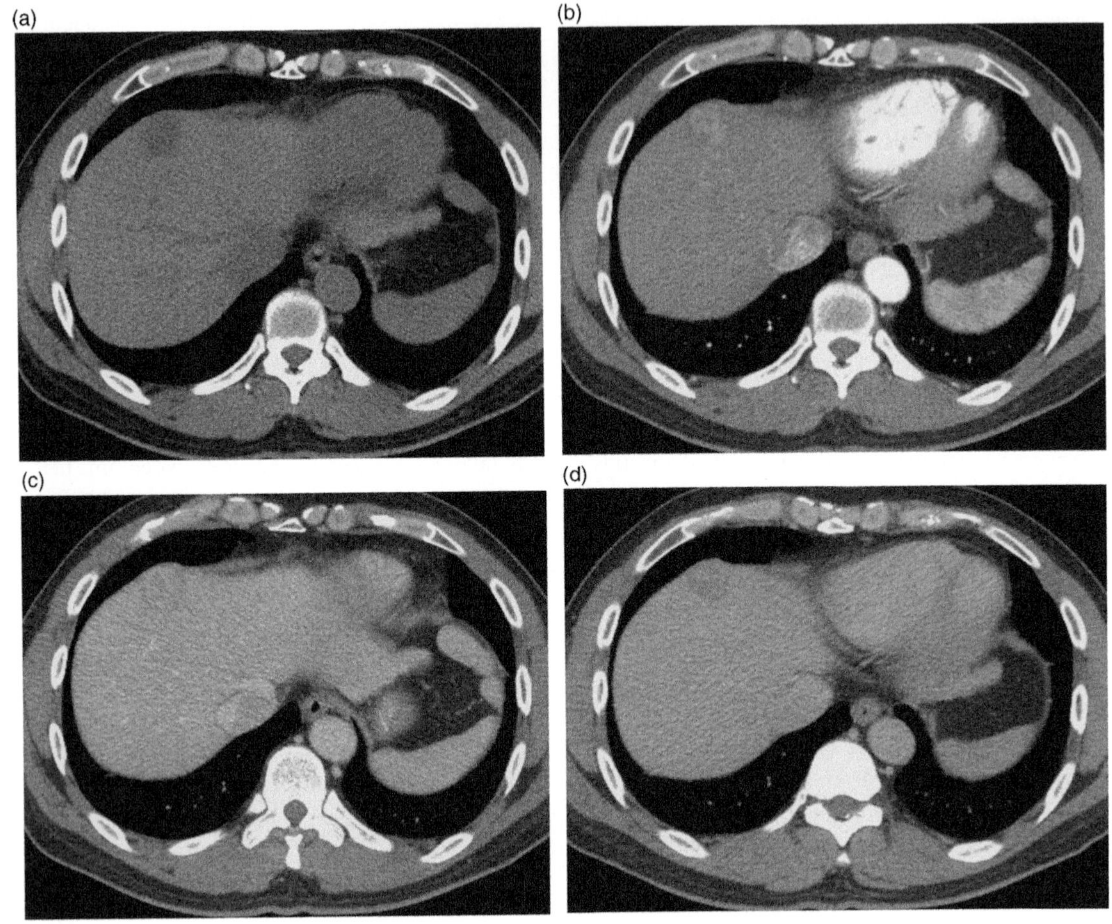

Figure 10.1 Four-phase, contrast-enhanced images of hepatocellular carcinoma from computed tomography (CT) scan. (a) Pre-contrast phase; (b) a hypervascular, enhancing nodule is observed in the anterior, superior right lobe of liver in the arterial phase; (c) the contrast has washed-out from the nodule in portal venous phase; (d) more wash-out is seen in delayed phase.

or dysplastic nodules. The diagnostic algorithm for HCC is presented in Figure 10.3. The use of CEUS in HCC diagnosis has been excluded from updated American Association for the Study of Liver Diseases (AASLD) guidelines for the reason that intrahepatic cholangiocarcinoma can be misdiagnosed as HCC [26]. However, this issue needs to be further studied.

It is important to assess the stage of HCC accurately and consistently at the time of diagnosis for stratifying patients to predict overall survival, facilitate treatment, and enable comparison of research outcomes. Because of the heterogeneity and complex clinicopathologic characteristics of HCC as well as cirrhotic background which is accompanied in most HCCs, various staging systems have been developed. The tumor–node–metastasis (TNM) staging system proposed by the American Joint Committee on Cancer (AJCC) is the most widely applied in solid cancers [27]. Although this staging was originally based on pathologic information after surgical operation, validation in HCC patients who underwent nonsurgical treatment has been tried according to advancement in imaging techniques [28]. As the overall survival of HCC patients is substantially affected by underlying liver function, several staging systems included Child–Pugh score or class. The Cancer of Liver Italian Program (CLIP) score combines tumor factors (tumor morphology, AFP, portal vein thrombosis) and Child–Pugh score to generate a simple scoring system [29]. Similarly, Japanese Integrated Staging (JIS) combines Japanese TNM system and Child–Pugh class to produce a score of 0–5 [30].

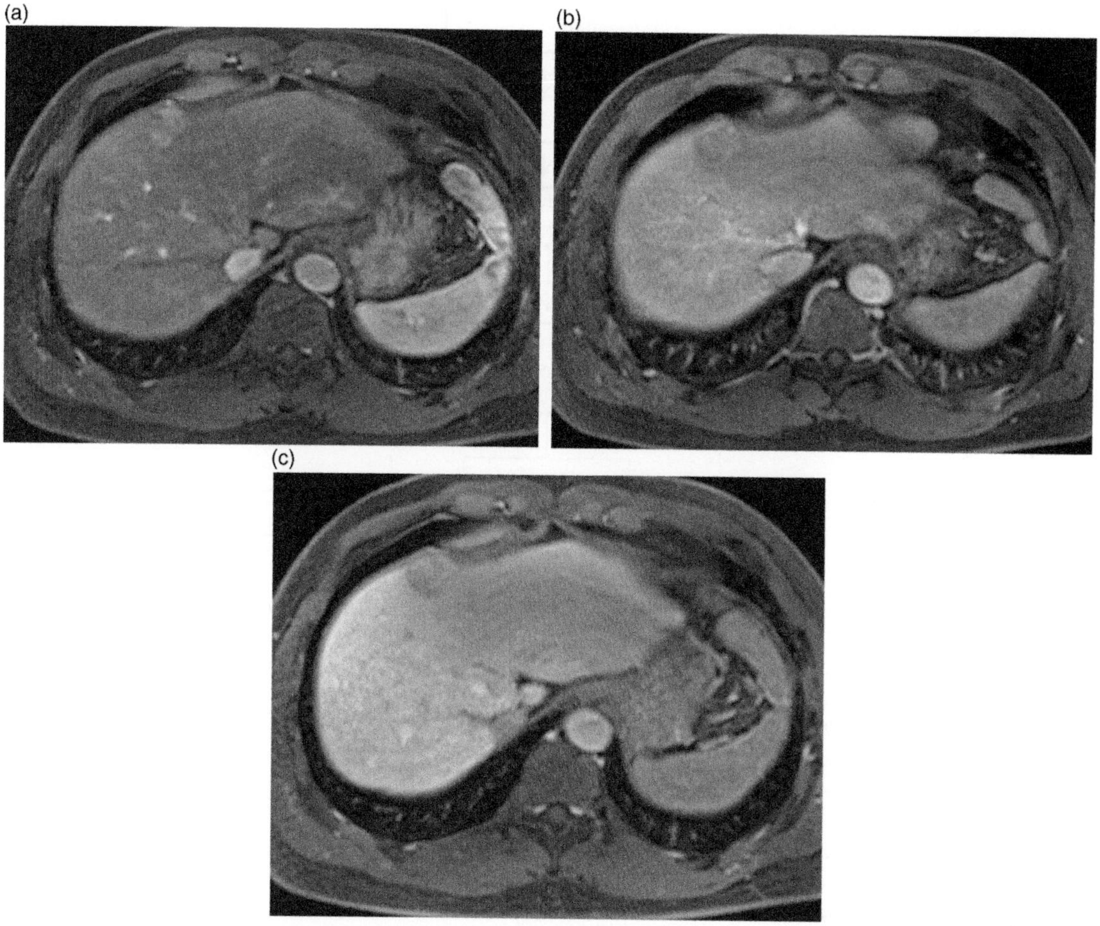

Figure 10.2 Features of dynamic magnetic resonance imaging (MRI) of hepatocellular carcinoma. (a) An enhancing nodule-in-nodule is noticed in arterial phase; (b) wash-out of contrast dye from the nodule in portal venous phase; (c) the nodule shows low signal intensity compared with the neighboring parenchyma in delayed phase.

The prognostic value of these staging systems has been validated internally or externally [31,32]. However, it appears that none can be recommended universally because of the lack of validation in both Western and Asia-Pacific populations. The Barcelona Clinic Liver Cancer (BCLC) staging system, proposed in 1999, is the only one that is endorsed by AASLD and the European Association for the Study of the Liver (EASL) [33]. This is unique in that it offers specific treatment recommendations for each stage. Four categories of A (early), B (intermediate), C (advanced), and D (end-stage) are based on the tumor stage (tumor size, number of tumors, presence of portal vein invasion), liver function (Child–Pugh class, bilirubin level, portal hypertension), performance status indicated by European Cooperative Oncology Group (ECOG) scale, and cancer-related symptoms (Figure 10.4). BCLC B and C stages have broad ranges of tumors resulting in a wide range of survival, which makes it challenging for this staging system to provide a fine stratification of patients for clinical trial design. Refinement of intermediate and advanced stages combined with molecular classification like other cancers such as breast cancer would be more helpful.

Treatment

Surgical treatment

Liver resection is the first option of curative treatment for patients who have early stage HCC and well-preserved

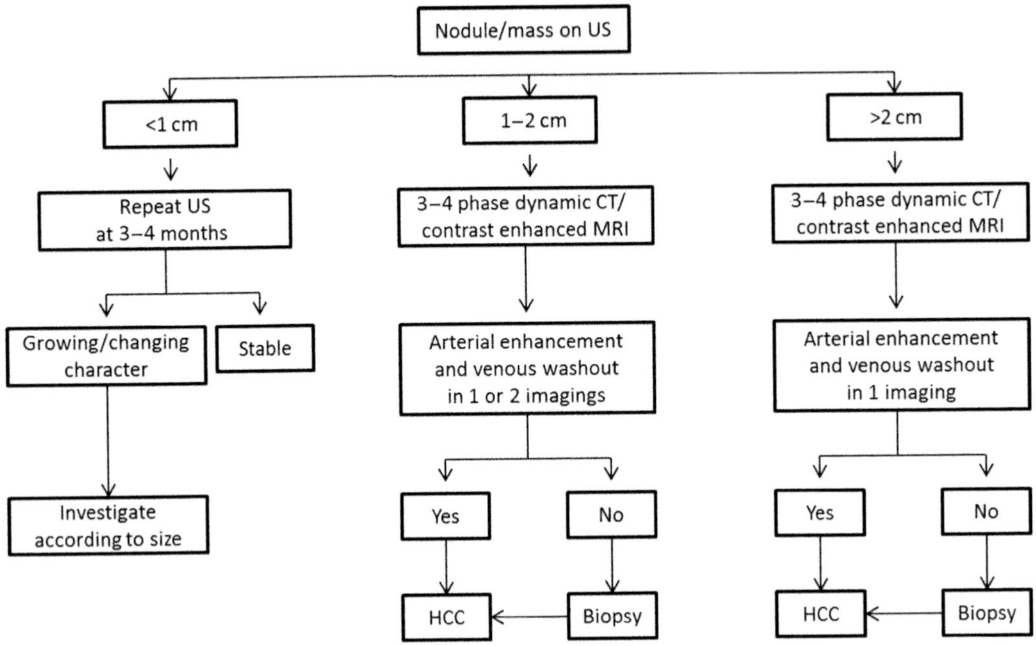

Figure 10.3 Diagnostic algorithm of hepatocellular carcinoma (HCC) (modified from AASLD and EASL guidelines). CT, computed tomography; MRI, magnetic resonance imaging; US, ultrasonography. Adapted from AASLD guidelines (www.aasld.org/practiceguidelines) and EASL guidelines (www.easl.eu/_clinical-practice-guideline).

liver function. Survival after resection has been increasing with the improvement of operative techniques, patient selection, and postoperative management. Anatomic resection is the standard technique to achieve complete removal of tumor in liver resection [34]. Preoperative measurement of liver function is important to avoid postoperative liver failure. Child–Pugh classification is a simple method to assess liver function, and patients with Child–Pugh class B or C are poor candidates for resection. However, this measure is insufficient to stratify the operative risk of patients with Child–Pugh A. The indocyanine green (ICG) clearance rate is commonly used in Asian countries to complement preoperative Child–Pugh classification. ICG-R15 up to 10–20% is generally necessary for a safe major hepatectomy [35]. The best candidate for surgical resection suggested by BCLC staging system is single HCC less than 2 cm in a patient with performance status 0, Child–Pugh class A, normal bilirubin level, and without portal hypertension [33]. The prognosis of HCC patients who receive a resection depends on underlying liver function and tumor factors including tumor size, vascular invasion, and presence of satellite nodules [36–38]. As recurrence of HCC even after apparently curative resection is quite common, careful monitoring is crucial.

Liver transplantation (LT) has the advantage that it would eliminate the tumor and cure the underlying liver disease. Early experiences of LT in HCC patients found that tumor burden determined success of LT. Patients with a solitary HCC of less than 5 cm or with up to three nodules less than 3 cm (the Milan criteria) have a 5-year survival of 70% after LT, with recurrence rates of less than 10% [39]. This survival is equal to that of most other indications for LT. The expansion of criteria for HCC patients requires a careful consideration about post-transplant outcomes in the context of absolute donor organ shortage. The University of California San Francisco (UCSF) criteria (one tumor ≤6.5 cm, three nodules at most with the largest ≤4.5 cm, and total tumor diameter ≤8 cm) is the only one which has been prospectively validated to be comparable to Milan criteria in terms of survival, even though the UCSF criteria were developed according to post-transplant pathologic findings [40]. Unlike deceased donor LT (DDLT) with organ

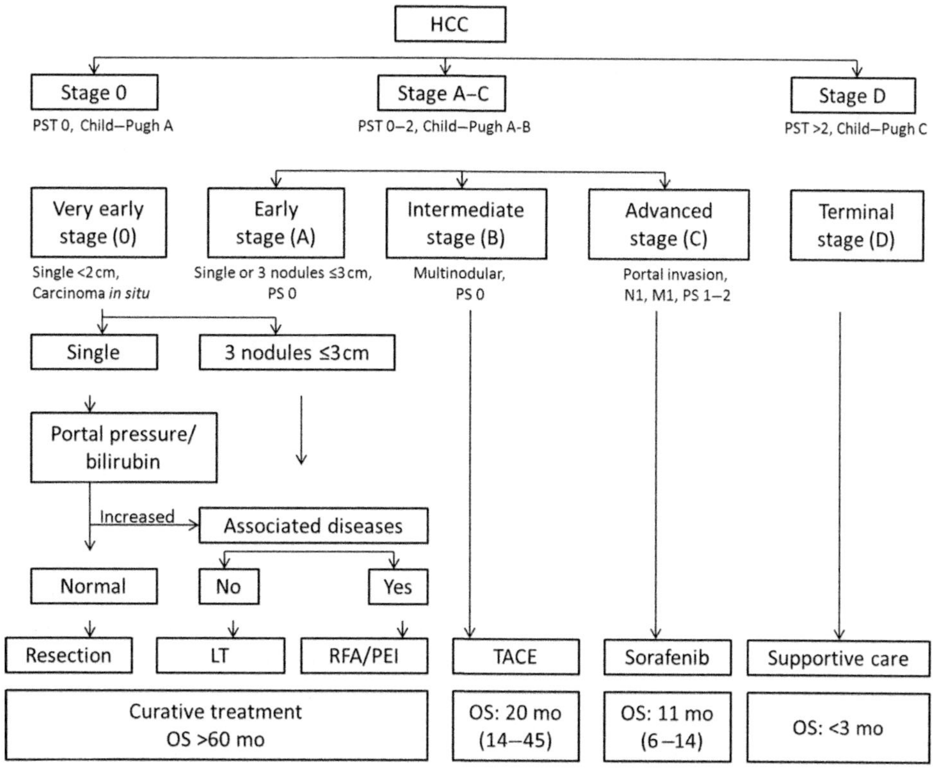

Figure 10.4 Barcelona Clinic Liver Cancer (BCLC) staging system. LT, liver transplantation; mo, month; OS, overall survival; PEI, percutaneous ethanol injection; PST, performance status; RFA, radiofrequency ablation; TACE, transarterial chemoembolization. Adapted from AASLD guidelines (www.aasld.org/practiceguidelines) and EASL guidelines (www.easl.eu/_clinical-practice-guideline).

donations from brain dead or non-heart-beating donors, living donor LT (LDLT) using the right or left lobe of a healthy donor is widely applied for the treatment of HCC in Asian countries including Korea and Japan, where there is limited or no availability of deceased-donor organs [41,42]. Post-transplant survival of patients seems to be similar between DDLT and LDLT although donor safety is one of the most important concerns in LDLT [43]. The decision which to choose as a primary modality between resection and LT needs to take several aspects into consideration including donor availability, tumor burden, liver function of recipient, and experience of the surgical team. Overall long-term survival is not different between LT and resection; however, HCC recurrence rate is higher after resection [44]. Given the limited availability of transplantable organs, resection remains the main curative modality especially for HCC patients with compensated liver function [45].

Local ablative therapy

Local ablative therapy (LAT) is a treatment modality for HCC, adopting physical or chemical tumor destruction by a needle inserted into the tumor. This technique is regarded as a curative method together with resection and LT, and includes percutaneous ethanol injection (PEI) and radiofrequency ablation (RFA). In a randomized controlled trial, RFA was superior to PEI with respect to overall survival, recurrence, and local tumor progression in the treatment of three or fewer lesions, each 3 cm or less in diameter [46]. In tumors ≤2 cm, there seems to be no difference in survival between RFA and PEI [47]. When performing RFA, there is a technical difficulty if a nodule is close to large vessels or bile duct, which act as heat sinks reducing thermal power. In addition, more meticulous sedation or analgesia is required to decrease procedure-related pain than with PEI [48].

Transarterial chemoembolization

The basic concept of transarterial chemoembolization (TACE) is that transarterial delivery of cytotoxic chemotherapeutic drugs combined with embolization of feeding arteries might cause enhanced local anticancer and ischemic effects to tumor tissue, reducing systemic adverse effects. The rationale for TACE is based on the predominant arterial blood supply to HCC in contrast with dual (portal vein and hepatic artery) supplies to the other liver tissue. In conventional TACE, administration of anticancer drugs mixed with lipiodol (iodinized poppy seed oil) is followed by occlusion of tumor feeding arteries with embolic material like gelfoam particles. This procedure requires advancement of a catheter into the hepatic artery and navigating it into the segmental and subsegmental branches to a point of administration that maximizes tumor exposure, and minimizes nontumor tissue damage [49]. Although TACE is the most commonly used locoregional modality for HCC, there is no standard protocol for this procedure and it remains unknown which drug or combination among doxurubicin, cisplatin, and mitomycin C exhibits the best therapeutic effect. The typical candidates for TACE are multiple tumors without vascular invasion or distant metastasis in patients whose liver function is Child–Pugh class A or B, which corresponds to BCLC stage B. However, HCC of intermediate stage includes a broad and heterogeneous population of patients who vary widely in terms of tumor burden and liver function. TACE was shown to provide a significant survival benefit compared to supportive care by two independent systematic reviews [50,51]. The most common adverse effect after TACE is fever which is a reflection of cytokine release in response to tumor necrosis and systemic exposure to chemotherapeutic drugs. Most patients undergoing TACE experience post-embolization syndrome which is self-limited and consists of fever, nausea, vomiting, and abdominal pain. More serious but less common adverse effects of TACE include renal failure, bone marrow aplasia, liver abscess, systemic infection, bile duct injury, cardiac toxicity due to doxorubicin, and hepatic failure. Furthermore, repeated sessions of TACE may result in hepatic arterial damage and deterioration of liver function.

The limitations of conventional TACE of inconsistency of techniques, size variation of gelfoam particles, and nonstandardized treatment schedule require improvement in catheter-based HCC management. Recently, TACE using DC Bead (Biocompatibles UK Ltd.), which is a novel drug delivery and embolic agent, may be preferred for TACE. TACE with DC Bead results in significantly higher rate of objective response with less systemic toxicity than conventional TACE [52–56]. However, it remains to be further studied whether DC Bead TACE could result in longer survival or decrease of recurrence after treatment compared with conventional TACE.

Systemic therapy

HCC displays a marked refractoriness to the currently available cytotoxic chemotherapy. Furthermore, this is usually aggravated because HCC readily develops drug resistance during systemic treatment [57]. Among the various underlying molecular mechanisms, multi-drug resistance-1 (*MDR-1*) gene expressed in HCC tissue may in part offer inherent resistance to cytotoxic agents [58]. Altered pharmacokinetics and metabolizing capability of liver, and variable drug binding and distribution are phenomena seen in HCC patients with cirrhosis, which are also limiting factors for selecting and dosing appropriate drugs. The response rate is low, and the duration of response is short. More importantly, survival benefit has been rarely documented for systemic administration of chemotherapeutic agents. Doxorubicin as a single agent showed a small but significant overall survival gain compared with supportive care. However, there was fatal toxicity in 25% of patients [59]. Combination regimen with cisplatin, interferon-α, doxorubicin, and 5-fluorouracil (PIAF) produced a promising result of 26% of response rate in a phase II study, but failed to show superior survival compared with doxorubicin alone in a phase III trial [60,61].

Among the complicated genetic and epigenetic alterations related to HCC pathogenesis, several signaling pathways have been implicated as key drivers for HCC development. Overactivation of Raf/MEK/ERK signaling pathway appears to be particularly important in this regard (Figure 10.5) [62]. Oncogenic mutation of *Ras* gene, overexpression of growth factors including platelet derived growth factor (PDGF) and vascular endothelial growth factor (VEGF), stimulation by HBV protein x (HBx), or HCV core protein can induce overactivation of Raf/MEK/ERK pathway, which in turn increases cell proliferation and survival [63]. Apart from tumor cell proliferation, angiogenesis is also involved in HCC invasion and metastasis [64]. Established pro-angiogenic

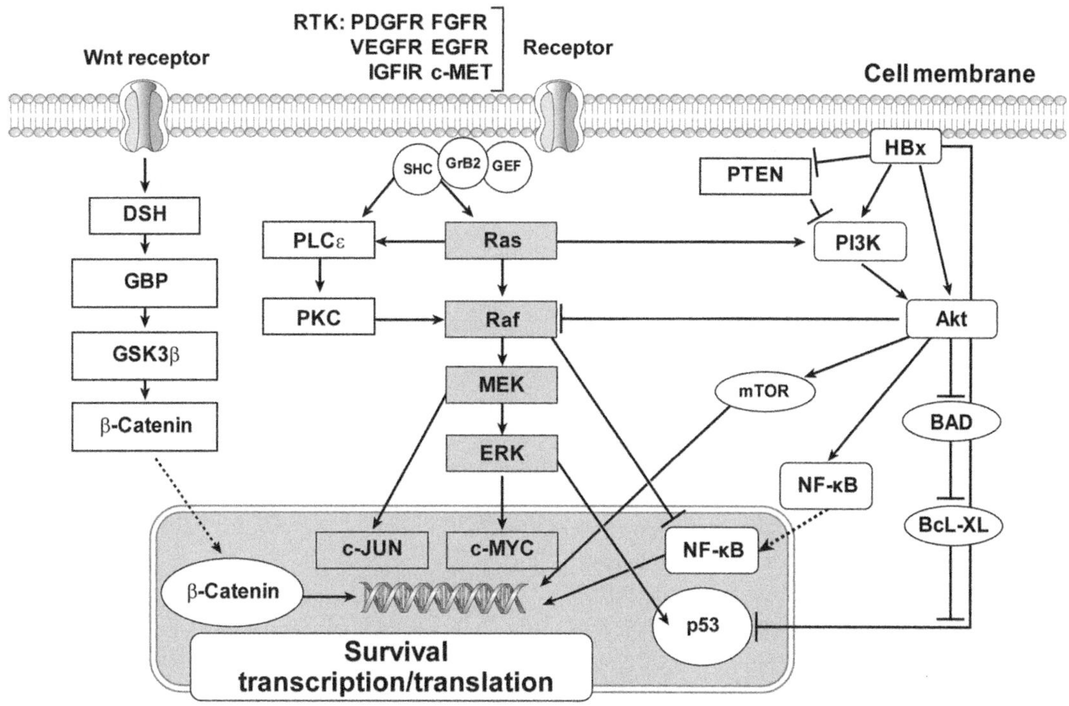

Figure 10.5 Signal transduction related with development of hepatocellular carcinoma. See text for abbreviations.

factors and their receptor signaling pathways in HCC include VEGF, fibroblast growth factor (FGF)-2, PDGF, and angiopoietin-2 [65].

Sorafenib is the first developed molecular targeted agent that blocks Raf/MEK/ERK pathway by inhibiting Raf serine/threonine kinase and also inhibiting the upstream receptor tyrosine kinases that are important in angiogenesis, such as VEGFR-2, VEGFR-3, PEGFR-β, and kit. In a phase III, multicenter, randomized trial of 602 patients with advanced stage HCC, median overall survival in the sorafenib group was 10.7 months versus 7.9 months in the placebo group (hazard ratio 0.69; 95% confidence interval 0.55–0.87; $P = 0.0001$). Survival benefit was preceded by a delay in time to progression: 5.5 months for sorafenib versus 2.8 months ($P < 0.001$) [66]. Based on these results, sorafenib was approved as the first systemic drug for patients with advanced HCC not amenable to other treatments including resection, ablation, and LT. Diarrhea and hand–foot skin reaction (HFSR) are consistently the most common adverse events in patients treated with sorafenib [66]. HFSR appears in the first 2–4 weeks of treatment as hyperkeratotic lesions with superficial blistering and callus formation usually affecting the flexural surfaces of the digits. The lesions typically have a peripheral halo of erythema and accompany symptoms of paresthesia, burning pain, and decreased tolerance to contact with hot objects [67]. Though the majority of HFSR cases are grade I or II, and manageable in Western patients, the incidence of HFSR was reported to be higher in Asian-Pacific patients [68]. Other sorafenib-related adverse effects include anorexia, alopecia, weight loss, dry skin, abdominal pain, and hypertension. Because of its adverse effects, relatively modest survival benefit (3 months in advanced HCC) and high cost, sorafenib is not widely used. However, as the era of molecular target therapy begins for HCC management, dozens of new tyrosine kinase inhibitors or monoclonal antibodies for HCC treatment are under clinical trials [69].

Other and emerging treatments

The heterogeneity of patient populations even in the same stage makes it difficult to obtain consistent outcomes after treatment. For example, post-TACE survival depends largely on tumor characteristics including tumor number and size in BCLC-B stage [70]. Therefore, there are several other treatment modalities that are used in clinical practice and they need to be compared with the current standard of care. With technical advancement, data regarding the anticancer efficacy of external beam radiation therapy have been accumulated in intermediate to advanced HCC [71,72]. Radioembolization with yttrium-90 represents a novel form of catheter-based, liver-directed radiotherapy. Although the precise indication for radioembolization is not established, a subset of patients with intermediate stage with multiple (>5) tumors, bilobar disease, and prior failure of TACE could be candidates, along with those with advanced HCC [73]. Hepatic arterial infusional chemotherapy (HAIC) is a kind of regional therapy to deliver chemotherapeutic agents directly to the tumor through supplying vessels, based on the first-pass effect of liver [74]. A randomized trial to compare HAIC with sorafenib in advanced HCC with portal vein invasion is ongoing. As recent studies have revealed that microRNA, which is endogenous ~22nt long single strand RNA, is closely related to HCC cell survival and metastasis, microRNA-based gene therapy is emerging as a novel and promising strategy in the treatment of HCC [75].

Conclusions

Recent progress in molecular biology has enabled deeper understanding of the pathogenesis of HCC and has resulted in more attention to this cancer, which had been called an "orphan disease." It has also made possible commencement of molecular targeted therapy. Apparently, heterogeneous tumor and patient characteristics make a multidisciplinary approach essential to the management of HCC. Also, clinical improvements in unsolved issues including early detection of HCC, more effective treatment of advanced HCC, and prevention of recurrence are necessary.

References

1 Perz JF, Armstrong GL, Farrington LA, et al. The contributions of hepatitis B virus and hepatitis C virus infections to cirrhosis and primary liver cancer worldwide. J Hepatol 2006;45:529–38.

2 Jemal A, Bray F, Center MM, et al. Global cancer statistics. Ca Cancer J Clin 2011;61:69–90.

3 Altekruse SF, McGlynn KA, Reichman ME. Hepatocellular carcinoma incidence, mortality, and survival trends in the United States from 1975 to 2005. J Clin Oncol 2009;27: 1485–91.

4 El-Serag HB, Rudolph KL. Hepatocellular carcinoma: epidemiology and molecular carcinogenesis. Gastroenterology 2007;132:2557–76.

5 Fattovich G. Natural history and prognosis of hepatitis B. Semin Liver Dis 2003;23:47–58.

6 Jung KS, Kim SU, Ahn SH, et al. Risk assessment of hepatitis B virus-related hepatocellular carcinoma development using liver stiffness measurement (FibroScan). Hepatology 2011;53:885–94.

7 Bolondi L. Screening for hepatocellular carcinoma in cirrhosis. J Hepatol 2003;39:1076–84.

8 Zhang BH, Yang HB, Tang ZY. Randomized controlled trial of screening for hepatocellular carcinoma. J Cancer Res Clin Oncol 2004;130:417–22.

9 Amarapurkar D, Han KH, Chan HL, et al. Asia-Pacific working party on prevention of hepatocellular carcinoma application of surveillance programs for hepatocellular carcinoma in the Asia–Pacific region. J Gastroenterol Hepatol 2009;24: 955–61.

10 Singal A, Volk ML, Waljee A, et al. Meta-analysis: surveillance with ultrasound for early-stage hepatocellular carcinoma in patients with cirrhosis. Aliment Pharmacol Ther 2009;30:37–47.

11 Bruix J, Sherman M. American Association for the Study of Liver Diseases. Management of hepatocellular carcinoma: an update. Hepatology 2011;53:1020–2.

12 European Association for the Study of the Liver, European Organisation for Research and Treatment of Cancer. EASL-EORTC Clinical Practice Guidelines: Management of hepatocellular carcinoma. J Hepatol 2012;56:908–43.

13 Lok AS, Sterling RK, Everhart JE, et al. Des-gamma-carboxy prothrombin and alpha-fetoprotein as biomarkers for the early detection of hepatocellular carcinoma. Gastroenterology 2010;138:493–502.

14 Singal AG, Conjeevaram HS, Volk ML, et al. Effectiveness of hepatocellular carcinoma surveillance in patients with cirrhosis. Cancer Epidemiol Biomarkers Prev 2012;21: 793–9.

15 Santi V, Trevisani F, Gramenzi A, et al. Semiannual surveillance is superior to annual surveillance for the detection of early hepatocellular carcinoma and patient survival. J Hepatol 2010;53:291–7.

16 Welch HG, Black WC. Overdiagnosis in cancer. J Natl Cancer Inst 2010;102:605–13.

17 Park YN. Update on precursor and early lesions of hepatocellular carcinoma. Arch Pathol Lab Med 2011;135:704–15.

18 Bialecki ES, Di Bisceglie AM. Diagnosis of hepatocellular carcinoma. HPB (Oxford) 2005;7:26–34.

19 Baek CK, Choi JY, Kim KA, et al. Hepatocellular carcinoma in patients with chronic liver disease: a comparison of gadoxetic acid-enhanced MRI and multiphasic MDCT. Clin Radiol 2012;67:148–56.
20 Kim SH, Lee J, Kim MJ, et al. Gadoxetic acid-enhanced MRI versus triple-phase MDCT for the preoperative detection of hepatocellular carcinoma. AJR Am J Roentgenol 2009;192: 1675–81.
21 Kim TK, Jang H-J. Contrast-enhanced ultrasound in the diagnosis of nodules in liver cirrhosis. World J Gastroenterol 2014;20:3590–6.
22 Zheng SG, Xu HX, Liu LN. Management of hepatocellular carcinoma: the role of contrast-enhanced ultrasound. World J Radiol 2014;6:7–14.
23 Roskams T, Kojiro M. Pathology of early hepatocellular carcinoma: conventional and molecular diagnosis. Semin Liver Dis 2010;30:17–25.
24 Forner A, Vilana R, Ayuso C, et al. Diagnosis of hepatic nodules 20 mm or smaller in cirrhosis: prospective validation of the noninvasive diagnostic criteria for hepatocellular carcinoma. Hepatology 2008;47:97–104.
25 Sangiovanni A, Manini MA, Iavarone M, et al. The diagnostic and economic impact of contrast imaging techniques in the diagnosis of small hepatocellular carcinoma in cirrhosis. Gut 2010;59:638–44.
26 Bruix J, Sherman M. Management of hepatocellular carcinoma: an update. Hepatology 2011;53:1020–2.
27 Edge SB, Carducci MA, Compton CC, et al. AJCC Cancer Staging Manual, 7th ed. Chicago: Springer; 2009. p. 237.
28 Chun YH, Kim SU, Park JY, et al. Prognostic value of the 7th edition of the AJCC staging system as a clinical staging system in patients with hepatocellular carcinoma. Eur J Cancer 2011;47:2568–75.
29 Cancer of the Liver Italian Program (CLIP) Investigators. A new prognostic system for hepatocellular carcinoma: a retrospective study of 435 patients. Hepatology 1998;28:751–5.
30 Kudo M, Chung H, Osaki Y. Prognostic staging system for hepatocellular carcinoma (CLIP score): its value and limitations, and a proposal for a new staging system, the Japan Integrated Staging score (JIS score). J Gastroenterol 2003;38:207–15.
31 Ueno S, Tanabe G, Sako K, et al. Discrimination value of the new western prognostic system (CLIP score) for hepatocellular carcinoma in 662 Japanese patients. Cancer of the Liver Italian Program. Hepatology 2001;34:529–34.
32 Kudo M, Chung, Haji S, et al. Validation of a new prognostic staging system for hepatocellular carcinoma: the JIS score compared with the CLIP score. Hepatology 2004;40:1396–405.
33 Llovet JM, Bru C, Bruix J. Prognosis of hepatocellular carcinoma: the BCLC staging classification. Semin Liver Dis 1999;19:329–38.
34 Hasegawa K, Kokudo N, Imamura H, et al. Prognostic impact of anatomic resection for hepatocellular carcinoma. Ann Surg 2005;242:252–9.
35 Rahbari NN, Mehrabi A, Mollberg NM, et al. Hepatocellular carcinoma: current management and perspectives for the future. Ann Surg 2011;253:453–69.
36 Han KH, Kudo M, Ye SL, et al. Asian consensus workshop report: expert consensus guideline for the management of intermediate and advanced hepatocellular carcinoma in Asia. Oncology 2011; 81 (Suppl 1): 158–64.
37 Kokudo N, Makuuchi M. Evidence-based clinical practice guidelines for hepatocellular carcinoma in Japan: the J-HCC guidelines. J Gastroenterol 2009;44 (Suppl 19): 119–21.
38 Choi GH, Park JY, Hwang HK, et al. Predictive factors for long-term survival in patients with clinically significant portal hypertension following resection of hepatocellular carcinoma. Liver Int 2011;31:485–93.
39 Mazzaferro V, Regalia E, Doci R, et al. Liver transplantation for the treatment of small hepatocellular carcinomas in patients with cirrhosis. N Engl J Med 1996;334:693–99.
40 Yao FY, Xiao L, Bass NM, et al. Liver transplantation for hepatocellular carcimoma: validation of the UCSF-expanded criteria based on preoperative imaging. Am J Transplant 2007;7:2587–96.
41 Tamura S, Sugawara Y, Kokudo N. Living donor liver transplantation for hepatocellular carcinoma: the Japanese experience. Oncology 2011;81 (Suppl 1): 111–5.
42 Clavien PA, Lesurtel M, Bossuyt PM, et al. Recommendations for liver transplantation for hepatocellular carcinoma: an international consensus conference report. Lancet Oncol 2012;13:e11–22.
43 Hwang S, Lee SG, Joh JW, et al. Liver transplantation for adult patients with hepatocellular carcinoma in Korea: comparison between cadaveric donor and living donor liver transplantations. Liver Transpl 2005;11:1265–72.
44 Ho CM, Lee PH, Chen CL, et al. Long-term outcomes after resection versus transplantation for hepatocellular carcinoma within UCSF criteria. Ann Surg Oncol 2012;19:826–33.
45 Koniaris LG, Levi DM, Pedroso FE, et al. Is surgical resection superior to transplantation in the treatment of hepatocellular carcinoma? Ann Surg 2011;254:527–37.
46 Shiina S, Teratani T, Obi S, et al. A randomized controlled trial of radiofrequency ablation with ethanol injection for small hepatocellular carcinoma. Gastroenterology 2005;129: 122–30.
47 Germani G, Pleguezuelo M, Gurusamy K, et al. Clinical outcomes of radiofrequency ablation, percutaneous ethanol and acetic acid injection for hepatocellular carcinoma: a meta-analysis. J Hepatol 2010;52:380–8.
48 Lencioni R, Crocetti L. Loco-regional treatment of hepatocellular carcinoma. Radiology 2012;262:43–58.
49 Meza-Junco J, Montano-Loza AJ, Liu DM, et al. Locoregional radiological treatment for hepatocellular carcinoma; which, when and how? Cancer Treat Rev 2012;38:54–62.
50 Llovet JM, Bruix J. Systematic review of randomized trials for unresectable hepatocellular carcinoma: chemoembolization improves survival. Hepatology 2003;37:429–42.

51 Marelli L, Stigliano R, Triantos C, et al. Transarterial therapy for hepatocellular carcinoma: which technique is more effective? A systematic review of cohort and randomized studies. Cardiovasc Intervent Radiol 2007;30:6–25.
52 Lewis AL, Gonzales MV, Lloyd AW, et al. DC Bead: in vitro characterisation of a drug-delivery device for transarterial chemoembolization. J Vasc Interv Radiol 2006;17: 335–42.
53 Lee KH, Liapi E, Vossen JA, et al. Distribution of iron oxide-containing embosphere particles after transcatheter arterial embolization in an animal model of liver cancer: evaluation with MR imaging and implication for therapy. J Vasc Interv Radiol 2008;19:1490–6.
54 Hong K, Khwaja A, Liapi E, et al. New intra-arterial drug delivery system for the treatment of liver cancer: preclinical assessment in a rabbit model of liver cancer. Clin Cancer Res 2006;12:2563–7.
55 Poon RT, Tso WK, Pang RW, et al. A phase I/II trial of chemoembolization for hepatocellular carcinoma using a novel intra-arterial drug-eluting bead. Clin Gastroenterol Hepatol 2007;5:1100–8.
56 Lammer J, Malagari K, Vogl T, et al. Prospective randomized study of doxorubicin-eluting-bead embolization in the treatment of hepatocellular carcinoma: results of the PRECISION V study. Cardiovasc Intervent Radiol 2010; 33:41–52.
57 Martin JJ, Romero MR, Blazquez AG, et al. Importance and limitations of chemotherapy among the available treatments for gastrointestinal tumours. Anticancer Agents Med Chem 2009;9:162–84.
58 Kato A, Miyazaki M, Ambiru S, et al. Multidrug resistance gene (MDR-1) expression as a useful prognostic factor in patients with human hepatocellular carcinoma after surgical resection. J Surg Oncol 2001;78:110–5.
59 Lai CL, Wu PC, Chan GC, et al. Doxorubicin versus no antitumor therapy in inoperable hepatocellular carcinoma: a prospective randomized trial. Cancer 1988;62:479–83.
60 Leung TW, Patt YZ, Lau WY, et al. Complete pathological remission is possible with systemic combination chemotherapy for inoperable hepatocellular carcinoma. Clin Cancer Res 1999;5:1676–81.
61 Yeo W, Mok TS, Zee B, et al. A randomized phase III study of doxorubicin versus cisplatin/interferon alpha-2b/doxorubicin/fluorouracil (PIAF) combination chemotherapy for unresectable hepatocellular carcinoma. J Natl Cancer Inst 2005;97:1532–8.
62 Calvisi DF, Ladu S, Gorden A, et al. Ubiquitous activation of Ras and Jak/stat pathways in human HCC. Gastroenterology 2006;130:1117–28.
63 Gollob JA, Wilhelm S, Carter C, et al. Role of Raf kinase in cancer: therapeutic potential of targeting the Raf/MEK/ERK signal transduction pathway. Semin Oncol 2006;33:392–406.
64 Aznavoorian S, Murphy AN, Stetler-Stevenson WG, et al. Molecular aspects of tumor cell invasion and metastasis. Cancer 1993;71:1368–83.
65 Ribatti D, Vacca A, Nico B, et al. Angiogenesis and anti-angiogenesis in hepatocellular carcinoma. Cancer Treat Rev 2006;32:437–44.
66 Llovet J, Ricci S, Mazzaferro V, et al. Sorafenib in advanced hepatocellular carcinoma. N Engl J Med 2008;359:378–90.
67 Autier J, Escudier B, Wechsler J, et al. Prospective study of the cutaneous adverse effects of sorafenib, a novel multi-kinase inhibitor. Arch Dermatol 2008;144:886–92.
68 Cheng AL, Kang YK, Chen Z, et al. Efficacy and safety of sorafenib in patients in the Asia-Pacific region with advanced hepatocellular carcinoma: a phase III randomized, double-blind, placebo-controlled trial. Lancet Oncol 2009;10:25–34.
69 Villanueva A, Llovet JM. Targeted therapies for hepatocellular carcinoma. Gastroenterology 2011;140:1410–26.
70 Kim DY, Ryu HJ, Choi JY, et al. Radiological response predicts survival following transarterial chemoembolization in patients with unresectable hepatocellular carcinoma. Aliment Pharmacol Ther 2012;35:1343–50.
71 Han KH, Seong J, Kim JK, et al. Pilot clinical trial of localized concurrent chemoradiation therapy for locally advanced hepatocellular carcinoma with portal vein thrombosis. Cancer 2008;113:995–1003.
72 Lee IJ, Seong J. Radiotherapeutic strategies in the management of hepatocellular carcinoma. Oncology 2011;81 (Suppl 1): 123–33.
73 Sangro B, Carpanese L, Cianni R, et al. Survival after yttrium-90 resin microsphere radioembolization of hepatocellular carcinoma across Barcelona clinic liver cancer stages: a European evaluation. Hepatology 2011;54:868–78.
74 Park JY, Ahn SH, Yoon YJ, et al. Repetitive short-course hepatic arterial infusion chemotherapy with high-dose 5-fluorouracil and cisplatin in patients with advanced hepatocellular carcinoma. Cancer 2007;110:129–37.
75 Kota J, Chivukula RR, O'Donnell KA, et al. Therapeutic microRNA delivery suppresses tumorigenesis in a murine liver cancer model. Cell 2009;137:1005–17.

CHAPTER 11
Hepatic encephalopathy

Piero Amodio
Department of Medicine (DIMED), University of Padova, Padova, Italy

Introduction

Cirrhosis, far from being an isolated disorder of the liver, has well known consequences on the whole body and, notably, on brain functioning. The influence of liver failure on the brain is clearly evidenced by mental and/or behavioral changes that have been known since Ancient Greek and Roman times. Hippocrates recognized a "symptomatic delirium" related to "jaundice and suppression of natural periodical evacuation" [1]. In the last centuries, the issue of mental and behavioral alterations in individuals with advanced liver disease was studied by many authors [2,3].

The neurological or psychiatric alterations occurring in severe liver failure were termed portosystemic encephalopathy (PSE) [4] and later included in the term hepatic encephalopathy (HE) [5].

Definition

HE can be defined as brain dysfunction caused by liver insufficiency and/or portosystemic shunting that produces a spectrum of neurologic and psychiatric abnormalities ranging from subclinical alterations to coma [6]. Consequently, the encephalopathies caused by isolated defects of liver metabolism (e.g., urea cycle disorders, Reye's syndrome) or valproate hyperammonemia are not implicated in the term HE.

Clinical manifestation

HE produces a wide and nonspecific spectrum of neurological and psychiatric abnormalities. In its mildest form, HE is detectable only by psychometric or neurophysiologic tools. It manifests clinically with personality changes, such as apathy or irritability, and inappropriate behavior that may be reported by patient's relatives; also, obvious mental changes and motor function are detectable on clinical examination. Mental changes progressively include disorientation to time and space, inappropriate behavior, delirium with agitation or somnolence, stupor and, finally, coma. Of motor changes, asterixis or "flapping tremor" is the most typical and can be detected in the early middle stages of HE, but not in coma. Actually, asterixis is not tremor, but negative myoclonus consisting of loss of postural tone that is easily elicited by the hyperextension of the wrists with separated fingers. However, it may involve other muscles. Rarely, transient focal neurologic signs may occur in severe HE [7].

In some patients, massive motor alterations occur. The label of non-Wilsonian hepatocerebral or hepatolenticular degeneration was given to persistent HE with prominent extrapyramidal and/or pyramidal signs in which postmortem brain examination proves the existence of relevant pathologic changes with brain atrophy [8]. Rare cases of paraplegia with progressive spasticity and weakness of lower limbs with hyperreflexia and relatively mild persistent or recurrent mental alterations that may or may not reverse with liver transplantation [9,10] are preferentially labelled as hepatic myelopathy [11].

Sleep disturbances were reported in subjects with cirrhosis [4,12,13]; daily somnolence is the one that has a proven relationship with HE [14]. Finally, it was recently recognized that HE is associated with falls; if this is caused by cognitive or motor abnormalities or by their combination, or even by cirrhosis per se, is not yet clear [15,16].

In brief, the manifestation of HE can be summarized into the five patterns in Table 11.1. The exact grading of the severity of mental alterations of HE is less relevant

Cirrhosis: A practical guide to management, First Edition. Edited by Samuel S. Lee and Richard Moreau.

Table 11.1 Clinical patterns of hepatic encephalopathy presentation.

Pattern		Description
Coma		The patient is eye closed, unresponsive even to pain stimulation
Abrupt confusional state	Inhibited	The patient is disoriented in time or/and space or/and identity and somnolent
	Agitated	The patient is disoriented in time or/and space or/and identity and agitated/ angry/restless
Almost continuous mental dysfunction with interspersed recurrent confusional episodes		The pattern is dementia-like
Predominant motor disorder with mild/ moderate mental dysfunction/confusion	Extrapyramidal	Parkinsonism, chorea, or athetosis
	Pyramidal	Spastic paraparesis with hyperyflexia
Minimal brain dysfunction		The patient is oriented and his/her mental activity seems perfectly normal or nearly normal; however, on psychometric testing cognitive alterations are detectable (concerning attention, working memory, visuopractical ability, inhibition). Other signs are the slowing of EEG activity and/or the reduction of critical flicker frequency

than the *pattern of HE presentation,* because this latter is of great importance both for HE recognition and for differential diagnosis. Staging of the severity of mental alteration is simple and can be easily done according to West Haven criteria (Table 11.2), possibly adopting operative criteria [17].

Recently, the term "covert" HE was coined for patients with grade 1 HE (barely discernible on clinical examination) or minimal HE (i.e., only detectable by specific tools) (Table 11.2) [18]. Other grading systems can be used (CHESS scale [19], HESS scale [20], Glasgow Coma Scale, Mo-log [21]), but there is no clear proof that they are better than the widely used West Haven classification, once operative definitions of staging are used.

Proper assessment of HE takes into account not only grading of the severity of mental alteration, but also the underlying condition producing HE, the time course of HE, and the existence of precipitating factors. Therefore, proper assessment of HE is multi-axial [24] (Table 11.3). Therefore, to properly HE in a single patient, all the four items should be mentioned. If possible, the information on treatment should be added, because this can provide cues for diagnosis (a mental disorder absolutely unresponsive to treatment for HE may be something other than HE) and for alternative or add-on treatment. For instance, a proper report for a single patient with a bout of HE is "type C episodic overt HE (grade 3) precipitated by paracentesis in a subject on lactulose treatment."

Epidemiology

The prevalence of HE is related to the severity of liver dysfunction and/or the extent of portosystemic shunting. The prevalence of overt HE is 10–14% in patients with cirrhosis and 16–21% in those with decompensated cirrhosis [25,26]. The prevalence in noncirrhotic portal hypertension is not defined. The prevalence of minimal HE varies according to: (i) the occurrence of previous bouts of overt HE [27,28]; and (ii) the tools used for its detection, because it escapes obvious identification. A conservative esteem is about 30% in inpatients with cirrhosis.

The incidence of overt HE was 9% at 5 years and 25% at 10 years in a cohort of subjects with virus-related hepatitis after the first diagnosis of cirrhosis [29]. Another study reported 25% cumulative incidence of HE at 5 years after the diagnosis of compensated cirrhosis of various etiologies [30]. Patients with decompensated viral cirrhosis have 38% risk of overt HE within 2 years [31]. Subjects with a previous bout of overt HE have a 40% cumulative risk of another bout of overt HE at 1 year [32], and subjects with more than one bout of overt HE in the previous 6 months have a 40% cumulative risk of another bout within 6 months, despite disaccharide treatment [33]. In individuals with minimal HE detected by cognitive or EEG criteria, the incidence of bouts of overt HE is 26–35 per 100 patient-years [34,35].

Subjects at higher risk for HE are those who underwent transjugular intrahepatic portosystemic shunt (TIPS) or surgical portosytemic shunt. The 1-year risk

Table 11.2 Grading of the severity mental alterations in hepatic encephalopathy.

ISHEN criteria [18]	West Haven grading [22], updated concerning the conditions "MHE" and "unaffected"		Operative criteria[b]
Unaffected			
Covert	Minimal	Psychometric and/or EEG alterations without mental changes on routine clinical examination	
	Grade 1	Trivial lack of awareness Euphoria or anxiety Shortened attention span Impairment of addition or subtraction	Lack of consensus on definition, low inter-rater reproducibility
Overt[a]	Grade 2	Lethargy or apathy Disorientation for time Obvious personality change Inappropriate behavior	**Disorientation for time** *(≥ three incorrect items)* • Day of the week • Day of the month • The month • The season • The year With or without other symptoms
	Grade 3	Somnolence to semi-stupor Responsive to stimuli Confused Gross disorientation Bizarre behavior	**Disorientation for place[c]** *(≥ three incorrect items)* • State/country • Region/county • City • Place • Floor/ward **Plus** Disorientation for time With or without other symptoms
	Grade 4	Coma, unable to test mental state	• Unresponsive to pain stimuli • Glasgow score <8

[a] The presence of asterixis (flapping tremor) is considered an independent marker of overt HE; note that it is absent in coma.
[b] Operative criteria were suggested to reduce misclassification caused by the colloquial and poorly defined terms used in West Haven classification [17].
[c] At variant from Folstein et al. [23], three items are required for disorientation in space, because hospitalized patients may reasonably ignore the floor.

for HE after the procedure is estimated to be about 10–50% [36,37]. At any rate, the incidence of HE after TIPS and after surgical portosystemic shunt [38] is greatly influenced by selection criteria [39]. HE accounts for approximately 100,000 hospitalizations each year in the United States [40].

Diagnostic tools and differential diagnosis

The diagnosis of HE is not always as simple as might be expected and this depends, in part, on poor insight into the concept of HE. This can lead to errors, ascribing uncritically to HE any neuropsychiatric disorder occurring in patients with liver disease, even without the evidence of a causal link to liver failure or portosystemic shunting. Consequently, brain disorders that only occasionally coexist with liver disease can be mislabeled as HE, preventing patients from receiving proper etiologic treatment.

Basically, the diagnosis of HE is based on the clinical findings; the differential diagnosis is based on the Bayes' theorem, which states that the probability of a disease is given by: (i) the *a priori* probability that the disease may exist; and (ii) the likelihood of symptoms and/or signs.

Table 11.3 The multi-axial classification of hepatic encephalopathy (HE).

Domain/ dimension	Name of the domain	Subdivision	Description
Underlying condition producing HE	Type	A	Caused by ALF
		B	Caused by PS without significant liver disease
		C	Caused by cirrhosis (both liver disease and PS shunting)
Severity of mental alterations	Grade	MHE	Covert HE (see Table 11.2)
		1	
		2	Overt HE (see Table 11.2)
		3	
		4	
Interval between bouts of HE	Time course	Episodic	An occasional bout of HE
		Recurrent	Bout of HE occurring ≤6 months from the previous one(s)
		Persistent	Patient is always more or less symptomatic
Presence of precipitating factors	Precipitation factors	Precipitated	There is an obvious factor that produced the occurrence of the bout of HE. If this the case it should be mentioned
		Not precipitated	Absence of a known factor to which to ascribe the occurrence of the bout of HE

ALF, acute liver failure; MHE minimal hepatic encephalopathy; PS, portosystemic shunting.

The probabilities of the occurrence of different diseases should then be compared. Therefore, the first step towards a diagnosis of HE is the detection of neurologic or psychiatric findings compatible with HE. The second step is the recognition that the patient has severe liver insufficiency and/or portosystemic shunting, because these conditions provide the *a priori* probability of HE.

The risk of HE is related to the severity of liver dysfunction, with the exception of the subgroup of individuals with large portosystemic shunting, as these risk factors are independent [41,42], so that patients with huge shunting can experience HE even without liver insufficiency. Hyperammonemia is a good marker of portosystemic shunting, even with negligible liver disease [43], because ammonia has high first-pass liver metabolism (about 70%) [44,45] and its plasma level increases if portal liver perfusion is reduced due to portosystemic shunting [46,47]. The value of hyperammonemia as a prerequisite for the occurrence of HE was emphasized by Conn [48], but was later neglected or even disputed [49], possibly due to confusion between two concepts:

1 Hyperammonemia as an element involved in the pathophysiology of HE.
2 Hyperammonemia as a marker of portosystemic shunting and advanced liver disease.

In fact, even admitting that the pathophysiology of HE is mutifactorial or uncertain, it is hardly conceivable that a patient with low plasma ammonia may have encephalopathy caused by liver disease and/or portosystemic shunting. In patients with low plasma ammonia, due to the very low *a priori* probability of HE, intense scrutiny for alternative causes of mental alteration is mandatory. In addition, recently it was clearly proven that high ammonia plasma level is a risk factor for the development of HE [50].

Of note, ammonia determination needs some precaution, because ammonia develops rapidly in blood maintained at room temperature. Therefore, blood samples should be immediately put in ice, rapidly delivered to the laboratory, and the determination should be performed as soon as possible. The use of venous blood is simpler, but arterial or capillary blood may be preferable.

The third step is the recognition of precipitating factors for HE (e.g., bleeding, constipation, and infections) or a history of previous bouts of HE, which further increase the risk of HE. However, HE can occur without their occurrence.

The fourth step is the exclusion of alternative causes or the detection of concomitant causes of brain alteration, depending on the clinical findings. However, the exclusion of alternative causes does not require always formal

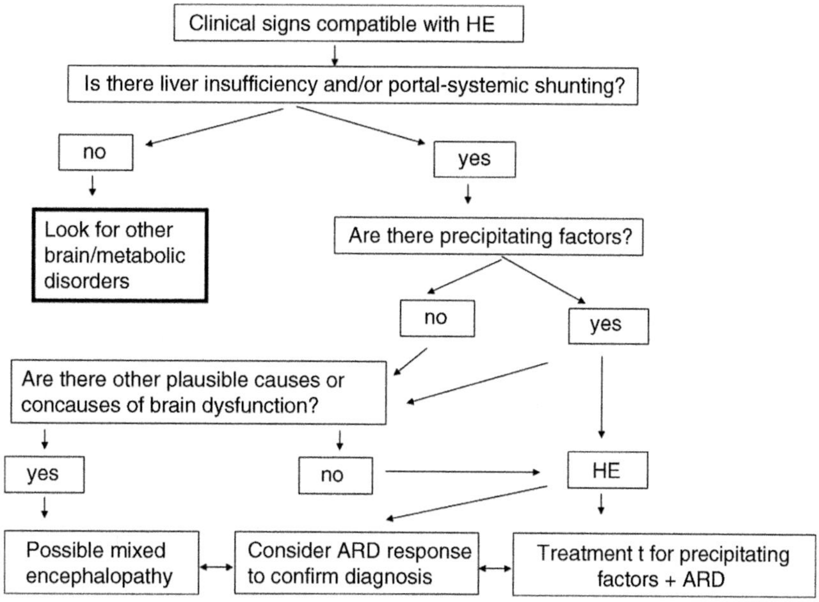

Figure 11.1 Flow chart for the diagnosis of hepatic encephalopathy (HE). ARD, ammonia reducing drugs (disaccharides/rifaximine or other antibiotics).

investigation because it can be obtained by the history and clinical manifestations together with probabilistic reasoning. Finally, the response to treatment should be considered to confirm the diagnosis or suggest the existence of alternative or concomitant neurologic disorders (Figure 11.1).

On closer inspection, for the patient with coma or confusion, the differential diagnosis between HE and other disorders is reported in Table 11.4 For the patient with almost continuous mild mental alterations interspersed with relapses of confusion or even coma, the differential diagnosis between relapsing and persistent HE and other disorders is reported in Table 11.5. Finally, for the patient with prominent motor disorder and mental/behavioral alterations, the differential diagnosis between HE and other disorders [51] is reported in Table 11.6.

Considering these alterative disorders that should be taken into account in the differential diagnosis of HE, the diagnostic procedures that are required for the diagnosis of patients with suspected HE are reported in Table 11.7. Particular problems are: (i) the association; and (ii) the interaction between HE and other neurologic and metabolic disorders that can produce encephalopathy per se, but can also interact in the pathophysiologic pathways producing HE. An example of the former is HE occurring in an individual who is already suffering from vascular dementia (stroke sequelae, Binswanger's disease), Alzheimer's disease, or post-traumatic brain sequelae. The clinical improvement – albeit incomplete – after treatment for HE orients towards a diagnosis of HE associated

Table 11.4 Differential diagnosis of HE for patients with acute confusion or coma.

1	Diabetic ketoacidosis or hyperosmolar coma
2	Drug intoxication (Bz, opioids, neuroleptics, valproate) or alcohol intoxication
3	Encephalitis/meningitis
4	Head trauma
5	Hypercalcemia
6	Hypercapnia
7	Hypoglycemia *(for coma)*
8	Malingering
9	Nonconvulsive epilepsy *(for coma)*
10	Sepsis*
11	Severe, acute hyponatremia*
12	Stroke (hemorragic/ischemic)
13	Wernike's encephalopathy (thiamine deficiency) *(for confusion)*

For agitated confusion state, consider drug intoxication and acute psychosis

* Sepsis, hyponatremia, and, to a lesser extent, thiamine deficiency are also implicated into the pathophysiology of HE, so that the conditions may overlap.

Table 11.5 Differential diagnosis of HE for patients with highly relapsing/persistent mental impairment.

1. Alcoholic dementia
2. Alzheimer's disease and other neurodegenerative dementias
3. Brain masses (subdural hematoma, slow-growing tumors)
4. Drug related encephalopathies
5. Hypercalcemia
6. Hyponatremia
7. Hypothyroidism
8. Korsakoff dementia (thymine deficiency) and other micronutrient deficiencies (e.g., B12)
9. Neurologic sequelae (trauma)
10. Obstructive sleep apnea syndrome
11. Renal failure (uremic encephalopathy/dialysis and disequilibrium syndrome)
12. Vascular dementia
    - Binswanger's disease
    - Hypoperfusion
    - Large stroke or multiple strokes
    - Stroke in strategic areas

Table 11.6 Differential diagnosis of HE for patients with prominent motor disorder with mild/moderate mental decay.

1. Cerebrovascular disorders
2. Dementia with Parkinsonism
3. Normotensive hydrocephalus
4. Extrapyramidal syndromes
5. Demyelinating disorders
6. Vitamin B12 deficiency
7. Wilson's disease

with another brain disease. An example of the latter is sepsis that can produce encephalopathy per se (septic encephalopathy) [52], but also interacts with the mechanisms producing HE and is therefore a cause of HE [53]. The same occurs for hyponatremia [54,55] and, possibly, thiamine deficiency [56].

The existence of concurrent causes of brain dysfunction should be considered, diagnosed, and properly treated, because mixed encephalopathies do exist and

Table 11.7 Diagnostic procedure for patients with suspected HE.

Clinical history
Clinical examination for hepatic stigmata, asterixis, and exclusion of neurologic focal signs, rigor, evidence of trauma
Body temperature (fever, hypothermia), blood pressure, pulse frequency, chest and abdomen clinical examination
Blood sample for:

- Red blood cell, WBC, and platelet counts
- INR, bilirubin (ammonia can be measured for its high negative predictive value; i.e., patients with normal ammonia level have so low probability, if any, of HE that alternative causes should be investigated. In addition, ammonia-reducing drugs are not a rational treatment for patients with low plasma ammonia level)
- Reactive C protein
- Glucose
- Na
- Ca
- Toxicologic screening (e.g., benzodiazepines, barbituriates, opioids, cannabinols, alcohol), *when needed*
- Blood gas analysis (O_2, CO_2 and CO) and pH
    - Vitamin B12 (*in dementia-like syndromes)*
    - thyroid stimulating hormone (*in dementia-like syndromes)*

Urine examination for WBC (*in confusion/coma)*
Polymorphonuclear leukocyte count in ascites, if there is ascites *(in confusion/coma)*
Brain CT scan *(in sudden coma, focal signs, or rigor)*
EEG *(if nonconvulsive epilepsy, herpes encephalitis, or malingering are suspected)*
Brain MRI (*in dementia-like syndromes)* + spinal MRI with FLAIR sequences *(in prominent motor manifestations)*
Cerebrospinal fluid examination (*if meningitis or encephalitis are suspected*)
Motor EP, electromyography, somatosensory EP (*in prominent motor manifestations)*
Splanchnic US Doppler study and/or CT scan with portal system reconstruction *(in highly recurrent HE, persistent HE, and in HE with relevant motor component)*

EP, evoked potential; INR, international normalized ratio; WBC, white blood cell.

neglecting to treat one of them can have deleterious consequences (e.g., coexisting thiamine deficiency). The response to treatment to disaccharides and rifaximin provide information on the role that HE can have in patients with overlapping disorders (e.g., Alzheimer disease or vascular dementia and HE) (Figure 11.1).

Diagnosis of minimal and covert HE

HE can occur without clinical evidence (minimal HE, MHE) or, at least, without clear disorientation (covert HE, CHE). Brain alteration in these patients is proven by neuropsychologic or neurophysiologic investigation. Cognitive alterations mainly regard attention, working memory, visuomotor abilities, speed in fine movements, and executive function. In contrast, verbal abilities and verbal memory, both short-term and long-term memory are preserved or relatively preserved, at odds with the amnestic mild cognitive impairment that frequently heralds Alzheimer's disease. As memory and verbal alterations are more easily noted by relatives and physicians, than attention disturbance subjects with MHE can be easily missed on routine clinical examination.

Paper and pencil tests that are suited for the detection of MHE are the ones comprising the Portal-Hepatic Psychometric Score (PHES; i.e., the Trial Making Test A, TMT-A) – also called number connection test (NCT) – the Trial Making Test B (TMT-B), the Digit Symbol test (DST), the Serial Dotting Test (SDT), and the Line Trait test (LTT) (Figure 11.2) [57,58]. Other tests exploring the same areas, such as the Block Design Test or the Figure Connection Test can be used; the latter can substitute for TMT-B in individuals who do not know the alphabet [59–61]. The use of more than one test is recommended [24]. There is consensus that the PHES is the preferable diagnostic tool based on paper and pencil tests [62]. It can be simplified using only three tests (i.e., DST, SDT, and LTT) [63]. Computerized tests exploring working memory or inhibition and attention [17,64,65] have also proven to be useful. They require some familiarity with computer usage.

The use of any neuropsychologic tests (paper and pencil or computerized) for the diagnosis of MHE require that:

1 The tests are standardized and adjusted by local norms for age and education; education adjustment is required in populations having individuals with less than 8–12 years of education.

Table 11.8 Differential diagnosis for minimal and covert HE.

1	Combined/overlapping conditions with or without HE
2	Drug-related encephalopathies
3	Hypercalcemia
4	Hyponatremia
5	Hypothyroidism
6	Low pre-morbid intellectual quotient, mental deficiency
7	Mild cognitive impairment related to Alzheimer's disease and other neurodegenerative or cerebrovascular dementias
8	Neurologic sequalae (trauma, alcohol, or drug abuse)
9	Obstructive apnea syndrome/respiratory failure
10	Subclinical renal encephalopathy
11	Vitamin B12 deficiency

2 Illiterate people are excluded from examination.
3 The patient cooperates with the evaluation (i.e., confused and uncooperative individuals cannot be tested, and malingering is possible).
4 Visual acuity, or hearing when needed, are adequate (also with correction).

In addition, it should be noted that psychometric information, as well as other functional data, is nonspecific. Therefore, other clinical conditions causing mild cognitive impairment should be considered in differential diagnosis (Table 11.8).

The study of critical flicker frequency (i.e., psychophysiologic measure of the threshold at which flickering light is perceived as a flickering and not as a continuous light) can be used to assess brain dysfunction because the threshold reduces in HE. This measure is valid to detect patients who correspond to grade 1 HE, according to West Haven classification [66]. The influence of alcohol misuse [66] and age [61] is not negligible on this technique which, like psychometric investigation, depends on the patient's cooperation and is an nonspecific marker of brain dysfunction.

Electrophysiologic techniques – electroencephalogram (EEG) and evoked potentials – provide functional assessment of the nervous system and are used to detect and monitor HE [67]. When compared with clinical examination, they provide more quantitative assessment of brain functioning. The EEG is a technique independent of the patient's cooperation that is potentially amenable for follow-up. The EEG is extremely sensitive to metabolic function, electrolyte homeostasis, and the effects of neurotoxic substances. Some 60 years ago, Parsons-Smith

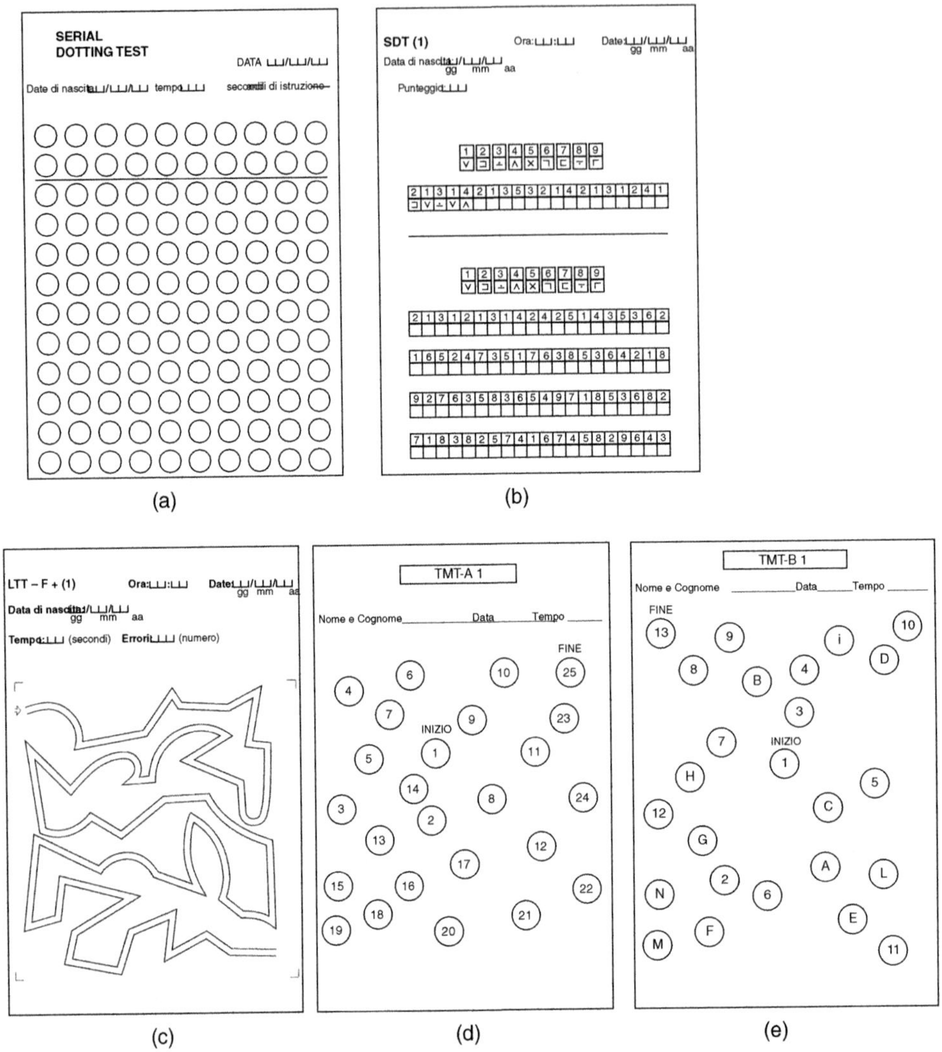

Figure 11.2 Pencil and paper psychometric tests useful for the detection of minimal hepatic encephalopathy (MHE). A, Serial Dotting Test; B, Digit Symbol Test; C, Line Trait Test; D, TMT-A; and E, TMT-B (Italian forms, based on Italian alphabet).

et al. [68] described slowing of the EEG rhythms in about 40% of individuals with cirrhosis without overt HE, thus proving the existence of MHE, even if they did not recognize the importance of their findings. Modern EEG equipment records digitized EEG that is easily analyzable by quantitative techniques. In adults, an increase in theta activity in parietal regions accounting for more than 35% indicates brain patterns compatible with MHE [69]. An index of higher HE affliction is the slowing of Mean Dominant Frequency [54]. At any rate, even without quantitative analysis, a slowing of eye-closed main resting rhythm at 8 Hz or lower is an index of encephalopathy [35], though nonspecific (Figure 11.3). The presence of triphasic waves (Figure 11.4), which is common – but nonspecific – in HE with confusion, is extremely rare in MHE/CHE.

An electrophysiologic technique to detect MHE/CHE is the prolongation of the latency of P300 wave (a cognitive potential evoked by the oddball paradigm). However, (i) it requires age-related standardization; (ii) it is not detectable in all individuals; and (iii) it requires considerable expertise by the clinician to be properly recorded and analyzed. Therefore, is not recommended for routine clinical use [67].

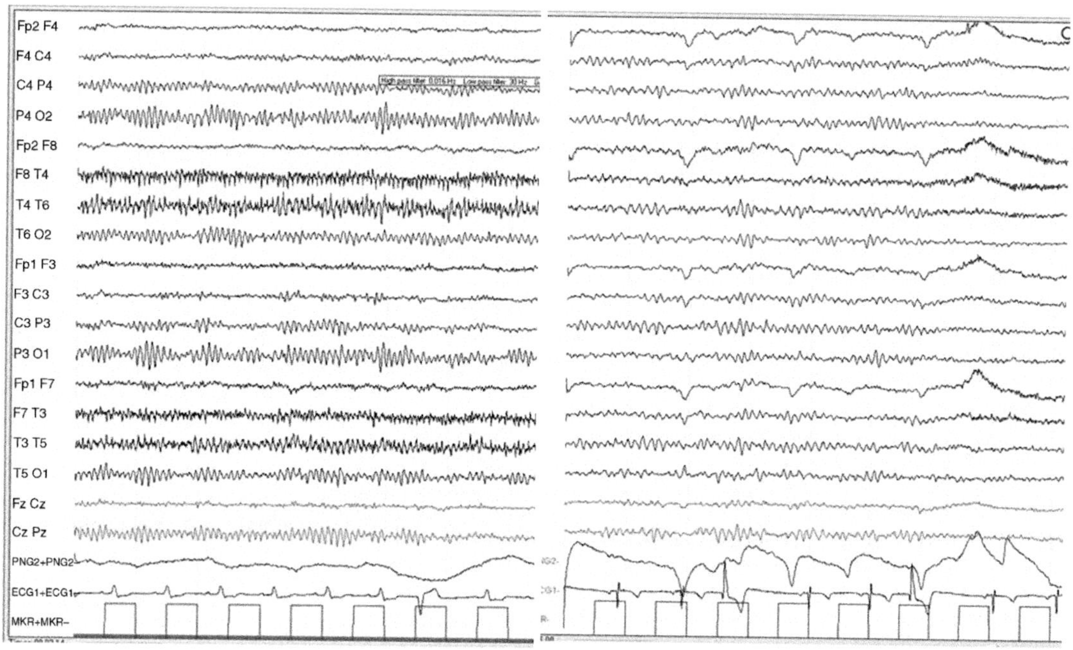

Figure 11.3 Eye closed EEG. On the left a normal tracing, on the right a tracing slowed down with interspersed theta activity (i.e., frequency <8 Hz) >35% in parietal derivation, suggesting MHE. (See colour plate section.)

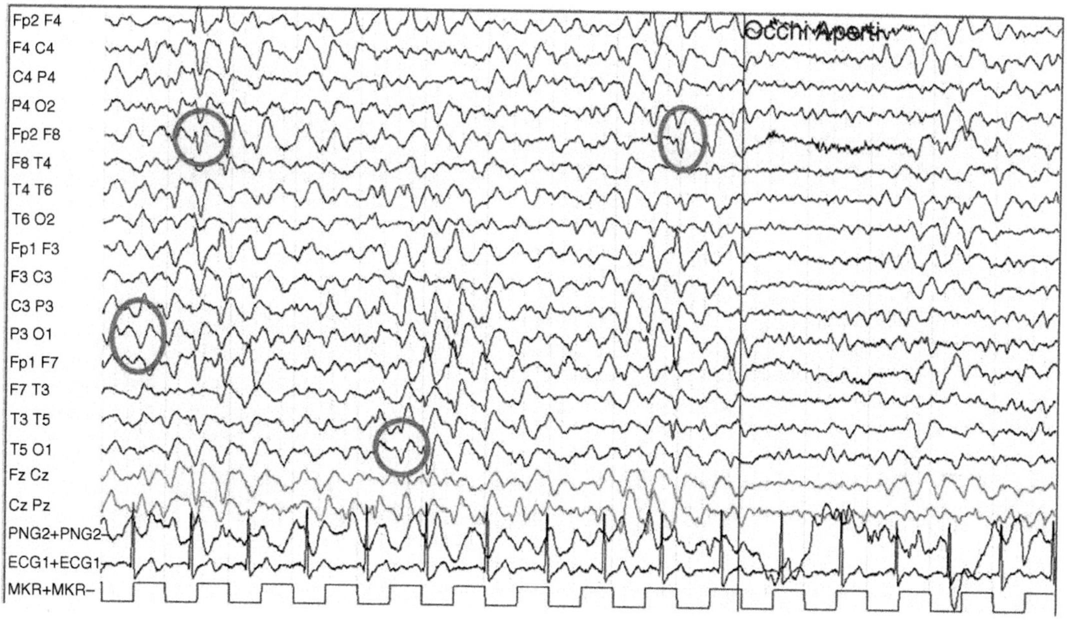

Figure 11.4 Severe (grade 3) HE in a subject with portosystemic shunt. Presence of triphasic waves (circles) and absence of block reaction on eye opening (on the right of the vertical blue line). (See colour plate section.)

In patients without overt HE, brain imaging techniques prove brain abnormalities that are related to cognitive findings, therefore highlighting some aspects of covert HE. Fludeoxyglucose positron emission tomography (FDG-PET) detects reduction of glucose oxidation mainly in prefrontal areas, cingulated gyrus, premotor areas, and parietal areas – with some inconsistencies concerning basal ganglia – which is related to cognitive dysfunction and impairment in movement initiation [70–74].

1H-magnetic resonance spectroscopy shows an increase in glutamine and/or glutamate signal intensity and a decrease in myo-inositol and choline in cirrhotic patients, independent of psychometric performance [75], therefore showing that this biochemical marker is not immediately related to brain function.

Imaging studies prove a relationship of psychometric performance with brain atrophy on computed tomography (CT) scanning [76], as well as white matter alterations on magnetic resonance imaging (MRI) [77]. Functional MRI allows the brain localization and characterization of abnormality in cortical activation during cognitive tasks in patients with MHE [78] and the measurement of resting state connectivity on MRI reveals alterations related to HE [79]. At any rate, these techniques are useful to highlight the pathophysiology of HE, but currently are not recommended for routine diagnostic purposes [80].

Etiology and pathogenesis

The pathophysiology of HE can be considered at the organism level and at organ level (i.e., at brain level) (Figure 11.5).

Organism level

It is clear that HE depends on liver insufficiency and/or portosystemic shunt, as elegantly described more than 50 years ago by Sherlock et al. [4]. In fact, both conditions produce HE in humans as well as in experimental models [81]. In addition, the disorder is elicited by substances

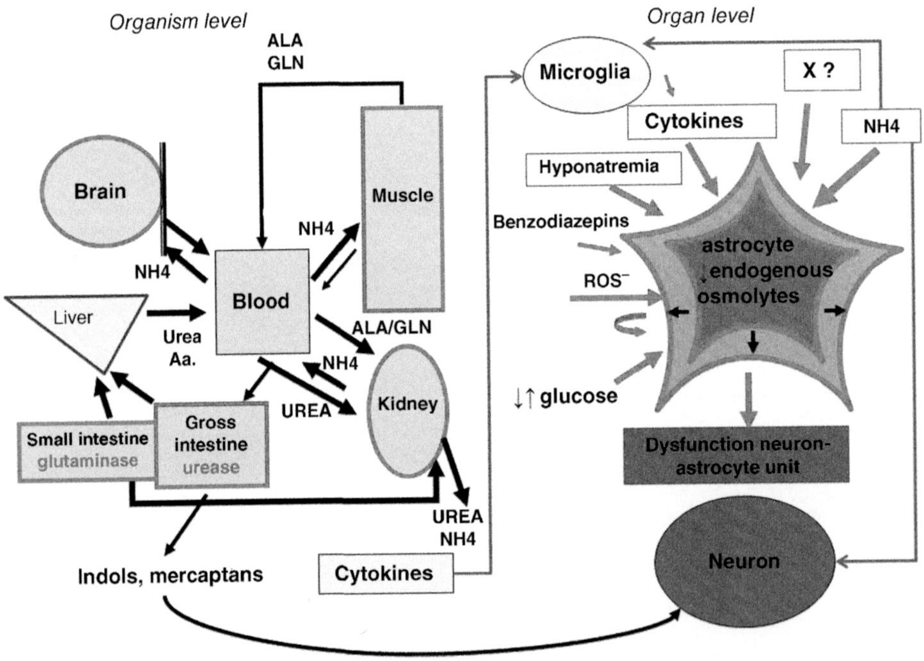

Figure 11.5 Sketch of the pathophysiology of HE. On the left, at organism level various organs concur to the occurrence of hyperammonemia that produces a proportional increase in brain ammonia metabolism; in addition, other toxic substaces are produced by gut dysbiosis, as well as cytokines. On the right, at organ level, in the brain peripheral cytokines and ammonia activate microglia, which amplifies cytokine reaction. This, together with ammonia and other substances, swell astrocytes, cause oxidative and nitrosative stress, and produce astrocyte–neuron dysfunction. Ammonia may also directly disturb neurotransmission.

coming from the gut and is facilitated by the action of gut bacteria. This has been proved since the 1930s, when it was observed that the administration of ammonia salt in patients with cirrhosis causes HE [82] and dogs with portosystemic shunt develop HE under the influence of ammoniagenic meat loads [83]. The beneficial action of disaccharides and oral antibiotics, both acting on gut bacteria, prove that the gut microbiota is implicated in the pathophysiology of HE [32,33,84,85].

Among the substances coming from the gut, the most important is ammonia, because the administration of ammonia salts causes HE, although inconstantly, thus suggesting interaction with other factors. Other gut-derived substances may have some neurotoxic effect. Among these, indole which can be converted into the neurotoxic oxyphenole in the brain; mercaptans, which, however, do not reach neurotoxic levels per se; short chain fatty acids, whose role has never been proven; gut-derived cytokines, and benzodiazepine-like substances [86–91].

In addition, profound metabolic changes occur in individuals with cirrhosis and in those with portosystemic shunt, causing changes in the profile of plasma amino acids [92], in fuel homeostasis after overnight fasting [93], in glucagon, insulin plasma levels and insulin sensitivity [94,95], in renal production of ammonia and ammonia utilization in muscle due to muscle wasting, as well as in brain ammonia utilization [96–98]. Some of these changes, such as the reduction in branched chain amino acids (BCAA) and the increase in aromatic amino acids (AAA) with reduction of the plasma molar ratio BCAA: AAA have been hypothesized to influence brain catecolaminergic neurotransmission [99,100]. However, neither the BCAA: AAA ratio is related to mental changes [101], nor catecholamine changes in the brain of subjects with HE [102]. Other changes, such as the sensitivity to fasting and the activation of gluconeogenesis after an overnight fast, can explain the reduction of fasting ammonia with glucose overnight infusion [103] and the rational of giving a bedtime snack of complex carbohydrates for the dietary management of patients with HE [104].

Organ level

HE is associated with reduction in brain glucose oxidation detectable by FDG-PET studies [74], with increase in water brain content, intracellular in acute liver failure and mainly extracellular and intracellular in cirrhosis, with increase in glutamine and reduction of myo-inositole and choline content in basal ganglia on spectral MRI [105,106]. Cerebral oxygen uptake and blood flow are reduced to two-thirds in cirrhotic patients with clinically overt HE but not in cirrhotic patients with minimal HE. Cerebral ammonia metabolism is enhanced because of increased blood ammonia level, but the kinetics of cerebral ammonia uptake and metabolism is not affected by hyperammonemia. Low grade cerebral edema is detectable not only in astrocytes but also in the white matter in cirrhotic patients with HE.

Hyperintensity of globus pallidus, and to a lesser extent of striatum and substatia nigra reticulata on T1-weighted MRI, is frequent in patients with HE and is related to brain manganese deposition, which, in turn, is caused by reduction of manganese clearance due to portosystemic shunting and liver failure [107]. Manganese is neurotoxic and may impair dopaminergic neurotransmission, as well as causing astrocyte oxidative stress [108]. However, hyperintensity of globus pallidus and basal ganglia is poorly related, if at all, to the cognitive symptoms of HE. In addition, after liver transplantation the time-course of globus pallidus hyperintensity is much longer than that of the symptoms of HE, therefore showing that the relationship of the two phenomena is poor at best [109]. Some association between brain atrophy and long long-lasting HE is likely [76,77].

Neurophysiologic studies have demonstrated that HE causes reduction of the oscillatory properties of neural networks [110,111] with movement of EEG alpha frequencies from the posterior cortical areas to the anterior ones (frontal cortex) in mild HE [112], and occurrence of triphasic waves in severe HE [67].

At the cellular level, the most striking events in HE are: (i) astrocyte changes (swelling in type A HE, and the occurrence of type 2 Alzheimer astrocytosis in type B and C HE); and (ii) microglia activation, at least in experimental models. Therefore, HE is primarily a glia disorder with secondary neuronal and/or neurotransmitter dysfunction [113,114]. Multiple pathways converge to alter astrocyte function, causing oxidative and/or nitrosative stress that ultimately amplify and maintain astrocyte dysfunction, and explain the clinical observation that the interaction of noxious events (e.g., hyperammonemia, hyponatremia, interleukins) correlate with the occurrence of bouts of HE [115].

The increased brain metabolism of ammonia, which is linearly related to hyperammonemia [96], can either cause HE per se or sensitize the brain to other noxious agents. The actions of ammonia on the brain, which are not yet completely elucidated, can be summarized as follows:

1 Impairment of brain energy metabolism via inhibition of the enzymes ketoglutarate dehydrogenase and pyruvate dehydrogenase, with ensuing tricarboxylic acid cycle dysfunction and increase in glycolytic activity [116,117].
2 Increased glutamine synthesis in astrocytes, activation of mitochondrial permeability transition, with ensuing mitochondrial dysfunction, oxidative stress, and osmotic swelling [118].
3 Interference with glutamatergic and GABAergic neurotransmission; the latter directly [119] or indirectly via promotion of the synthesis of inhibitory neurosteroids [120].
4 Interference of ammonium ions on inhibitory and excitatory neurotransmission [121].
5 Activation of microglia and induction of neuroinflammation [122].

Finally, evidence for alterations in serotoninergic, histaminergic, and dopaminergic neurotransmission does exist [123,124].

Treatment

Treatment for HE has some mild differences, depending on the pattern of HE. In patients with an acute episode of HE (coma or confusion) the following treatments are indicated.

1 Any effort should be done *to recognize and treat the precipitating event(s)*, if any, that have caused the episode of HE (Table 11.9). In the case of gastrointestinal bleeding, in addition to treatments oriented to stop bleeding and correct acute anemia, two other treatments are recommended:
   - Systemic antibiotics are indicated to increase survival in patients with cirrhosis and gastrointestinal bleeding [125]; in addition, it is reasonable that they reduce the production of ammonia and enterotoxins by gut microbiota, and thus might also prevent HE [126].
   - Osmotic catharsis aiming at rapidly removing blood from the gut. This was proven to reduce the occurrence of HE, reducing post-bleeding hyperammonemia [127,128]. In principle, osmotic catharsis with acidifying agents given orally or by nasogastric tube (disaccharides, mannitol, sorbitol) traps ammonia into the intestinal lumen and acts as a prebiotic, therefore this is is preferred over saline cathartics. Care should be taken to avoid hypernatremia which is a side effect of injudicious osmotic catharsis [129].
2 Ammonia reducing drugs (ARD):
   - Non-selective
     (a) Disaccharides (lactulose or lactitole, 10–120 g/day, so as to produce 2–3 bowel movements of soft faeces)
     (b) Nonabsorbable oral antibiotics (e.g., rifaximine, neomicine, paramomicine, vancomicine). Also metranidazole was used, but it is not recommended for its collateral effects. Note that the utility of oral nonabsorbable antibiotics in patients already on systemic antibiotic treatment is unproven. In addition, the rationale of using nonabsorbable oral antibiotics in patients with constipation is poor at best.
   - Selective
     (a) L-ornithine-L-aspartate (LOLA)
     (b) Non-ureic nitrogen scavengers (NUNS; sodium benzoate, sodium phenylacetate, ornitine phenylacetate, glycerol phenylbutyrate) are under study for this indication.

Nonselective ARD act on microbiota, therefore reduce the production of ammonia and other enterotoxins. The inhibition of ammonia production by antibiotics is due to reduction of ammoniogenic bacteria activity. Reduced production of inflammatory cytokines by the gut and laxative effect may have additional role. Nonabsorbable disaccharides act as prebiotics on gut microbioma, acidify the intestinal

Table 11.9 Principal precipitating factors for HE.

Infections	Urinary infections Spontaneous bacterial peritonitis Respiratory infections Cutaneous infections Biliary infections Others
Hypovolemia/dehydration	Overdiuresis Paracentesis Thirst Diarrhea Hyperemesis
Gastrointestinal bleeding	
Electrolyte imbalance	Hyponatremia
Constipation	

lumen – so trapping ammonia – and produce osmotic catharsis; thus, eventually reducing blood ammonia level.

Disaccharides can be given orally or by enema. Enemas have immediate cathartic effect, although their pharmacologic action is limited to the distal colon. Therefore, in constipated patients, enemas, which rapidly remove stools – a major source of toxins causing HE – quickly improve HE.

Selective ARD acts by: (i) increasing nitrogen/ammonia detoxification either stimulating urea cycle activity (e.g. LOLA); or (ii) causing the urinary excretion of nitrogen via soluble nitrogen-containing molecules different from urea that are excreted by urine (NUNS).

Adjuvant therapy with LOLA, which was proven to reduce ammonia plasma level [130], might shorten hospitalization due to episodes of overt HE [131].

3 Nutritional support is preferably given intravenously in patients with risk of food aspiration or unable to ingest a sufficient energy and/or nitrogen amount. The utility of the administration of solutions enriched by BCAA versus standard solutions has not been proven [132]. BCAA were introduced into therapy: (i) to correct plasma amino acid imbalance (low BCAA: AAA ratio) of patients with cirrhosis; (ii) in the hypothesis that this imbalance might produce weak catecholaminergic neurotransmitters in the brain that could reduce excitatory catecholaminergic tone and thus causing HE. This assumption is false, because no relation exists between plasma amino acid imbalance and brain function [101]. However, other mechanisms can explain the action of BCAA: (i) plasma ammonia levels decrease during glucose + BCAA-enriched solutions [133]; and (ii) a direct effect on the brain is plausible [134], possibly by supporting brain energy production [135]. Therefore, the utilization of BCAA-enriched solution to hydrate and nourish individuals with severe overt HE in addition to standard treatments [136] cannot be excluded by the absence of proof of BCAA efficacy in a single meta-analysis [132] based on small trials that were neither based on an "add on treatment" design, nor oriented to measure the velocity of HE recovery.

4 Flumazenil bolus infusion (1–2 mg) was found to improve briefly mental state in about one-fifth of patients with advanced HE [137]. The transience and unpredictability of the effect discourages the use of flumazenil in the treatment of HE, unless there is suspicion of intoxication by benzodiazepines.

5 Patients with agitated delirium can be difficult to treat. Benzodiazepines are contraindicated in these patients because they interact with the mechanisms producing HE. It is preferable to use neuroleptics, such as haloperidol or promazine (the latter is more sedative) [138]. Severely agitated patients may require ICU hospitalization and IV propofol sedation [139,140]. Obviously, treatment of the precipitating event, ARD treatment, and nutrition and hydration are mandatory while the patient is sedated.

In patients with persistent HE, or highly recurrent HE, the treatment is based on ARD and removal of concurrent disorders, if any. Theoretically, ARD acting by different mechanisms could be associated (e.g., disaccharides + rifaximine or other oral antibiotics). In addition to ARD, other treatments that can be considered on a "add-on" basis are as follow:

1 Reduction of huge portosystemic shunting (either spontaneous or not, as in the case of TIPS) [43,141];

2 Dietetic treatment [104]:
- optimization of energy supply and introduction of snacks and a bedtime snack;
- reduction of meat protein, which can be substituted by vegetable protein (e.g. from pulses);
- increase of dietary fiber (for its prebiotic and laxative effect);
- use of pre/probiotics;
- supplementation with oral BCAA; and
- liberal short courses of vitamin supplementation, if micronutrient lack is suspected.

Other treatments that can be utilized in these patients are as follow:

1 Acarbose can be used in the subgroup of patients with HE and diabetes. This drug inhibits the intestinal enzyme alpha-glucosidase that converts carbohydrates into monosaccharides. Therefore, it produces an overall effect similar to that of nonabsorbable disaccharides, by modifying the microbiota, acidifying intestinal lumen, and producing a cathartic effect. It was proven to be effective in improving cognition and lowering blood ammonia in low grade HE [142].

2 Carnitine and acetylcarnitine supplementation might reduce hyperammonemia and improve HE [143,144].

3 Zinc carnosine was shown to improve long-term cognitive performance; however, without significant

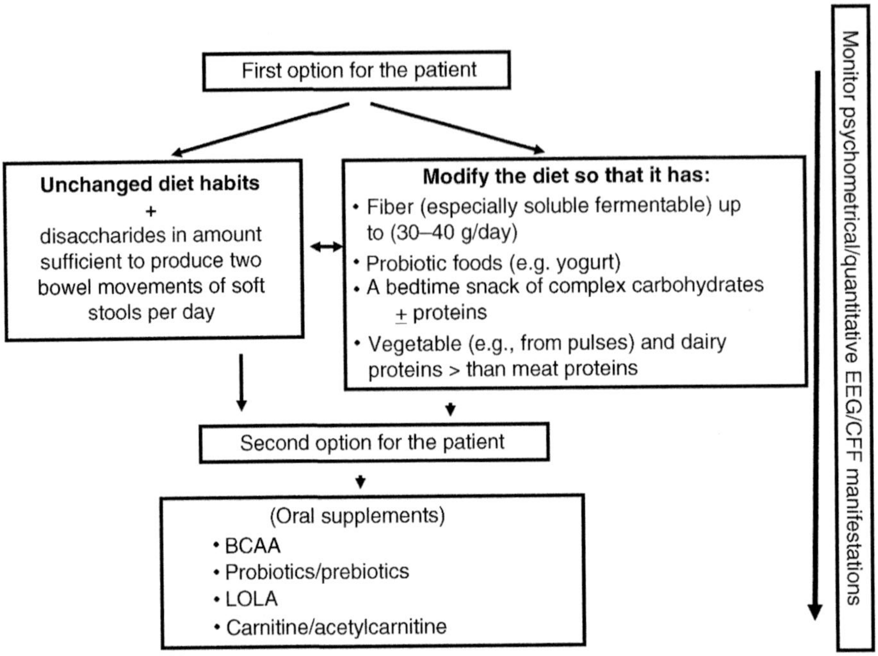

Figure 11.6 Treatment strategy for MHE based on the minimization of drug use. BCAA, branched chain amino acids; CFF, Critical Flicker Frequency; LOLA, L-ornithine-L-aspartate.

reduction of episodes of overt HE in follow-up [145]. Notably, a large trial on zinc sulfate did not demonstrate reduction of episodes of overt HE in follow-up [146].

4 Theoretically, NUNS might have a rational role in these patients, but no evidence-based information exists.

The patients with severe motor alterations (i.e., hepatic myelopathy or non-Wilsonian hepatocerebral degeneration) respond only partially to drug treatment, but may recover completely after liver transplantation [9,10]. The efficacy of dopaminergic drugs on motor symptoms in these patients is uncertain. For the patient with minimal or covert HE, there is evidence that they improve with disaccharides [147] and rifaximin [148], as well as LOLA [149], pre/probiotics [150], and acetylcarnitine [151]. However, because MHE has a less severe clinical impact on patients and their caregivers than overt HE [152], a reasonable approach aiming at minimizing drug use and reducing costs is shown in Figure 11.6.

Prophylaxis

Primary prophylaxis for HE coincides with prevention of cirrhosis decompensation. Therefore, depending on the etiology of cirrhosis, of paramount importance is alcohol abstinence and treatment of HBV, HCV, steatohepatitis, and iron overload. In addition, prevention of gastrointestinal bleeding and spontaneous bacterial peritonitis, and avoidance of malnutrition are recommended.

Secondary prophylaxis concerns those individuals who had at least one bout of HE in the previous 6 months. The higher the number of episodes of HE in the past, the higher the risk to develop HE in the future. In addition, patients with recurrent HE have a high risk of residual minimal HE in between the overt episodes [27,28,54] so in the patient with recurrent HE the distinction between prophylaxis and treatment is disputable.

After one episode of HE, disaccharides are indicated and were found to about halve the recurrence of HE at 1 year (from 40% to 20%) [32]. In those patients who had more than one episode of HE in the previous 6 months, the use of rifaximine (550 mg bid), with or without disaccharides, was found to further about halve the risk of a new episode of HE within 6 months (from 40% to 20%) [33]. Finally, in a phase II trial, the NUNS glycerol-phenylbutyrate reduced by about 40% the recurrence of HE in patients who experienced recurrent HE; this effect was found to be higher in patients that were not on rifaximine treatment [50].

There is no agreement on the rules for stopping HE prophylaxis. It can reasonably be stopped if liver function improves because of virus treatment, nutrition, or alcohol abstinence.

References

1 Moffat J. Prognostics and Prorrhetics of Hippocrates, translated from the original Greek. London, UK: Bensley, 1788.
2 Walshe JM. Observations on the symptomatology and pathogenesis of hepatic coma. Q J Med 1951;20:421–38.
3 Adams RD, Foley JM. The neurological disorder associated with liver disease. Res Publ Assm Res Nerv Ment Dis 1953;32:198–237.
4 Sherlock S, Summerskill WHJ, White LP, Phear EA. Portal-systemic encephalopathy: neurological complications of liver disease. Lancet 1954;267:454–7.
5 Fazekas JE, Ticktin HE, Shea JG. effects of L-arginine on hepatic encephalopathy. Am J Med Sci 1957;234:462–7.
6 Vilstrup H, Amodio P, Bajaj J, et al. Hepatic encephalopathy in chronic liver disease: 2014 Practice Guideline by the American Association for the Study of Liver Diseases and the European Association for the Study of the Liver. Hepatology 2014;60:715–35.
7 Cadranel JF, Lebiez E, Di Martino V, et al. Focal neurological signs in hepatic encephalopathy in cirrhotic patients: an underestimated entity? Am J Gastroenterol 2001;96:515–8.
8 Victor M, Adams RD, Cole M. The acquired (non Wilsonian) type of chronic hepatocerebral degeneration. Medicine 1965;44:345–96.
9 Baccarani U, Zola E, Adani GL, et al. Reversal of hepatic myelopathy after liver transplantation: fifteen plus one. Liver Transpl 2010;16:1336–7.
10 Weissenborn K, Tietge UJ, Bokemeyer M, et al. Liver transplantation improves hepatic myelopathy: evidence by three cases. Gastroenterology 2003;124:346–51.
11 Mendoza G, Marti-Fabregas J, Kulisevsky J, Escartin A. Hepatic myelopathy: a rare complication of portacaval shunt. Eur Neurol 1994;34:209–12.
12 Cordoba J, Cabrera J, Lataif L, Penev P, Zee P, Blei AT. High prevalence of sleep disturbance in cirrhosis. Hepatology 1998;27:339–45.
13 Mostacci B, Ferlisi M, Baldi AA, et al. Sleep disturbance and daytime sleepiness in patients with cirrhosis: a case control study. Neurol Sci 2008;29:237–40.
14 Montagnese S, Middleton B, Skene DJ, Morgan MY. Night-time sleep disturbance does not correlate with neuropsychiatric impairment in patients with cirrhosis. Liver Int 2009;29:1372–82.
15 Roman E, Cordoba J, Torrens M, Guarner C, Soriano G. Falls and cognitive dysfunction impair health-related quality of life in patients with cirrhosis. Eur J Gastroenterol Hepatol 2013;25:77–84.
16 Soriano G, Roman E, Cordoba J, et al. Cognitive dysfunction in cirrhosis is associated with falls: a prospective study. Hepatology 2012;55:1922–30.
17 Amodio P, Montagnese S, Gatta A, Morgan MY. Characteristics of minimal hepatic encephalopathy. Metab Brain Dis 2004;19:253–67.
18 Bajaj JS, Cordoba J, Mullen KD, et al. Review article: the design of clinical trials in hepatic encephalopathy - an International Society for Hepatic Encephalopathy and Nitrogen Metabolism (ISHEN) consensus statement. Aliment Pharmacol Ther 2011;33:739–47.
19 Ortiz M, Cordoba J, Doval E, et al. Development of a clinical hepatic encephalopathy staging scale. Aliment Pharmacol Ther 2007;26:859–67.
20 Hassanein TI, Hilsabeck RC, Perry W. Introduction to the Hepatic Encephalopathy Scoring Algorithm (HESA). Dig Dis Sci 2008;53:529–38.
21 Salam M, Matherly S, Farooq IS, et al. Modified-orientation log to assess hepatic encephalopathy. Aliment Pharmacol Ther 2012;35:913–20.
22 Conn HO, Leevy CM, Vlahcevic ZR, et al. Comparison of lactulose and neomycin in the treatment of chronic portal-systemic encephalopathy: a double blind controlled trial. Gastroenterology 1977;72:573–83.
23 Folstein MF, Folstein SE, McHugh PR. "Mini-mental state": a practical method for grading the cognitive state of patients for the clinician. J Psychiatr Res 1975;12:189–98.
24 Ferenci P, Lockwood A, Mullen K, Tarter R, Weissenborn K, Blei AT. Hepatic encephalopathy: definition, nomenclature, diagnosis, and quantification. Final report of the working party at the 11th World Congresses of Gastroenterology, Vienna, 1998. Hepatology 2002;35:716–21.
25 D'Amico G, Morabito A, Pagliaro L, Marubini E. Survival and prognostic indicators in compensated and decompensated cirrhosis. Dig Dis Sci 1986;31:468–75.
26 Coltorti M, Del Vecchio-Blanco C, Caporaso N, Gallo C, Castellano L. Liver cirrhosis in Italy: a multicentre study on presenting modalities and the impact on health care resources. National Project on Liver Cirrhosis Group. Ital J Gastroenterol 1991;23:42–8.
27 Bajaj JS, Schubert CM, Heuman DM, et al. Persistence of cognitive impairment after resolution of overt hepatic encephalopathy. Gastroenterology 2010;138:2332–40.
28 Riggio O, Ridola L, Pasquale C, et al. Evidence of persistent cognitive impairment after resolution of overt hepatic encephalopathy. Clin Gastroenterol Hepatol 2011;9:181–3.
29 Gentilini P, Laffi G, La Villa G, et al. Long course and prognostic factors of virus-induced cirrhosis of the liver. Am J Gastroenterol 1997;92:66–72.
30 Gines P, Quintero E, Arroyo V, et al. Compensated cirrhosis: natural history and prognostic factors. Hepatology 1987; 7:122–8.

31 Jmaa A, Ksiaa M, Ben SA, et al. The natural history of hepatitis B virus cirrhosis after the first hepatic decompensation in Tunisia. Tunis Med 2012;90:172–6.
32 Sharma BC, Sharma P, Agrawal A, Sarin SK. Secondary prophylaxis of hepatic encephalopathy: an open-label randomized controlled trial of lactulose versus placebo. Gastroenterology 2009;137:885–91, 891.
33 Bass NM, Mullen KD, Sanyal A, et al. Rifaximin treatment in hepatic encephalopathy. N Engl J Med 2010;362: 1071–81.
34 Prasad S, Dhiman RK, Duseja A, Chawla YK, Sharma A, Agarwal R. Lactulose improves cognitive functions and health-related quality of life in patients with cirrhosis who have minimal hepatic encephalopathy. Hepatology 2007;45:549–59.
35 Amodio P, Pellegrini A, Ubiali E, et al. The EEG assessment of low-grade hepatic encephalopathy: comparison of an artificial neural network-expert system (ANNES) based evaluation with visual EEG readings and EEG spectral analysis. Clin Neurophysiol 2006;117:2243–51.
36 Boyer TD, Haskal ZJ. The role of transjugular intrahepatic portosystemic shunt (TIPS) in the management of portal hypertension: update 2009. Hepatology 2010;51:306
37 Riggio O, Angeloni S, Salvatori FM, et al. Incidence, natural history, and risk factors of hepatic encephalopathy after transjugular intrahepatic portosystemic shunt with polytetrafluoroethylene-covered stent grafts. Am J Gastroenterol 2008;103:2738–46.
38 Spina G, Santambrogio R. The role of portosystemic shunting in the management of portal hypertension. Bailliere Clin Gastroenterol 1992;6:497–515.
39 Bai M, Qi X, Yang Z, et al. Predictors of hepatic encephalopathy after transjugular intrahepatic portosystemic shunt in cirrhotic patients: a systematic review. J Gastroenterol Hepatol 2011;26:943–51.
40 Stepanova M, Mishra A, Venkatesan C, Younossi ZM. In-hospital mortality and economic burden associated with hepatic encephalopathy in the United States from 2005 to 2009. Clin Gastroenterol Hepatol 2012;10:1034–41.
41 Del Piccolo F, Sacerdoti D, Amodio P, et al. Central nervous system alterations in liver cirrhosis: the role of portal-systemic shunt and portal hypoperfusion. Metab Brain Dis 2002;17:347–58.
42 Garcia-Martinez R, Simon-Talero M, Cordoba J. Prognostic assessment in patients with hepatic encephalopathy. Dis Markers 2011;31:171–9.
43 Watanabe A. Portal-systemic encephalopathy in non-cirrhotic patients: classification of clinical types, diagnosis and treatment. J Gastroenterol Hepatol 2000;15:969–79.
44 Keiding S, Munk OL, Roelsgaard K, Bender D, Bass L. Positron emission tomography of hepatic first-pass metabolism of ammonia in pig. Eur J Nucl Med 2001;28:1770–5.
45 Aldrete JS. Quantification of the capacity of the liver to remove ammonia from the circulation of dogs with portacaval transposition. Surg Gynecol Obstet 1975;141: 399–404.
46 Riggio O, Mannaioni G, Ridola L, et al. Peripheral and splanchnic indole and oxindole levels in cirrhotic patients: a study on the pathophysiology of hepatic encephalopathy. Am J Gastroenterol 2010;105:1374–81.
47 Nomura F, Ohnishi K, Terabayashi H, et al. Effect of intrahepatic portal-systemic shunting on hepatic ammonia extraction in patients with cirrhosis. Hepatology 1994;20: 1478–81.
48 Conn HO. Hepatic encephalopathy. In: Schiff L, Schiff ER (eds) Diseases of the Liver, 7th edn. Philadelphia: Lippicott, 1993. pp. 1036–60.
49 Arora S, Martin CL, Herbert M. Myth: interpretation of a single ammonia level in patients with chronic liver disease can confirm or rule out hepatic encephalopathy. CJEM 2006;8:433–5.
50 Rockey DC, Vierling JM, Mantry P, et al. Randomized, double-blind, controlled study of glycerol phenylbutyrate in hepatic encephalopathy. Hepatology 2014;59:1073–83.
51 Fahn S. Classification of movement disorders. Mov Disord 2011;26:947–57.
52 Comim CM, Constantino LC, Barichello T, Streck EL, Quevedo J, Dal-Pizzol F. Cognitive impairment in the septic brain. Curr Neurovasc Res 2009;6:194–203.
53 Shawcross D, Jalan R. The pathophysiologic basis of hepatic encephalopathy: central role for ammonia and inflammation. Cell Mol Life Sci 2005;62:2295–304.
54 Amodio P, Del Piccolo F, Petteno E, et al. Prevalence and prognostic value of quantified electroencephalogram (EEG) alterations in cirrhotic patients. J Hepatol 2001;35:37–45.
55 Angeli P, Wong F, Watson H, Gines P. Hyponatremia in cirrhosis: results of a patient population survey. Hepatology 2006;44:1535–42.
56 Butterworth RF. Thiamine deficiency-related brain dysfunction in chronic liver failure. Metab Brain Dis 2009;24:189–96.
57 Schomerus H, Hamster W. Neuropsychological aspects of portal-systemic encephalopathy. Metab Brain Dis 1998;13: 361–77.
58 Weissenborn K, Ennen JC, Schomerus H, Ruckert N, Hecker H. Neuropsychological characterization of hepatic encephalopathy. J Hepatol 2001;34:768–73.
59 Amodio P, Wenin H, Del Piccolo F, et al. Variability of trail making test, symbol digit test and line trait test in normal people: a normative study taking into account age-dependent decline and sociobiological variables. Aging Clin Exp Res 2002;14:117–31.
60 Dhiman RK, Saraswat VA, Verma M, Naik Sr. Figure connection test: a universal test for assessment of mental state. J Gastroenterol Hepatol 1995;10:14–23.
61 Dhiman RK, Kurmi R, Thumburu KK, et al. Diagnosis and prognostic significance of minimal hepatic encephalopathy in patients with cirrhosis of liver. Dig Dis Sci 2010;55:2381–90.

62 Randolph C, Hilsabeck R, Kato A, et al. Neuropsychological assessment of hepatic encephalopathy: ISHEN practice guidelines. Liver Int 2009;29:629–35.

63 Riggio O, Ridola L, Pasquale C, et al. A simplified psychometric evaluation for the diagnosis of minimal hepatic encephalopathy. Clin Gastroenterol Hepatol 2011;9: 613–6.

64 Amodio P, Ridola L, Schiff S, et al. Improving the inhibitory control task to detect minimal hepatic encephalopathy. Gastroenterology 2010;139:510–8.

65 Bajaj JS, Hafeezullah M, Franco J, et al. Inhibitory control test for the diagnosis of minimal hepatic encephalopathy. Gastroenterology 2008;135:1591–600.

66 Kircheis G, Wettstein M, Timmermann L, Schnitzler A, Haussinger D. Critical flicker frequency for quantification of low-grade hepatic encephalopathy. Hepatology 2002;35:357–66.

67 Guerit JM, Amantini A, Fischer C, et al. Neurophysiological investigations of hepatic encephalopathy: ISHEN practice guidelines. Liver Int 2009;29:789–96.

68 Parsons-Smith BG, Summerskill WHJ, Dawson AM, Sherlock S. The electroencephalograph in liver disease. Lancet 1957;273:867–71.

69 Amodio P, Marchetti P, Del Piccolo F, et al. Spectral versus visual EEG analysis in mild hepatic encephalopathy. Clin Neurophysiol 1999;110:1334–44.

70 Kato A, Suzuki K, Kaneta H, Obara H, Fujishima Y, Sato S. Regional differences in cerebral glucose metabolism in cirrhotic patients with subclinical hepatic encephalopathy using positron emission tomography. Hepatol Res 2000;17: 237–45.

71 Senzolo M, Pizzolato G, Ferronato C, Chierichetti F, Boccagni P, Dam M, Burra P. Long-term evaluation of cognitive function and cerebral metabolism in liver transplanted patients. Transplant Proc 2009;41:1295–6.

72 Giewekemeyer K, Berding G, Ahl B, Ennen JC, Weissenborn K. Bradykinesia in cirrhotic patients with early hepatic encephalopathy is related to a decreased glucose uptake of frontomesial cortical areas relevant for movement initiation. J Hepatol 2007;46:1034–9.

73 Lockwood AH, Weissenborn K, Bokemeyer M, Tietge U, Burchert W. Correlations between cerebral glucose metabolism and neuropsychological test performance in non-alcoholic cirrhotics. Metab Brain Dis 2002;17:29–40.

74 Weissenborn K, Bokemeyer M, Ahl B, et al. Functional imaging of the brain in patients with liver cirrhosis. Metab Brain Dis 2004;19:269–80.

75 Kostler H. Proton magnetic resonance spectroscopy in portal-systemic encephalopathy. Metab Brain Dis 1998;13: 291–301.

76 Amodio P, Pellegrini A, Amista P, et al. Neuropsychological-neurophysiological alterations and brain atrophy in cirrhotic patients. Metab Brain Dis 2003;18:63–78.

77 Guevara M, Baccaro ME, Gomez-Anson B, et al. Cerebral magnetic resonance imaging reveals marked abnormalities of brain tissue density in patients with cirrhosis without overt hepatic encephalopathy. J Hepatol 2011;55:564–73.

78 Zhang LJ, Yang G, Yin J, Liu Y, Qi J. Neural mechanism of cognitive control impairment in patients with hepatic cirrhosis: a functional magnetic resonance imaging study. Acta Radiol 2007;48:577–87.

79 Zhang LJ, Qi R, Zhong J, et al. Disrupted functional connectivity of the anterior cingulate cortex in cirrhotic patients without overt hepatic encephalopathy: a resting state fMRI study. PLoS One 2013;8:e53206.

80 Berding G, Banati RB, Buchert R, et al. Radiotracer imaging studies in hepatic encephalopathy: ISHEN practice guidelines. Liver Int 2009;29:621–8.

81 Butterworth RF, Norenberg MD, Felipo V, Ferenci P, Albrecht J, Blei AT. Experimental models of hepatic encephalopathy: ISHEN guidelines. Liver Int 2009;29:783–8.

82 Van Caulert C, Deviller C, Halff M. Troubles provoques par l'ingestion de sels ammoniacaux chez l'homme atteint de cirrhose de Laennec. Comptes Rendus Soc Biol 1932;111:739–40.

83 Balo J, Korpassy B. The encephalitis of the dog with Eck fistula fed on meat. Arch Pathol 1932;13:80–7.

84 Stormont JM, Mackie JE, Davidson CS. Observations on antiobiotics in the treatment of hepatic coma and on factors contributing to prognosis. N Engl J Med 1958;259:1145–50.

85 Bircher J, Muller J, Guggenheim P, Haemmerli UP. Treatment of chronic portal-systemic encephalopathy with lactulose. Lancet 1966;1:890–2.

86 Baraldi M, Avallone R, Corsi L, Venturini I, Baraldi C, Zeneroli ML. Natural endogenous ligands for benzodiazepine receptors in hepatic encephalopathy. Metab Brain Dis 2009;24:81–93.

87 Felipo V, Urios A, Montesinos E, et al. Contribution of hyperammonemia and inflammatory factors to cognitive impairment in minimal hepatic encephalopathy. Metab Brain Dis 2012;27:51–8.

88 Mannaioni G, Carpenedo R, Corradetti R, et al. Tryptophan metabolism and hepatic encephalopathy. Studies on the sedative properties of oxindole. Adv Exp Med Biol 1999;467:155–67.

89 Montagnese S, Biancardi A, Schiff S, et al. Different biochemical correlates for different neuropsychiatric abnormalities in patients with cirrhosis. Hepatology 2011;53:558–66.

90 Odeh M. Pathogenesis of hepatic encephalopathy: the tumour necrosis factor-alpha theory. Eur J Clin Invest 2007;37:291–304.

91 Zieve L. The mechanism of hepatic coma. Hepatology 1981;1:360–5.

92 Campollo O, Sprengers D, McIntyre N. The BCAA/AAA ratio of plasma amino acids in three different groups of cirrhotics. Rev Invest Clin 1992;44:513–8.

93 Owen OE, Reichle FA, Mozzoli MA, et al. Hepatic, gut, and renal substrate flux rates in patients with hepatic cirrhosis. J Clin Invest 1981;68:240–52.

94 Petrides AS, Stanley T, Matthews DE, Vogt C, Bush AJ, Lambeth H. Insulin resistance in cirrhosis: prolonged reduction of hyperinsulinemia normalizes insulin sensitivity. Hepatology 1998;28:141–9.

95 Sherwin RS, Fisher M, Bessoff J, et al. Hyperglucagonemia in cirrhosis: altered secretion and sensitivity to glucagon. Gastroenterology 1978;74:1224–8.

96 Keiding S, Sorensen M, Bender D, Munk OL, Ott P, Vilstrup H. Brain metabolism of 13N-ammonia during acute hepatic encephalopathy in cirrhosis measured by positron emission tomography. Hepatology 2006;43:42–50.

97 Olde Damink SW, Deutz NE, Dejong CH, Soeters PB, Jalan R. Interorgan ammonia metabolism in liver failure. Neurochem Int 2002;41:177–88.

98 Olde Damink SW, Dejong CH, Deutz NE, et al. Kidney plays a major role in ammonia homeostasis after portasystemic shunting in patients with cirrhosis. Am J Physiol Gastrointest Liver Physiol 2006;291:G189–94.

99 Fischer JE, Baldessarini RJ. False neurotransmitters and hepatic failure. Lancet 1971;2:75–80.

100 Fischer JE, Rosen HM, Ebeid AM, James JH, Keane JM, Soeters PB. The effect of normalization of plasma amino acids on hepatic encephalopathy in man. Surgery 1976;80:77–91.

101 Morgan MY, Milsom JP, Sherlock S. Plasma ratio of valine, leucine and isoleucine to phenylalanine and tyrosine in liver disease. Gut 1978;19:1068–73.

102 Cuilleret G, Pomier-Layrargues G, Pons F, Cadilhac J, Michel H. Changes in brain catecholamine levels in human cirrhotic hepatic encephalopathy. Gut 1980;21:565–9.

103 Mpabanzi L, Deutz N, Hayes PC, Dejong CH, Olde Damink SW, Jalan R. Overnight glucose infusion suppresses renal ammoniagenesis and reduces hyperammonaemia induced by a simulated bleed in cirrhotic patients. Aliment Pharmacol Ther 2012;35:921–8.

104 Amodio P, Bemeur C, Butterworth R, et al. The nutritional management of hepatic encephalopathy in patients with cirrhosis: International Society for Hepatic Encephalopathy and Nitrogen Metabolism Consensus. Hepatology 2013;58:325–36.

105 McPhail MJ, Patel NR, Taylor-Robinson SD. Brain imaging and hepatic encephalopathy. Clin Liver Dis 2012;16:57–72.

106 Rovira A, Alonso J, Cordoba J. MR imaging findings in hepatic encephalopathy. AJNR Am J Neuroradiol 2008;29:1612–21.

107 Rose C, Butterworth RF, Zayed J, et al. Manganese deposition in basal ganglia structures results from both portal-systemic shunting and liver dysfunction. Gastroenterology 1999;117:640–4.

108 Rama Rao KV, Reddy PV, Hazell AS, Norenberg MD. Manganese induces cell swelling in cultured astrocytes. Neurotoxicology 2007;28:807–12.

109 Weissenborn K, Ehrenheim C, Hori A, Kubicka S, Manns MP. Pallidal lesions in patients with liver cirrhosis: clinical and MRI evaluation. Metab Brain Dis 1995;10:219–31.

110 Marchetti P, D'Avanzo C, Orsato R, et al. Electroencephalography in patients with cirrhosis. Gastroenterology 2011;141:1680–9.

111 Timmermann L, Butz M, Gross J, et al. Impaired cerebral oscillatory processing in hepatic encephalopathy. Clin Neurophysiol 2008;119:265–72.

112 Montagnese S, Jackson C, Morgan MY. Spatio-temporal decomposition of the electroencephalogram in patients with cirrhosis. J Hepatol 2007;46:447–58.

113 Butterworth RF. Altered glial-neuronal crosstalk: cornerstone in the pathogenesis of hepatic encephalopathy. Neurochem Int 2010;57:383–8.

114 Butterworth RF. Hepatic encephalopathy: a central neuroinflammatory disorder? Hepatology 2011;53:1372–6.

115 Haussinger D, Gorg B. Interaction of oxidative stress, astrocyte swelling and cerebral ammonia toxicity. Curr Opin Clin Nutr Metab Care 2010;13:87–92.

116 Hertz L, Kala G. Energy metabolism in brain cells: effects of elevated ammonia concentrations. Metab Brain Dis 2007;22:199–218.

117 Lai JC, Cooper AJ. Brain alpha-ketoglutarate dehydrogenase complex: kinetic properties, regional distribution, and effects of inhibitors. J Neurochem 1986;47:1376–86.

118 Rama Rao KV, Jayakumar AR, Norenberg MD. Glutamine in the pathogenesis of acute hepatic encephalopathy. Neurochem Int 2012;61:575–80.

119 Leke R, Bak LK, Anker M, et al. Detoxification of ammonia in mouse cortical GABAergic cell cultures increases neuronal oxidative metabolism and reveals an emerging role for release of glucose-derived alanine. Neurotox Res 2011;19:496–510.

120 Norenberg MD, Itzhak Y, Bender AS. The peripheral benzodiazepine receptor and neurosteroids in hepatic encephalopathy. Adv Exp Med Biol 1997;420:95–111.

121 Szerb JC, Butterworth RF. Effect of ammonium ions on synaptic transmission in the mammalian central nervous system. Prog Neurobiol 1992;39:135–53.

122 Rodrigo R, Cauli O, Gomez-Pinedo U, et al. Hyperammonemia induces neuroinflammation that contributes to cognitive impairment in rats with hepatic encephalopathy. Gastroenterology 2010;139:675–84.

123 Corenblum B, Shaffer EA. Hyperprolactinemia in hepatic encephalopathy may result from impaired central dopaminergic neurotransmission. Horm Metab Res 1989;21:675–7.

124 Lozeva V, Montgomery JA, Tuomisto L, et al. Increased brain serotonin turnover correlates with the degree of shunting and hyperammonemia in rats following variable portal vein stenosis. J Hepatol 2004;40:742–48.

125 Chavez-Tapia NC, Barrientos-Gutierrez T, Tellez-Avila F, et al. Meta-analysis: antibiotic prophylaxis for cirrhotic

patients with upper gastrointestinal bleeding - an updated Cochrane review. Aliment Pharmacol Ther 2011;34: 509–18.
126 Alexander T, Thomas K, Cherian AM, Kanakasabapathy. Effect of three antibacterial drugs in lowering blood and stool ammonia production in hepatic encephalopathy. Indian J Med Res 1992;96:292–6.
127 Rolachon A, Zarski JP, Lutz JM, Fournet J, Hostein J. [Is the intestinal lavage with a solution of mannitol effective in the prevention of post-hemorrhagic hepatic encephalopathy in patients with liver cirrhosis? Results of a randomized prospective study]. Gastroenterol Clin Biol 1994;18:1057–62.
128 Sharma P, Agrawal A, Sharma BC, Sarin SK. Prophylaxis of hepatic encephalopathy in acute variceal bleed: a randomized controlled trial of lactulose versus no lactulose. J Gastroenterol Hepatol 2011;26:996–1003.
129 American Academy of Clinical Toxicology and European Association of Poison Centers and Clinical Toxicologists. Position paper: cathartics. J Toxicol Clin Toxicol 2004;42: 243–53.
130 Soarez PC, Oliveira AC, Padovan J, Parise ER, Ferraz MB. A critical analysis of studies assessing L-ornithine-L-aspartate (LOLA) in hepatic encephalopathy treatment. Arq Gastroenterol 2009;46:241–7.
131 Abid S, Jafri W, Mumtaz K, et al. Efficacy of L-ornithine-L-aspartate as an adjuvant therapy in cirrhotic patients with hepatic encephalopathy. J Coll Physicians Surg Pak 2011; 21:666–71.
132 Gluud LL, Dam G, Borre M, et al. Lactulose, rifaximin or branched chain amino acids for hepatic encephalopathy: what is the evidence? Metab Brain Dis 2013;28:221–5.
133 Rossi-Fanelli F, Riggio O, Cangiano C, et al. Branched-chain amino acids vs lactulose in the treatment of hepatic coma: a controlled study. Dig Dis Sci 1982;27:929–35.
134 Higuchi K, Shimizu Y, Nambu S, et al. Effects of an infusion of branched-chain amino acids on neurophysiological and psychometric testings in cirrhotic patients with mild hepatic encephalopathy. J Gastroenterol Hepatol 1994;9:366–72.
135 Ott P, Clemmesen O, Larsen FS. Cerebral metabolic disturbances in the brain during acute liver failure: from hyperammonemia to energy failure and proteolysis. Neurochem Int 2005;47:13–8.
136 Plauth M, Cabre E, Campillo B, et al. ESPEN Guidelines on Parenteral Nutrition: hepatology. Clin Nutr 2009;28:436–44.
137 Barbaro G, Di Lorenzo G, Soldini M, et al. Flumazenil for hepatic coma in patients with liver cirrhosis: an Italian multicentre double-blind, placebo-controlled, crossover study. Eur J Emerg Med 1998;5:213–8.
138 Prabhakar S, Bhatia R. Management of agitation and convulsions in hepatic encephalopathy. Indian J Gastroenterol 2003;22 (Suppl 2): S54–8.
139 Hoetzel A, Ryan H, Schmidt R. Anesthetic considerations for the patient with liver disease. Curr Opin Anaesthesiol 2012;25:340–7.
140 Sharma P, Singh S, Sharma BC, et al. Propofol sedation during endoscopy in patients with cirrhosis, and utility of psychometric tests and critical flicker frequency in assessment of recovery from sedation. Endoscopy 2011;43: 400–5.
141 Clarke B, Ellis MJ, Leung V, et al. Reversal of hepatic encephalopathy and alteration in amino acid profiles after blocking a surgical splenorenal shunt by interventional radiological techniques. J Hepatol 1989;8:325–9.
142 Gentile S, Guarino G, Romano M, Alagia IA, et al. A randomized controlled trial of acarbose in hepatic encephalopathy. Clin Gastroenterol Hepatol 2005;3:184–91.
143 Malaguarnera M, Pistone G, Elvira R, Leotta C, Scarpello L, Liborio R. Effects of L-carnitine in patients with hepatic encephalopathy. World J Gastroenterol 2005;11:7197–202.
144 Malaguarnera M, Vacante M, Motta M, et al. Acetyl-L-carnitine improves cognitive functions in severe hepatic encephalopathy: a randomized and controlled clinical trial. Metab Brain Dis 2011;26:281–9.
145 Takuma Y, Nouso K, Makino Y, Hayashi M, Takahashi H. Clinical trial: oral zinc in hepatic encephalopathy. Aliment Pharmacol Ther 2010;32:1080–90.
146 Bresci G, Parisi G, Banti S. Management of hepatic encephalopathy with oral zinc supplementation: a long-term treatment. Eur J Med 1993;2:414–6.
147 Luo M, Li L, Lu CZ, Cao WK. Clinical efficacy and safety of lactulose for minimal hepatic encephalopathy: a meta-analysis. Eur J Gastroenterol Hepatol 2011;23:1250–7.
148 Sidhu SS, Goyal O, Mishra BP, Sood A, Chhina RS, Soni RK. Rifaximin improves psychometric performance and health-related quality of life in patients with minimal hepatic encephalopathy (the RIME Trial). Am J Gastroenterol 2011;106:307–16.
149 Mittal VV, Sharma BC, Sharma P, Sarin SK. A randomized controlled trial comparing lactulose, probiotics, and L-ornithine L-aspartate in treatment of minimal hepatic encephalopathy. Eur J Gastroenterol Hepatol 2011;23:725–32.
150 Shukla S, Shukla A, Mehboob S, Guha S. Meta-analysis: the effects of gut flora modulation using prebiotics, probiotics and synbiotics on minimal hepatic encephalopathy. Aliment Pharmacol Ther 2011;33:662–71.
151 Malaguarnera M, Bella R, Vacante M, et al. Acetyl-L-carnitine reduces depression and improves quality of life in patients with minimal hepatic encephalopathy. Scand J Gastroenterol 2011;46:750–9.
152 Montagnese S, Amato E, Schiff S, et al. A patients' and caregivers' perspective on hepatic encephalopathy. Metab Brain Dis 2012;27:567–72.

CHAPTER 12

Malnutrition and nutritional support

Jian-Gao Fan and Hai-Xia Cao

Department of Gastroenterology, Shanghai Key Laboratory of Pediatric, Gastroenterology and Nutrition, Xinhua Hospital Affiliated to Shanghai Jiaotong University School of Medicine, Shanghai, China

Introduction

Malnutrition is a condition that results from an unbalanced diet in which certain nutrients are lacking, in excess (too high an intake), or in the wrong proportions. There are several types of malnutrition including undernutrition and obesity, depending on which nutrients are under or overabundant in the diet (Table 12.1). Because the major form of malnutrition in patients with cirrhosis is undernutrition or protein–calorie malnutrition, malnutrition in the current chapter only refers to protein–calorie malnutrition. Malnutrition is a frequent and integral component of acute and chronic diseases. Patients with advanced liver disease commonly have malnutrition but its assessment is confounded by many of the usual indicators of nutritional status. Although a clear consensus on the criteria of malnutrition in cirrhosis is still lacking at present, malnutrition is extremely common in cirrhotic patients worldwide.

The working definition of malnutrition in cirrhosis in most studies is decreased lean body mass as well as diminished skeletal muscle weight and reduced fat mass. On one hand, malnutrition is the single reversible prognostic marker in cirrhosis that accelerates deteriorating liver function and adversely affects clinical outcome both before and after liver transplantation, including increased morbidity and prolonged hospital stay [1,2]. Mortality increases in direct proportion to the extent of malnutrition, approaching 80% in patients with severe malnutrition (i.e., less than 50% of normal body weight) [3]. On the other hand, adequate nutrition is a fundamental component of survival and quality of life in cirrhotic patients, and correction of malnutrition might improve the clinical outcome of these patients. Therefore, nutritional assessment should be routinely performed in cirrhotic patients, and aggressive nutritional management might be useful in patients with malnutrition. However, the mechanism leading to malnutrition is not fully understood yet, and the logistic challenges of identifying patients in need of nutritional therapy and determining the type, duration, and quantity of nutritional supplements remain problematic.

Etiologies of malnutrition in cirrhosis

Malnutrition, characterized by protein and calorie deficiency, is defined as a state of nutrition in which a deficiency of energy, protein, and other nutrients causes measurable adverse effects on tissue and body form and function and on clinical outcome (Table 12.2). There are three forms of malnutrition: kwashiorkor (protein malnutrition predominant), marasmus (deficiency in calorie intake), and marasmic kwashiorkor (both marked protein deficiency and calorie insufficiency signs are present). Marasmic kwashiorkor is sometimes referred to as the most severe form of malnutrition and is more commonly seen in the context of a wide variety of diseases that lead to depletion of body fat, muscle wasting, and multiple signs of micronutrient deficiencies.

As the liver is the most important metabolic organ that regulates a complex array of physiologic and biochemical processes including protein and energy metabolism, malnutrition may commonly be secondary to chronic liver disease, especially advanced cirrhosis in which protein

Cirrhosis: A practical guide to management, First Edition. Edited by Samuel S. Lee and Richard Moreau.

Table 12.1 Classification of malnutrition.

Form	Interpretation
Undernutrition	Underweight, protein–calorie malnutrition
Kwashiorkor	Selective protein malnutrition with edema and fatty liver
Marasmus	Deficiency in calorie intake with loss of body fat and protein
Marasmic kwashiorkor	Marked protein deficiency and marked calorie insufficiency signs present
Obesity	Overweight, central obesity

Table 12.2 The usual indicators of protein–calorie malnutrition.

If the patients meet one or more of the following criteria, they should be considered at risk for malnutrition:
Unintentional loss >10% of usual body weight in the preceding 3 months
Body weight <90% of ideal for height
- <80% of ideal constitutes mild malnutrition
- <70% of ideal represents severe malnutrition

BMI <18.5 kg/m^2

BMI, body mass index (the weight in kilograms divided by the height in square meters).

energy wasting may occur. Malnutrition in patients with cirrhosis is multifactorial (Table 12.3), including reduced food intake, maldigestion, and malabsorption. Many of these factors can be treated successfully if the nutritional status is recognized.

Decreased nutrient intake The majority of cirrhotic patients have inadequate dietary intake which is attributed to several factors. Anorexia is a frequent symptom in patients with cirrhosis, with an incidence as high as 90% [4]. Many patients with advanced liver disease have an altered sense of taste, which might be related to vitamin A and/or zinc deficiency [5]. Patients with cirrhosis often experience early satiety that is related to mechanical compression from massive ascites [6]. Patients with chronic liver diseases experience abdominal pain, nausea, and bloating [7], and are found to have altered gut motility [8], all of which lead to the development of functional dyspepsia. The dietary restrictions that are commonly recommended to these patients, such as restriction of sodium, protein, and water, can discourage adequate oral intake. In addition, weakness, fatigue, and low-grade encephalopathy can contribute to decreased oral intake. Other iatrogenic causes for protein and caloric loss include multiple hospitalizations which may lead to loss of regular meals for reasons of pending examinations and procedures.

Malabsorption Cholestatic liver disease is one of the reasons for impaired absorption, especially of fat-soluble

Table 12.3 Factors contributing to malnutrition in cirrhosis.

Outpatients with cirrhosis	Inpatients with cirrhosis
Decreased diet intake • Anorexia, nausea/vomiting, abdominal pain, dysphagia • Iatrogenic or restriction of prorein, fluid/salt • Poverty due to inadequate income	Fasting status and accelerated starvation • Frequently diagnostic testing • Gastrointestinal bleeding • Altered neurologic status
Decreased assimilation of diet • Impaired digestion of diet, e.g., pancreatic and bile salt deficiency • Intestinal malabsorption of dietary constituents, e.g., portal hypertension, enteropathy, gastrointestinal infections, bacterial overgrowth, chronic alcoholism, chronic diarrhea, use of either neomycin or lactulose	Use of either neomycin or lactulose for hepatic encephalopathy Routine or prophylactic protein restriction Stress or critical acute illness (hypermetabolism)
Abnormal metabolism of protein and energy • Increased protein breakdown and reduced protein synthesis • Accelerated lipolysis and reduced lipogenesis • Increased resting energy expenditure	• Acute sepsis • Major surgery • Renal failure • Acute or chronic inflammation
Effects of chronic alcoholism on protein and energy metabolism	

vitamins such as A, D, E, and K, due to reduced intraluminal bile salt concentrations [9,10]. Chronic alcohol drinking impairs gastrointestinal mucosal absorption of nutrients, especially folate and vitamin B12. Furthermore, conditions such as small intestine bacterial overgrowth, coexistent small intestinal disease (i.e., inflammatory bowel disease and celiac sprue), pancreatic insufficiency, mucosal congestion, and villus atrophy contribute to the impaired absorption and utilization of nutrients [8,11,12]. The presence of portal hypertension has also been implicated as a cause of malabsorption and gastrointestinal protein loss [13,14]. An additional factor is the administration of medications that lead to malabsorption, such as neomycin, which has been used in the treatment of hepatic encephalopathy [15].

Inadequate synthesis of protein Other important factors in the loss of body protein are the inadequate synthesis of various proteins by the affected liver. It has been observed that among cirrhotic patients, an early switch to gluconeogenesis from amino acids originating from body proteins after an overnight fast is often the rule. Deficiency in vitamins and trace minerals is often observed in advanced cirrhosis. The most common iatrogenic interventions are the use of diuretics in order to cope with ascites and fluid retention. Last but not least, the occult or overt blood loss from esophageal and gastric varices and the intestinal lumen due to ulcerations or portal enteropathy are some of the main reasons for protein loss [16].

Hypermetabolic state Another factor that might contribute to malnutrition, around which there has been considerable debate, is increased energy expenditure. The well-recognized hyperdynamic circulation in cirrhosis is associated with a systematic vasodilatation and an expanded intravascular blood volume leading to an increased cardiac stroke volume. Therefore, greater use of macro- and micro-nutrients is one of the most common causes of high energy demand and expenditure. In fact, it has been suggested that up to 30% of patients with cirrhosis are actually hypermetabolic [17–19].

Nutritional assessment in cirrhosis

Malnutrition is common in patients with cirrhosis and increase the severity of disease [20,21]. Therefore, every hospitalized patient should have an assessment of their nutritional status. Severely malnourished patients have poorer outcomes, regardless of the disease entity or reason for hospitalization. The usual evaluation of malnutrition includes the following.

1 The patient's history and etiologies of malnutrition, such as diet and weight change, socioeconomic conditions, and symptoms unique to each clinical setting.
2 Physical findings of malnutrition: unintentional loss of >10% of usual body weight in the past 3 months, anthropometry of triceps skinfold and mid-arm muscle circumference (decreased temporal and proximal extremity muscle mass (muscle wasting), and decreased skinfold thickness by "pinch test" (loss of subcutaneous fat)), mouth and mucus membranes (i.e., nasolabial seborrhea for deficiency of essential fatty acids, and glossitis for deficiency of riboflavin, niacin, vitamin B12, pyridoxine, folate), skin rashes, ocular changes, and neurologic changes.
3 Laboratory assessment of malnutrition, such as serum albumin and other visceral proteins, assess blood vitamins (A, E, 25(OH)D, B12, folic acid) and minerals (zinc, magnesium, phosphorus), and immune function (reduced total lymphocyte count and delayed hypersensitivity skin reaction).
4 Specialized procedures for nutritional assessment (i.e., bioelectric impedance analysis, resting and total energy expenditure, and urine nitrogen excretion and nitrogen balance).
5 Integrated bedside assessment, such as subjective global assessment (SGA) and prognostic nutritional assessment.

In 2006, the European Society for Parenteral and Enteral Nutrition (ESPEN) suggested a simple and practical method to assess nutritional status. The methods that are universally used to evaluate nutritional status and to detect the presence of malnutrition are SGA, and some anthropometric parameters and laboratory tests [22]. The algorithm for assessing the nutitional state is seen in Figure 12.1.

Subjective global assessment SGA is recommended by ESPEN as a practical bedside method that combines multiple elements of nutritional assessment to classify the severity of malnutrition [22]. These components are weight loss during the previous 6 months, changes in dietary intake, gastrointestinal symptoms, functional capacity, metabolic demands, signs of muscle wasting,

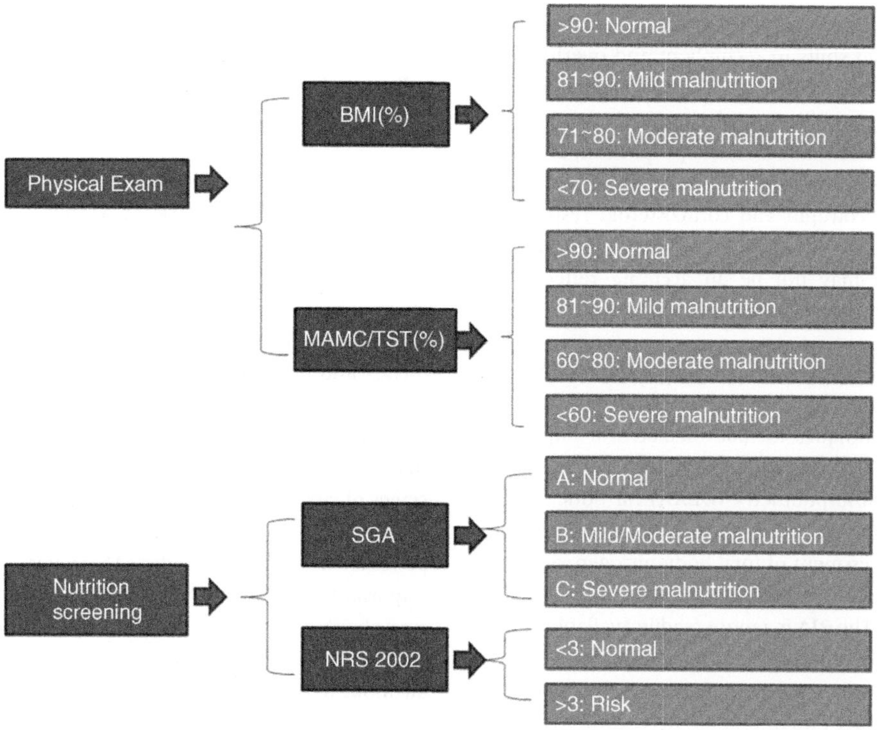

Figure 12.1 Algorithm for assessing nutritional state in cirrhotic patients. BMI, body mass index; MAMC, mid-arm muscle circumference; NRS, nutrition risk screening; SGA, subjective global assessment; TST, tricep skinfold thickness.

and the presence of presacral or pedal edema. The SGA is scored from 0 to 3 as well nourished (0), mild malnutrition (1), moderate malnutrition (2), and severe malnutrition (3). Of the various components, muscle wasting is weighted the most [23,24], and the change of body weight is the least reliable because it can be confounded by the fluid retention frequently seen in these patients. As it calculates recent body weight loss or gain, the SGA is considered reliable, and it is not affected by fluid retention or the formation of ascites. The SGA has been shown to have an interobserver reproducibility rate of 80% [25,26].

Anthropometric parameters Apart from the data that are collected by the SGA questionnaire, the ESPEN guidelines recommend the use of simple anthropometric parameters in evaluating malnutrition which are also not affected by the presence of ascites and peripheral edema. These parameters consist of body mass index corrected for fluid retention (BMIc), mid-arm muscle circumference (MAMC) or mid-arm circumference (MAC), and triceps skinfold thickness (TST). However, it is suggested that they should be performed by experienced clinicians in order to avoid intra- and interobserver variabilities. The BMIc is calculated as estimated dry body weight/(height)^2 (in kg/m^2). The BMIc cutoff values are used to indicate malnutrition, for example, 22, 23, and 25 kg/m^2 in patients without, with mild, and with tense ascites, respectively. Diagnosis of malnutrition is established on values of MAMC and/or TST below the fifth percentile in patients aged 18–74 years, or the tenth percentile in patients aged over 74 years [27]. The assessment of muscle function measuring hand-grip strength and respiratory-muscle strength has also been used in nutritional evaluation; these are more useful when taken serially.

Laboratory tests The visceral proteins such as albumin, pre-albumin, retinol-binding protein, and transferrin are produced in the liver and correlate better with severity of the underlying liver disease than with malnutrition status [28]. As we know, the laboratory markers of malnutrition are capricious. Hypoalbuminemia may result from protein–calorie malnutrition but is equally likely to result from fluid shifts in recumbent and overhydrated patients; from losses in the urine, gastrointestinal tract, or the third space; and from cytokine effects or inflammation that reduces hepatic albumin production. Similarly, lymphopenia has causes other than malnutrition, particularly the corticotropin and corticosteroid response to acute biologic stress. Serum creatinine confounded by renal function may not be an accurate reflection of muscle mass in patients with renal insufficiency.

Specialized procedures for nutritional assessment Body cell mass is a useful estimation of nutritional status. The assessment techniques include bioelectrical impedance analysis (BIA) for determination of fat-free mass, dual-energy X-ray absorptiometry (DEXA) for bone mineral density and fat-free mass, *in vivo* neutron activation analysis for assessment of total body nitrogen, and deuterium oxide dilution for determination of total body water [29,30]. The BIA is a more readily available tool for estimating body cell mass; it is reliable in many patient populations. Furthermore, the BIA-derived phase angle is also a useful evaluating tool in chronic liver diseases [31]. However, the accuracy of BIA in patients with cirrhosis can be affected by fluid retention [32] and it does not accurately reflect changes in body composition associated with chronic liver disease. Although abnormalities of nutritional parameters are highly prevalent among patients with end-stage liver disease, most parameters of nutritional status do not correlate with body cell mass. Quantification of body composition changes in cirrhosis requires the use of direct methods such as *in vivo* neutron activation analysis, DEXA, or deuterium oxide dilution. However, these techniques are cumbersome, expensive, and not routinely used in clinical practice. In addition, MAMC and hand-grip strength might be the most sensitive markers of body cell mass depletion in patients with end-stage liver disease, so we prefer these simple and easy measurements.

Prevalence of malnutrition in cirrhosis

On one hand, malnutrition is often underdiagnosed in cirrhosis, as advanced liver disease – especially with ascites and edema – can affect the results of many of the traditional techniques currently used to evaluate nutritional status. On the other hand, clinically obvious malnutrition is uncommon in the pre-cirrhotic and early stages of cirrhosis, and the prevalence of obesity and the metabolic syndrome has increased sharply in these patients in the past decades. Moreover, obesity is an important risk factor for the progression of nonalcoholic steatohepatitis (NASH) and risk for the development of cirrhosis and hepatocellular carcinoma in patients with alcoholic and viral liver diseases.

However, malnutrition is frequently seen in decompensated cirrhosis or end-stage liver disease. The reported prevalence in cirrhotic patients varies widely (from 20% to 100%), mainly depending on the methods used for nutritional assessment in studies and the severity of cirrhosis (Table 12.4) [33–38]. There is a direct correlation between the severity of liver disease defined by the Child–Turcotte–Pugh score and the prevalence of malnutrition. Malnutrition commonly develops in all forms of cirrhosis irrespective of the etiology of disease, and there is no difference in the prevalence of malnutrition between alcoholic and nonalcoholic cirrhosis [39–42].

Table 12.4 Prevalence of malnutrition in cirrhotic patients in different countries.

Author	Year	Country	No.	Malnutrition (%)	Malnutrition in Child A	Malnutrition in Child C	*P*-value
Huisman	2011	Netherlands	84	56 (67%)	57%	100%	0.047
Houissa	2010	Tunis	44	35 (79.5%)	66.6%	100%	0.003
Castellanos	2008	Spain	121	55 (45%)	21%	90%	<0.001
Carvalho	2006	Brazil	300	226 (75.3%)	21%	58%	<0.05
Guglielmi	2005	Italy	334	83 (25%)	16%	44%	<0.05
Maio	2004	Portugal	117	74 (63%)	44%	68%	>0.05

Regarding the degree of muscle wasting, loss of fat stores, and synthetic function, there are indeed disease-specific patterns of malnutrition in different forms of cirrhosis. Moderate or severe malnutrition occurs in 70–80% of patients with cirrhosis awaiting liver transplantation according to different parameters [43]. It has been demonstrated that patients with cirrhosis who are malnourished have a higher rate of hepatic encephalopathy, infection, ascites, and variceal bleeding [24,44,45] and it can severely compromise the results of liver transplantation [46]. Therefore, physicians need to be aware that malnutrition is common in cirrhosis, with reversible prognostic significance.

Table 12.5 Nutritional supplement guidelines in cirrhosis.

Calories	35–40 kcal/kg/day
Protein	1.2–1.5 g/kg/day
Carbohydrate	50–60% of total calories
Fat	40–50% of total calories
Water	40–50 mL/kg/day
Salt (sodium)	2–3 g/day
Calcium	1200–1500 mg/day
Vitamin D	400–800 IU/day
Vitamin A	100 000–200 000 IU every 4 weeks
Vitamin K	10 mg every 4 weeks

Nutritional support in patients with cirrhosis

Indications for nutritional support

As malnutrition is prevalent in advanced liver disease and it has prognostic value, it is of great importance to improve the nutritional status in cirrhotic patients. First, patients who have recently lost >10% of their body weight and those >30% below ideal body weight are considered candidates for nutritional support. Second, any hospitalized patients with predicated severe inadequate nutrition for >7 days should be supported from the time of admission. Finally, patients with a variety of specific disease entities have quicker recoveries and shorter hospital stays if nutritional needs are met. Such patients include severely malnourished patients about to undergo surgery, patients with acute or chronic renal failure, alcoholic hepatitis or cirrhosis, and chronic extrahepatic biliary obstruction.

Goals for nutritional support

Recent studies suggest that improvements in nutritional status, infection rates, immune function, nitrogen balance, and perioperative morbidity are seen in cirrhotic patients receiving nutritional therapy. Nutritional support is most effective when used for longer periods or in certain subgroups such as in those with severe malnutrition, chronic hepatic encephalopathy, or decompensated liver disease. Regarding goals specific for cirrhosis, nutritional therapy needs to correct pre-existing protein–calorie malnutrition by supplying the basic requirements of nitrogen and calories, while simultaneously providing sufficient vitamins and minerals to encourage hepatic regeneration and normalization of liver function without precipitating hepatic encephalopathy and ascites (Table 12.5).

Route of nutritional support

When nutritional support is indicated, it should be initiated by the enteral route unless specific contraindications are present. Actually, most critically ill patients can tolerate enteral feeding. In general, oral intake should be encouraged when the gastrointestinal tract is functional. If patients are unable to maintain adequate intake orally, a nasogastric, nasoduodenal, or nasojejunal tube should be inserted for 4–6 weeks of enteral feeding. Parenteral nutrition is a less desirable option than enteral nutrition and should be reserved for patients in whom enteral feeding cannot be achieved. In fact, clinicians frequently have limited options in selecting the route of nutritional support.

Enteral nutrition The goals of nutritional therapy are to improve nutritional status and correct nutrient deficiencies. This can be accomplished via oral, enteral, or parenteral methods, or a combination of these modalities. Intervention in the early stages of malnutrition can improve outcome. The presence of nonbleeding esophageal varices is not a contradiction to the use of enteral feeding tubes in these patients. However, feeding tubes should not be used if there is active esophageal variceal bleeding. The placement of a gastrotomy tube in cirrhotic patients with ascites is not recommended because of the possible complications of peritonitis or ascitic fluid leakage. Enteral nutrition is preferred to parenteral nutrition because of its low cost, decreased risk of infection, maintenance of gut mucosal integrity, and prevention of bacterial translocation. In patients with cirrhosis, enteral nutrition improves nutritional status and liver function, reduces the rate of complications and even prolongs survival [47–51]. The ESPEN guidelines show that enteral supplements improved nutritional status and immune function in outpatients with alcoholic cirrhosis.

Parenteral nutrition The parenteral route is used whenever the enteral or oral routes are not safe or possible or when patients need to stay fasting for 72 hours or more [52,53]. Peripheral parenteral nutrition may be used to provide partial or total nutrition for up to 2 weeks, while central parenteral nutrition is good for long-term therapy or in patients with fluid restriction. However, central parenteral nutrition is plagued by mechanical complications of catheter insertion in 4–6% of cases. Infectious complications occur in about 5% of patients receiving peripheral parenteral nutrition. Moreover, severe hyperglycemia and fluid, acid–base, and electrolyte disturbances, as well as nutritional deficiencies, are more common with parenteral nutrition. However, recent clinical trials showed that patients with parenteral nutrition had a decreased incidence of ascites and infection [54].

Hepatobiliary complications are common in patients on parenteral nutrition. Parenteral nutrition-associated liver disease (PNALD) is a complex disease that is diagnosed by clinical presentation, biochemical markers of liver injury, concurrent use of total parenteral nutrition, and negative work-up for other causes of liver disease. As liver biopsy is invasive, the diagnosis of PNALD is usually made by a rise in serum conjugated bilirubin of 2 mg/dL or more, which may be accompanied by increasing gamma-glutamyl transpeptidase, alkaline phosphatase, and aminotransferases. The spectrum of PNALD can range from parenteral nutrition-associated cholestasis, parenteral nutrition-associated liver injury, to intestinal failure-associated liver disease. PNALD is reported to occur in 50–66% of children receiving long-term total parenteral nutrition, with a higher incidence in premature neonates [55]. Although the incidence of PNALD is much higher in children, PNALD also occurs in adult patients but may present with cholestasis, hepatosteatosis, or cholelithiasis [55].

Parenteral nutrition-associated cholestasis usually improves after cessation of parenteral nutrition [56]. PNALD may be prevented or reversed if enteral feeding can be established. If enteral nutrition is impossible, reducing the duration of daily parenteral nutrition or using cyclic infusions may be useful. The other preventive measures include maintaining the calories at less than 25 kcal/kg/day and using lipid emulsions with long and medium-chain triglycerides or omega-9 monounsaturated fatty acids [56,57]. Moreover, metronidazole, ursodeoxycholic acid, and S-adenosylmethionine can be used.

Parenteral nutrition is thus a less desirable option than enteral nutrition and should be reserved for patients in whom enteral feeding cannot be achieved [58]. The ESPEN guidelines indicate that parenteral nutrition should be considered in patients with higher grade hepatic encephalopathy, particularly in hepatic encephalopathy IV with malfunction of swallowing and cough reflexes, and unprotected airways. After liver transplantation, patients should receive early postoperative nutrition, and then parenteral nutrition is the secondary option after enteral nutrition.

Practical implementation

In general, nonstressed patients should be provided a daily total energy of 30 kcal/kg ideal body weight, and protein should constitute at least 4 kcal/kg/day or 1 g/kg/day. Stressed patients may require increased protein up to 1.5 g/kg/day to avoid catabolism of muscle protein. The ESPEN guidelines recommend that cirrhotic patients should achieve an energy intake of 35–40 kcal/kg/day (147–168 kJ/kg/day) and a protein intake of 1.2–1.5 g/kg/day. In addition, during intermittent acute illness or exacerbations of the underlying chronic liver disease, an above-normal protein intake (1.5 g/kg/day) and kilocalorie intake (40 kcal/kg/day) might improve protein–calorie malnutrition, and should be considered in the treatment of these patients.

Protein supplementation A protein intake of 1.2–1.5 g/kg/day is safe in patients with cirrhosis. For those with compensated cirrhosis, this goal can be achieved with a normal diet without any restrictions in carbohydrates, proteins, or fat. In the case of decompensated cirrhosis, supplementary meals are often recommended and prescribed. It was previously believed that protein should be restricted for patients with cirrhosis to avoid precipitation of hepatic encephalopathy. Later studies, however, showed that patients undergoing protein restriction may develop muscle catabolism, leading to a rise in ammonia and worsening of hepatic encephalopathy. A randomized clinical trial has demonstrated that an intake

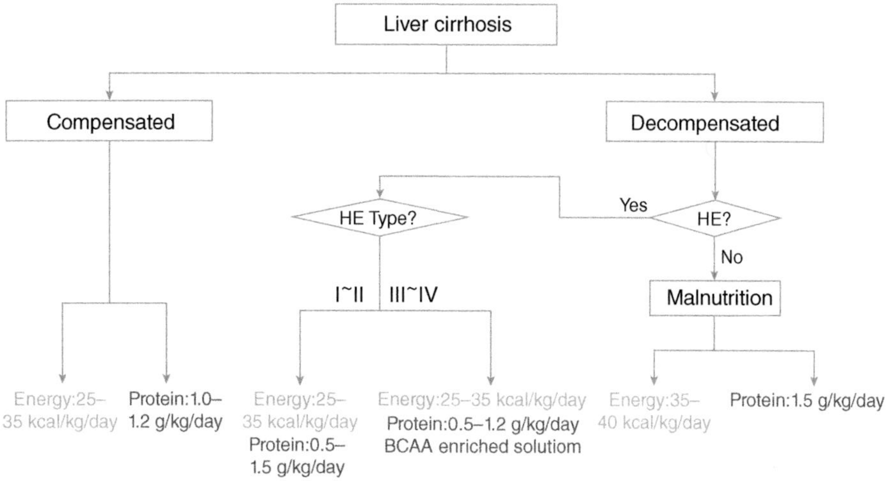

Figure 12.2 Algorithm for the recommendations of European Society for Parenteral and Enteral Nutrition (ESPEN) in liver cirrhosis. BCAA, branched chain amino acid; HE, hepatic encephalopathy.

of 1.2 g/kg/day protein prevents muscle catabolism and does not precipitate hepatic encephalopathy [59]. According to the ESPEN guidelines, low-grade hepatic encephalopathy (grades I and II) is not regarded as a reason for diet or protein restriction, underscoring that malnutrition is certainly considered a negative prognostic factor. There is an exception, however, for those patients with severe hepatic encephalopathy (grades III and IV) who should have a restricted protein intake (Figure 12.2).

Carbohydrates and fat In the prescribed diets there should be no restriction on carbohydrate intake, even in patients with diabetes mellitus or who belong to the subgroup of patients with insulin resistance. In fact, 40–50% of all patients with end-stage liver disease develop insulin-resistant diabetes mellitus. The exact cause differs from patient to patient, with the most prominent being chronic hyperinsulinemia, pancreatic insufficiency due to alcohol toxicity, diminished glycogen storage capacity of the liver, and impaired glucose uptake from the skeletal muscles. Four to six meals daily containing foods rich in carbohydrates are recommended [60]. Carbohydrate intake should exclusively be provided by glucose and cover 50–60% of nonprotein energy requirements, with the other 40–50% of nonprotein energy requirements provided by lipid intake. Most of the calories in parenteral nutritional formulations are derived from dextrose and fat, and lipid emulsions can be used to advantage to provide 20–40% of total calories.

Vitamin and mineral requirements Nutritional therapy in patients with chronic liver disease should not only focus on treatment of protein energy malnutrition, but should also aim to correct specific nutrient deficiencies. Patients with advanced liver disease commonly develop micronutrient deficiencies. One of the most common complications of cirrhosis is osteoporosis. Prescription of 1200–1500 mg calcium and 400–800 IU vitamin D, especially in patients with cholestasis, is advised. Biphosphonates are also recommended [61]. Lack of vitamin A results in nyctotyphlosis and dry cornea and so the use of 100 000–200 000 IU every 4 weeks is advisable [62]. Parenteral administration of 10 mg vitamin K every 4 weeks is recommended as well. A diet low in sodium of <2–3 g/day NaCl is generally advised in end-stage liver disease in patients with ascites and fluid retention. Most commercially available enteral feeding formulas also contain about 1 kcal/mL energy and sufficient vitamins, electrolytes, and trace minerals to guarantee adequate nutrition when provided in 2–3 L volumes each day. The majority contain less than 2 g sodium and are acceptable when salt intake must be limited. Parenteral solutions routinely have water-soluble and miscible vitamins as well as standard additions of trace minerals. In addition, adults daily require about 30 mL of water per kilogram of body weight, or approximately 1 mL/kcal of energy. However, patients with ascites, edema, heart failure, or intrinsic kidney disease may have low urine output and require less water.

Amino acids Both peripheral and central parenteral nutrition solutions are formulated with amino acids rather than proteins. Two liters of a 5% amino acid solution is equivalent to about 80 g protein. Disease-specific amino acid mixtures are commercially available for parenteral nutrition, but their superiority over balanced mixtures of essential and nonessential amino acids is uncertain. Branched chain amino acids (BCAAs), such as valine, leucine, and isoleucine, have a branched side chains instead of an aromatic group in aromatic amino acids, such as phenylalanine, histidine, and tryptophan. BCAAs help protein synthesis and turnover in the peripheral muscles with subsequent generation of energy. This leads to reduced BCAA levels in patients with cirrhosis [62]. An initial randomized clinical trial of 37 cirrhotic patients showed that BCAA supplementation compared with conventional protein supplementation (80 g/day protein intake in both groups) was superior in improving hepatic encephalopathy without any effect on the serum ammonia levels [63]. A much larger study 646 of patients showed benefit of BCAA granule supplementation (12 g/day for 2 years) in 314 patients to reduce the composite primary endpoint of death or transplantation compared with standard protein intake in 308 patients, due to reduced progression to liver failure. Also, BCAA supplementation resulted in improved quality of life. There was no difference, however, in the occurrence of esophageal variceal rupture, liver cancer, and death. The use of a more palatable form of BCAAs as granules instead of powder in the previous study resulted in improved patient compliance, with 86% of patients taking the full amount of recommended doses throughout the study [64].

However, other studies have failed to show a clinical benefit of BCAA supplementation. Kanematsu et al. [65] reported that there was no significant difference in rate of occurrence of hepatic encephalopathy between BCAA and control groups during a 14-day follow-up. Furthermore, in patients with severe decompensated cirrhosis, the timing of oral BCAA administration is an important issue because BCAA granules take time to take effect. The available basic research and clinical trials about BCAA in cirrhosis were carried out mainly in Japanese subjects and more research is needed to explore the novel effects of BCAA in the prognosis of cirrhosis. Because oral BCAA granules are unavailable in China, we usually use an intravenous amino acid solution enriched with more BCAA to treat patients with hepatic encephalopathy. In other parts of the world, the high cost and unpalatability may limit the potential applicability of this treatment [66]. In summary, the use of BCAA supplementation in decompensated cirrhosis remains a controversial issue [67], and it is clear that further trials are needed before this strategy can be routinely recommended to treat hepatic encephalopathy.

Specific patient populations for nutritional support

Alcoholic liver disease Alcoholic liver disease (ALD) is the most prevalent form of liver disease in North America and Europe, and is an emerging problem in developing countries including China. It encompasses a spectrum of liver injury, ranging from simple hepatic steatosis through alcoholic steatohepatitis to frank cirrhosis and hepatocellular carcinoma. The presence of significant malnutrition is a common finding in alcoholics, as are deficiencies in a number of vitamins and trace minerals, including vitamins A, D, thiamine, folate, pyridoxine, and zinc. The reasons for malnutrition in alcoholism include the finding that alcohol has profound effects on protein and energy metabolism, and direct effects on small bowel mucosal function and absorption. Malnutrition due to impaired caloric intake and increased catabolism is very common in patients with ALD [68–71], is associated with an increased rate of major complications of severe alcoholic hepatitis and cirrhosis, and indicates a poor prognosis. Therefore, the presence and extent of malnutrition and micronutrient deficiencies have an important role in determining the outcome of patients with ALD, and nutrition status should be carefully evaluated. In 2010, the ALD practice guideline by the American Association for the Study of Liver Disease (AASLD) and the American College of Gastroenterology (ACG) recommended that all patients with alcoholic hepatitis or advanced ALD should be assessed for nutritional deficiencies, as well as vitamin and mineral deficiencies.

Current clinical management of patients with ALD focuses on alcohol abstinence, aggressive nutritional therapy rich in calories and proteins, and early treatment of alcohol abuse or dependence, and liver-related complications. Long-term aggressive nutritional therapy by the enteral or oral route in patients with alcoholic cirrhosis is supported by several studies that have shown improved nutritional status [72,73]. However, a recent meta-analysis showed that nutritional supplementation provided no mortality benefit in patients with ALD, while patients with hepatic encephalopathy should be encouraged to have nutritional supplementation [74].

Considering the potential risk of Wernicke's encephalopathy, supplementation with B-complex vitamins is recommended. Independent from hepatic encephalopathy, a daily protein intake of 1.2–1.5 g/kg of body weight and 35–40 kcal/kg for energy should be ensured. Lipid-soluble vitamin deficiency should be compensated. The AASLD/ACG ALD guideline [75] recommends that patients with alcoholic cirrhosis should receive feedings at frequent intervals, including a nighttime snack and morning feeding, to improve their nitrogen balance. As the recommended protein–caloric intake is often difficult to achieve orally in a significant proportion of patients with severe alcoholic hepatitis, those with severe disease should thus be treated aggressively with enteral nutritional therapy. Many recommendations [52], based on the results of the study by Cabre et al. [76], suggest that enteral nutritional support might increase survival in patients with severe alcoholic hepatitis. However, double-blinded randomized controlled and larger multi-center clinical trials are still needed to guide clinical practice.

Hepatic encephalopathy More than 25% of cirrhotic patients will eventually develop some grade of hepatic encephalopathy [77]. Hepatic encephalopathy is a wide spectrum of neuropsychiatric abnormalities occurring in patients with significant liver dysfunction due to an as yet uncertain mechanism. Nutritional factors have a major role both in the pathogenesis and the management of hepatic encephalopathy. The neuropsychiatric alterations may range from mild behavior changes to deep coma. Various measures are used to treat hepatic encephalopathy [78,79]. First, identify and correct the precipitating factors including electrolyte abnormalities, constipation, and so on. Second, initiate empiric therapy including gut cleaning with enemas, use of non-absorbable disaccharide and/or a nonabsorbable antibiotic. Third, institute a low or zero protein diet only for immediate management of overt encephalopathy, and a vegetable-based protein diet and BCAA-enriched oral diet are recommended for long-term treatment [80]. However, information regarding improvement in hepatic encephalopathy after BCAA supplementation is still controversial [77,81]. A recent systematic review by Gluud et al. [81] show that oral BCAA supplements improve manifestations of hepatic encephalopathy but have no effect on survival. Actually, more than 95% of cirrhotic patients can tolerate diets containing as much as 1.5 g/kg/day of mixed proteins. For those few patients with protein intolerance, BCAA might be better than standard amino acid supplements.

Liver transplantation Malnutrition is a common problem for patients waiting for orthotopic liver transplantation, and poses a major risk factor for postoperative morbidity and mortality [82–84]. Recipients' malnutrition is associated with increased operative blood loss, length of stay in the intensive care unit, mortality, and total hospital charges after liver transplantation [84,85]. Whether the presence of a compromised nutritional status has a role as an independent risk factor for the outcome of liver transplantation is still a matter of debate, although, interestingly, current opinion is that malnutrition should not be considered as a contraindication to liver transplantation [58]. Results from Singal et al. [43] support the feasibility of liver transplantation for patients with alcoholic cirrhosis with obesity or malnutrition. However, there is no uniform approach among transplant centers regarding the management of nutrition in transplant patients [86]. Particular attention should be focused on these patients, by evaluating their nutritional status and by planning possible nutritional corrections.

Recently, the Council of the British Transplant Society issued guidelines for the management of NASH before and after liver transplantation. According to the guidelines [3,87], the criteria for listing of patients for liver transplantation for those with NASH cirrhosis, either due to end-stage liver disease or presence of hepatocellular carcinoma, should be in line with standard national criteria; there are no data to support an absolute cutoff for BMI and liver transplantation. BMI should be corrected for the presence of ascites and peripheral edema. Weight loss should not be recommended in patients with decompensated end-stage liver disease because of the risk of protein–calorie malnutrition. All potential NASH transplant recipients, including those with an elevated BMI, should be assessed by a dietitian and supplemental feeding considered if protein–calorie malnutrition is present. Dietary assessment of patients being assessed for liver transplantation should include use of hand-grip strength, anthropometry, and/or SGA to assess the patient's nutritional status and allow supplementation if required. Dietary assessment of patients should be repeated on an annual basis while they remain on the waiting list for liver transplantation.

Conclusions

As malnutrition is prevalent in advanced liver disease and it has prognostic value, it is of great importance to assess the nutritional status of cirrhotic patients. Malnutrition in cirrhosis can be defined as the loss of both visceral and skeletal muscle protein stores and fat mass. However, it is sometimes difficult to evaluate the nutritional status in these patients as many have ascites and edema. In addition, a number of aspects of nutritional assessment are controversial. Further studies are needed to explore the effects of malnutrition on liver disease, and clinicians need to realize that malnutrition is ubiquitous in all kinds of cirrhosis. The treatment of malnutrition may improve the clinical outcome as it has prognostic significance.

References

1 Koretz RL. The evidence for the use of nutrition support in liver disease. Curr Opin Gastroenterol 2014;30:208–14.

2 Juakiem W, Torres DM, Harrison SA. Nutrition in cirrhosis and chronic liver disease. Clin Liver Dis 2014;18:179–190.

3 Newsome PN, Allison ME, Andrews PA, et al. Guidelines for liver transplantation for patients with non-alcoholic steatohepatitis. Gut 2012;61:484–500.

4 Achord JL. Malnutrition and the role of nutritional support in alcoholic liver disease. Am J Gastroenterol 1987;82:1–7.

5 Garrett-Laster M, Russell RM, Jacques RF. Impairment of taste and olfaction in patients with cirrhosis: the role of vitamin A. Hum Nutr Clin Nutr 1984;38:203–14.

6 Plauth M, Schutz ET. Cachexia in liver cirrhosis. Int J Cardiol 2002;85:83–7.

7 Kalaitzakis E, Simren M, Olsson R, et al. Gastrointestinal symptoms in patients with liver cirrhosis: associations with nutritional status and health-related quality of life. Scand J Gastroenterol 2006;41:1464–72.

8 Gunnarsdottir SA, Sadik R, Shev S, et al. Small intestinal motility disturbances and bacterial overgrowth in patients with liver cirrhosis and portal hypertension. Am J Gastroenterol 2003;98:1362–70.

9 Gundling F, Teich N, Strebel HM, Schepp W, Pehl C. Nutrition in liver cirrhosis. Med Klin 2007;102:435–44.

10 Moscatiello S, Manini R, Marchesini G. Diabetes and liver disease: an ominous association. Nutr Metab Cardiovasc Dis 2007;17:63–70.

11 Vlahcevic ZR, Buhac I, Farrar JT, et al. Bile acid metabolism in patients with cirrhosis. I. Kinetic aspects of cholic acid metabolism. Gastroenterology 1971;60:491–8.

12 Sanchez E, Casafont F, Guerra A, et al. Role of intestinal bacterial overgrowth and intestinal motility in bacterial translocation in experimental cirrhosis. Rev Esp Enferm Dig 2005;97:805–14.

13 Romiti A, Merli M, Martorano M, et al. Malabsorption and nutritional abnormalities in patients with liver cirrhosis. Ital J Gastroenterol 1990;22:118–23.

14 Conn HO. Is protein-losing enteropathy a significant complication of portal hypertension. Am J Gastroenterol 1998;93:127–8.

15 Thompson GR, Barrowman J, Gutierrez L, et al. Action of neomycin on intraluminal phase of lipid absorption. J Clin Invest 1971;50:319–23.

16 Kondrup J. Nutrition in end stage liver disease. Best Pract Res Clin Gastroenterol 2006;20:547–60.

17 Muller MJ, Bottcher J, Selberg O, et al. Hypermetabolism in clinically stable patients with liver cirrhosis. Am J Clin Nutr 1999;69:1194–201.

18 Muller MJ, Boker KH, Selberg O. Are patients with liver cirrhosis hypermetabolic? Clin Nutr 1994;13:131–44.

19 Madden AM, Morgan M. Resting energy expenditure should be measured in patients with cirrhosis, not predicted. Hepatology 1999;30:655–64.

20 Vieira PM, De-Souza DA, Oliveira LC. Nutritional assessment in hepatic cirrhosis; clinical, anthropometric, biochemical and hematological parameters. Nutr Hosp 2013; 28:1615–21.

21 Johnson TM, Overgard EB, Cohen AE, et al. Nutrition assessment and management in advanced liver disease. Nutr Clin Pract 2013;28:15–29.

22 Plauth M, Cabre E, Riggio O, et al. ESPEN guidelines on enteral nutrition: liver disease. Clin Nutr 2006;25:285–94.

23 Detsky AS, McLaughlin JR, Baker JP, et al. What is subjective global assessment of nutritional status? J Parenter Enteral Nutr 1987;11:8–13.

24 Pikul J, Sharpe MD, Lowndes R, et al. Degree of preoperative malnutrition is predictive of postoperative morbidity and mortality in liver transplant recipients. Transplantation 1994;57:469–72.

25 Steenson J, Vivianti A, Isenring E. New clinicians require ongoing training to ensure high inter-rater reliability of the Subjective Global Assessment. Nutrition 2013;29: 361–2.

26 Hasse J, Strong S, Gorman MA. Subjective global assessment: alternative nutrition-assessment technique for liver-transplant candidates. Nutrition 1993;9:339–43.

27 Campillo B, Richardet JP, Bories PN. Enteral nutrition in severely malnourished and anorectic cirrhotic patients in clinical practice. Gastroenterol Clin Biol 2005;29:645–51.

28 Merli M, Romiti A, Riggio O, Capocaccia L. Optimal nutritional indexs in chronic liver disease. J Parenter Enteral Nutr 1987;11:130S–4S.
29 Figueiredo FA, Dickson ER, Pasha TM, et al. Utility of standard nutritional parameters in detecting body cell mass depletion in patients with end-stage liver disease. Liver Transpl 2000;6:575–81.
30 Prijatmoko D, Strauss BJ, Lambert JR, et al. Early detection of protein depletion in alcoholic cirrhosis: role of body composition analysis. Gastroenterology 1993;105:1839–45.
31 Peres WA, Lento DF, Baluz K, et al. Phase angle as a nutritional evaluation tool in all stages of chronic liver disease. Nutr Hosp 2012;27:2072–8.
32 Schloerb PR, Forster J, Delcore R. Bioelectrical impedance in the clinical evaluation of liver disease. Am J Clin Nutr 1996;64:510S–4S.
33 Huisman EJ, Trip EJ, Siersema PD, et al. Protein energy malnutrition predicts complications in liver cirrhosis. Eur J Gastroenterol Hepatol 2011;23:982–9.
34 Houissa F, Salem M, Debbeche R, et al. Evaluation of nutritional status in patients with liver cirrhosis. Tunis Med 2010;88:76–9.
35 Castellanos Fernández M, Santana Porbén S, García Jordá E, et al. Influence of hyponutrition on occurrence of complications and mortality among cirrhosis patients. Nutr Hosp 2008;23:68–74.
36 Carvalho L, Parise ER. Evaluation of nutritional status of nonhospitalized patients with liver cirrhosis. Arq Gastroenterol 2006;43:269–74.
37 Guglielmi FW, Panella C, Buda A, et al. Nutritional state and energy balance in cirrhotic patients with or without hypermetabolism. Multicentre prospective study by the Nutritional Problems in Gastroenterology Section of the Italian Society of Gastroenterology (SIGE). Dig Liver Dis 2005;37:681–8.
38 Maio R, Dichi JB, Burini RC. Sensibility of anthropometric-laboratory markers of protein-energy malnutrition in cirrhotic patients. Arq Gastroenterol 2004;41:93–9.
39 DiCecco SR, Wieners EJ, Wiesner RH, et al. Assessment of nutritional status of patients with end-stage liver disease undergoing liver transplantation. Mayo Clin Proc 1989;64:95–102.
40 Roongpisuthipong C, Sobhonslidsuk A, Nantiruj K, et al. Nutritional assessment in various stages of liver cirrhosis. Nutrition 2001;17:761–5.
41 Sarin SK, Dhingra N, Bansal A, et al. Dietary and nutritional abnormalities in alcoholic liver disease: a comparison with chronic alcoholics without liver disease. Am J Gastroenterol 1997;92:777–83.
42 Lolli R, Marchesini G, Bianchi G, et al. Anthropometric assessment of the nutritional status of patients with liver cirrhosis in an Italian population. Ital J Gastroenterol 1992;24:429–35.
43 Singal AK, Kamath PS, Francisco Ziller N, et al. Nutritional status of patients with alcoholic cirrhosis undergoing liver transplantation: time trends and impact on survival. Transpl Int 2013;26:788–94.
44 Moller S, Bendtsen F, Christensen E, et al. Prognostic variables in patients with cirrhosis and oesophageal varices without prior bleeding. J Hepatol 1994;21:940–6.
45 Lautz HU, Selberg O, Korber J, et al. Protein-calorie malnutrition in liver cirrhosis. Clin Investig 1992;70:478–86.
46 Selberg O, Bottcher J, Tusch G, et al. Identification of high- and low-risk patients before liver transplantation: a prospective cohort study of nutritional and metabolic parameters in 150 patients. Hepatology 1997;25:652–7.
47 Bunout D, Aicardi V, Hirsch S, et al. Nutritional support in hospitalized patients with alcoholic liver disease. Eur J Clin Nutr 1989;43:615–21.
48 Cabre E, Gonzalez-Huix F, Abad-Lacruz A, et al. Effect of total enteral nutrition on the short-term outcome of severely malnourished cirrhotics: a randomized controlled trial. Gastroenterology 1990;98:715–20.
49 Hirsch S, Bunout D, de la Maza P, et al. Controlled trial on nutrition supplementation in outpatients with symptomatic alcoholic cirrhosis. J Parenter Enteral Nutr 1993;17:119–24.
50 Kearns PJ, Young H, Garcia G, et al. Accelerated improvement of alcoholic liver disease with enteral nutrition. Gastroenterology 1992;102:200–5.
51 Dupont B, Dao T, Joubert C, et al. Randomised clinical trial: enteral nutrition does not improve the long-term outcome of alcoholic cirrhotic patients with jaundice. Aliment Pharmacol Ther 2012;35:1166–74.
52 Plauth M, Cabre E, Campillo B, et al. ESPEN Guidelines on parenteral nutrition: hepatology. Clin Nutr 2009;28:436–44.
53 Van Gossum A, Cabre E, Hebuterne X, et al. ESPEN Guidelines on parenteral nutrition: gastroenterology. Clin Nutr 2009;28:415–27.
54 Koretz RL, Avenell A, Lipman TO. Nutritional support for liver disease. Cochrane Database Syst Rev 2012;5:CD008344.
55 Tillman EM. Review and clinical update on parenteral nutrition-associated liver disease. Nutr Clin Pract 2013;28:30–9.
56 Guglielmi FW, Regano N, Mazzuoli S, et al. Cholestasis induced by total parenteral nutrition. Clin Liver Dis 2008;12:97–110.
57 Kelly DA. Preventing parenteral nutrition liver disease. Early Hum Dev 2010;86:683–7.
58 Plauth M, Merli M, Kondrup J, et al. ESPEN guidelines for nutrition in liver disease and transplantation. Clin Nutr 1997;16:43–55.
59 Cordoba J, Lopez-Hellin J, Planas M, et al. Normal protein diet for episodic hepatic encephalopathy: results of a randomized study. J Hepatol 2004;41:38–43.
60 Nakaya Y, Okita K, Suzuki K, et al. BCAA-enriched snack improves nutritional state of cirrhosis. Nutrition 2007;23:113–20.
61 Tsiaousi ET, Hatzitolios AI, Trygonis SK, et al. Malnutirion in end stage liver disease: recommendation and nutritional support. J Gastroenterol Hepatol 2008;23:527–33.

62 Yamauchi M, Takeda K, Sakamoto K, et al. Effect of oral branched-chain amino acid supplements in the late evening on the nutritional state of patients with liver cirrhosis. Hepatol Res 2001;21:199–204.
63 Horst D, Grace ND, Conn HO, et al. Comparison of dietary protein with an oral, branched chain-enriched amino acid supplement in chronic portalsystemic encephalopathy: a randomized controlled trial. Hepatology 1984;4:279–87.
64 Muto Y, Sato S, Watanabe A, et al. Effects of oral branched-chain amino acid granules on event-free survival in patients with liver cirrhosis. Clin Gastroenterol Hepatol 2005;3: 705–13.
65 Kanematsu T, Koyanagi N, Matsumata T, et al. Lack of preventive effect of branched-chain amino acid solution on postoperative hepatic encephalopathy in patients with cirrhosis: a randomized prospective trial. Surgery 1988;104:482–8.
66 Cheung K, Less SS, Raman M. Prevalence and mechanisms of malnutrition in patients with advanced liver disease, and nutrition managenment strategies. Clin Gastroenterol Hepatol 2012;10:117–25.
67 Charlton M. Branched-chain amino-acid granules: can they improve survival in patients with liver cirrhosis? Nat Clin Pract Gastroenterol Hepatol 2006;3:72–3.
68 Mezey E. Interaction between alcohol and nutrition in the pathogenesis of alcoholic liver disease. Semin Liver Dis 1991;11:340–8.
69 Mendenhall CL, Anderson S, Weesner RE, et al. Protein-calorie malnutrition associated with alcoholic hepatitis. Veterans Administration Cooperative Study Group on Alcoholic Hepatitis. Am J Med 1984;76:211–22.
70 Mendenhall C, Roselle GA, Gartside P, et al. Relationship of protein calorie malnutrition to alcoholic liver disease: a reexamination of data from two Veterans Administration Cooperative Studies. Alcohol Clin Exp Res 1995;19:635–41.
71 Leevy CM, Moroianu SA. Nutritional aspects of alcoholic liver disease. Clin Liver Dis 2005;9:67–81.
72 Mathurin P, Lucey MR. Management of alcoholic hepatitis. J Hepatol 2012;56:S39–45.
73 European Association for the Study of Liver. EASL clinical practical guidelines: management of alcoholic liver disease. J Hepatol 2012;57:399–420.
74 Antar R, Wong P, Ghali P. A meta-analysis of nutritional supplementation for management of hospitalized alcoholic hepatitis. Can J Gastroenterol 2012;26:463–7.
75 O'Shea RS, Dasarathy S, McCullough AJ. Alcoholic liver disease. AASLD practice guideline. Hepatology 2010;51:307–28.
76 Cabre E, Rodriguez-Iglesias P, Caballeria J, et al. Short- and long-term outcome of severe alcohol-induced hepatitis treated with steroids or enteral nutrition: a multicenter randomized trial. Hepatology 2000;32:36–42.
77 Moctezuma-Velázquez C, García-Juárez I, Soto-Solís R, et al. Nutritional assessment and treatment of patients with liver cirrhosis. Nutrition 2013;29:1279–85.
78 Jalan R, Seery JP, Taylor-Robinson SD. Review article: pathogenesis and treatment of chronic hepatic encephalopathy. Aliment Pharmacol Ther 1996;10:681–97.
79 Merli M, Riggio O. Dietary and nutritional indications in hepatic encephalopathy. Metab Brain Dis 2009;24:211–21.
80 Marchesini G, Dioguardi FS, Bianchi GP, et al. Long-term oral branched chain amino acid treatment in chronic hepatic encephalopathy: a randomized double-blind casein-controlled trial. The Italian Multicenter Study Group. J Hepatol 1990;11:92–101.
81 Gluud LL, Dam G, Borre M, et al. Oral branched-chain amino acids have a beneficial effect on manifestations of hepatic encephalopathy in a systematic review with meta-analyses of randomized controlled trials. J Nutr 2013;143: 1263–8.
82 Merli M, Nicolini G, Angeloni S, Riggio O. Malnutrition is a risk factor in cirrhotic patients undergoing surgery. Nutrition 2002;18:978–86.
83 Millwala F, Nguyen GC, Thuluvat PJ. Outcomes of patients with cirrhosis undergoing non-hepatic surgery: risk assessment and management. World J Gastroenterol 2007;13: 4056–63.
84 Pikul J, Sharpe MD, Lowndes R, Ghent CN. Degree of preoperative malnutrition is predictive of postoperative morbidity and mortality in liver transplant recipients. Transplantation 1994;57:469–72.
85 Harrison J, McKiernan J, Neuberg JM. A prospective study on the effect of recipient nutritional status on outcome in liver transplantation. Transplant Int 1997;10:369–74.
86 De Luis DA, Izaola O, Velicia MC, et al. Impact of dietary intake and nutritional status on outcomes after liver transplantation. Rev Esp Enferm Gig 2006;98:6–13.
87 Fan JG, Cao HX. The role of diet and nutritional management of nonalcoholic fatty liver diseases. J Gastroenterol Hepatol 2013;28(Suppl 4):81–7.

CHAPTER 13

Varices, portal hypertensive gastropathy and GAVE

Isabelle Colle,[1] Xavier Verhelst,[2] Anja Geerts,[2] and Hans Van Vlierberghe[2]

[1]*Department of Hepatology and Gastroenterology, Algemeen Stedelijk Ziekenhuis (ASZ), Aalst, Belgium and Ghent University,*
[2]*Department of Hepatology and Gastroenterology, Ghent University Hospital, Ghent, Belgium*

Variceal bleeding

Acute variceal bleeding is a notorious complication of portal hypertension with a high morbidity and mortality. When the portal pressure (measured by the hepatic venous pressure gradient, HVPG) is ≥10 mmHg, porto-systemic collaterals and varices begin to form. These varices subsequently grow in size and the wall becomes thinner with increasing wall tension according to Laplace's law. Finally, the wall ruptures resulting in a variceal bleed [1]. Acute variceal bleeding occurs in 25–40% of patients with cirrhosis [2] and mortality rates vary from 10% to 50% per episode [3–5]. Up to one-third of survivors will experience rebleeding within 6 weeks [6] and up to 62% at 2 years [1]. Variceal hemorrhage generally occurs in patients diagnosed with end-stage chronic liver disease but it can be the first presentation of an unknown underlying liver cirrhosis. Rarely, it is a consequence of noncirrhotic portal hypertension or portal vein thrombosis. The typical clinical presentation is a patient with liver cirrhosis presenting with hematemesis, coffee-ground emesis, melena, or rectorrhagia. Severity of bleeding and prognosis are associated with several factors. Patients with high portal pressures (HVPG ≥20 mmHg) have worse outcomes. Advanced liver failure is a bad prognostic factor. In Child–Pugh A patients, mortality is close to zero, in Child–Pugh B it is 10%, and in Child–Pugh C patients almost one in three will die. Patients with massive bleeding presenting with hemorrhagic shock and patients with several comorbidities such as hepatocellular carcinoma, portal vein thrombosis, acute alcoholic hepatitis, sepsis, and organ failure have a worse outcome [1].

Diagnosis and management

Initial evaluation

Endoscopy is the gold standard for diagnosing upper variceal bleeding and should be performed within 12 hours [7,8]. Before endoscopy can be performed, a clinical approach is essential to establish a tentative diagnosis. The following questions should be answered during this initial evaluation [7].

1. Rule out an aorto-enteric fistula. Suspicion should be raised in patients with a history of aortic aneurysm with or without past surgery [9].
2. Are there anamnestic or clinical signs suggestive of portal hypertension and cirrhosis? You should actively look for stigmata of portal hypertension such as ascites, spider nevi, palmar erythema, and so on. The family should be questioned about chronic alcohol abuse and risk factors for hepatitis B or C virus infection. If the answer is yes, vasoactive medication must immediately be started [1,7,8].
3. Are there signs of impaired vital functions (Airway, Breathing, Circultation, altered consciousness, and so on)? If the answer is positive, the patient should immediately be transferred to a monitored environment and examined by an emergency physician or intensive care specialist [10].
4. Is the patient taking anticoagulant or antiplatelet therapy?

Cirrhosis: A practical guide to management, First Edition. Edited by Samuel S. Lee and Richard Moreau.

General management

The first goals in the management of acute variceal bleeding are to control the bleeding, prevent early rebleeding, and treat concomitant complications, thus allowing the patient to survive the 5-day acute bleeding period [1]. Acute variceal bleeding should be managed by a multidisciplinary team involving experienced medical intensive care staff, well-trained nurses, clinical hepatologists, endoscopists, interventional radiologists, and surgeons [10]. An algorithm is proposed in Figure 13.1.

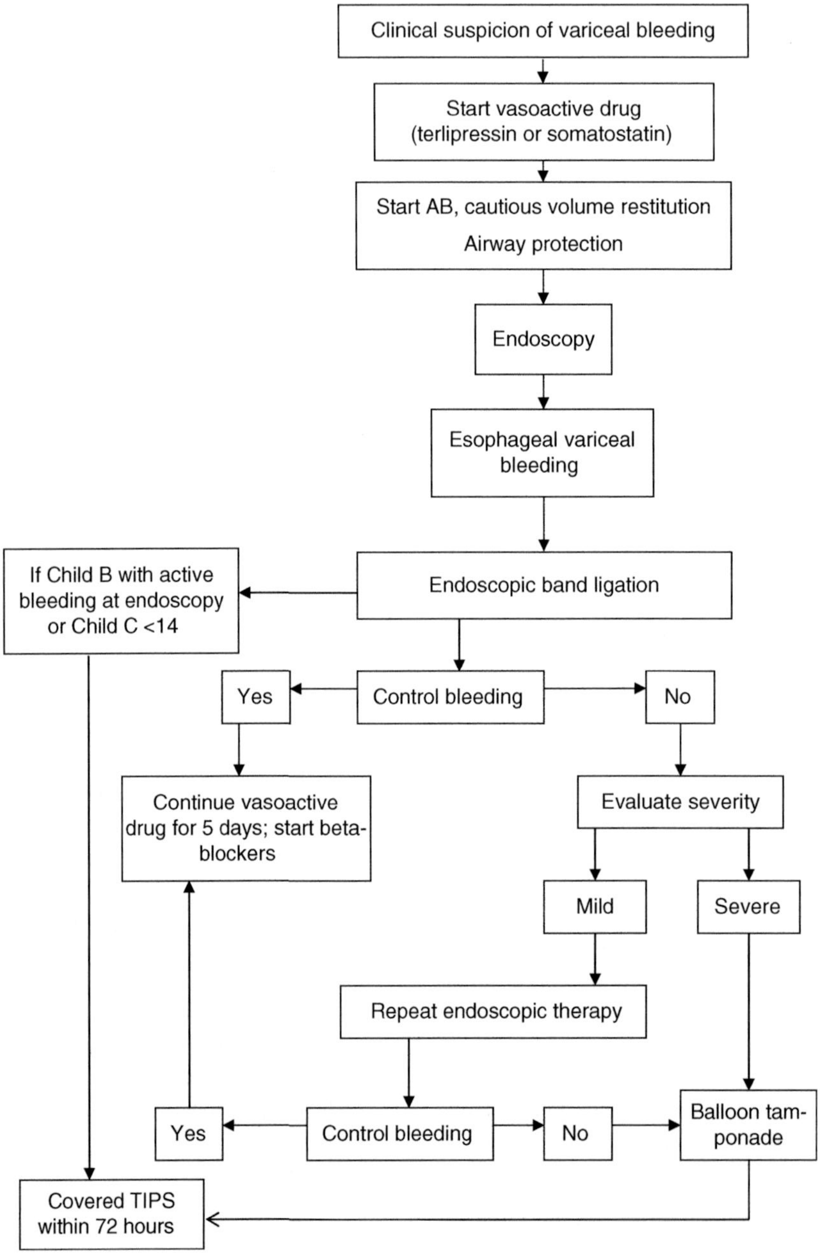

Figure 13.1 Algorithm for esophageal variceal bleeding based on the Baveno V guidelines. AB, antibiotic; EBL, endoscopic band ligation; TIPS, transjugular intrahepatic portosystemic shunt.

The management of a patient with acute variceal bleeding includes resuscitation, vasoactive medication, and endoscopy.

Resuscitation

Resuscitation is guided by the classic mnemonic ABC (Airway, Breathing, Circulation). Any doubt about airway safety should lead to prompt endotracheal intubation [11].

Fluid resuscitation should be initiated as soon as possible in patients with signs of shock (tachycardia >100/minute, systolic blood pressure <100 mmHg, or increased lactate levels) with a target of mean arterial pressure (MAP) >65 mmHg [12]. Albumin 5% is the preferred volume expander. After reaching hemodynamic stability, volume replacement at 30 mL/kg/24 hours can be performed in the absence of cardiac or renal contraindications. Transfusion of packed red blood cells above 8 g/dL is not appropriate, unless the patient has a history of coronary or cerebrovascular disease [13,14], as blood transfusion can induce a rebound increase in portal pressure, cause rebleeding or sustained bleeding [15].

Vasoactive medication

Vasoactive drugs (terlipressin and somatostatin) aim to cause splanchnic vasoconstriction, thereby decreasing portal pressure and reducing or even stopping bleeding from varices. Bleeding is stopped in 75–80% of patients and the risk of rebleeding is reduced. Therefore, vasoactive medication should be started as early as possible when a variceal bleeding is presumed [16]. Vasoactive medication should be continued for 5 days according to the most recent Baveno V guidelines [8].

Different vasoactive drugs are locally available around the world. The first choice should be terlipressin because it is the only drug that has been proved to bring about a reduction in mortality in acute variceal bleeding [17,18]. Somatostatin and its analogs are second choice considering that they have not demonstrated a reduction in mortality [19]. However, a recent meta-analysis claimed to show no difference in efficacy among octreotide, somatostatin, terlipressin, vasopressin, and vapreotide [20] including in mortality, but there were some methodologic issues. Vasoactive drugs should always be used in combination with endoscopic treatment.

Terlipressin is a long-acting triglyl lysine derivative of vasopressin. It is started as an intravenous (IV) bolus (<50 kg = 1 mg; 50–70 kg = 1.5 mg; >70 kg = 2 mg) followed by an IV bolus of 1–2 mg every 4 hours for 48 hours and then 1 mg every 4 hours until day 5. Terlipressin improves the rates of bleeding and survival [21]. Fewer side effects seem to appear when it is given in a continuous IV infusion (6 mg/24 hours) as proposed in hepatorenal syndrome [22]. It is contraindicated in patients with coronary insufficiency, peripheral vascular disease, pregnancy, heart rhythm disease, severe bronchial asthma, uncontrolled arterial hypertension, or epilepsy.

If terlipressin cannot be used, somatostatin is a good alternative. Somatostatin treatment starts with a continuous IV infusion of 6 mg over 24 hours followed immediately by a bolus of 250 μg within 5 minutes. The bolus can be repeated up to three times during the first hour if bleeding is uncontrolled. The dosage can be increased to 12 mg over 24 hours in cases of active bleeding. There are no important side effects or contraindications [1,19]. Minor complications are seen in up to 30% of patients and include nausea, vomiting, and hyperglycemia [19,23]. Somatostatin is also used in children; however, large clinical trials are not available. It is started with a continuous IV infusion of 3.5 μg/kg/hour immediately followed by a bolus of 3.5 μg/kg IV over 5 minutes [24].

A second alternative is octreotide. This somatostatin analog has a longer half-life than somatostatin [25]. The safety profile is similar to that of somatostatin. However, clinical trials are limited and could not demonstrate a reduction in mortality [26]. This may be because of the rapid development of tachyphylaxis [25]. Octreotide only showed a reduction in rebleeding after sclerotherapy [27].

There is no evidence for the use of proton pump inhibitors [8] or antifibrinolytics [28] in these patients.

Antibiotics

The use of prophylactic antibiotics is mandatory in patients with variceal bleeding, as they decrease infectious complications and reduce mortality [29–31]. Patients with variceal bleeding need an active search for infections, including blood, ascites, and urine culture. Empiric antibiotic regimens should be based on local resistance patterns. Proposed first line antibiotics are amoxicillin-clavulanic acid, quinolones, or third line cephalosporins. In patients with advanced cirrhosis, a third line cephalosporin may be advised (e.g., ceftriaxone 1 g/day), especially in inpatients with high quinolone resistance or those chronically taking norfloxacin for prevention of spontaneous bacterial peritonitis [32]. The duration should be limited to 7 days according to the American Association for the Study of Liver Diseases (AASLD) guidelines [30].

Coagulation disorders

Many cirrhotic patients present with coagulation disorders, low platelet counts, and intake of antiplatelet or antivitamin K drugs. However, we should remind that prothrombin time/international normalized ratio is not a reliable indicator of the coagulation status in these patients [8]. For this, the use of coagulation factors, fresh frozen plasma, and platelets is not encouraged, as these could increase portal pressure and maintain the bleeding. However, when the platelet count is lower than 30 000/µL, platelet transfusion can be advised in cases of persistent bleeding. Withdrawal of antiplatelet drugs and antivitamin K medication can cause thrombotic events and should only be stopped after consultation with a cardiologist [7].

Endoscopy

Endoscopy should be performed as soon as possible but within 12 hours [8,16,33]. Hemodynamically unstable and high risk patients should be transferred to an intensive care unit to perform endoscopy in a safe environment. Prophylactic endotracheal intubation should be performed in patients with active hematemesis, hemodynamic instability in spite of adequate volume loading, absence of cooperation, or Glasgow Coma Scale (GCS) <8.

Stomach cleansing can be performed by administrating 250 mg erythromycin IV over 5 minutes, 20 minutes before endoscopy [34–36]. This may help to improve the endoscopic view and hence lead to a better therapeutic performance.

Endoscopic diagnostic criteria for variceal bleeding are active bleeding from a varix, presence of a white nipple (fibrin clot) on a varix, or the presence of varices without other potential source of bleeding and fresh blood in the stomach [1,11,37]. Endoscopic therapy should be performed during the same procedure by a skilled endoscopist.

Esophageal varices

Endoscopic band ligation (EBL) is preferred for esophageal varices as it is superior for bleeding control and rebleeding compared to sclerotherapy and has fewer adverse events. However, sclerotherapy can be a valuable alternative if EBL is not available or cannot be performed for technical reasons [1].

Gastric varices

Gastric varices are responsible for 5–10% of variceal bleeds, but are more severe and have a higher mortality [38].

Gastric varices can be divided into four types according to the Sarin classification (Figure 13.2) [38]. This classification is based upon their relation with esophageal varices and location. Gastroesophageal varices (GOV) are associated with esophageal varices along the lesser curvature (GOV1) or along the fundus (GOV2). Isolated gastric varices (IGV) appear in the fundus (IGV1) or on other sites in the stomach or the first part of the duodenum (IGV2). If these appear after endoscopic obliteration of esophageal varices, they are classified as secondary gastric varices. Gastric varices are more frequent in individuals with portal hypertension resulting from extrahepatic portal vein thrombosis. Gastric varices located in the fundus have a higher bleeding incidence. Other risk factors for a first hemorrhage are advancing Child–Pugh stage, presence of red spots, and increasing size of the varices [39].

The therapeutic approach remains empirical, as large randomized controlled trials (RCTs) are not available.

Acute bleeding from gastric varices is challenging. Based on the extrapolation of data from esophageal varices, the use of vasoactive drugs is recommended [40]. GOV1 are the most common type of gastric varices (74%) [38] and can endoscopically be treated like "conventional" esophageal varices with EBL. The other types of gastric varices require a patient-tailored approach but most of them will need injection of glue agents such as *N*-butyl-2-cyanoacrylate (Histoacryl©) or isobutyl-2-cyanoacrylate (Bucrylate©). This procedure can be technically demanding during active bleeding. It should be performed by a skilled and experienced endoscopist. Major complications can occur because obturation can extend beyond the varices and pulmonary and cerebrovascular embolization has been reported [40]. A small series reports successful treatment of gastric varices by thrombin injection [41]; however, these findings have not been confirmed in larger trials.

Rescue treatment in esophageal and gastric variceal bleeding

Failure to control bleeding was defined by the Baveno V guidelines as a fresh hematemesis ≥2 hours after the start of a drug treatment, or therapeutic endoscopy; a 3 g/dL drop in hemoglobin if no transfusion is administered; or death. This should lead to a change of treatment options.

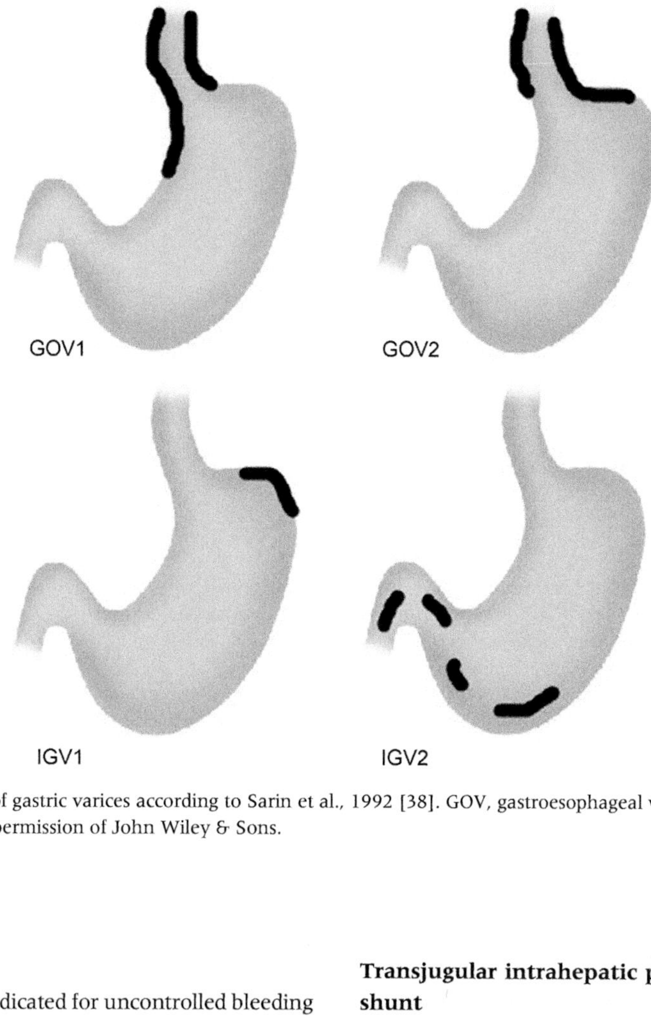

Figure 13.2 Classification of gastric varices according to Sarin et al., 1992 [38]. GOV, gastroesophageal varices; IGV, isolated gastric varices. Reproduced with permission of John Wiley & Sons.

Balloon tamponade

Balloon tamponade is indicated for uncontrolled bleeding as a bridge to a definitive therapy within 24 hours. Two types are available: a Linton tamponade (Figure 13.3) can treat esophageal and gastric varices, whereas a Sengstaken–Blakemore tamponade (containing two balloons) will only compress esophageal and cardiac varices (Figure 13.4). The Linton type is easier to use in daily practice. It is effective in bleeding control but rebleeding after balloon deflation is very common. Complications can be serious and include aspiration pneumonia, laceration of the esophagus, malposition in the airway, and can be lethal [8,11,42]. Presence of the balloon for more than 24 hours can cause necrosis of the esophageal or the stomach wall [40].

A covered removable esophageal stent has been developed for esophageal varices but has not yet been validated in large trials [43].

Transjugular intrahepatic portosystemic stent shunt

Transjugular intrahepatic portosystemic shunt (TIPS) is an intrahepatic stent that is placed via a transjugular approach creating a portosystemic venous shunt. It was first described in 1987 for the use of variceal bleeding [44]. However, the complication rate was high with mortality rates approaching 50%. Nowadays, polytetrafluoroethylene (PTFE) covered TIPS are available. These are very effective in controlling variceal bleeding and have a low rate of obliteration. The goal of TIPS placement in variceal bleeding is to reduce hepatic venous pressure gradient below 12 mmHg or obtain a reduction of more than 20% from baseline [45]. TIPS placement is preferred over surgical shunts. Although shunts are extremely effective in controlling variceal bleeding, they have higher morbidity and mortality rates. TIPS placement may induce encephalopathy and deterioration of liver function.

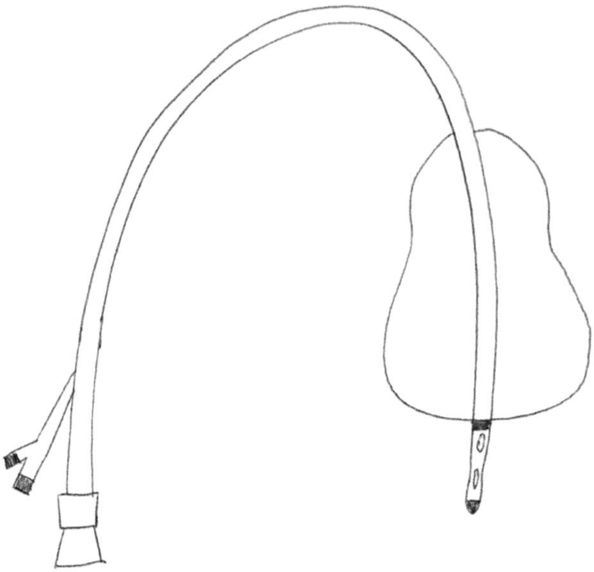

Figure 13.3 Linton balloon tamponade. A Linton balloon is made of a pear-formed balloon placed over a tube with three lumens. At the proximal side of the tube, three ports are visible: one for inflation of the gastric balloon, one for the esophageal port, and one for the gastric port. Inflate the balloon to check for leaks. Deflate the balloon. Lubricate the tube. Insert the tube, in a ventilated patient, through the nasal (or oral) passage and advance it until it reaches the stomach. Inflate the balloon with 200 mL of air. Withdraw the balloon gently until resistance is felt. This indicates that the gastric balloon is positioned against the cardioesophageal juncture and held by the diaphragm. Now, correct position must be confirmed by a chest X-ray (including the subdiaphragmatic region). If the balloon is in a correct position (under the diaphragm), inflate the Linton balloon to 500 mL. Record the amount of air inflated in the patient's file. The insufflation port should be clamped to avoid uncontrolled air loss. Finally, attach a rope to the tube and adjust a serum bag of 200 mL on this rope. Place this over a pulley system to ensure traction on the rope and ascertain the correct position of the balloon against the gastroesophageal junction by another chest X-ray. The gastric balloon should not be maintained for more than 24 hours.

Two recent studies [46,47] have shown that high risk patients for rebleeding have a survival benefit when early PTFE-covered TIPS is placed (within 72 hours of admission) compared with a combination of vasoactive drugs and endoscopic therapy (1 year survival of 86% vs. 60%, respectively). These data were confirmed in a post-RCT surveillance study [48]. Moreover, TIPS had a higher bleeding control rate and less early rebleeding. Based on these studies, the Baveno V consensus meeting states that early, covered TIPS placement should be considered in high risk patients. High risk patients are defined as Child B cirrhotic patients with active bleeding at the moment of endoscopy or Child C patients with less than 14 points after optimal medical and endoscopic treatment.

Surgical shunt

Surgical splenorenal, portacaval, and Rex shunts are highly effective in controlling variceal bleeding. However, they should be reserved for patients with well-preserved liver function in which bleeding control is not achieved with vasoactive drugs and endoscopic therapy, and without complications from the bleeding or the endoscopy. It should be performed by a well-trained and experienced surgeon. According to the Baveno V consensus statement, decompressive surgery should be considered for patients with portal vein thrombosis and failure of endoscopic therapy. In patients who are not eligible for TIPS or shunt operation, for example those with extensive portal vein thrombosis with extension in the splenic and superior mesenteric veins, a Sugiura procedure can be used. A Sugiura procedure consists of an esogastric devascularization, a splenectomy, and an esophageal transection [49].

Rebleeding

In cases of rebleeding, a second-look endoscopy is allowed for esophageal varices, but not for gastric varices.

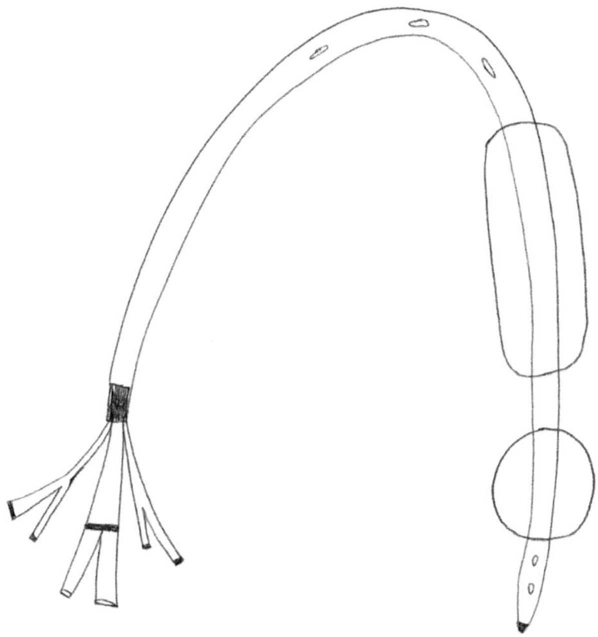

Figure 13.4 Sengstaken–Blakemore tamponade. A Sengstaken–Blakemore balloon contains two balloons (one esophageal balloon and one gastric balloon) placed over a tube with four lumens: one lumen for every balloon, and two lumens that aspirate the gastric and esophageal contents at the proximal end. Inflate the balloons to check for leaks. Deflate the balloon. Lubricate the tube. Insert the tube in a ventilated patient through the nasal (or oral) passage and advance it until the stomach. Inflate the gastric balloon with 50 mL of air. Withdraw the balloon gently until resistance is felt. This indicates that the gastric balloon is positioned against the cardioesophageal juncture and hold by the diaphragm. The correct position now must be confirmed by a chest X-ray including the subdiaphragmatic region. If the balloon is in the correct position, inflate the esophageal balloon to 150 mL of air maximum and the gastric balloon to 250 mL of air maximum. A manometer can be used to check the air pressure in the esophageal ballon, which should not exceed 40 mmHg [87]. Record the amount of air inflated in the patient's file. All insufflation ports should be clamped to avoid uncontrolled air loss. Finally, attach a rope to the tube and adjust a serum bag of 200 mL to this rope. Place this over a pulley system to ensure traction on the rope and ascertain the correct position of the balloons in the esophagus and against the gastroesophageal junction by another chest X-ray. The gastric balloon should not be maintained for more than 24 hours. The esophageal balloon may be deflated every 8 hours for 30–60 minutes to prevent esophageal mucosal necrosis. Evidence-based guidelines are lacking.

In case of failure or severe bleeding, again TIPS should be considered before a further deterioration of the patient's condition. Increasing the dose of vasoactive medication to maximal levels can be tried, but is not based on hard evidence. Again, balloon tamponnade can be used as a bridge to TIPS or shunt surgery. Esophageal covered stents and Sengstaken–Blakemore cannot be used in gastric varices.

Antibiotic prophylaxis

Antibiotic prophylaxis should be started at admission for 5–7 days. In cases of a confirmed infection, the duration and the choice of antibiotics should be tailored to the individual patient. Patients who have spontaneous bacterial peritonitis should be given a secondary prophylaxis with oral norfloxacine 400 mg/day life-long, until transplantation, or until complete resolution of ascites [50].

Secondary prophylaxis

Risk of rebleeding after a first episode of variceal bleeding ranges between 30% and 40% during the first 6 weeks; 40% will occur during the first 5 days [6,51]. Secondary prophylaxis is mandatory. The preferred option is a combination of beta-blockade with EBL [8]. Nonselective beta-blockers (e.g., propranolol) should be given in the maximum tolerated dose, aiming for a heart rate of 50–60beats per minute [8,33]. The aim of EBL is eradication of varices,

Table 13.1 Summary of Baveno V guidelines regarding secondary prophylaxis for variceal bleeding [8].

Patient	Recommendation
Patient with cirrhosis	• Nonselective beta-blocker + EBL • Hemodynamic response to drug therapy provides information about rebleeding risk and survival • In nonresponders, addition of isosorbide mononitrate can improve efficacy
Patients with cirrhosis who are unable or unwilling to be treated with EBL	Nonselective beta-blocker + isosorbide mononitrate
Patients with cirrhosis who have contraindications or intolerance to beta-blockers	EBL
Patients who fail endoscopic and pharmacologic treatment for the prevention of rebleeding	TIPS with PTFE-covered stents Surgical shunt in Child–Pugh A and B patients if TIPS is unavailable Transplantation in Child–Pugh C patients TIPS can be used as a bridge to transplantation
Patients who have bled from IGV1 or GOV2	Tissue adhesive (*N*-butyl-cyanoacrylate) or TIPS
Patients who have bled from GOV1	Tissue adhesive, nonselective beta-blocker, or EBL
Patients who have bled from portal hypertensive gastropathy	Nonselective beta-blocker
Patients in whom beta-blockers are contraindicated or fail and who cannot be managed by non-shunt therapy	TIPS or surgical shunt

EBL, endoscopic band ligation; GOV, gastroesophageal varices; IGV, isolated gastric varices; PTFE, polytetrafluoroethylene; TIPS, transjugular intrahepatic portosystemic stent shunt.

Source: de Franachis & Baveno, 2010 [8]. Reproduced with permission of Elsevier.

so it should be repeated every 2–3 weeks until this goal is reached, usually after 2–4 sessions. Repeat endoscopy is advocated after 1–3 months and then 1–2 times per year [11,30].

The Baveno V guidelines (2010) for specific patient groups are summarized in Table 13.1.

A relatively new tool for rescue after a first bleeding or for secondary prophylaxis of gastric variceal bleeding in patients with splenorenal shunts is balloon retrograde transvenous obliteration of varices (BRTO). During this procedure a catheter is placed under fluoroscopic guidance in the splenorenal shunt (Figure 13.5). The shunt is blocked with a balloon and glue is injected in the varices in order to achieve obliteration [52,53].

Primary prophylaxis

Preprimary prophylaxis aims to prevent the formation of varices. According to the most recent Baveno V guidelines [8], all cirrhotic patients should be screened for varices at the moment of diagnosis. The first step is to treat underlying liver disease to reduce portal hypertension and its complications. Beta-blockers are not indicated to prevent the formation of varices. These patients should undergo gastroscopy every 2–3 years [54].

Esophageal varices

The goal of primary prevention is to prevent bleeding in patients diagnosed with varices. In patients with small varices with red wale marks or Child C cirrhosis, nonselective beta-blockers should be started. In patients with small varices without red spots, red whale marks, or advanced cirrhosis, the role of nonselective beta-blockers is not totally clear yet.

In patients with medium or large varices with a high risk of bleeding (Child B or C and/or red signs), nonselective beta-blockers or EBL can be recommended. For patients with medium or large varices without these risk factors (Child A and no red signs), nonselective beta-blockers are preferred and EBL should be only considered in those patients with intolerance, noncompliance, or with contraindications to beta-blockers (AASLD guidelines) [30].

According to the Baveno V guidelines, patients with medium or large varices should be treated by either nonselective beta-blockers or endoscopic band ligation, according to local resources and expertise, patient characteristics, and contraindications [8]. Carvedilol is a promising drug but requires further exploration in this setting. Shunt therapy, endoscopic sclerotherapy, and isosorbide mononitrate are not indicated for primary prevention.

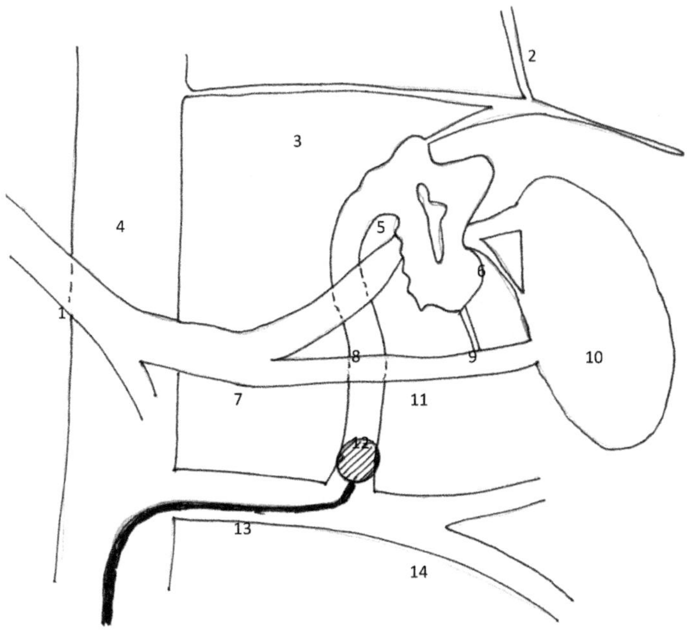

Figure 13.5 Schematic overview of balloon-occluded retrograde transvenous obliteration of gastric varices (BRTO). A balloon catheter is inserted from the right femoral (or right internal jugular) vein and wedged into the left adrenal vein. When the balloon is occluded, a venogram should be performed. Collaterals are first occluded with glue according to their importance. When gastric varices are well opacified, glue is injected slowly with fluoroscopic monitoring until complete filling of the varix. Clot formation is tested by a final venogram. 1, Portal vein; 2, pericardiophrenic vein; 3, inferior phrenic vein; 4, inferior vena cava; 5, gastric varix; 6, short gastric vein; 7, coronary vein; 8, gastrorenal shunt; 9, posterior gastric vein; 10, spleen; 11, splenic vein; 12, adrenal vein; 13, balloon catheter; 14, renal vein. (Based on Hirota et al., 1999 [53]).

Gastric varices

For primary prophylaxis of gastric varices, Baveno V guidelines [8] propose the use of nonselective beta-blockers. However, a recent RCT comparing cyanoacrylate injection with beta-blockers with no primary preventive measures in high risk patients (GOV2 and IGV1 with size of gastric varix >20 mm, MELD score ≥17, and presence of portal hypertensive gastropathy) demonstrated a survival benefit in the cyanoacrylate group [55]. This should be validated in larger trials to elucidate the clinical significance of these interesting findings and might support the eradication of gastric varices in these high risk patients [40].

Portal hypertensive gastropathy

Endoscopic findings

Portal hypertensive gastropathy (PHG) is characterized by typical mucosal lesions mimicking a snakeskin mosaic pattern easily identified during endoscopy. This is caused by a dilatation of the mucosal capillaries and submucosal veins in the stomach [56,57]. According to the Baveno III consensus, mucosal injury can be classified into mild and severe. Mild lesions show a mosaic-like pattern (Figure 13.6), whereas severe lesions show red markings (Figure 13.7) [54].

Pathogenesis

The pathogenesis of PHG has not totally been elucidated. It is related to high portal pressure and can be seen in patients with liver cirrhosis and those with noncirrhotic portal hypertension. Independent risk factors are Child–Pugh C cirrhosis, large variceal size, and HVPG >12 mmHg [58].

Epidemiology

PHG has a prevalence of 20–80% according to patient characteristics and is more frequent in patients with severe liver disease [59,60] and in patients with cirrhosis who had a previous endoscopic treatment for varices [38,57]. This is because of redistribution of the blood

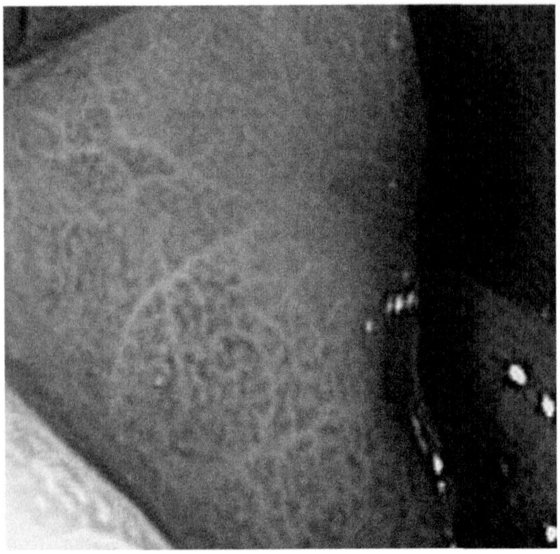

Figure 13.6 Mild portal hypertensive gastropathy. Note the snakeskin mosaic pattern. (See colour plate section.)

flow into the gastric mucosa previously drained through the esophageal varices.

Portal hypertensive gastropathy and hemorrhage

PHG accounts for less than 3% of acute bleedings but can be responsible for chronic blood loss in cirrhotic patients [57]. PHG is predominantly observed in the fundus of the stomach, but patients with diffuse PHG bleed much more than those with isolated PHG in the antrum or fundus [57].

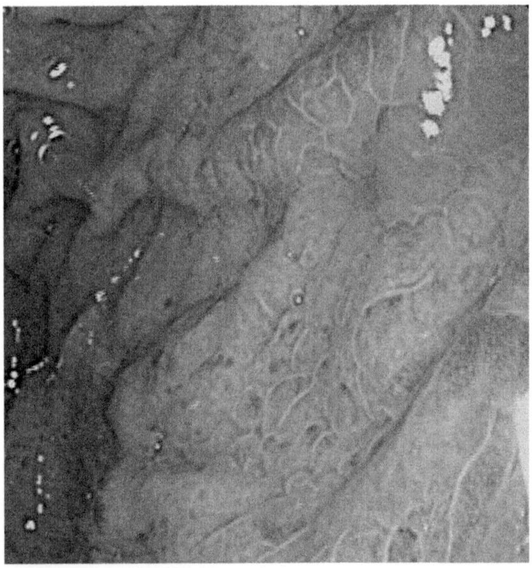

Figure 13.7 Severe portal hypertensive gastropathy. Note the snakeskin mosaic pattern with dark spots. (See colour plate section.)

Acute bleeding from portal hypertensive gastropathy

Acute bleeding from PHG is defined as the presence of melena or hematemesis associated with an actively bleeding mucosal lesion endoscopy [58]. Bleeding from PHT related jejunopathy should be considered and assessed by capsule endoscopy [61,62]. Treatment of acute bleeding from PHG is based on decreasing gastric blood flow with vasoactive agents such as terlipressin, somatostatin, or nonselective beta-blockers [63]. Secondary prophylaxis after a first bleeding episode from PHG with nonselective beta-blockade is indicated [33]. In uncontrolled bleeding, covered TIPS placement can be considered to achieve a reduction of PHG [45]. For selected patients, shunt surgery [64] or liver transplantation is the right option [40]. In patients with uncontrolled bleeding who are not eligible for TIPS or transplantation, endoscopic therapy with argon plasma coagulation might become an alternative; however, this has not been validated in large RCTs [65].

The use of hemospray (a hemostatic powder that can cover the mucosa) licensed for endoscopic hemostasis may be of benefit in acute PHG bleeding. However, larger studies should be set up [66].

Chronic bleeding from portal hypertensive gastropathy

Chronic bleeding from PGH is defined by a decrease of 2 g/dL or more in hemoglobin in the absence of nonsteroidal anti-inflammatory drug (NSAID) use in the previous 6 months. These patients should be offered iron replacement therapy [40,67]. If the patient becomes transfusion dependent, TIPS or shunt surgery must be considered [64]. In treatment refractory patients with advanced liver disease, a liver transplantation can be the only option [40]. Primary prophylaxis for asymptomatic patients with PHG without concomitant varices and without past or present bleeding is not advocated [67].

Gastric antral vascular ectasia

Gastric antral vascular ectasia (GAVE) is a distinct clinical entity and should not be confused with PHG.

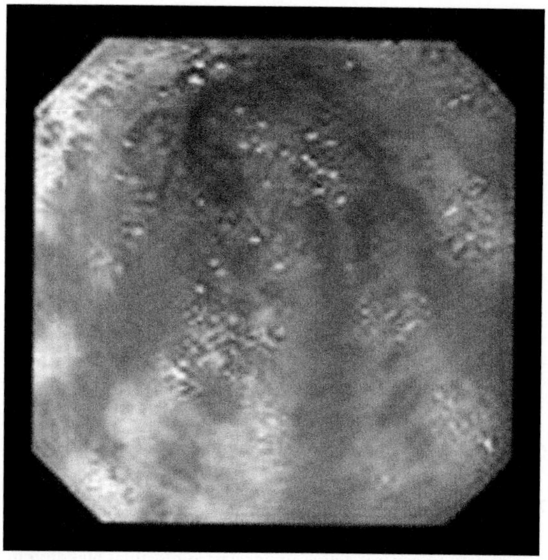

Figure 13.8 Gastric antral vascular ectasia (GAVE). Note the typical watermelon-like pattern. (See colour plate section.)

In contrast to PHG, GAVE is present in cirrhotic patients, but can also be seen in patients with non-hepatic chronic diseases such as diabetes, heart failure, atrophic gastritis, chronic renal failure, autoimmune connective tissue disorders, and after bone marrow transplantation [68–73]. However, liver insufficiency seems to have an important role as GAVE is more frequently seen in patients with severe liver disease and resolves after liver transplantation [74].

Diagnosis is established by endoscopy. Patients with GAVE present with flat red spots without a background mosaic pattern. These red spots can merge into red lines, which converge to the pylorus, creating a typical "watermelon stomach" image (Figure 13.8). These lesions are only observed in the stomach [67]. Differentiating GAVE from PHG, which are two distinct conditions, can be hard.

Histopathologic differentiation can also be challenging, as both GAVE and PHG show mucosal capillary dilatation. The standard microscopic characteristics of both include capillary ectasia, regenerative mucosal changes, and increased lamina propria smooth muscle, with the presence of fibrin thrombi being a cardinal attribute for GAVE [75]. Furthermore, GAVE appears to be characterized by more extensive ectasia, thrombi, and spindle cell proliferation. Fibrohyalinosis is an important lesion for differentiating GAVE from severe PHG [76].

Patients with GAVE often are asymptomatic and diagnosis can be an accidental finding during routine endoscopy. Some patients will present with a chronic iron deficiency anemia. Only those patients require treatment. The mainstay of treatment is endoscopy. Different thermoablative techniques have been studied. Argon plasma coagulation (APC) is the most studied and has the best results. APC is based on thermal coagulation by applying a high frequency electric current that is passed through with argon gas without direct contact with the mucosa. Multiple sessions are needed to achieve a reduction of mucosal lesions in GAVE and hence a reduction of bleeding, most often with a 2–6 week interval [67].

An alternative to APC is the neodymium:yttrium-aluminium-garnet (Nd:YAG) laser which can be applied to a large surface area in a single session. It has proven effective in reducing rebleeding and the need for transfusion in GAVE [68,71,77]. A major drawback is the higher risk for perforation.

Another, less well documented, method is cryotherapy. Compressed nitrous oxide is rapidly expanded in the stomach resulting in a local rapid decrease of the temperature with a freezing of the gastric mucosa [78,79]. However, this technique needs further validation.

Some pharmacologic therapies have shown a beneficial effect when endoscopy fails, such as estrogen–progesterone [80], corticosteroid [81], tranexamic acid [82], thalidomide [83], octreotide [84], and a serotonin antagonist [85]. Most of them are small series or anecdotal case reports. In refractory patients, surgical treatment with antrectomy can be considered [86]. Contrary to the case for PHG, TIPS or shunt surgery are *not* effective for GAVE.

Conclusions

Acute variceal bleeding is a major complication of portal hypertension with high mortality rates and a high risk for rebleeding. These patients require a proper multidisciplinary approach by experienced clinical emergency care doctors, intensive care medicine specialists, clinical hepatologists, interventional radiologistst, and hepatobiliary surgeons. The mainstay of therapy is vasoactive therapy (terlipressin or somatostatin), to be started as early as possible and endoscopy (EBL for esophageal varices, glue injection for independent gastric varices) to be performed as soon as possible and certainly within 12 hours. In Child B patients with severe active bleeding at endoscopy or Child C <14 patients, and in patients with therapy refractory bleeding TIPS is a valuable new strategy. Balloon tamponade can be a bridging therapy in patients with uncontrolled bleeding.

PHG is a rare cause of acute bleeding but can be a source of chronic intestinal blood loss. Therapy is based upon the use of vasoactive medication (e.g., somatostatin or terlipressin) to reduce gastric blood flow. APC of focal bleeding lesions can be a valuable alternative.

GAVE, not to be confused with PHG, is a cause of chronic blood loss and iron deficiency anemia. In symptomatic patients, the mainstay of treatment is APC.

References

1 Bosch J. Management of Active Variceal Hemorrhage. AASLD Postgraduate Course 2009.

2 Grace ND. Prevention of initial variceal hemorrhage. Gastroenterol Clin North Am 1992;21:149–61

3 D'Amico G, De Franchis R. Upper digestive bleeding in cirrhosis. Post-therapeutic outcome and prognostic indicators. Hepatology 2003;38:599–612.

4 Carbonell N, Pauwels A, Serfaty L, Fourdan O, Lévy VG, Poupon R. Improved survival after variceal bleeding in patients with cirrhosis over the past two decades. Hepatology 2004;40:652–9.

5 Hearnshaw SA, Logan RF, Lowe D, Travis SP, Murphy MF, Palmer KR. Acute upper gastrointestinal bleeding in the UK: patient characteristics, diagnoses and outcomes in the 2007 UK audit. Gut 2011;60:1327–35.

6 Graham DY, Smith JL. The course of patients after variceal hemorrhage. Gastroenterology 1981;80:800–9.

7 Colle I, Wilmer A, Le Moine O, et al. Upper gastrointestinal tract bleeding management: Belgian guidelines for adults and children. Acta Gastroenterol Belg 2011;74:45–66.

8 de Franchis R, Baveno VF. Revising consensus in portal hypertension: report of the Baveno V consensus workshop on methodology of diagnosis and therapy in portal hypertension. J Hepatol 2010;53:762–8.

9 Debonnaire P, Van Rillaer O, Arts J, Ramboer K, Tubbax H, Van Hootegem P. Primary aorto enteric fistula: report of 18 Belgian cases and literature review. Acta Gastroenterol Belg 2008;71:250–8.

10 Abraldes JG, Bosch J. The treatment of acute variceal bleeding. J Clin Gastroenterol 2007;41(Suppl 3):S312–7.

11 Garcia-Tsao G, Lim JK, Members of Veterans Affairs Hepatitis CRCP. Management and treatment of patients with cirrhosis and portal hypertension: recommendations from the Department of Veterans Affairs Hepatitis C Resource Center Program and the National Hepatitis C Program. Am J Gastroenterol 2009;104:1802–29.

12 Dellinger RP, Levy MM, Carlet JM, et al. Surviving Sepsis Campaign: international guidelines for management of severe sepsis and septic shock: 2008. Intensive Care Med 2008;34:17–60.

13 Taylor RW, Manganaro L, O'Brien J, Trottier SJ, Parkar N, Veremakis C. Impact of allogenic packed red blood cell transfusion on nosocomial infection rates in the critically ill patient. Crit Care Med 2002;30:2249–54.

14 Carson JL, Duff A, Poses RM, et al. Effect of anaemia and cardiovascular disease on surgical mortality and morbidity. Lancet 1996;348:1055–60.

15 Castaneda B, Debernardi-Venon W, Bandi JC, et al. The role of portal pressure in the severity of bleeding in portal hypertensive rats. Hepatology 2000;31:581–6.

16 Garcia-Tsao G, Bosch J. Management of varices and variceal hemorrhage in cirrhosis. N Engl J Med 2010;362:823–32.

17 Levacher S, Letoumelin P, Pateron D, Blaise M, Lapandry C, Pourriat JL. Early administration of terlipressin plus glyceryl trinitrate to control active upper gastrointestinal bleeding in cirrhotic patients. Lancet 1995;346:865–8.

18 Ioannou G, Doust J, Rockey DC. Terlipressin for acute esophageal variceal hemorrhage. Cochrane Database Syst Rev 2003;1:CD002147.

19 Gotzsche PC, Hrobjartsson A. Somatostatin analogues for acute bleeding oesophageal varices. Cochrane Database Syst Rev 2008;3:CD000193.

20 Wells M, Chande N, Adams P, et al. Meta-analysis: vasoactive medications for the management of acute variceal bleeds. Aliment Pharmacol Ther 2012;35:1267–78.

21 Ioannou GN, Doust J, Rockey DC. Systematic review: terlipressin in acute oesophageal variceal haemorrhage. Aliment Pharmacol Ther 2003;17:53–64.

22 Gerbes AL, Huber E, Gulberg V. Terlipressin for hepatorenal syndrome: continuous infusion as an alternative to iv bolus administration. Gastroenterology 2009;137:1179; authorreply, 81.

23 Moitinho E, Planas R, Banares R, et al. Multicenter randomized controlled trial comparing different schedules of somatostatin in the treatment of acute variceal bleeding. J Hepatol 2001;35:712–8.

24 Lacroix J, Nadeau D, Laberge S, Gauthier M, Lapierre G, Farrell CA. Frequency of upper gastrointestinal bleeding in a pediatric intensive care unit. Crit Care Med 1992;20:35–42.

25 Escorsell A, Bandi JC, Andreu V, et al. Desensitization to the effects of intravenous octreotide in cirrhotic patients with portal hypertension. Gastroenterology 2001;120:161–9.

26 International Octreotide Varices Study Group BA. Double blind RCT of 5 day octreotide versus placebo, associated with sclerotherapy for trial failures. Hepatology 1996;24:352A.

27 Corley DA, Cello JP, Adkisson W, Ko WF, Kerlikowske K. Octreotide for acute esophageal variceal bleeding: a meta-analysis. Gastroenterology 2001;120:946–54.

28 Gluud LL, Klingenberg SL, Langholz SE. Systematic review: tranexamic acid for upper gastrointestinal bleeding. Aliment Pharmacol Ther 2008;27:752–8.

29 Goulis J, Armonis A, Patch D, Sabin C, Greenslade L, Burroughs AK. Bacterial infection is independently associated with failure to control bleeding in cirrhotic patients with gastrointestinal hemorrhage. Hepatology 1998;27:1207–12.

30 Garcia-Tsao G, Sanyal AJ, Grace ND, Carey W, Practice Guidelines Committee of the American Association for the Study of Liver Diseases, Practice Parameters Committee of the American College of Gastroenterology. Prevention and management of gastroesophageal varices and variceal hemorrhage in cirrhosis. Hepatology 2007;46:922–38.

31 Bernard B, Grange JD, Khac EN, Amiot X, Opolon P, Poynard T. Antibiotic prophylaxis for the prevention of bacterial infections in cirrhotic patients with gastrointestinal bleeding: a meta-analysis. Hepatology 1999;29:1655–61.

32 Fernandez J, Ruiz del Arbol L, Gomez C, et al. Norfloxacin vs ceftriaxone in the prophylaxis of infections in patients with advanced cirrhosis and hemorrhage. Gastroenterology 2006;131:1049–56; quiz, 285.

33 de Franchis R. Evolving consensus in portal hypertension. Report of the Baveno IV consensus workshop on methodology of diagnosis and therapy in portal hypertension. J Hepatol 2005;43:167–76.

34 Carbonell N, Pauwels A, Serfaty L, Boelle PY, Becquemont L, Poupon R. Erythromycin infusion prior to endoscopy for acute upper gastrointestinal bleeding: a randomized, controlled, double-blind trial. Am J Gastroenterolo 2006;101:1211–5.

35 Coffin B, Pocard M, Panis Y, et al. Erythromycin improves the quality of EGD in patients with acute upper GI bleeding: a randomized controlled study. Gastrointest Endosc 2002;56:174–9.

36 Frossard JL, Spahr L, Queneau PE, et al. Erythromycin intravenous bolus infusion in acute upper gastrointestinal bleeding: a randomized, controlled, double-blind trial. Gastroenterology 2002;123:17–23.

37 de Franchis R, Pascal JP, Ancona E, et al. Definitions, methodology and therapeutic strategies in portal hypertension. A Consensus Development Workshop, Baveno, Lake Maggiore, Italy, April 5 and 6, 1990. J Hepatol 1992;15:256–61.

38 Sarin SK, Lahoti D, Saxena SP, Murthy NS, Makwana UK. Prevalence, classification and natural history of gastric varices: a long-term follow-up study in 568 portal hypertension patients. Hepatology 1992;16:1343–9.

39 Kim T, Shijo H, Kokawa H, et al. Risk factors for hemorrhage from gastric fundal varices. Hepatology 1997;25:307–12.

40 Sarin SK. Gastric Varices and Portal Hypertensive Gastropathy. AASLD Postgraduate Course. 2009.

41 Ramesh J, Limdi JK, Sharma V, Makin AJ. The use of thrombin injections in the management of bleeding gastric varices: a single-center experience. Gastrointest Endosc 2008;68:877–82.

42 Avgerinos A, Klonis C, Rekoumis G, Gouma P, Papadimitriou N, Raptis S. A prospective randomized trial comparing somatostatin, balloon tamponade and the combination of both methods in the management of acute variceal haemorrhage. J Hepatol 1991;13:78–83.

43 Hubmann R, Bodlaj G, Czompo M, et al. The use of self-expanding metal stents to treat acute esophageal variceal bleeding. Endoscopy 2006;38:896–901.

44 Gordon JD, Colapinto RF, Abecassis M, et al. Transjugular intrahepatic portosystemic shunt: a nonoperative approach to life-threatening variceal bleeding. Can J Surg 1987;30:45–9.

45 Boyer TD, Haskal ZJ, American Association for the Study of Liver Diseases. The role of transjugular intrahepatic portosystemic shunt (TIPS) in the management of portal hypertension: update 2009. Hepatology 2010;51:306

46 Monescillo A, Martinez-Lagares F, Ruiz-del-Arbol L, et al. Influence of portal hypertension and its early decompression by TIPS placement on the outcome of variceal bleeding. Hepatology 2004;40:793–801.

47 Garcia-Pagan JC, Caca K, Bureau C, et al. Early use of TIPS in patients with cirrhosis and variceal bleeding. N Engl J Med 2010;362:2370–9.

48 Garcia-Pagan JC, Di Pascoli M, Caca K, et al. Use of early-tips for high-risk variceal bleeding: results of a post-RCT surveillance study. J Hepatol 2013;58:45–50.

49 Sugiura M, Futagawa S. A new technique for treating esophageal varices. J Thorac Cardiovasc Surg 1973;66:677–85.

50 European Association for the Study of the Liver. EASL clinical practice guidelines on the management of ascites, spontaneous bacterial peritonitis, and hepatorenal syndrome in cirrhosis. J Hepatol 2010;53:397–417.

51 Garcia-Pagan JC, Reverter E, Abraldes JG, Bosch J. Acute variceal bleeding. Semin Respir Crit Care Med 2012;33:46–54.

52 Matsumoto A, Yamauchi H, Inokuchi H. Balloon occluded retrograde transvenous obliteration: a feasible alternative to transjugular intrahepatic portosystemic stent shunt. Gut 2003;52:611–2.

53 Hirota S, Matsumoto S, Tomita M, Sako M, Kono M. Retrograde transvenous obliteration of gastric varices. Radiology 1999;211:349–56.

54 de Franchis R. Updating consensus in portal hypertension: report of the Baveno III Consensus Workshop on definitions, methodology and therapeutic strategies in portal hypertension. J Hepatol 2000;33:846–52.

55 Mishra SR, Sharma BC, Kumar A, Sarin SK. Primary prophylaxis of gastric variceal bleeding comparing cyanoacrylate injection and beta-blockers: a randomized controlled trial. J Hepatol 2011;54:1161–7.

56 McCormack TT, Sims J, Eyre-Brook I, et al. Gastric lesions in portal hypertension: inflammatory gastritis or congestive gastropathy? Gut 1985;26:1226–32.

57 Primignani M, Carpinelli L, Preatoni P, et al. Natural history of portal hypertensive gastropathy in patients with liver cirrhosis. The New Italian Endoscopic Club for the study and treatment of esophageal varices (NIEC). Gastroenterology 2000;119:181–7.

58 Kumar A, Mishra SR, Sharma P, Sharma BC, Sarin SK. Clinical, laboratory, and hemodynamic parameters in portal hypertensive gastropathy: a study of 254 cirrhotics. J Clin Gastroenterol 2010;44:294–300.
59 Merli M, Nicolini G, Angeloni S, Gentili F, Attili AF, Riggio O. The natural history of portal hypertensive gastropathy in patients with liver cirrhosis and mild portal hypertension. Am J Gastroenterol 2004;99:1959–65.
60 Fontana RJ, Sanyal AJ, Mehta S, et al. Portal hypertensive gastropathy in chronic hepatitis C patients with bridging fibrosis and compensated cirrhosis: results from the HALT-C trial. Am J Gastroenterol 2006;101:983–92.
61 Evrard S, Le Moine O, Deviere J, et al. Unexplained digestive bleeding in a cirrhotic patient. Gut 2004;53:1771; quiz answer, 80.
62 Urbain D, Vandebosch S, Hindryckx P, et al. Capsule endoscopy findings in cirrhosis with portal hypertension: a prospective study. Dig Liver Dis 2008;40:392–3.
63 Perez-Ayuso RM, Pique JM, Bosch J, et al. Propranolol in prevention of recurrent bleeding from severe portal hypertensive gastropathy in cirrhosis. Lancet 1991;337:1431–4.
64 Kamath PS, Lacerda M, Ahlquist DA, McKusick MA, Andrews JC, Nagorney DA. Gastric mucosal responses to intrahepatic portosystemic shunting in patients with cirrhosis. Gastroenterology 2000;118:905–11.
65 Herrera S, Bordas JM, Llach J, et al. The beneficial effects of argon plasma coagulation in the management of different types of gastric vascular ectasia lesions in patients admitted for GI hemorrhage. Gastrointest Endosc 2008;68:440–6.
66 Smith LA, Morris AJ, Stanley AJ. The use of hemospray in portal hypertensive bleeding: a case series. J Hepatol 2014;60:457–60.
67 Ripoll C, Garcia-Tsao G. The management of portal hypertensive gastropathy and gastric antral vascular ectasia. Dig Liver Dis 2011;43:345–51.
68 Gostout CJ, Viggiano TR, Ahlquist DA, Wang KK, Larson MV, Balm R. The clinical and endoscopic spectrum of the watermelon stomach. J Clin Gastroenterol 1992;15:256–63.
69 Ingraham KM, O'Brien MS, Shenin M, Derk CT, Steen VD. Gastric antral vascular ectasia in systemic sclerosis: demographics and disease predictors. J Rheumatol 2010;37:603–7.
70 Kim MY, Choi H, Baik SK, et al. Portal hypertensive gastropathy: correlation with portal hypertension and prognosis in cirrhosis. Dig Dis Sci 2010;55:3561–7.
71 Liberski SM, McGarrity TJ, Hartle RJ, Varano V, Reynolds D. The watermelon stomach: long-term outcome in patients treated with Nd:YAG laser therapy. Gastrointest Endosc 1994;40(5):584–7.
72 Tobin RW, Hackman RC, Kimmey MB, et al. Bleeding from gastric antral vascular ectasia in marrow transplant patients. Gastrointest Endosc 1996;44:223–9.
73 Raja K, Kochhar R, Sethy PK, Dutta U, Bali HK, Varma JS. An endoscopic study of upper-GI mucosal changes in patients with congestive heart failure. Gastrointest Endosc 2004;60:887–93.
74 Vincent C, Pomier-Layrargues G, Dagenais M, et al. Cure of gastric antral vascular ectasia by liver transplantation despite persistent portal hypertension: a clue for pathogenesis. Liver Transpl 2002;8:717–20.
75 Westerhoff M, Tretiakova M, Hovan L, Miller J, Noffsinger A, Hart J. CD61, CD31, and CD34 improve diagnostic accuracy in gastric antral vascular ectasia and portal hypertensive gastropathy: an immunohistochemical and digital morphometric study. Am J Surg Pathol 2010;34:494–501.
76 Payen JL, Cales P, Voigt JJ, et al. Severe portal hypertensive gastropathy and antral vascular ectasia are distinct entities in patients with cirrhosis. Gastroenterology 1995;108:138–44.
77 Labenz J, Borsch G. Bleeding watermelon stomach treated by Nd-YAG laser photocoagulation. Endoscopy 1993;25:240–2.
78 Cho S, Zanati S, Yong E, et al. Endoscopic cryotherapy for the management of gastric antral vascular ectasia. Gastrointest Endosc 2008;68:895–902.
79 Kantsevoy SV, Cruz-Correa MR, Vaughn CA, Jagannath SB, Pasricha PJ, Kalloo AN. Endoscopic cryotherapy for the treatment of bleeding mucosal vascular lesions of the GI tract: a pilot study. Gastrointest Endosc 2003;57:403–6.
80 Tran A, Villeneuve JP, Bilodeau M, et al. Treatment of chronic bleeding from gastric antral vascular ectasia (GAVE) with estrogen-progesterone in cirrhotic patients: an open pilot study. Am J Gastroenterol 1999;94:2909–11.
81 Bhowmick BK. Watermelon stomach treated with oral corticosteroid. J R Soc Med 1993;86:52.
82 McCormick PA, Ooi H, Crosbie O. Tranexamic acid for severe bleeding gastric antral vascular ectasia in cirrhosis. Gut 1998;42:750–2.
83 Dunne KA, Hill J, Dillon JF. Treatment of chronic transfusion-dependent gastric antral vascular ectasia (watermelon stomach) with thalidomide. Eur J Gastroenterol Hepatol 2006;18:455–6.
84 Nardone G, Rocco A, Balzano T, Budillon G. The efficacy of octreotide therapy in chronic bleeding due to vascular abnormalities of the gastrointestinal tract. Aliment Pharmacol Ther 1999;13:1429–36.
85 Cabral JE, Pontes JM, Toste M, et al. Watermelon stomach: treatment with a serotonin antagonist. Am J Gastroenterol 1991;86:927–8.
86 Mann NS, Rachut E. Gastric antral vascular ectasia causing severe hypoalbuminemia and anemia cured by antrectomy. J Clin Gastroenterol 2002;34:284–6.
87 Christensen T. The treatment of oesophageal varices using a Sengstaken–Blakemore tube: considerations for nursing practice. Nurs Crit Care 2004;9:58–63.

CHAPTER 14
Ascites

Andrés Cárdenas,[1] Isabel Graupera,[2] and Pere Ginès[2]
[1]*GI Unit, Hospital Clínic and University of Barcelona, Institut d'Investigacions Biomèdiques August Pi-Sunyer (IDIBAPS), Ciber de Enfermedades Hepaticas y Digestivas (CIBERHED)*
[2]*Liver Unit, Hospital Clínic and University of Barcelona, Institut d'Investigacions Biomèdiques August Pi-Sunyer (IDIBAPS), Ciber de Enfermedades Hepaticas y Digestivas (CIBERHED), Instituto Reina Sofía de Investigación Nefrológica (IRSIN), Barcelona, Spain*

Cirrhosis is the twelfth leading cause of mortality in the United States, accounting for nearly 32 000 deaths in 2010 [1]. Ascites is the most common complication of cirrhosis resulting in poor quality of life, high risk of development of other complications, increased morbidity and mortality associated with surgical interventions, and poor long-term outcome [2–6]. Cirrhotic patients with first onset ascites have survival rates of 85% at 1 year and 56% at 5 years without liver transplantation [3].

The practical management of ascites involves a proper evaluation of the patient with a thorough history and physical examination. In addition, complete laboratory, ascitic fluid, radiologic, endoscopic, and, in some cases, histologic tests should be performed. One of the most important steps in the initial assessment of patients with ascites is referral of appropriate candidates for liver transplantation as this offers a definitive cure of cirrhosis and its complications.

Taking proper care of patients with ascites can be challenging because they are prone to complications such as spontaneous bacterial peritonitis (SBP), hypervolemic hyponatremia, hepatic hydrothorax, hepatorenal syndrome (HRS) and hepatocellular carcinoma, bleeding from esophageal or gastric varices, and hepatic encephalopathy. While the initial management of uncomplicated ascites with low sodium diet and diuretic treatment is straightforward in the majority of patients, there is a group of patients that fails to respond to diuretics and become a real therapeutic challenge. This chapter focuses on the practical aspects of the evaluation and treatment of patients with ascites and cirrhosis.

Pathophysiology of ascites

The major factor contributing to ascites formation is splanchnic vasodilatation resulting in a decreased effective arterial blood volume [7]. Increased hepatic resistance to portal flow due to cirrhosis causes a progressive increase in portal pressure with collateral vein formation and shunting of blood to the systemic circulation. As portal hypertension develops, splanchnic arterial vasodilatation occurs due to the enhanced local production of nitric oxide and other vasodilators including carbon monoxide and endogenous cannabinoids as a consequence of endothelial stretching and bacterial translocation [8–10]. Evidence indicates that bacterial translocation to mesenteric lymph nodes with increased production of bacterial products and subsequent stimulation of cytokine synthesis has a major role in the pathogenesis of arterial vasodilatation and the associated circulatory abnormalities that occur in cirrhosis [10,11]. In the early stages of cirrhosis, splanchnic arterial vasodilation is moderate and has no major effect on effective arterial blood volume, which is maintained within normal limits due to an increase in plasma volume and cardiac output [7]. In advanced stages, splanchnic arterial vasodilatation is so intense that effective arterial blood

Grant support: some of the studies reported in this manuscript and performed in the authors' Unit have been supported by research grants from the Instituto de Salud Carlos III (FIS PI08/0126 and EC07/90077). Isabel Graupera is partly supported by a grant from the Reina Sofia d'Investigación en Nefrologia (IRSIN).

Cirrhosis: A practical guide to management, First Edition. Edited by Samuel S. Lee and Richard Moreau.

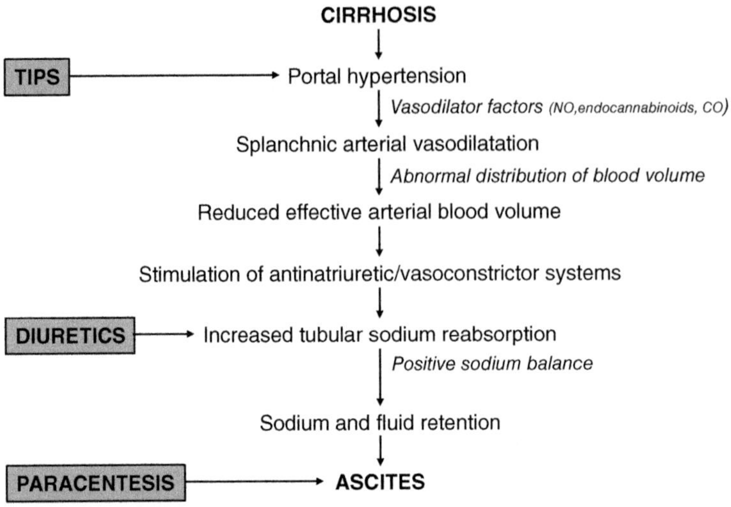

Figure 14.1 Pathogenesis of ascites formation in cirrhosis and current therapeutic options for ascites and dilutional hyponatremia. Portal hypertension is the main factor responsible for the development of splanchnic vasodilation and a decrease in effective arterial blood volume (NO, nitric oxide; CO, carbon moxide). The transjugular intrahepatic portosystemic shunt (TIPS) by reducing portal pressure is an effective treatment of ascites, particularly in patients with refractory ascites. The compensatory homeostatic response occurs secondary to a reduced effective arterial blood volume and leads to the activation of antinatriuretic factors (mainly the angiotensin–aldosterone system) with subsequent sodium retention. The use of diuretics (spironolactone) that promote natriuresis are the preferred therapy for patients with sodium retention and fluid accumulation. Patients with large-volume ascites should be treated with therapeutic paracentesis and albumin administration followed by diuretics as tolerated.

volume becomes markedly reduced and arterial pressure falls. A reduction in cardiac output occurs in the late stages of cirrhosis and also contributes to the impairment in effective arterial blood volume [12–14]. As a consequence of the impairment in effective arterial blood volume, there is homeostatic activation of vasoconstrictor and antinatriuretic factors to maintain arterial pressure, resulting in renal sodium and fluid retention. The combination of portal hypertension and splanchnic arterial vasodilation alters intestinal capillary pressure and permeability, which facilitates the accumulation of the retained fluid in the abdominal cavity. With disease progression, there is a marked impairment in renal solute-free water excretion and renal vasoconstriction, leading to hypervolemic hyponatremia and hepatorenal syndrome, respectively. The pathophysiologic rationale for the treatment of patients with cirrhosis and ascites is described in Figure 14.1.

Patients' history

Patients with cirrhosis presenting with ascites must always be questioned about precipitating events such as excessive salt intake, alcohol consumption, infections, medications such as nonsteroidal anti-inflammatory drugs or steroids, and noncompliance with diuretic therapy if they previously had ascites. Worsening liver disease, portal vein thrombosis, parenchymal renal failure (i.e., glomerular diseases), and development of hepatocellular carcinoma (most often associated with tumor invasion of the portal vein) may also precipitate the development of ascites. More commonly, ascites develops insidiously over the course of weeks.

The main symptoms are an increase in abdominal girth often accompanied by lower extremity edema [15]. In patients with a large amount of ascites, respiratory function and physical activity may be impaired. Dyspnea may occur as a consequence of increasing abdominal distention and/or accompanying pleural effusions. Patients with SBP can present with fever, chills, abdominal pain, encephalopathy, renal failure, and rebound abdominal tenderness. However, patients with SBP may be asymptomatic and the diagnosis relies on the examination of peritoneal fluid.

Other common manifestations of patients with ascites include colicky abdominal pain, anorexia, malaise, weakness, malnutrition, and/or jaundice. Increased intrabdominal pressure favors the formation of abdominal hernias in patients with cirrhosis and long-standing ascites [15]. Umbilical hernias increase in size if ascites is not treated and sometimes cause significant complications such as strangulation and rupture due to previous ulcer formation on the surface. Rupture may be complicated with infection of the ascitic fluid and delayed wound healing. Inguinal hernias can also be problematic in patients with ascites. The best treatment is prevention of ascites because surgical treatment is usually not recommended in those with advanced cirrhosis. Muscle cramps are a common clinical feature in patients with cirrhosis and ascites. The prevalence of muscle cramps (>3 episodes per week) in cirrhotic patients is approximately 50–60% and is related to the duration of cirrhosis and severity of impairment in circulatory function and presence of ascites. Muscle cramps commonly occur in the lower extremities and can significantly impair the patients' quality of life. Painful gynecomastia may occur in patients with cirrhosis and ascites. The exact mechanisms are unknown; however, it is postulated that estrogen excess in cirrhotic patients and the estrogenic effects of the spironolactone are possible causes [15].

Physical examination

Most patients are malnourished and have signs of muscle wasting and atrophy. Other common findings are palmar erythema, spider nevi, jaundice, loss of body hair, white nails (Terry nails), splenomegaly, inguinal and umbilical hernias, and lower extremity edema [15]. The physical examination is not completely reliable for detecting fluid in abdominal cavity. Patients must have approximately 1500 mL of fluid to be detected reliably by examination [16]. The abdomen is distended with bulging flanks; dullness to percussion in these areas indicates ascites. When free fluid is present in the abdominal cavity, it moves to the flanks and the intestines float upward when the patient is supine. The air–fluid level is higher than that normally found on the lateral aspect of the abdomen, if the patient is turned on his/her side the dullness will shift and percussion over the uppermost part becomes tympanic, because that area is occupied by intestines as fluid shifts to the other side. This maneuver is called shifting dullness and is very sensitive for detecting ascites [16]. Mild or moderate pleural effusions are also common in patients with ascites. Large pleural effusions, usually greater than 500 mL, in cirrhotic patients without cardiopulmonary disease are uncommon and are known as hepatic hydrothorax. The current quantitative classification of ascites divides patients into three groups. In grade 1 ascites, fluid is detected only by ultrasound, in grade 2, ascites is moderate with symmetrical distention of the abdomen, and in grade 3, ascites is large or tense with marked abdominal distention [17,18].

Patient evaluation

The evaluation of patients with ascites should include standard hematology, electrolyte, renal (serum creatinine and blood urea nitrogen, and urinary sodium), coagulation (prothrombin time, PT, or international normalized ratio, INR), and liver tests (aminotransferases, bilirubin, albumin, total protein, alkaline phosphatase, gamma-glutamyl transferase) [17–19]. An abdominal ultrasonography to rule out hepatocellular carcinoma and evaluate the patency of the portal venous system should be performed in all patients. In addition, an upper gastrointestinal endoscopy to assess the presence and characteristics of esophageal and gastric varices is recommended. In patients with renal failure (serum creatinine >1.5 mg/dL), urine sediment, and 24-hour urine protein should be assessed and the kidneys examined by ultrasonography. Evaluation of circulatory function should include measurement of arterial pressure and heart rate.

A diagnostic paracentesis (30 mL of fluid) is required in all patients presenting with their first episode of ascites, and all patients with any evidence of clinical deterioration such as fever, abdominal pain, gastrointestinal bleeding, hepatic encephalopathy, hypotension, or renal failure. The ascitic fluid in cirrhotics is mostly transparent and yellow–amber in color. Tests on the ascitic fluid should include cell count, albumin, total protein and cultures in blood culture bottles (10 mL of fluid injected at the bedside) [17–20]. The cell count is the most helpful test in determining bacterial infection. In patients without infection of the ascitic fluid, the ascitic fluid white blood cell count is $<100/mm^3$ with a predominance of mononuclear cells (>75%) and a low number of neutrophils. An increased number of white blood cells with predominance of neutrophils indicates peritoneal infection [18,21]. The diagnosis of SBP is made when the fluid sample has >250/mm^3 neutrophils and there are no signs of peritonitis due to perforation or inflammation of intra-abdominal organs. The difference between serum albumin concentration and ascites albumin concentration (serum–ascites albumin gradient) in patients with cirrhosis and ascites is usually >11 g/L, values <11 g/L suggest a cause of ascites other than cirrhosis [22]. A low total protein concentration in ascitic fluid (<15 g/L) is associated with an increased risk of SBP and in selected patients may indicate a need for antibiotic prophylaxis with oral quinolones to reduce the risk of SBP and HRS. Finally, cultures of ascitic fluid of patients with ascitic fluid infection in blood culture bottles increase the probability of isolating an organism to approximately 50% of cases if the fluid is inoculated into the bottles at the bedside [21,23].

Management of patients with ascites

General measures

A low sodium diet of approximately 80–120 mmol/day (i.e., no added salt and no preprocessed meals) facilitates the elimination of ascites and delays the reaccumulation of fluid [18]. However, a reduction in sodium intake alone only achieves a negative sodium balance and complete elimination of ascites in only 10% of patients unless diuretics are given. Fluid restriction is not necessary unless patients have hypervolemic hyponatremia (defined as serum sodium <130 mEq/L together with ascites and/or edema). An evaluation by a nutritionist is of utmost importance for appropriate education regarding an appropriate caloric and salt intake. Improvement of the nutritional status is essential because patients with advanced liver disease have decreased intake and absorption of nutrients, increased energy expenditure, and altered fuel metabolism with an accelerated starvation metabolism [24,25]. Nutritional therapy in cirrhotic patients can improve nutritional status, reduce infection rates, and decrease perioperative morbidity [24]. The goal is for nutritional supplementation to correct the underlying protein energy malnutrition. In advanced cases of malnutrition, supplemental enteral nutrition in cirrhotic patients with ascites may improve liver function and hepatic encephalopathy [24–27].

Table 14.1 Management practice points in patients with ascites and cirrhosis.

A	Treatment strategy for patients with cirrhosis and moderate-volume (grade 2) ascites Start with a low-sodium diet (90 mmol/day) and spironolactone (50–100 mg/day) to reach goal of weight loss: 300–500 mg/day. If needed, doses to be increased every 7 days up to 400 mg/day spironolactone. Furosemide can be added at a starting dose of 20–40 mg/day and subsequently increased to 160 mg/day if needed
B	Treatment strategy for patients with cirrhosis and large-volume (grade 3) ascites Total paracentesis plus intravenous albumin (8 g/L of ascites removed) followed by a low-sodium diet (90 mmol/day) and diuretics if patient tolerated them beforehand
C	Treatment strategy for refractory ascites Total paracentesis plus intravenous albumin can be performed as needed. Consider use of TIPS in patients with very frequent recurrent ascites, very rapid recurrence of ascites, and preserved liver function (bilirubin <3 mg/dL, platelet count >75 000, serum sodium level >130 mEq/L, Child–Pugh score <13, model for end-stage liver disease (MELD) score <18), aged <70 years, without hepatic encephalopathy, central or large hepatocellular carcinoma or cardiopulmonary disease

Specific measures

Patients with grade 1 ascites do not require any specific treatment but they should be cautioned about avoiding foods with large amounts of salt. Patients with grade 2 ascites are usually treated with sodium restriction and diuretics. Patients with grade 3 ascites are managed with large-volume paracentesis along with diuretics. Patients with refractory ascites do not respond to high doses of diuretics or develop side effects that preclude their use. The discussion of the management of ascites may therefore be divided in three parts: moderate-volume ascites (grade 2 ascites), large-volume ascites (grade 3), and refractory ascites. A summary of recommendations for the management of ascites is included in Table 14.1.

Moderate-volume ascites

Patients with moderate ascites usually accumulate fluid slowly, such that they typically do not develop large-volume ascites unless their sodium intake is very high or they do not seek medical attention for long periods of time. Renal solute-free water excretion and glomerular filtration rates are normal in most cases; therefore, serum sodium and creatinine concentration are usually within normal limits. These patients typically can be managed as outpatients and do not require admission unless they have other complications of cirrhosis. A negative sodium balance with loss of ascites is obtained in most cases with low doses of diuretics. Diuretics eliminate the excess extracellular fluid presenting as ascites and edema by increasing renal sodium excretion together with fluid excretion. The diuretics most frequently used in patients with cirrhosis and ascites are aldosterone antagonists, mainly spironolactone and potassium canrenoate, drugs that selectively antagonize the sodium-retaining effects of aldosterone in the renal collecting tubules, and loop diuretics, especially furosemide, that inhibit the Na^{+}-K^{+}–$2Cl^{-}$ cotransporter in the loop of Henle. Diuretic therapy is effective in the elimination of ascites in 80–90% of patients with ascites, a percentage that increases up to 95% if only patients without renal failure are considered [18].

Diuretics are indicated for all patients with grade 2 ascites. Patients with their first episode of ascites usually respond with spironolactone 50–100 mg/day [18,19,28–30]. Patients with recurrent episodes of ascites should receive the combination of spironolactone 100 mg/day with furosemide 40 mg/day. If there is no response, compliance with diet and medications should be confirmed and diuretics may then be increased every 7 days by doubling doses (1 : 1 ratio) to a maximal dose of spironolactone (400 mg/day) and a maximal dose of furosemide (160 mg/day).

The goal of treatment is to produce an average weight loss of 500 g/day in patients without peripheral edema and 800–1000 g/day in those with peripheral edema until ascites has decreased markedly and afterwards diuretic dosage can be reduced. This is in order to avoid overdiuresis and side effects. In patients who do not respond, compliance with low sodium diet and diuretics should always be assessed. In these cases, measurement of urine sodium, which provides an accurate assessment of the response to diuretics, may help in deciding whether there is a need to increase dosage.

Diuretics should be used judiciously in patients with cirrhosis as they can precipitate disturbances in fluid and electrolyte balance including hyponatremia, dehydration, renal impairment, hyperkalemia, or hypokalemia. Patients should be closely followed and serum and urine eletrolytes need to be measured within the first 2 weeks after starting or modifying dosage. Diuretics should be stopped or their dosage reduced if any of the abovementioned effects appear. Moreover, patients should be instructed to monitor their weight and reduce the diuretic dosage and seek medical advice if there is an excessive decrease in body weight. An excessive weight loss over several days may be associated with dehydration and renal failure. Hepatic encephalopathy may occur, particularly in those patients with advanced liver disease. Whether diuretics are responsible for episodes of hepatic encephalopathy in a particular patient is very difficult to establish. So, as a rule of thumb, if there is a chronologic relationship between the use diuretics and an episode of hepatic encephalopathy in at least two distinct time points, then diuretics should be considered the trigger of encephalopathy and treatment discontinued. Spironolactone may cause tender gynecomastia in some patients and in most instances the dosage needs to be reduced or the medication needs to be stopped. Alternative treatments to spironolactone in those patients who require discontinuation are amiloride and eplerenone [31,32]. However, both drugs have less natriuretic potency than that of spironolactone and their use may be associated with recurrence of ascites [31,32]. Tamoxifen (20 mg orally, two times daily) may be useful in reducing pain in some cases; however, information is very limited [33]. Muscle cramps, which also may appear with diuretic therapy, may require a reduction in diuretic dosage. Isolated reports indicate that quinidine (quinidine sulfate 400 mg/day) [34,35] and intravenous albumin administration (25 g/week) [36] reduce the frequency and intensity of muscle cramps in cirrhotic patients with ascites treated with diuretics. An algorithm explaining the treatment of grade 2 ascites is depicted in Figure 14.2.

Large-volume ascites

Patients with large-volume ascites can be treated as outpatients unless they have associated complications. The majority of these patients have intense sodium retention (urine sodium frequently <10 mEq/L), so that ascites accumulates rapidly even under sodium restriction. Serum creatinine levels are normal or only moderately increased indicating normal or moderately reduced glomerular filtration rate. Patients should be treated with large-volume paracentesis followed by diuretics. Complete removal of ascites with one session of large-volume paracentesis with intravenous albumin (8 g per liter tapped) is a faster and more effective measure in controlling tense ascites and associated with a lower

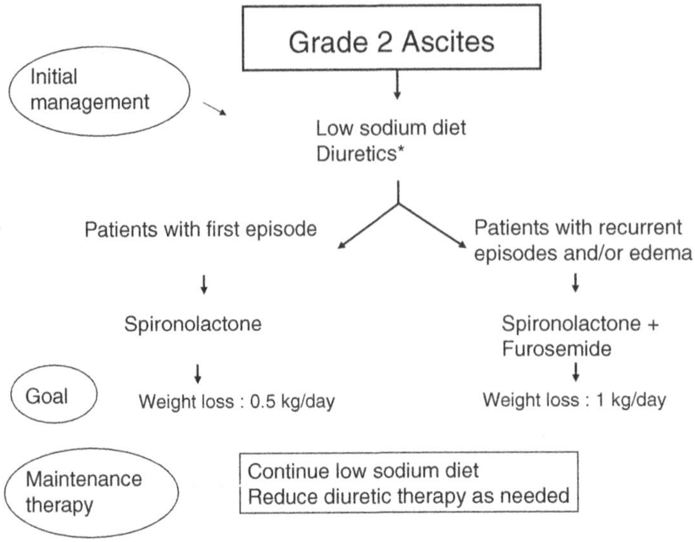

Figure 14.2 Treatment strategy for patients with cirrhosis and grade 2 ascites. *Recommended diuretics are described in Table 14.1.

number of complications than conventional diuretic therapy [37–39]. Current guidelines establish paracentesis followed by diuretics as the method of choice to treat large-volume ascites [17,18]. Large-volume paracentesis without plasma expanders is associated with a derangement in circulatory function characterized by reduction of effective arterial blood volume with subsequent activation of vasoconstrictor and antinatriuretic factors [39,40]. Circulatory dysfunction after large-volume paracentesis is associated with a high ascites recurrence rate, development of renal failure and/or hyponatremia in 20% of cases, and shortened survival [39–41]. This disorder can be effectively prevented with the administration of plasma expanders [37–44]. When less than 5 L of ascites is removed, artificial plasma expanders, saline, and albumin are equally effective [41,43]. However, if more than 5 L is removed, albumin is recommended [37–44]. As ascites will invariably recur after paracentesis, patients need to be started or continued on diuretics in order to prevent a positive sodium balance and recurrence of ascites [45]. Although the use of albumin after paracentesis is controversial due to the lack of data proving a survival benefit and high cost in some countries, a recent meta-analysis of 17 trials with a total of 1225 patients showed that albumin reduced morbidity and mortality among patients with tense ascites undergoing large-volume paracentesis, as compared with alternative treatments [44]. Therefore, the protective effect of albumin on the circulatory system compared with other expanders favors its use in this setting. An algorithm explaining the treatment of grade 3 ascites in depicted in Figure 14.3.

Complications related to paracentesis, such as bleeding, infection, or intestinal perforation, are exceedingly rare if paracentesis is performed under sterile conditions and with an appropriate technique and needle. The recommended location for performing paracentesis is the left lower quadrant, two finger breadths cephalad and two finger breadths medial to the anterior superior iliac spine. In this area, the skin is thin and there is a larger pool of fluid than the midline [20,46]. The risk of bleeding in cirrhotic patients when performing a paracentesis is extremely low; the frequency of severe hemorrhage after a tap is approximately 0.20% and a lethal outcome occurs is less than 0.01% of cases [47]. In some cases, severe hemorrhage due to a paracentesis may occur due to trauma of the inferior hypogastric artery. Thus, when performing paracentesis, the area of the inferior hypogastric arteries (midway between the pubis and anterior superior iliac spines) should be avoided. Most clinical trials in patients with cirrhosis and ascites have excluded patients with an elevated PT greater than 21 seconds or INR greater than 1.6 or platelet count below 50 000/μL. Therefore, the risk of bleeding complications in patients with more severe coagulopathy is

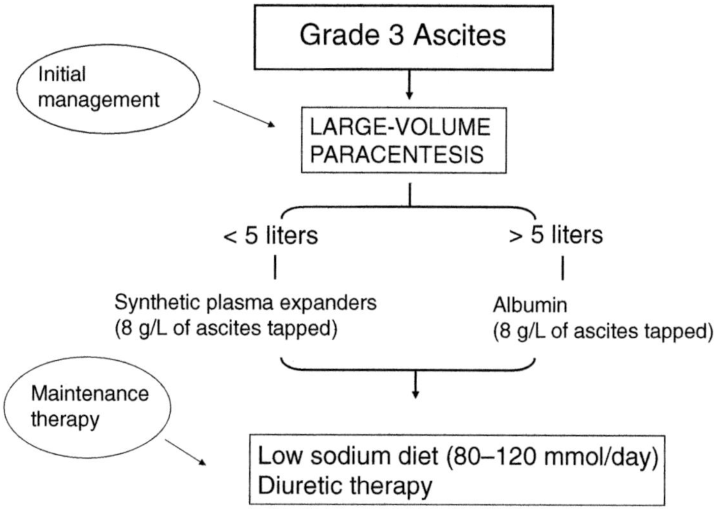

Figure 14.3 Treatment strategy for patients with cirrhosis and grade 3 ascites.

unknown and deserves investigation. Nonetheless, consensus meetings, guidelines, and expert opinion consider that the abnormal coagulation profile of the cirrhotic patient (mild prolonged PT and low platelets with a value >50 000/μL) is not an absolute contraindication for paracentesis and the routine administration of platelets or fresh frozen plasma as prophylaxis for bleeding is not recommended [48]. In patients with severe thrombocytopenia with a platelet count <30 000/μL, transfusion of platelets should be considered prior to the procedure [48]. Patients with suspected disseminated intravascular coagulopathy should not undergo a paracentesis.

Refractory ascites

This condition occurs in nearly 10% of patients with cirrhosis and ascites [49,50]. The difference from non-refractory ascites patients is that in the latter patients, sodium excretion may be increased with the use of diuretics, whereas in patients with refractory ascites, sodium excretion cannot be increased with diuretics either because patients do not respond to high doses of diuretics (spironolactone 400 mg/day plus furosemide 160 mg/day) or they develop side effects with lower doses that preclude their use (Table 14.2). In general, these patients have features of advanced liver disease, a high recurrence rate of ascites after large-volume paracentesis, an increased risk of HRS, and a poor prognosis. Patients can be treated with either repeated large-volume

Table 14.2 Definition and diagnostic criteria for refractory ascites in cirrhosis.

Diuretic-resistant ascites: ascites that cannot be mobilized or the early recurrence of which cannot be prevented because of a lack of response to sodium restriction and diuretic treatment

Diuretic-intractable ascites: ascites that cannot be mobilized or the early recurrence of which cannot be prevented because of the development of diuretic-induced complications that preclude the use of an effective diuretic dosage

Requisites:

1. *Treatment duration*: patients must be on intensive diuretic therapy (spironolactone 400 mg/day and furosemide 160 mg/day) for at least 1 week and on a salt-restricted diet of less than 90 mmol/day
2. *Lack of response*: mean weight loss of <0.8 kg over 4 days and urinary sodium output less than the sodium intake
3. *Early ascites recurrence*: reappearance of grade 2 or 3 ascites within 4 weeks of initial mobilization
4. *Diuretic-induced complications*: diuretic-induced hepatic encephalopathy is the development of encephalopathy in the absence of any other precipitating factor. Diuretic-induced renal impairment is an increase of serum creatinine by >100% to a value >2 mg/dL in patients with ascites responding to treatment. Diuretic-induced hyponatremia is defined as a decrease of serum sodium by >10 mEq/L to a serum sodium of <125 mEq/L. Diuretic induced hypo- or hyperkalemia is defined as a change in serum potassium to <3 or >6 mEq/L despite appropriate measures

Adapted from Moore et al., 2003 [17]. Reproduced with permission of John Wiley & Sons.

paracentesis with plasma expansion or transjugular intrahepatic portosystemic shunts (TIPS). Repeated large-volume paracentesis plus albumin is the recommended initial therapy for refractory ascites [18]. Patients generally require paracentesis every 2–4 weeks, which can be done in the outpatient setting. This approach is therefore easy to perform and relatively inexpensive. The main drawback is early recurrence of ascites because paracentesis does not modify the mechanisms responsible for ascites formation.

In contrast to paracentesis, TIPS, a nonsurgical method of portal decompression that consists of the insertion of an intrahepatic stent between one hepatic vein and the portal vein using a transjugular approach, is effective in preventing ascites recurrence because by reducing portal pressure ascites disappears in most patients [51–56]. Uncovered TIPS are very effective in relieving ascites, but frequently complicated by stenosis of the prosthesis (18–78%) [51–56]. Polytetrafluoroethylene-covered prostheses seem to improve TIPS patency and decrease the number of clinical relapses and reinterventions without increasing the risk of encephalopathy [57,58]. Randomized clinical trials comparing uncovered TIPS with repeated paracentesis demonstrate that TIPS controls ascites effectively and is associated with a lower rate of ascites recurrence [51–55]. Hepatic encephalopathy may occur in approximately 30–50% of patients. Two studies showed a survival benefit with TIPS [52,55], but two other studies demonstrated no difference in survival [53,54]. Three meta-analyses of these randomized controlled studies conclude that TIPS is better at controlling ascites but does not improve survival compared with paracentesis [59–61]. Another meta-analysis that reviewed individual patient data of three trials [52,54,55] indicates that TIPS significantly improves transplant-free survival of cirrhotic patients with refractory ascites [62]. Although meta-analysis using individual data is in theory a more reliable tool than standard meta-analysis, it cannot overcome deficiencies of individual studies, such as inclusion of patients who did not all have refractory ascites in two of the studies, use of large-volume paracentesis without albumin in one study, and use of TIPS as rescue therapy in a large proportion of patients treated with large-volume paracentesis in another study. Thus, given these results and the higher frequency of hepatic encephalopathy as well as the higher cost of TIPS than large-volume paracentesis plus albumin, in the context of a lack of survival benefit, this leaves TIPS as a second line strategy in the management of refractory ascites. TIPS placement certainly should be considered an option for patients with loculated ascites, those with very rapid recurrence of ascites and preserved liver function (bilirubin <3 mg/dL, platelet count >75 000, serum sodium level >130 meq/L, Child–Pugh score <13, model for end-stage liver disease (MELD) score <18), aged <70 years, without hepatic encephalopathy, central or large hepatocellular carcinoma or cardiopulmonary disease [18,50,56,63,64]. An algorithm explaining the treatment of refractory ascites is depicted in Figure 14.4.

Evaluation for liver transplantation

Patients with cirrhosis developing their first episode of ascites have a relatively good mid-term prognosis (probability of survival of 85% at 1 year) [3]. This prognosis is somewhat similar to the outcome of liver transplant recipients (probability of survival of 87% at 1 year) (www.unos.org). Several factors associated with poor prognosis have been described in patients with cirrhosis and ascites. These factors, which are usually not present at the time of development of the first episode of ascites, may occur later in the course of the disease. These include low serum sodium concentration, low arterial pressure, high serum creatinine, intense sodium retention (urine sodium <10 mEq/day), and high Child–Pugh scores [65,66]. Thus, patients with cirrhosis and the first episode of ascites without associated poor prognostic factors may not necessarily benefit from liver transplantation, particularly if they have a MELD score <15 (A. Cárdenas, P. Ginès, unpublished data). Nevertheless, whenever some of the abovementioned factors are present, patients should be promptly referred for evaluation for liver transplantation [67].

Other therapies

New treatments for ascites are being evaluated based on two approaches. The first stems from what is known regarding the underlying pathophysiologic abnormalities that cause sodium and water retention. In this approach the use of new agents (V2 vasopressin receptor antagonists, known as vaptans) that act on the kidney and promote solute-free water diuresis can be combined with diuretics in order to improve mobilization of ascites and edema. Animal and human studies suggest that these drugs, apart from causing solute-free water

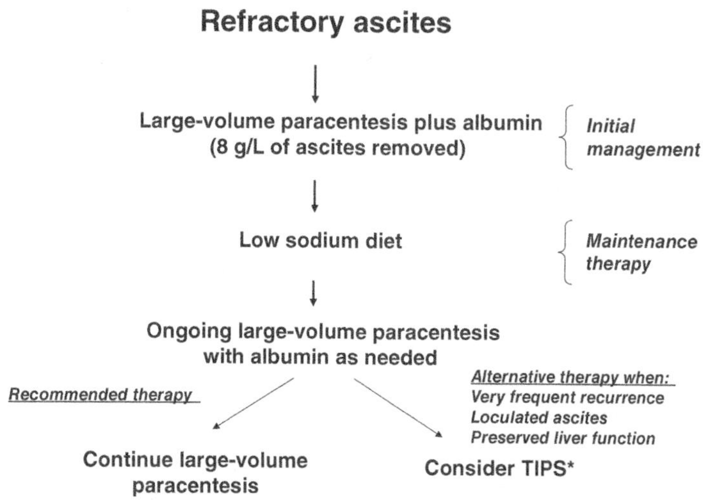

Figure 14.4 Treatment strategy for patients with refractory ascites. Consider TIPS for those with very rapid recurrence of ascites and preserved liver function (bilirubin <3 mg/dL, platelet count >75 000, serum sodium level >130 meq/L, Child–Pugh score <13, model for end-stage liver disease (MELD) score <18), aged <70, without hepatic encephalopathy, central hepatocellular carcinoma, or cardiopulmonary disease.

excretion, enhance sodium excretion [68,69]. The second approach relates to the use of vasoconstrictor drugs that are able to improve the underlying hemodynamic derangements that lead to ascites formation in cirrhosis, thereby reducing the activity of antinatriuretic factors. These drugs may theoretically improve the action of diuretics in order to maximize ascites mobilization.

The use of specific antagonists of the vasopressin receptor (V2 receptor antagonists) on the distal tubule of the kidney by means of counteracting AVP and increasing the excretion of solute-free water has been evaluated for the management of ascites in cirrhosis. These drugs are not yet approved for patients with cirrhosis and ascites; however, an intravenous V1–V2 receptor antagonist (conivaptan) and a V2 receptor antagonist (tolvaptan) are approved by the Food and Drug Administration and the European Medication Agency for the treatment of hypervolemic and euvolemic hyponatremia. Other V2 receptor antagonists such as satavaptan have been evaluated for the treatment of ascites in association with diuretics with the rationale that by increasing diuresis the vaptan would help manage ascites and prevent its recurrence. Although results of phase 2 studies were promising [70], phase 3 long-term treatment studies in three different populations of patients with cirrhosis and ascites demonstrated a lack of efficacy in both ascites management and prevention of its recurrence [71]. Furthermore, use of satavaptan was associated with an increased mortality and the drug was withdrawn from development. The reason for this increased mortality could not be elucidated. A small study in 18 patients with cirrhosis and ascites without hyponatremia showed that the administration of tolvaptan dose-dependently decreased body weight and improved ascites and edema; however, the results of this observation need to be further studied in large cohorts of patients before considering this agent a treatment for patients with ascites [72].

Other potential therapies for patients with ascites stem from data on the use of vasoconstrictors (midodrine and terlipressin) with plasma expansion in patients with cirrhosis and HRS. These agents improve renal function, urinary sodium excretion, and serum sodium levels and decrease the levels of vasoctive/antinatriuretic systems in patients with advanced cirrhosis and HRS. Therefore, the use of an oral vasoconstrictor is an attractive approach in the treatment of patients with ascites without HRS who do not respond to diuretics.

In a study of 39 patients with cirrhosis, oral midodrine (an α_1-adrenergic agonist) 10 mg, three times daily, was given to 11 patients without ascites and 12 with ascites and compared with placebo in eight patients without ascites and eight patients with ascites for 7 days [73]. In the midodrine group there was a moderate increase in urine sodium excretion in patients with ascites (urinary sodium from 30 ± 15 to 49 ± 16 meq/L) as well as glomerular filtration rate (from 80 ± 23 to 92 ± 27 mL/min) and urine volume (from 0.98 ± 0.26 to 1.15 ± 0.34 L) and significant decreases in plasma renin activity and aldosterone. Nonetheless, in this study neither body weight nor abdominal girth as measures of an effect on ascites were recorded.

A more recent study also demonstrated that oral midodrine (7.5 mg every 8 hours) plus standard medical therapy (sodium restriction plus diuretics) was significantly superior to standard medical therapy alone in the control of ascites ($P = 0.013$) at 3 months [74]. The mortality rate in the standard medical therapy group was significantly higher than the midodrine group ($P < 0.046$). There was no significant difference in the frequency of complications at the end of follow-up. Clonidine, a centrally acting α_2-agonist and sympatholitic agent, was evaluated as an adjunct treatment in patients with cirrhosis and ascites. In a randomized study, oral clonidine (0.075 mg, two times daily) led to a more rapid mobilization of ascites with fewer complications than placebo in patients with cirrhosis, ascites, and a plasma norepinephrine level of >300 pg/mL [75]. This medication was also evaluated in a randomized study of clonidine plus diuretics versus diuretics alone which showed that the highest efficacy was obtained in patients who had high serum levels of norepinephine and the presence of two specific genetic polymorphisms that predicted clonidine response in cirrhotic patients [76]. Although the results are interesting, the study was not a double-blind placebo-controlled trial, the medication was administered for only 3 months, and in practice genetic polymorphisms cannot be easily performed to ensure adequate response. More studies from other centers confirming the efficacy and safety of clonidine need to be carried out before considering this drug a therapeutic agent for patients with refractory ascites.

Intravenous terlipressin has also been evaluated as a potential therapy for patients with nonrefractory and refractory ascites. There is very limited information; however, available data indicate that it improves glomerular filtration rate and natriuresis in both types of ascites, but a clinical effect on weight or abdominal girth was not recorded [77]. The use of these drugs in cirrhosis and ascites is limited to a small number of reports; therefore, more controlled studies are needed to evaluate their efficacy and safety in treating patients with ascites.

References

1 Murphy SL, Xu J, Kochanek KD. Deaths: final data for 2010. Centers for Disease Control and Prevention. www.cdc.gov/nchs/data/nvsr/nvsr61/nvsr61_04.pdf. Updated May 8, 2013 (accessed August 28, 2014).
2 Ginès P, Quintero E, Arroyo V, et al. Compensated cirrhosis: natural history and prognostic factors. Hepatology 1987;7: 122–8.
3 Planas R, Montoliu S, Ballesté B, et al. Natural history of patients hospitalized for management of cirrhotic ascites. Clin Gastroenterol Hepatol 2006;4:1385–94.
4 Ginès A, Escorsell A, Ginès P, et al. Incidence, predictive factors, and prognosis of hepatorenal syndrome in cirrhosis. Gastroenterology 1993;105:229–36.
5 Fernández-Esparrach G, Sánchez-Fueyo A, Ginès P, et al. A prognostic model for predicting survival in cirrhosis with ascites. J Hepatol 2001;34:46–52.
6 Nazal L, Cárdenas A. Prognostic markers in patients with ascites and hepatorenal syndrome. Dis Markers 2011;31: 139–46.
7 Schrier RW, Arroyo V, Bernardi M, Epstein M, Henriksen JH, Rodés J. Peripheral arterial vasodilation hypothesis: a proposal for the initiation of renal sodium and water retention in cirrhosis. Hepatology 1988;8:1151–7.
8 Iwakiri Y. Endothelial dysfunction in the regulation of cirrhosis and portal hypertension. Liver Int 2012;32:199–213.
9 Caraceni P, Domenicali M, Giannone F, Bernardi M. The role of the endocannabinoid system in liver diseases. Best Pract Res Clin Endocrinol Metab 2009;23:65–77.
10 Wiest R, Garcia-Tsao G. Bacterial translocation (BT) in cirrhosis. Hepatology 2005;41:422–33.
11 Riordan S, Williams R. The intestinal flora and bacterial infection in cirrhosis. J Hepatol 2006;45:744–57.
12 Ruiz-del-Arbol W, Urman J, Fernandez J, et al. Systemic, renal, and hepatic hemodynamic derangement in cirrhotic patients with spontaneous bacterial peritonitis. Hepatology 2003;38:1210–8.
13 Ruiz del Arbol L, Monescillo A, Arocena C, et al. Circulatory function and hepatorenal syndrome in cirrhosis. Hepatology 2005;42:439–47.
14 Krag A, Bendtsen F, Henriksen JH, Møller S. Low cardiac output predicts development of hepatorenal syndrome and survival in patients with cirrhosis and ascites. Gut 2010;59:105–10.
15 Ascites. In: Sherlock S, Dooley J (eds). Diseases of the Liver and Biliary System, 11th edn. Oxford, UK: Blackwell Science, 2002. pp. 127–46.

16 Williams JW Jr, Simel DL. Does this patient have ascites? How to divine fluid in the abdomen. J Am Med Assoc 1992;267:2645–48.
17 Moore KP, Wong F, Ginès P, et al. The management of ascites in cirrhosis: report on the consensus conference of the International Ascites Club. Hepatology 2003;38:258–66.
18 European Association for the Study of the Liver (EASL). EASL clinical practice guidelines on the management of ascites, spontaneous bacterial peritonitis, and hepatorenal syndrome in cirrhosis. J Hepatol 2010;53:397–417.
19 Ginès P, Cárdenas, A, Arroyo V, Rodés J. Management of cirrhosis and ascites. N Engl J Med 2004;350:1646–54.
20 Cárdenas A, Guevara M, Ginés P. Paracentesis. In: Weinstein W, Hawkey CJ, Bosch J (eds) Clinical Gastroenterology and Hepatology. Elsevier Science, 2005. pp. 1097–100.
21 Wong CL, Holroyd-Leduc J, Thorpe KE, Straus SE. Does this patient have bacterial peritonitis or portal hypertension? How do I perform a paracentesis and analyze the results? J Am Med Assoc 2008;299:1166–78.
22 Runyon BA, Montano AA, Akriviadis EA, Antillon MR, Irving MA, McHutchison JG. The serum-ascites albumin gradient is superior to the exudate-transudate concept in the differential diagnosis of ascites. Ann Intern Med 1992; 117:215–20.
23 Runyon BA, Antillon MR, Akriviadis EA, McHutchison JG. Bedside inoculation of blood culture bottles is superior to delayed inoculation in the detection of spontaneous bacterial peritonitis. J Clin Microbiol 1990;28:2811–2.
24 Henkel AS, Buchman AL. Nutritional support in patients with chronic liver disease. Nat Clin Pract Gastroenterol Hepatol 2006;3:202–9.
25 McCullough AJ. Nutrition and malnutrition in liver disease. In: Wolfe MM, Davis GL, Farraye F, Giannella RA, Malagelada JR, Steer ML (eds) Therapy of Digestive Disorders, 2nd edn. Saunders, 2006. pp. 67–83.
26 Kearns PJ, Young H, Garcia G, et al. Accelerated improvement of alcoholic liver disease with enteral nutrition. Gastroenterology 1992;102:200–5.
27 Cabrè E, Gonzalez-Hux F, Abad-Lacruz A, et al. Effect of total enteral nutrition on the short-term outcome of severely malnourished cirrhotics: a randomized controlled trial. Gastroenterology 1990;98:715–20.
28 Perez-Ayuso RM, Arroyo V, Planas R, et al. Randomized comparative study of efficacy of furosemide versus spironolactone in nonazotemic cirrhosis with ascites: relationship between the diuretic response and the activity of the renin-aldosterone system. Gastroenterology 1983;84: 961–8.
29 Santos J, Planas R, Pardo A, et al: Spironolactone alone or in combination with furosemide in the treatment of moderate ascites in nonazotemic cirrhosis: a randomized comparative study of efficacy and safety. J Hepatol 2003;39:187–92.
30 Angeli P, Fasolato S, Mazza E, et al. Combined versus sequential diuretic treatment of ascites in nonazotemic patients with cirrhosis: results of an open randomized clinical trial. Gut 2010;59:98–104.
31 Angeli P, Pria MD, De Bei E, et al. Randomized clinical study of the efficacy of amiloride and potassium canreonate in nonazotemic cirrhotic patients with ascites. Hepatology 1994;19:72–9.
32 Mimidis K, Papadopoulos V, Kartalis G. Eplerenone relieves spironolactone-induced painful gynaecomastia in patients with decompensated hepatitis B-related cirrhosis. Scand J Gastroenterol 2007;42:1516–7.
33 Li CP, Lee FY, Hwang SJ, et al. Treatment of mastalgia with tamoxifen in male patients with liver cirrhosis: a randomized crossover study. Am J Gastroenterol 2000;95:1051–5.
34 Lee FY, Lee SD, Tsai YT, et al. A randomized controlled trial of quinidine in the treatment of cirrhotic patients with muscle cramps. J Hepatol 1991;12:236–40.
35 Corbani A, Manousou P, Calvaruso V, Xirouchakis I, Burroughs AK. Muscle cramps in cirrhosis: the therapeutic value of quinine. Is it underused? Dig Liver Dis 2008;40:794–9.
36 Angeli P, Albino G, Carraro P, et al. Cirrhosis and muscle cramps: evidence of a causal relationship. Hepatology 1996;23:264–73.
37 Ginès P, Arroyo V, Quintero E, et al. Comparison of paracentesis and diuretics in the treatment of cirrhotics with tense ascites: results of a randomized study. Gastroenterology 1987;93:234–41.
38 Salerno F, Badalamenti S, Incerti P, et al. Repeated paracentesis and i.v. albumin infusion to treat 'tense' ascites in cirrhotic patients: a safe alternative therapy. J Hepatol 1987; 5:102–8.
39 Ginès P, Tito L, Arroyo V, et al. Randomized comparative study of therapeutic paracentesis with and without intravenous albumin in cirrhosis. Gastroenterology 1988;94: 1493–502.
40 Ruiz-del-Arbol L, Monescillo A, Jiménez W, et al. Paracentesis-induced circulatory dysfunction: mechanism and effect on hepatic hemodynamics in cirrhosis. Gastroenterology 1997;113:579–86.
41 Ginès A, Fernández-Esparrach G, Monescillo A, et al. Randomized trial comparing albumin, dextran 70, and polygeline in cirrhotic patients with ascites treated by paracentesis. Gastroenterology 1996;111:1002–110.
42 Moreau R, Valla DC, Durand-Zaleski I, et al. Comparison of outcome in patients with cirrhosis and ascites following treatment with albumin or a synthetic colloid: a randomised controlled pilot trail. Liver Int 2006;26:46–54.
43 Sola-Vera J, Minana J, Ricart E, et al. Randomized trial comparing albumin and saline in the prevention of paracentesis-induced circulatory dysfunction in cirrhotic patients with ascites. Hepatology 2003;37:1147–53.
44 Bernardi M, Caraceni P, Navickis RJ, Wilkes MM. Albumin infusion in patients undergoing large-volume paracentesis: a meta-analysis of randomized trials. Hepatology 2012;55: 1172–81.

45 Fernández-Esparrach G, Guevara M, Sort P, et al. Diuretic requirements after therapeutic paracentesis in non-azotemic patients with cirrhosis: a randomized double-blind trial of spironolactone versus placebo. J Hepatol 1997;26: 614–20.
46 Thomsen TW, Shaffer RW, White B, Setnik GS. Videos in clinical medicine. Paracentesis. N Engl J Med 2006;355: e21.
47 Pache I, Bilodeau M. Severe haemorrhage following abdominal paracentesis for ascites in patients with liver disease. Aliment Pharmacol Ther 2005;21:525–9.
48 Caldwell S, Hoffmann M, Lisman B, et al. Coagulation disorders and hemostasis in liver disease: pathophysiology and critical assessment of current management. Hepatology 2006;44:1039–46.
49 Arroyo V, Ginès P, Gerbes A, et al. Definition and diagnostic criteria of refractory ascites and hepatorenal syndrome in cirrhosis. Hepatology 1996;23:164–76.
50 Salerno F, Guevara M, Bernardi M, et al. Refractory ascites: pathogenesis, definition and therapy of a severe complication in patients with cirrhosis. Liver Int 2010;30:937–47.
51 Lebrec D, Giuily N, Hadengue A, et al. Transjugular intrahepatic portosystemic shunts: comparison with paracentesis in patients with cirrhosis and refractory ascites – a randomized trial. J Hepatol 1996;25:135–44.
52 Rossle M, Ochs A, Gulberg V, et al. A comparison of paracentesis and transjugular intrahepatic portosystemic shunting in patients with ascites. N Engl J Med 2000;342:1701–7.
53 Ginès P, Uriz J, Calahorra B, et al. Transjugular intrahepatic portosystemic shunting versus paracentesis plus albumin for refractory ascites in cirrhosis. Gastroenterology 2002;123: 1839–47.
54 Sanyal A, Genning C, Reddy RK, et al. The North American Study for Treatment of Refractory Ascites. Gastroenterology 2003;124:634–41.
55 Salerno F, Merli M, Riggio O, et al. Randomized controlled study of TIPS versus paracentesis plus albumin in cirrhosis with severe ascites. Hepatology 2004;40:629–35.
56 Boyer TD, Haskal ZJ. American Association for the Study of Liver Diseases. The role of transjugular intrahepatic portosystemic shunt (TIPS) in the management of portal hypertension: update 2009. Hepatology 2010;51: 306.
57 Bureau C, García-Pagan JC, Otal P, et al. Improved clinical outcome using polytetrafluoroethylene-coated stents for TIPS: results of a randomized study. Gastroenterology 2004;126:469–75.
58 Bureau C, Pagan JC, Layrargues GP, et al. Patency of stents covered with polytetrafluoroethylene in patients treated by transjugular intrahepatic portosystemic shunts: long-term results of a randomized multicentre study. Liver Int 2007;27:742–7.
59 Delterne P, Mathurin P, Dharancy S, et al. Transjugular intrahepatic portosystemic shunt in refractory ascites: a meta-analysis. Liver Int 2005;25:349–56.
60 Albillos A, Banares R, Gonzales M, et al. A meta-analysis of transjugular intrahepatic portosystemic shunt versus paracentesis for refractory ascites. J Hepatol 2005;43: 990–6.
61 Dámico G, Luca A, Morabito A, et al. Uncovered transjugular intrahepatic portosystemic shunt for refractory ascites: a meta-analysis. Gastroenterology 2005;129:1282–93.
62 Salerno F, Camma C, Enea M, et al. Transjugular intrahepatic portosystemic shunt for refractory ascites: a meta-analysis of individual patient data. Gastroenterology 2007; 133:825–34.
63 Cárdenas A, Ginès P. Management of refractory ascites. Clin Gastroenterol Hepatol 2005;3:1187–91.
64 Bureau C, Métivier S, D'Amico M, et al. Serum bilirubin and platelet count: a simple predictive model for survival in patients with refractory ascites treated by TIPS. J Hepatol 2011;54:901–7.
65 Llach J, Ginès P, Arroyo V, et al. Prognostic value of arterial pressure, endogenous vasoactive systems, and renal function in cirrhotic patients admitted to the hospital for the treatment of ascites. Gastroenterology 1988;94:482–7.
66 Guevara M, Cárdenas A, Uriz J, Ginés P. Prognosis of patients with ascites and cirrhosis. In: Ginès P, Arroyo V, Rodes J, Schrier R (eds) Ascites and Renal Dysfunction in Liver Disease, 2nd edn. Blackwell Publishing, Oxford: 2005. pp. 260–70.
67 Kamath P, Wiesner R, Malinchoc M, et al. A model to predict survival in patients with end-satge liver disease. Hepatology 2001;33:464–70.
68 Fernandez-Varo G, Ros J, Cejudo-Martin P, et al. Effect of the V1a/V2-AVP receptor antagonist, Conivaptan, on renal water metabolism and systemic hemodynamics in rats with cirrhosis and ascites. J Hepatol 2003;38:755–61.
69 Decaux G. Difference in solute excretion during correction of hyponatremic patients with cirrhosis or syndrome of inappropriate secretion of antidiuretic hormone by oral vasopressin V2 receptor antagonist VPA-985. J Lab Clin Med 2001;138:18–21.
70 Wong F, Ginès P, Watson H, et al. Effects of a selective vasopressin V2 receptor antagonist, satavaptan, on ascites recurrence after paracentesis in patients with cirrhosis. J Hepatol 2010;53:283–90.
71 Wong F, Watson H, Gerbes A, et al. Satavaptan Investigators Group. Satavaptan for the management of ascites in cirrhosis: efficacy and safety across the spectrum of ascites severity. Gut 2012;61:108–16.
72 Okita K, Sakaida I, Okada M, et al. A multicenter, open-label, dose-ranging study to exploratively evaluate the efficacy, safety, and dose–response of tolvaptan in patients with decompensated liver cirrhosis. J Gastroenterol 2010;45: 979–87.
73 Kalambokis G, Fotopoulos A, Economou M, et al. Effects of a 7-day treatment with midodrine in non-azotemic cirrhotic patients with and without ascites. J Hepatol 2007;46: 213–21.

74 Singh V, Dhungana SP, Singh B, et al. Midodrine in patients with cirrhosis and refractory or recurrent ascites: a randomized pilot study. J Hepatol 2012;56:348–54.
75 Lenaerts A, Codden T, Meunier JC, et al. Effects of clonidine on diuretic response in ascitic patients with cirrhosis and activation of sympathetic nervous system. Hepatology 2006;44:844–9.
76 Yang YY, Lin HC, Lee WP, et al. Association of the G-protein and α2-adrenergic receptor gene and plasma norepinephrine level with clonidine improvement of the effects of diuretics in patients with cirrhosis with refractory ascites: a randomised clinical trial. Gut 2010;59:1545–53.
77 Krag A, Møller S, Henriksen JH, Holstein-Rathlou NH, Larsen FS, Bendtsen F. Terlipressin improves renal function in patients with cirrhosis and ascites without hepatorenal syndrome. Hepatology 2007;46:1863–71.

CHAPTER 15

Spontaneous bacterial peritonitis and other infections

Thierry Gustot[1,2,3] and Richard Moreau[4,5,6]
[1]*Department of Gastroenterology and Hepato-Pancreatology, Erasme Hospital, Brussels, Belgium*
[2]*Laboratory of Experimental Gastroenterology, Université Libre de Bruxelles, Brussels, Belgium*
[3]*INSERM, U773, Centre de Recherche Biomédicale Bichat-Beaujon CRB3, Paris, France*
[4]*INSERM, U1149, Centre de Recherche sur l'Inflammation (CRI), Paris, France*
[5]*UMR S 1149, Université Paris Diderot-Paris 7, Faculté de Médecine Bichat, Paris, France*
[6]*Département Hospitalo-Universitaire (DHU) UNITY, Service d'Hépatologie, Hôpital Beaujon, Assistance Publique-Hôpitaux de Paris, Clichy, France*

General considerations

In cirrhosis, bacterial infection is defined as a pathologic process caused by invasion of normally sterile tissue, fluid, or cavity by pathogenic or potentially pathogenic bacteria. Bacterial infection is present at admission or develops during hospitalization in about 30% of patients with cirrhosis [1].

Infections may be classified as follow:

1 Community-acquired if the diagnosis is made at the admission or during the first 48 hours after hospitalization;
2 Healthcare-associated in the same conditions but with a history of previous contact with a healthcare environment (hospitalization or short-term admission for at least 2 days in the previous 90–180 days, residence in a nursing home or a long-term care facility, or chronic hemodialysis); and
3 Nosocomial infection if the diagnosis is made after 48 hours of hospitalization (Table 15.1) [2].

Approximatively one-third of bacterial infections are community-acquired, one-third healthcare-associated, and one-third nosocomial. Spontaneous bacterial peritonitis (SPB) and urinary tract infections (UTI) are the most frequent infections observed, followed by pneumonia, skin and soft tissue infections (SSTI), spontaneous bacteremia and catheter-related infections [3]. Clinical risk factors associated with occurrence of bacterial infections in cirrhosis are high Child–Pugh score, variceal bleeding, low ascitic protein levels, and prior episode of SBP [4–7].

Infection induces a systemic inflammatory host response with three stages of severity: sepsis, severe sepsis (when an acute organ failure occurs), and septic shock (when hypotension does not respond to adequate fluid resuscitation). Patients with cirrhosis have increased risk to develop bacterial infection, sepsis, sepsis-induced organ failure, and death [8]. A recent prospective European study defined the acute-on-chronic liver failure syndrome characterized by organ failures (defined by an adapted Sequential Organ Failure Assessment (SOFA) score, the Chronic Liver Failure (CLIF)-SOFA score; Table 15.2), requirement of intensive care management and high 28-day mortality (between 23% and 74%) [9]. The mortality of infected patients with cirrhosis reaches 38% [10]. Cirrhotic patients are two times more likely to die from sepsis than individuals without cirrhosis [11]. In-hospital mortality of cirrhotic patients with severe sepsis without shock or with septic shock is 41% and 71%, respectively [12].

The diagnostic approach

The early diagnosis of bacterial infections and the prompt initiation of adequate antibiotherapy are critical in the management of cirrhotic patients. The diagnosis of bacterial infection in cirrhosis is very difficult for several reasons.

Cirrhosis: A practical guide to management, First Edition. Edited by Samuel S. Lee and Richard Moreau.

Table 15.1 Types of bacterial infection.

Type	Definition
Community-acquired infection	Diagnosis at the admission or during the first 48 hours after hospitalization
Nosocomial infection	Diagnosis after 48 hours of hospitalization
Healthcare associated infection	Diagnosis at the admission or during the first 48 hours after hospitalization with an history of previous contact with a healthcare environment (hospitalization or short-term admission for at least 2 days in the previous 90 (−180) days, residence in a nursing home or a long-term care facility, or chronic hemodialysis)

First, in the early phase of infection, cirrhotic patients may be totally asymptomatic. Second, the classic parameters assessing the inflammatory host response to infection (systemic inflammatory response syndrome (SIRS)) are not specific for the diagnosis of infection in cirrhosis. SIRS is defined as the presence of at least two of four clinical criteria: body temperature ≥38 °C or ≤36 °C, heart rate ≥90 beats/min, respiratory rate ≥20 breaths/min or hyperventilation with a PaCO2 ≤32 mmHg, white blood cell count ≥12 000/mm^3, ≤4000/mm^3, or with >10% immature neutrophils [13]. Decompensated cirrhosis may be associated with some degree of encephalopathy-related tachypnea, tachycardia, or hypersplenism-related leukopenia. SIRS has a low sensitivity for the diagnosis of infection (57–70% of infected patients with decompensated cirrhosis) and is not specific (10–30% of patients without infection) [14,15]. On the other hand, the presence of SIRS in decompensated cirrhotic patients is a marker of poor prognosis. Thus, SIRS is associated with higher in-hospital mortality (31% vs. 4%). Moreover, common early markers of infection used in the general population, such as C-reactive protein (CRP) and procalcitonin, are not sufficient to distinguish infected cirrhotic patients. Indeed, CRP >2 mg/dL has only a sensitivity of 78% and specificity of 68% and procalcitonin >3 ng/mL has a sensitivity and specificity of 73%. This poor diagnostic accuracy could be explained by the decreased production of acute-phase proteins by the liver, especially CRP. Particularly, low CRP values should be interpreted with caution in patients with severe liver insufficiency.Infection should be suspected in any decompensated cirrhotic patient, when a hospitalized patient deteriorates (worsening of liver function, hepatic encephalopathy, shock, renal failure, or gastrointestinal bleeding), or when there are

Table 15.2 Definition of organ failures in patients with cirrhosis (in gray). Organ/systems whose functions are assessed by the Chronic Liver Failure (CLIF) Sequential Assessment of Organ Failure (SOFA) score.

Organ/system	0	1	2	3	4
Lungs					
(PaO_2/FiO_2)	>400	≤400	≤300	≤200	≤100
or SpO_2/FiO_2	>512	>357–≤512	>214–≤357	>89–≤214	≤89
Coagulation					
INR	<1.1	1.1–1.25	1.26–1.5	1.51–2.5	>2.5 or platelets ≤20 × 10^3/μL
Liver					
Bilirubin, mg/dL	<1.2	1.2–1.9	2–5.9	6–11.9	>12
Circulation					
MAP (mmHg)	≥70	<70	Dopamine ≤5 or dobutamine or terlipressin	Dopamine >5, epinephrine ≤0.1, or norepinephrine ≤0.1	Dopamine >15, epinephrine >0.1, or norepinephrine >0.1
Cerebral					
HE grade	No HE	1	2	3	4
Kidney					
Creatinine (mg/dL)	<1.2	1.2–1.9	2–3.4	3.5–4.9	≥5

Adrenergic agents were administred for at least 1 hour (doses are expressed as μg/kg per minute).

FiO_2 denotes fraction of inspired oxygen.

HE, hepatic encephalopathy; MAP, mean arterial pressure.

signs of systemic inflammation (hyper- or hypothermia, chills, altered blood cell count, tachycardia, and/or tachypnea). Therefore, a complete check-up, including urinary sediment and culture, diagnostic paracentesis and ascitic fluid culture, blood culture, and chest X-ray, must be made in order not to delay diagnosis and the administration of empiric antibiotics (for the therapeutic strategy see Figure 15.1). The choice of empiric antibiotics based on the site is proposed in Table 15.3. When the bacteria has been identified, we must potentially shift to a more specific antibiotic to avoid the occurrence of antibiotic resistance.

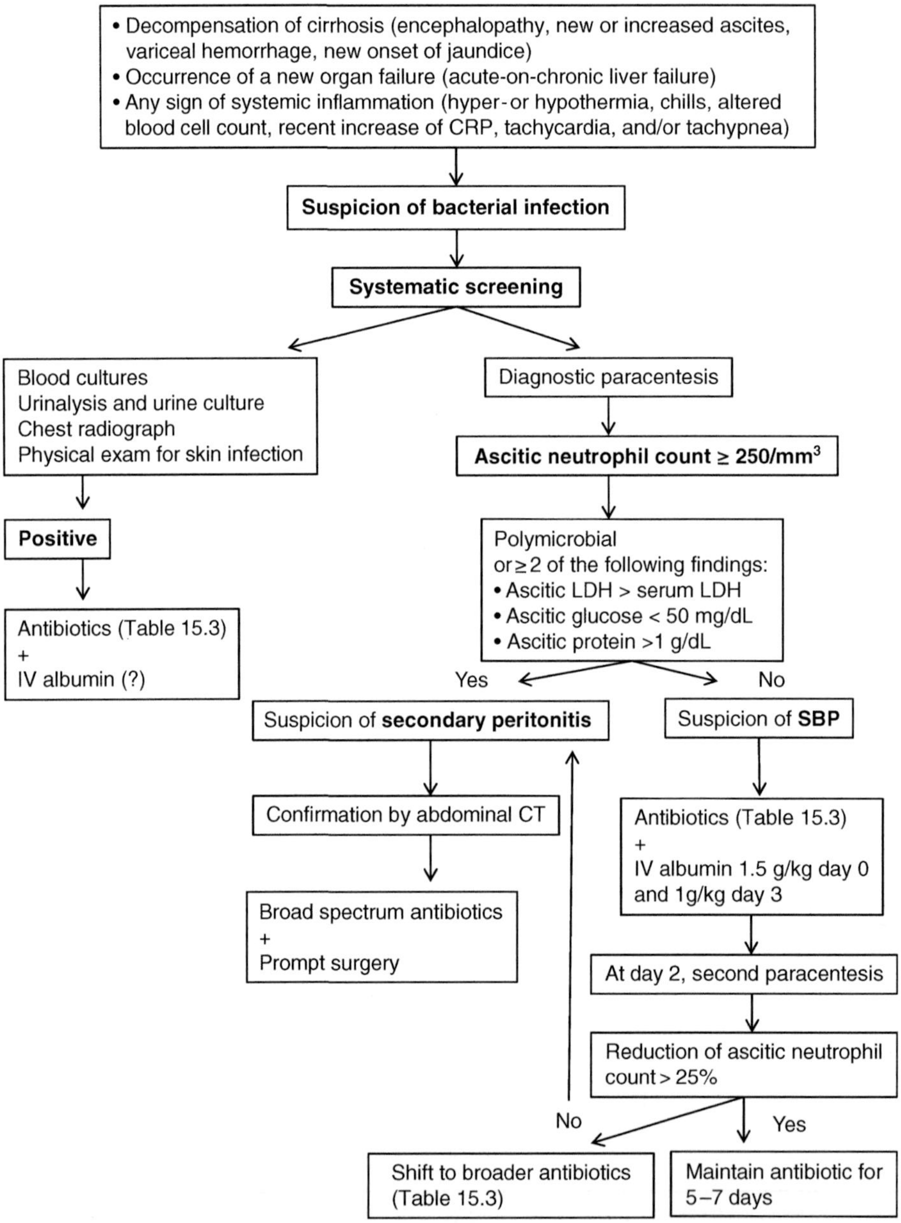

Figure 15.1 Therapeutic strategy for suspected bacterial infection. CRP, C-reactive protein; CT, computed tomography; LDH, lactic dehydrogenase; SBP, spontaneous bacterial peritonitis.

Table 15.3 Empiric antibiotic therapy for common bacterial infections in cirrhosis.

Sites	Types	Antibiotics
SBP, SBE, and spontaneous bacteremia	Community-acquired	Cefotaxime (2 g/6 h or 2 g/12 h IV) Ceftriaxone (1 g/24 h IV) Amoxicillin/clavulanic acid (1–0.2 g/8 h then 0.5–0.125 g/8 h PO)
	Nosocomial	Piperacillin/tazobactam (4 g/6 h IV) Meropenem (1 g/8 h IV)[a]
UTI	Community-acquired	Ciprofloxacin (500 mg/12 h PO) or cotrimoxazole (160–800 mg/12 h PO) if uncomplicated UTI Cefotaxime (2 g/6 h or 2 g/12 h IV) or Amoxicillin/clavulanic acid (1–0.2 g/8 h IV) if sepsis
	Nosocomial	Nitrofurantoin (50 mg/6 h PO) if uncomplicated UTI Piperacillin/tazobactam (4 g/6 h IV) or Meropenem (1 g/8 h IV)[a] if sepsis
Pneumonia[b]	Community-acquired	Amoxicillin/clavulanic acid (1–0.2 g/8 h IV) or ceftriaxone (1 g/24 h IV) and macrolide or levofloxacin (500 mg/24 h PO) Or moxifloxacin (400 mg/24 h PO)
	Nosocomial	Piperacillin/tazobactam (4 g/6 h IV) or Meropenem (1 g/8 h IV)[a] + vancomycine (15 mg/kg/12 h IV) or teicoplanin (first dose 18 mg/kg followed by 6 mg/kg/24 h IV) in patients with risk factors for MRSA
SSTI	Community-acquired/ nosocomial	Amoxicillin/clavulanic acid (1–0.2 g/8 h IV) or Ceftazidim (2 g/8 h IV) in patients with risk factors of *Pseudomonas spp.* or meropenem (1 g/8 h IV)[a] + Oxacillin (2 g/6 h IV); or vancomycine (15 mg/kg/12 h IV) or teicoplanin (first dose 18 mg/kg followed by 6 mg/kg/24 h IV) in patients with risk factors for MRSA

[a] In nosocomial infections in geographic areas with high prevalence of ESBL-producing bacteria.
[b] Liver disease is considered as severe comorbidity for community-acquired pneumonia in guidelines.
ESBL, extended-spectrum β-lactamase; MRSA, methycillin-resistant *Staphylococcus aureus*; SBE, spontaneous bacterial empyema; SBP, spontaneous bacterial peritonitis; SSTI, skin and soft tissue infections; UTI, urinary tract infection.

Spontaneous bacterial peritonitis

SBP is defined as an ascitic fluid infection without an evident abdominal source. It is the most frequent infection in cirrhotic patients (20–25% of all infections) [3]. In outpatients without symptoms the prevalence is low (<3%) [16,17] but it increases to 8–36% in hospitalized patients. The mortality for the first episode ranges from 10% to 25% [18]. Importantly, the 1-year mortality rate after the first SBP episode is reported to be at least 30%, suggesting that the deterioration of liver function accelerates [19].

Diagnosis

Patients with SBP may have one of the following: local symptoms and/or signs of peritonitis (abdominal pain, abdominal tenderness, Blumberg sign, vomiting, diarrhea, ileus). SBP may be asymptomatic, particularly in outpatients. The diagnosis of SBP is based on ascitic neutrophil count $\geq 250/mm^3$ [20]. Ascitic fluid neutrophil count is obtained by centrifugation of the ascitic fluid and then stained with Giemsa and differential cell counts are made with an optical microscope. For faster and cheaper results, reagent strips have been assessed, but a high rate of false negative results (around 50%) prevents their use [21]. Ascitic fluid lactoferrin measurement seems to be an alternative to ascitic fluid neutrophil count in the diagnosis of SBP. Indeed, a cutoff value of 242 ng/mL had a sensitivity and specificity in the diagnosis of SBP of 95% and 97%, respectively, in one study [22]. These results must be replicated before the method can be recommended for use in clinical practice. Pleural ascites could be also a site of infection. This infection is then called spontaneous bacterial empyema (SBE) and the diagnostic criteria are the same as in SBP.

Microbiology

Ascitic fluid cultures (10 mL into aerobic and anaerobic blood cultures), direct ascitic microscopic examination (rapid assessment for polymicrobial infection in the case of secondary peritonitis), and blood cultures (50% of SBP are associated with bacteremia) should also be obtained when SBP is suspected. The ascitic fluid culture is positive in 40% of cases. The most common pathogens are Gram-negative bacteria (GNB) (mainly *Escherichia coli, Klebsiella pneumoniae, Enterobacter* spp.) and Gram-positive cocci (GPC) (mainly *Streptococcus* spp. and *Enterococci*). In Spain, 20% of GNB are resistant to quinolones and 70% of these are also resistant to trimethoprim-sulfamethoxazole [1]. Long-term norfloxacin administration (see prevention section) increases the rate of quinolone resistance to 60% and the proportion of GPC. The rate of cephalosporin-resistant GNB is low in community-acquired SBP regardless of long-term norfloxacin prophylaxis. On the other hand, in Spain, extended-spectrum β-lactamase (ESBL)-producing *Enterobacteriacae* are isolated in 30% of nosocomial SBP and methicillin-resistant *Staphylococcus aureus* in 10% of healthcare-associated SBP [3].

Some patients have bacterascites in which cultures are positive but there is an ascitic neutrophil count of <250/mm^3. When this bacterascites is monomicrobial, it usually represents the colonization phase of ascitic fluid infection. It may progress to SBP or, in the majority of cases (62–86%), resolve spontaneously [23,24]. Bacterascites with microorganisms similar to those of the skin flora are probably due to contaminants. If symptoms are present, a second paracentesis is recommended.

Antibiotics

For community-acquired SBP, third-generation cephalosporins (cefotaxime, ceftriaxone) are the gold standard for empirical antibiotic treatment (Table 15.2) [25]. Amoxicillin-clavulanic acid and ciprofloxacin show similar results [26,27]. However, quinolones are not yet recommended in patients receiving long-term norfloxacin prophylaxis and in geographic areas with a high prevalence of quinolone-resistant bacteria. For nosocomial and healthcare-associated SBP, there are no clear recommendations at this time and the choice of empirical antibiotics depends on the local epidemiologic patterns of resistance. Where ESBL-producing *Enterobacteriaceae* are frequent, carbapenems or tigecycline could be good choice for the treatment of nosocomial SBP. Another strategy is a step-by-step protocol consisting of a first line antibiotic (e.g., piperacillin-tazobactam) followed by an assessment of response (defined by a reduction in the ascitic neutrophil count of >25% at day 2 of antibiotic therapy) and, in the case of nonresponders, to a shift to a broader antibiotic (e.g., carbapenems).

Special case: secondary peritonitis

Secondary peritonitis is infrequent (5–10% of all peritonitis) but is associated with a higher mortality rate (66%) [28]. Secondary peritonitis is suggested when at least two of the following parameters are present in ascites: glucose levels <50 mg/dL, protein concentration >10 g/dL, lactic dehydrogenase (LDH) concentration > normal serum levels, but these criteria only have a sensitivity of 67%. In the case of gut perforation, ascitic amylase or bilirubin levels could be high. In the case of secondary peritonitis, the ascitic culture is frequently positive and polymicrobial. Abdominal computed tomography (CT) imaging without contrast is diagnostic in 90%. Prompt treatment with broad-spectrum antibiotics with anti-anaerobic activity (amoxicillin/clavulanic acid, piperacillin/tazobactam or ceftazidime/metronidazole) and an early decision for surgery are key in the management of secondary peritonitis.

Other infections

Pneumonia

Deterioration of consciousness secondary to hepatic encephalopathy and basal atelectasia due to tense ascites contributes to the high frequency of lung infections in cirrhotic patients. When we consider cirrhotic patients with severe sepsis, lung infections are the most frequent infectious foci, suggesting that pneumonia is a severe infection in cirrhosis [29]. Indeed, community-acquired pneumonia (CAP) in cirrhotic patients is more frequently associated with septic shock and higher 1-month mortality rates than those in the noncirrhotic population (14% vs. 7%) [30]. The mortality of cirrhotic patients with community-acquired pneumococcal pneumonia requiring hospitalization increases to 34% (sixfold higher than in the general population) despite adequate antibiotic therapy [31]. Acute respiratory distress syndrome (ARDS) is a more severe form of lung infection defined by the association of severe hypoxemia, bilateral lung infiltration, and the absence of signs of left heart failure. The mortality of ARDS in the general population is 65% and in cirrhosis is independently associated with mortality, with a very high odds ratio of 27 [32].

Diagnosis

In the case of pneumonia, patients may have cough, pleuritic chest pain, dyspnea, sputum production but may be asymptomatic. Pulmonary auscultation may show audible rales or consolidation. A chest radiograph may show lobar consolidation, interstitial infiltrates, and/or cavitation. If there is high clinical suspicion of pneumonia with a negative chest radiograph, CT scan should be performed. Pneumococcal and legionella urinary antigen tests should be performed.

Microbiology

Only 28% of CAP are culture positive, with 75% GPC and 25% GNB [1]. The proportion of GNB and polymicrobial cultures (GNB + GPC) increases in nosocomial infections. Isolated microorganisms, in order of frequency, are *Streptococcus pneumonia, Staphylococcus aureus, Pseudomonas aeruginosa,* and *Escherichia coli. P. aeruginosa* and ESBL producing *Enterobacteriacae* are isolated in nosocomial and healthcare-associated pneumonia [3]. Cirrhosis seems also to be a predisposing condition of atypical infections such as *Legionella* spp [33].

Antibiotics

The recommendations for the empiric treatment for CAP do not differ from those of the general population. As detailed previously, cirrhosis is considered as a major comorbidity in the case of CAP. Some experts suggest the combination of antibiotics against typical and atypical bacteria [34]. The possibilities are a respiratory quinolone (moxifloxacin, levofloxacin) or the combination of a β-lactam (amoxicillin-clavulanate or a third generation cephalosporin) plus a macrolide. For nosocomial and healthcare-associated pneumonia, the use of empiric antibiotics should follow local guidelines.

Urinary tract infection

UTIs are frequent in cirrhotic patients and, as in the general population, more frequent in women and in those with a urinary catheter. UTIs are frequently asymptomatic in cirrhotic patients. The in-hospital mortality rate of UTIs is around 10% which increases to 18% in those with multiresistant bacteria [3].

Diagnosis

UTI may be asymptomatic in cirrhotic patients or associated with dysuria, frequency, urgency, or suprapubic pain. Patients with pyelonephritis frequently describe flank pain. If UTI is suspected, urinalysis and urine culture must be performed. The diagnosis is based on ≥10 urinary leukocytes/mm^3 or positive urinary leukocyte esterase. If cirrhotic patients have persistent symptoms of uncomplicated UTI after 48 hours of appropriate antibiotic therapy or symptoms of pyelonephritis, renal ultrasound or abdominal CT should be performed to detect stones, papillary necrosis, obstruction, and/or abscess.

Microbiology

In cirrhotic patients, 80% of UTIs are culture-positive with the large majority being GNB (76%) in community-acquired UTIs. The proportion of GPC increases in nosocomial infections. *Escherichia coli* is the most frequently isolated microorganism followed by *Enterococcus faecalis, Klebsiella pneumonia,* and *Enterococcus faecium.*

Antibiotics

Third-generation cephalosporins, amoxicillin-clavulanic acid, quinolones, or trimethoprim-sulfamethoxazole are the first choice for community-acquired UTIs. For uncomplicated UTIs, an oral antibiotic may be used. Quinolones and trimethoprim-sulfamethoxazole are not recommended in patients receiving long-term norfloxacin prophylaxis and in geographic areas with a high prevalence of quinolone-resistant bacteria. In nosocomial infections, nitrofurantoin could be a good option in uncomplicated UTI. In some regions, because of the high prevalence of ESBL-producing bacteria, carbapenems should be used. In the case of severe sepsis or septic shock secondary to UTI, a glycopeptide must be added to anti-GNB antibiotic to cover *Enterococcus faecium.*

Skin and soft tissue infection

SSTIs, in particular those of the lower limb or abdominal wall, are observed in 2–11% of cirrhotic patients with peripheral edema and/or ascites [35,36]. In a Spanish cohort, the mortality rate from SSTIs is 4% [37]. This rate could increase to 56% with GNB-related SSTIs [38].

Diagnosis

The most common symptoms of cellulitis are pain, tenderness, swelling, warmth, and redness in a distinct area of the skin. For SSTI, ultrasound of the region is an useful tool for excluding occult abscesses, to guide microbiologic sampling and/or surgical drainage, and for making the differential diagnosis from deep venous thrombosis. CT scan should be performed if necrotizing fascitis is suspected.

Microbiology

Skin cultures are positive in 50% of cases. GPC are isolated more frequently than GNB, but up to one-third of cultures yield GNB. Classically, the most isolated GPC are *Staphylococcus aureus, Streptococcus pyogenes,* and *Enterococcus faecalis*. GNB are represented by *E. coli, Pseudomonas aeruginosa,* and *Enterobacter cloacae*.

Antibiotics

Amoxicillin-clavulanic acid or ceftriaxone and oxacillin, which covers *Staphylococcus*, are the first choice for community-acquired cellulitis. These antibiotics are ineffective for *Pseudomonas* spp. Ceftazidime and oxacillin or piperacillin-tazobactam could be a better choice for those with a high risk of *Pseudomonas* spp.

Prevention of organ failure

Use of albumin

Spontaneous bacterial peritonitis

In patients with cirrhosis, an open-label unblinded randomized clinical trial (RCT) in patients with SBP (without shock) treated with cefotaxime showed that the intravenous administration of a 20% albumin solution reduced the incidence of renal failure and decreased mortality rates from 29% to 10% [39]. In this trial, albumin was given at an arbitrary dose of 1.5 g/kg body weight at the time of diagnosis, followed by 1 g/kg body weight on day 3. This effect was not observed in patients with low risk of mortality (total bilirubin <4 mg/dL and creatinine <1 mg/dL) [40]. A recent small unblinded RCT suggested that a 20% albumin solution improved systemic hemodynamics better than a 6% hydroxyethylstarch solution in SBP [41].

Infections other than SBP

The data are less clear. Only a small RCT showed no survival difference between patients treated with IV albumin at the classic dose but suggested a survival benefit in the multivariate per protocol analysis [42]. Albumin seemed to improve renal function but larger studies are needed before recommending the use of albumin in non-SBP infections in cirrhotic patients.

Use of nonselective beta-blockers

Based on a case–control study, nonselective beta-blockers (NSSBs) increased the risk of renal dysfunction and death in cirrhotic patients with SBP, suggesting that these patients should not receive NSBBs [43]. At this time, because of the lack of prospective data, we cannot recommend stopping NSSBs systematically in the case of SBP.

Management of organ failure, severe sepsis, and septic shock

In the general population with septic shock, each hour of delay before administration of antibiotics decreases the survival rate by 7.6% [44]. The choice of an adequate empiric antimicrobial treatment improves the outcome of patients and misuse doubles the mortality rate [45]. The same results are observed in cirrhotic patients with septic shock [46].

Hemodynamic therapy

Early hemodynamic therapy

In the general population, during the first 6 hours of severe sepsis and septic shock it may be beneficial to maintain mean arterial pressure ≥65 mmHg, central venous pressure at 8–12 mmHg, central venous oxygen saturation ≥70%, and urinary output ≥5 mL/kg/h [47]. These goals are achieved using fluids, vasopressors, inotropes, and blood transfusion. Patients with cirrhosis and septic shock have a lower baseline arterial pressure, are more hyperdynamic, have higher central venous oxygen saturation [48], and lower hematocrit than noncirrhotic patients with severe sepsis. Therefore, specific goals for early hemodynamic therapy should be established in cirrhotic patients with severe sepsis and septic shock.

Fluid therapy and vasopressors

At this time, we have no evidence-based data to aid in the choice of optimal fluid resuscitation and type of vasopressor in the management of severe sepsis and septic shock in the specific population of cirrhotic patients. Norepinephrine and dopamine remain first line vasopressors to correct hypotension in septic shock [49]. Dopamine seems to induce more cardiac arrhythmias than norepinephrine in the general population [50].

Stress dose steroids

Current guidelines only recommend stress dose steroids in patients with vasopressor-unresponsive septic shock in the general population [51]. Patients with cirrhosis and septic shock may have a high incidence of adrenal insufficiency (51–68%) which may be related to a reduction in adrenal blood flow and high cytokine expression [52]. A small uncontrolled study assessing severely cirrhotic patients (mean Child–Pugh scores of 11) with septic shock who were nonresponders to corticotropin suggested that hydrocortisone could shorten the duration of shock resolution and improve survival compared with a retrospective matched cirrhotic cohort [53]. A large double-blind RCT is needed to evaluate hydrocortisone therapy in cirrhotic patients with septic shock.

Other therapeutic modalities

Data about the type of renal replacement therapy, glucose control, protective ventilation strategy, selective digestive tract decontamination in cirrhotic patients with severe sepsis and septic shock are lacking. Further studies are needed in this specific population of patients to make clear recommendations.

Prevention of bacterial infection in cirrhosis

Bacterial infections are common and severe in patients with cirrhosis. Thus, it is important to try to prevent infections in patients who are at risk. Because infection is frequently caused by translocation of GNB of intestinal origin, prevention is based on selective intestinal decontamination with a fluoroquinolone (e.g., norfloxacin). The restriction of antibiotic prophylaxis to high-risk patients is essential to prevent the development of antibiotic resistance.

Patients with acute gastrointestinal hemorrhage

In this context, bacterial infections are frequent. A meta-analysis of trials in patients with variceal hemorrhage has shown that antibiotic prophylaxis reduced the incidence of severe infection (SBP and/or septicemia) and decreased mortality [4]. There is a decrease in mortality from variceal hemorrhage from 43% to 15% over a 20-year period and antibiotic prophylaxis is independently associated with improved survival. A beneficial effect of antibiotic prophylaxis on control of bleeding and prevention of rebleeding has also been observed [55]. Oral norfloxacin (800 mg/day for 7 days) is commonly used [56]. However, an RCT has shown that intravenous ceftriaxone (1 g/day for 7 days) was more effective than oral norfloxacin in preventing severe infections in patients with advanced cirrhosis (at least two of the following: ascites, severe malnutrition, encephalopathy, or bilirubin >3 mg/dL) and varieal bleeding [57]. Baveno V consensus guidelines recommend starting antibiotics at admission, ideally before or immediately after endoscopy, and to continue this treatment for 7 days [58].

Patients with low protein ascitic levels and no prior SBP: primary prophylaxis

Oral norfloxacin administration (400 mg/day) in patients with low protein ascitic levels (<1.5 g/dL) and advanced cirrhosis (Child–Pugh score ≥9 points with serum bilirubin level ≥3 mg/dL or impaired renal function (serum creatinine level ≥1.2 mg/dL, blood urea nitrogen level ≥25 mg/dL, or serum sodium level ≤130 mEq/L)) without prior SBP episode reduces the probability of SBP and HRS and improved the 3-month survival rate [59]. Similarly, oral ciprofloxacin (500 mg/day) reduces the 1-year mortality rate in patients with ascitic protein levels <1.5 g/dL and without prior SBP episode [60]. This primary prophylaxis is indicated until liver transplantation or until improvement of liver function.

Patients with prior SBP: secondary prophylaxis

After an episode of SBP, the cumulative recurrence rate at 1 year is 70% [61]. Oral norfloxacin decreases the recurrence of SBP from ~70% to 20% [62].

Issues with long-term antibiotic therapy

There is no consensus on the duration of long-term use of oral antibiotic therapy to prevent first SBP or its recurrence. However, antibiotic therapy is associated with the emergence of drug-resistant organisms.

Nonantibiotic strategy to prevent bacterial infections in cirrhotic patients

Restriction of the use of proton pump inhibitors

Several studies suggest an association between proton pump inhibitor (PPI) use and the occurrence of SBP [63,64]. Thus, we suggest stopping the PPI if there is no clear indication, especially in patients with ascites.

Pentoxifylline

A large double-blind RCT showed that oral pentoxifylline administration (1200 mg/day) decreased modestly but significantly the risk of bacterial infection in patients with advanced cirrhosis (Child–Pugh C) [65].

Prophylactic use of enoxaparin

A nonblinded RCT designed to evaluate the efficacy of enoxaparin (4000 IU/day subcutaneously) in preventing portal vein thrombosis in cirrhotic outpatients (Child–Pugh classes B7–C10) shows that this prophylaxis reduces significantly the occurrence of SBP and bacteremia (9% vs. 33% at 1 year) [66]. The mechanisms of this prevention is incompletely understood but the study suggests a reduction in bacterial translocation under enoxaparin treatment.

Catheter-related infections

These infections are common in critically ill cirrhotic patients. These patients may benefit from the following: appropriate hand hygiene, use of chlorhexidine for skin preparation, use of full-barrier precautions during the insertion of central venous catheters, use of the subclavian vein as the preferred site for insertion of the catheter, and the removal of unnecessary central venous catheters [67].

Conclusions

Bacterial infections have become the primary cause of death in cirrhosis. The outcome remains poor despite progress in understanding the pathogenesis of sepsis in cirrhosis. Multicenter RCTs are needed to improve the prognosis of this severe complication.

References

1 Fernandez J, Navasa M, Gomez J, et al. Bacterial infections in cirrhosis: epidemiologicalchanges with invasive procedures and norfloxacin prophylaxis. Hepatology 2002;35:140–8.

2 Friedman ND, Kaye KS, Stout JE, et al. Health care-associated bloodstream infections in adults: a reason to change the accepted definition of CA infections. Ann Intern Med 2002;137:791–7.

3 Fernandez J, Acevedo J, Castro M, et al. Prevalence and risk factors of infections by multiresistant bacteria in cirrhosis: a prospective study. Hepatology 2012;55:1551–61.

4 Bernard B, Grangé JD, Khac EN, Amiot X, Opolon P, Poynard T. Antibiotic prophylaxis for the prevention of bacterial infections in cirrhotic patients with gastrointestinal bleeding: a meta-analysis. Hepatology 1999;29:1655–61.

5 Yoshida H, Hamada T, Inuzuka S, Ueno T, Sata M, Tanikawa K. Bacterial infection in cirrhosis, with and without hepatocellular carcinoma. Am J Gastroenterol 1993;88:2067–71.

6 Llach J, Rimola A, Navasa M, et al. Incidence and predictive factors of first episode of spontaneous bacterial peritonitis in cirrhosis with ascites: relevance of ascitic fluid protein concentration. Hepatology 1992;16:724–7.

7 Ginès P, Rimola A, Planas R, et al. Norfloxacin prevents spontaneous bacterial peritonitis recurrence in cirrhosis: results of a double-blind, placebo-controlled trial. Hepatology 1990;12:716–24.

8 Gustot T, Durand F, Lebrec D, Vincent JL, Moreau R. Severe sepsis in cirrhosis. Hepatology 2009;50:2022–33.

9 Moreau R, Jalan R, Gines P, et al. Acute-on-chronic liver failure is a distinct syndrome that develops in patients with acute decompensation of cirrhosis. Gastroenterology 2013;144:1426–37.

10 Arvaniti V, D'Amcio G, Fede G, et al. Infections in patients with cirrhosis increase mortality four-fold and should be used in determining prognosis. Gastroenterology 2010;139:1246–56.

11 Foreman MG, Mannino DM, Moss M. Cirrhosis as a risk factor for sepsis and death: analysis of the National Hospital Discharge Survey. Chest 2003;124:1016–20.

12 Gustot T, Felleiter P, Pickkers P, et al. Impact of infection on the prognosis of critically ill cirrhotic patients: results from a large worldwide study. Liver Int 2014; in press.

13 American College of Chest Physicians/Society of Critical Care Medicine Consensus Conference: definitions for sepsis and organ failure and guidelines for the use of innovative therapies in sepsis. Crit Care Med 1992;20:864–74.

14 Cazzaniga M, Dionigi E, Gobbo G, Fioretti A, Monti V, Salerno F. The systemic inflammatory response syndrome in cirrhotic patients: relationship with their in-hospital outcome. J Hepatol 2009;51:475–82.

15 Thabut D, Massard J, Gangloff A, et al. Model for end-stage liver disease score and systemic inflammatory response are major prognostic factors in patients with cirrhosis and acute functional renal failure. Hepatology 2007;46:1872–82.

16 Evans LT, Kim WR, Poterucha JJ, et al. Spontaneous bacterial peritonitis in asymptomatic outpatients with cirrhotic ascites. Hepatology 2003;37:897–901.

17 Castellote J, Girbau A, Maisterra S, et al. Spontaneous bacterial peritonitis and bacterascites prevalence in asymptomatic cirrhotic outpatients undergoing large-volume paracentesis. J Gastroenterol Hepatol 2008;23:256–9.

18 Garcia-Tsao G. Spontaneous bacterial peritonitis: a historical perspective. J Hepatol 2004;41:522–7.

19 Silvain C, Besson I, Ingrand P, et al. Prognosis and long-term recurrence of spontaneous bacterial peritonitis in cirrhosis. J Hepatol 1993;19:188–9.

20 European Association for the Study of the Liver. EASL clinical practice guidelines on the management of ascites, spontaneous bacterial peritonitis, and hepatorenal syndrome in cirrhosis. J Hepatol 2010;53:397–417.

21 Nousbaum JB, Cardanel JF, Nahon P, et al. Diagnostic accuracy of the Multistix 8 SG reagent strip in diagnosis of spontaneous bacterial peritonitis. Hepatology 2007;45:1275–81.

22 Parsi MA, Saadeh SN, Zein NN, et al. Ascitic fluid lactoferrin for diagnosis of spontaneous bacterial peritonitis. Gastroenterology 2008;135:803–7.

23 Runyon BA. Monomicrobial nonneutrocytic bacterascites: a variant of spontaneous bacterial peritonitis. Hepatology 1990;12:710.

24 Pelletier G, Lesur G, Ink O, et al. Asymptomatic bacterascites: is it spontaneous bacterial peritonitis. Hepatology 1991;14:112.

25 European Association for the Study of the Liver. EASL clinical practice guidelines on the management of ascites, spontaneous bacterial peritonitis, and hepatorenal syndrome in cirrhosis. J Hepatol 2010;53:397–417.

26 Ricart E, Soriano G, Novella MT, et al. Amoxicillin-clavulanic acid versus cefotaxime in the therapy of bacterial infections in cirrhotic patients. J Hepatol 2000;32:596–602.

27 Angeli P, Guarda S, Fasolato S, et al. Switch therapy with cirpofloxacin vs. intraveinous ceftazidime in the treatment of spontaneous bacterial peritonis in patients with cirrhosis: similar efficacy at lower cost. Aliment Pharmacol Ther 2006;23:75–84.

28 Soriano G, Castellote J, Alvarez C, et al. Secondary bacterial peritonitis in cirrhosis: a retrospective study of clinical and analytical characteristics, diagnosis and management. J Hepatol 2010;52:39–44.

29 Plessier A, Denninger MH, Consigny Y, et al. Coagulation disorders in patients with cirrhosis and severe sepsis. Liver Int 2003;23:440–8.

30 Viasus D, Garcia-Vidal C, Castellote J, et al. Community-acquired pneumonia in patients with liver cirrhosis: clinical features, outcomes, and usefulness of severity scores. Medicine (Baltimore) 2011;90:110–8.

31 Feikin DR, Schuchat A, Kolczak M, et al. Mortality from invasive pneumococcal pneumonia in the era of antibiotic resistance, 1995–1997. Am J Public Health 2000;90:223–9.

32 Monchi M, Bellenfant F, Cariou A, et al. Early predictive factors of survival in the acute respiratory distress syndrome: a multivariate analysis. Am J Respir Care Med 1998;158:1076–81.

33 Qin T, Xia J, Ren H, Zhou H, Tang B, Shao Z. Liver cirrhosis as a predisposing condition for Legionnaires' disease: a report of four laboratory-confirmed cases from China. J Med Microbiol 2012;61:1023–8.

34 Mandell LA, Wunderink RG, Anzueto A, et al. Infectious Diseases Society of America/American Thoracic Society consensus guidelines on the management of community-acquired pneumonia in adults. Clin Infect Dis 2007; 44 (Suppl 2): S27.

35 Caly WR, Strauss E. A prospective study of bacterial infections in patients with cirrhosis. J Hepatol 1993;18:353–8.

36 Corredoira JM, Ariza J, Pallares R, et al. Gram-negative bacillary cellulitis in patients with hepatic cirrhosis. Eur J Clin Microbiol Infect Dis 1994;13:19–24.

37 Pereira G, Guevara M, Faqundes C, et al. Renal failure and hyponatremia in patients with cirrhosis and skin and soft tissue infection: a retrospective study. J Hepatol 2012;56:1040–6.

38 Horowitz Y, Sperber AD, Almog Y. Gram-negative cellulitis complicating cirrhosis. Mayo Clin Proc 2004;79:247–50.

39 Sort P, Navasa M, Arroyo V, et al. Effect of intravenous albumin on renal impairment and mortality in patients with cirrhosis and spontaneous bacterial peritonitis. N Engl J Med 1999;341:403–9.

40 Casas M, Soriano G, Ayala E, et al. Intravenous albumin is not necessary in cirrhotic patients with spontaneous bacterial peritonitis and low-risk mortality. J Hepatol 2007;76:S91.

41 Fernandez J, Monteagudo J, Bargallo X, et al. A randomized unblinded pilot study comparing albumin versus hydroxyethyl starch in spontaneous bacterial peritonitis. Hepatology 2005;42:627–34.

42 Guevara M, Terra C, Nazar A, et al. Albumin for bacterial infections other than spontaneous bacterial peritonitis in cirrhosis: a randomized, controlled study. J Hepatol 2012;57:759–65.

43 Mandorfer M, Bota S, Schwabl P, et al. Nonoselective β blockers increase risk for hepatorenal syndrome and death in patients with cirrhosis and spontaneous bacterial peritonitis. Gastroenterology 2014;146:1680–90.

44 Kumar A, Roberts D, Wood KE, et al. Duration of hypotension before initiation of effective antimicrobial therapy is the critical determinant of survival in human septic shock. Crit Care Med 2006;34:1589–96.

45 Ibrahim EH, Sherman G, Ward S, Fraser VJ, Kollef MH. The influence of inadequate antimicrobial treatment of bloodstream infections on patient outcomes in the ICU setting. Chest 2000;118:146–55.

46 Arabi YM, Dara SI, Memish Z, et al. Antimicrobial therapeutic determinants of outcomes from septic shock among patients with cirrhosis. Hepatology 2012;56:2305–15.

47 Rivers E, Nguyen B, Havstad S, et al. Early Goal-Directed Therapy Collaborative Group. Early goal-directed therapy in the treatment of severe sepsis and septic shock. N Engl J Med 2001;345:1368–77.

48 Moreau R, Hadengue A, Soupison T, et al. Septic shock in patients with cirrhosis: hemodynamic and metabolic characteristics and intensive care unit outcome. Crit Care Med 1992;20:746–50.

49 Dellinger RP, Levy MM, Carlet JM, et al. Surviving Sepsis Campaign: international guidelines for management of severe sepsis and septic shock: 2008. Crit Care Med 2008;36:296–327.

50 De Backer D, Biston P, Devriendt J, et al. SOAP II Investigators. Comparison of dopamine and norepinephrine in the treatment of shock. N Engl J Med 2010;362:779–89.
51 Marik PE, Pastores SM, Annane D, et al. Recommendations for the diagnosis and management of corticosteroid insufficiency in critically ill adult patients: consensus statements from an international task force by the American College of Critical Care Medicine. Crit Care Med 2008;36:1937–49.
52 Tsai MH, Peng YS, Chen YC, et al. Adrenal Insufficiency in patients with cirrhosis, severe sepsis and septic shock. Hepatology 2006;43:673–81.
53 Fernández J, Escorsell A, Zabalza M, et al. Adrenal insufficiency in patients with cirrhosis and septic shock: effect of treatment with hydrocortisone on survival. Hepatology 2006;44:1288–95.
54 Carbonell N, Pauwels A, Serfaty L, Fourdan O, Lévy VG, Poupon R. Improved survival after variceal bleeding in patients with cirrhosis over the past two decades. Hepatology 2004;40:652–9.
55 Chavez-Tapia NC, Barrientos-Gutierrez T, Tellez-Avila FI, Soares-Weiser K, Uribe M. Antibiotic prophylaxis for cirrhotic patients with upper gastrointestinal bleeding. Cochrane Database Syst Rev 2010;9: CD002907.
56 Rimola A, Garcia-Tsao G, Navasa M, et al. Diagnosis, treatment and prophylaxis of spontaneous bacterial peritonitis: a consensus document. International Ascites Club. J Hepatol 2000;32:142–53.
57 Fernández J, Ruiz del Arbol L, Gómez C, et al. Norfloxacin vs ceftriaxone in the prophylaxis of infections in patients with advanced cirrhosis and hemorrhage. Gastroenterology 2006;131:1049–56.
58 de Francis R, Baveno V. Faculty. Revising consensus workshop on methodology and therapy in portal hypertension. J Hepatol 2010;53:762–8.
59 Fernández J, Navasa M, Planas R, et al. Primary prophylaxis of spontaneous bacterial peritonitis delays hepatorenal syndrome and improves survival in cirrhosis. Gastroenterology 2007;133:818–24.
60 Terg R, Fassio E, Guevara M, et al. Ciprofloxacin in primary prophylaxis of spontaneous bacterial peritonitis: a randomized, placebo-controlled study. J Hepatol 2008;48:774–9.
61 Garcia-Tsao G. Current management of the complications of cirrhosis and portal hypertension: variceal hemorrhage, ascites, and spontaneous bacterial peritonitis. Gastroenterology 2001;120:726–48.
62 Gines P, Rimola A, Planas R, et al. Norfloxacin prevents spontaneous bacterial peritonitis recurrence in cirrhosis: results of a double-blind, placebo-controlled trial. Hepatology 1990;12:716–24.
63 Bajaj JS, Zadvornova Y, Heuman DM, Hafeezullah M, Hoffmann RG, Sanyal AJ. Association of proton pump inhibitor therapy with spontaneous bacterial peritonitis in cirrhotic patients with ascites. Am J Gastroenterol 2009; 104:1130–4.
64 Goel GA, Deshpande A, Lopez R, Hall GS, van Duin D, Carey WD. Increased rate of spontaneous bacterial peritonitis among cirrhotic patients receiving pharmacologic acid suppression. Clin Gastroenterol Hepatol 2012;10:422–7.
65 Lebrec D, Thabut D, Oberti F, et al; Pentocir Group. Pentoxifylline does not decrease short-term mortality but does reduce complications in patients with advanced cirrhosis. Gastroenetrology 2010;138:1755–62.
66 Villa E, Camma C, Marietta M, et al. Enoxaparin prevents portal vein thrombosis and liver decompensation in patients with advanced cirrhosis. Gastroenterology 2012;143:1253–60.
67 Provonost P, Needham D, Berenholtz S, et al. An intervention to decrease catheter-related bloodstream infections in the ICU. N Engl J Med 2006;355:2725–32.

CHAPTER 16

Hepatorenal syndrome and acute kidney injury

Florence Wong
Division of Gastroenterology, Department of Medicine, Toronto General Hospital, University of Toronto, Ontario, Canada

Renal dysfunction is a common complication of liver cirrhosis, estimated to occur in approximately 20% of patients with advanced cirrhosis and ascites admitted to hospital [1]. Although the prevalence of chronic kidney disease (CKD) is rising, related to an increasing number of patients worldwide affected by viral hepatitis, obesity, diabetes, and hypertension, the majority of cases of renal dysfunction are related to acute kidney injury (AKI), whether occurring *de novo* or superimposed on a background of CKD [1,2]. While structural renal disease can occur in patients with cirrhosis, leading to acute renal dysfunction, most of the AKI cases in cirrhosis are functional in nature, that is, there is no underlying structural abnormality in the kidneys; rather, the renal dysfunction is the result of hemodynamic changes that are prevalent in advanced cirrhosis. There is splanchnic and systemic arterial vasodilatation, which leads to an apparent decrease in the intravascular volume, the so-called reduction in the effective arterial blood volume. The physiologic response is an activation of various vasoconstrictor systems in an attempt to reduce the extent of vasodilatation, and to improve the intravascular volume by increasing renal sodium and water retention [3]. The renal circulation is very sensitive to the vasoconstrictive effects of these vasoconstrictor systems and therefore is susceptible to the development of renal vasoconstriction with renal impairment. Most episodes of functional renal disorder are responsive to intravascular volume replacement, with return of the renal function to the baseline level [1]. Hepatorenal syndrome (HRS) is the most severe form of functional renal failure and it is not responsive to intravascular volume challenge. The exact prevalence of AKI is unknown, as many cases of mild AKI are outpatients and therefore may escape medical attention. Amongst hospitalized patients, AKI including cases of structural renal disease and functional renal failure, has been reported to have a prevalence of 19% [1]. In a series of 263 cirrhotic patients with ascites admitted to two large tertiary centers in Barcelona for management of ascites, 27.4% of patients developed prerenal renal failure (volume-responsive functional renal failure, FRF), 14.1% developed infection-related FRF, and 7.6% developed HRS during a mean follow-up period of 41 months [4]. Interestingly, 7.6% of patients also developed renal failure due to structural renal diseases during follow-up [4]. Because the development of AKI in cirrhosis is associated with increased morbidity and mortality, even before patients reach the stage of established HRS [5,6], significant efforts have been made in recent years to better our understanding of the pathophysiology, and to update the various definitions and diagnostic criteria.

Hepatorenal syndrome

HRS is the most clearly defined and best studied amongst all the AKI entities in cirrhosis. It used to be an invariably fatal condition with a median survival of several days without treatment [7]. With the introduction of effective treatments, HRS is no longer a terminal condition. Therefore, it is paramount that early and accurate diagnosis is made, so as to implement treatment to improve the outcome for these patients.

Definition

In 2007, the International Ascites Club, an organization consisting of experts in hepatology, renal physiology, hemodynamics, electrolyte disorders, cardiopulmonary function, and transplant medicine, revised the definition of HRS. The group wanted to emphasize the functional nature of the condition, which is consequent upon the systemic vasodilatory hemodynamic changes that occur

Cirrhosis: A practical guide to management, First Edition. Edited by Samuel S. Lee and Richard Moreau.

Table 16.1 Pathophysiologic processes that have been implicated in the development of hepatorenal syndrome (HRS).

Pathophysiologic process	Underlying etiology	Consequence
Splanchnic and systemic arterial vasodilatation [3]	• Production of excess vasodilators [8] • Inability of the cirrhotic liver to clear excess vasodilators • Hyporesponsiveness of the arterial circulation to the vasoconstrictive effects of various vasoconstrictors • Increased mesenteric angiogenesis [9] • Post-receptor defect at the level of the smooth muscle cells [10]	• Increase in vascular capacitance • Reduction in effective arterial blood volume • Activation of various vasoconstrictor systems • Renal vasoconstriction and sodium retention
Cardiac dysfunction	• Cirrhotic cardiomyopathy, with systolic dysfunction, that is, there is inability of the heart to mount an increased cardiac output in the presence of significant systemic vasodilatation [14,15]	• Decreased cardiac output • Decreased renal perfusion pressure
Altered renal autoregulation	• Increased sympathetic activity with progression of cirrhosis [12]	• Progressive reduction in renal blood flow with advancing cirrhosis even when there is no reduction in renal perfusion pressure • Patients are predisposed to the development of HRS with smaller further reduction in renal blood flow

in advanced cirrhosis [8–10]. The group also recognized that changes in cardiac function and renal physiology contributed to the development of HRS (Table 16.1). For example, patients who developed renal failure with an episode of bacterial peritonitis had significantly lower cardiac output at the time of infection resolution when compared with baseline, and also when compared with those who did not develop HRS at the time of infection resolution [11]. Changes in renal autoregulation with progression of liver cirrhosis also has a role in the development of HRS. Autoregulation is a physiologic response that maintains renal blood flow despite alterations in renal perfusion pressure. However, increasing levels of sympathetic nervous activity with advancement of cirrhosis can lead to progressive reduction in renal blood flow even with adequate renal perfusion pressure, thus predisposing the patient to the development of renal failure [12].

Thus, the current definition of HRS states that:

> HRS is a potentially reversible syndrome occurring in patients with cirrhosis, ascites and liver failure. It is characterized by impaired renal function, marked alterations in the cardiovascular function and over-activity of the endogenous vasoactive systems. Marked vasoconstriction in the kidney causes low glomerular filtration, whereas in the systemic circulation, there is decreased vascular resistance due to splanchnic and peripheral arterial vasodilatation. A similar syndrome can also occur in acute liver failure and acute alcoholic hepatitis. [13]

A recent report has confirmed that patients with lower cardiac output had worse renal function as indicated by a lower glomerular filtration rate, lower renal blood flow, and higher serum creatinine, indicating a link between cardiac function and renal function [14]. Furthermore, those who went on to develop HRS had a lower cardiac index, as did those who died from their HRS [14]. Indeed, a cardiorenal interaction has been proposed in patients with advanced cirrhosis where cardiac dysfunction in cirrhosis is a major determinant of kidney function [15]. Therefore, there may be further refinement of the definition in the future as new pathophysiologic processes are recognized.

Diagnostic criteria

Table 16.2 sets out the most recent criteria for the diagnosis of HRS, which continues to mandate a diagnosis of exclusion [13]. These diagnostic criteria have been simplified to improve the diagnostic accuracy of HRS, thereby allowing application of effective treatment options according to a standard set of rules. Of note, HRS can be diagnosed in the setting of a bacterial infection, provided septic shock is not present. In addition, urinary electrolyte or creatinine clearance is not

Table 16.2 Diagnostic criteria for hepatorenal syndrome.

- Cirrhosis with ascites
- Serum creatinine >1.5 mg/dL (133 μmol/L)
- No improvement of serum creatinine (decrease to a level of 1.5 mg/dL or less) after at least 2 days of diuretic withdrawal and volume expansion with albumin. The recommended dose of albumin is 1 g/kg of body weight per day up to a maximum of 100 g/day
- Absence of shock
- No current or recent treatment with nephrotoxic drugs
- Absence of parenchymal kidney disease as indicated by proteinuria >500 mg/day, microhematuria (>50 red blood cells per high power field), and/or abnormal renal ultrasonography

Source: Adapted from Salerno et al., 2007 [13]. Reproduced with permision of BMJ Group.

required for the diagnosis of HRS, thereby obviating the need for a 24-hour urine collection. Despite its limitations as an accurate index of renal function [16,17], especially in advanced cirrhosis, serum creatinine is still the parameter used to diagnose HRS, because it is widely available and easy to measure. The diagnosis of HRS requires a serum creatinine level of >1.5 mg/dL (133 μmol/L). Clinically, HRS can be divided into two types: the acute form or type 1 HRS which is characterized by a rapidly progressive renal failure defined by doubling of the initial serum creatinine to a level greater than 2.5 mg/dL (221 μmol/L) in less than 2 weeks; whereas the chronic form or type 2 HRS is characterized by moderate renal failure (serum creatinine of 1.5–2.5 mg/dL or 133–221 μmol/L), which follows a steady or slowly progressive course, often associated with refractory ascites. Despite the emergence of several promising markers of renal dysfunction such as cystatin C, neutrophil gelatinase-associated lipocalin, interleukin-18, and liver type fatty acid binding protein [18], there are as yet no specific diagnostic markers for HRS. Many of these biomarkers are more specific for renal tubular damage and are therefore more appropriate for separating acute tubular necrosis from functional renal disorders rather than diagnosing hepatorenal syndrome per se.

Differential diagnosis of renal dysfunction in cirrhosis

Despite setting down the diagnostic criteria, the accurate diagnosis of HRS may not always be easy in daily clinical practice [19]. This is especially true for patients with rapidly deteriorating renal dysfunction, many of whom may be oliguric or anuric, thus making exclusion of structural renal disease on urinary criteria difficult. The volume replacement may not have followed strictly the criteria required for the diagnosis of HRS or the diuretic withdrawal may not have been complete before starting definitive treatment for HRS, as many physicians are unwilling to take a wait-and-see approach until the diagnostic serum creatinine level of >2.5 mg/dL (221 μmol/L) is reached. In a recent report of 263 consecutive patients with cirrhosis and renal failure admitted into 21 Italian hospitals, the cases of presumed diagnosis of HRS responded to treatment with vasoconstrictors with similar outcomes when compared with patients who fulfilled all the diagnostic criteria for HRS [19]. Therefore, physicians are encouraged to follow the diagnostic criteria for HRS, but should not delay or withhold treatment in cases of presumed HRS diagnosed on clinical grounds. Figure 16.1 sets out the diagnostic approach to a patient with cirrhosis, ascites, and renal dysfunction.

The most frequent differential diagnosis for HRS is acute tubular necrosis (ATN) and differentiating the two conditions is not always easy. Patients with ATN may not always provide a history of hypotension, or nephrotoxic drug use. Likewise, patients with a prolonged course of HRS may also develop ATN, related to intense renal arteriolar vasoconstriction, causing tubular damage [20]. Granular casts may be seen in both HRS and ATN. Urinary parameters such as urinary sodium excretion and urinary: plasma osmolality ratio are of no value in differentiating the two conditions [21]. The fact that patients who had abnormal serum creatinine but no proteinuria nor hematuria all showed structural renal changes on transvenous renal biopsy further adds to the confusion [22]. The recent report of the differential capability of various renal biomarkers holds promise in separating ATN from HRS [23], but this needs to be confirmed. Until then, physicians who lean towards the diagnosis of HRS should institute treatment for HRS, as renal dysfunction will invariably progress while waiting for clear differentiation, thus diminishing the likelihood of response to treatment [24].

Treatment of type 1 hepatorenal syndrome

Type 1 HRS is usually part of a multi-organ failure picture of the acute-on-chronic liver failure syndrome in a very

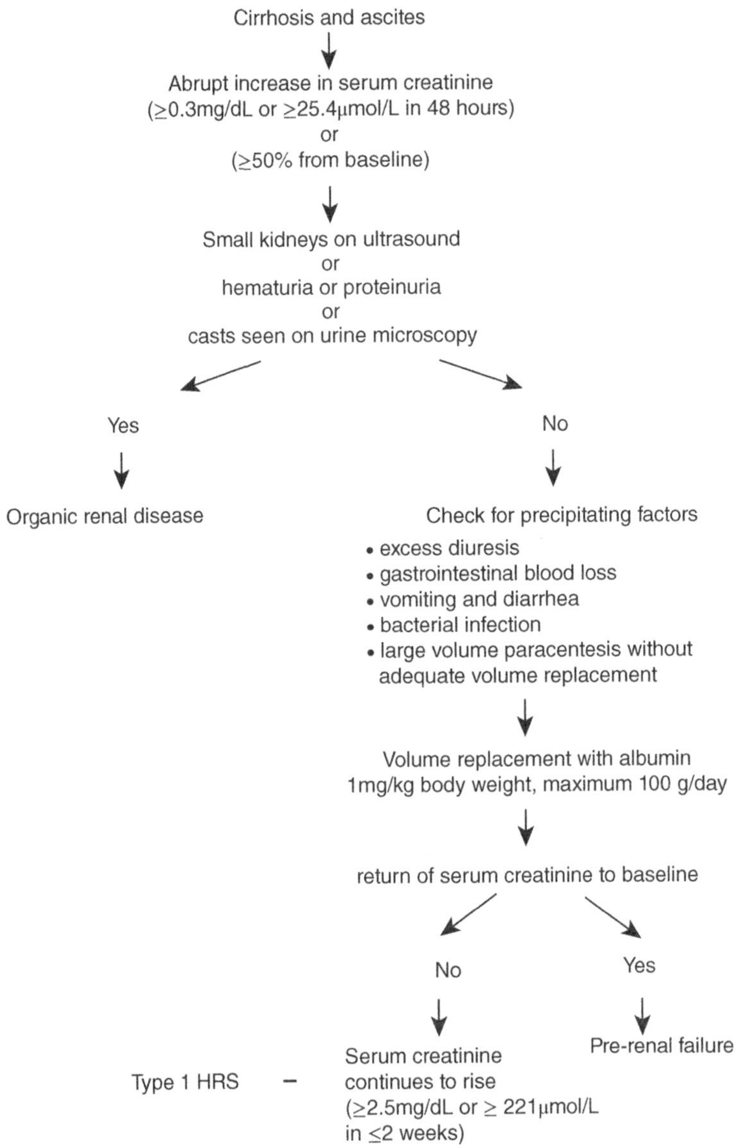

Figure 16.1 Approach to a patient with cirrhosis and ascites who presents with an acute rise in serum creatinine fulfilling the diagnostic criteria for acute kidney injury.

ill patient with advanced cirrhosis [25]. Although type 1 HRS can develop spontaneously, it usually is precipitated by an acute event that perturbs the already precarious hemodynamic state of the patient. Therefore, treatment for type 1 HRS involves managing the precipitating event, the associated systemic inflammatory response syndrome, and the renal failure as well as the global organ malfunction of the patient.

Treatment of precipitating event

The most common precipitating event for type 1 HRS is bacterial infection [26]. The myriads of inflammatory cytokines released by the bacteria can induce various changes in the microcirculation including microthrombi in capillaries, endothelial dysfunction, and capillary leaks in many organs including the kidneys, leading to organ dysfunction [27]. Although spontaneous bacterial peritonitis is the most frequent precipitating event for type 1 HRS [26,28], all bacterial infections can cause renal failure [29]. In addition, any event that disturbs the volume status or exaggerates the reduction of intravascular volume such as gastrointestinal blood loss, overdiuresis, or large-volume paracentesis without adequate intravascular volume replacement can also precipitate type 1 HRS.

Given that type 1 HRS is potentially reversible, it is imperative that the precipitating event is recognized early and treated accordingly. Volume replacement in the form of blood or blood products is given in cases of blood or blood volume loss. Diuretics and nephrotoxic drugs need to be withdrawn. In patients suspected of having an episode of bacterial infection, early and empirical use of antibiotics is recommended [30]. In those patients who have one of these precipitating events and who have not yet developed type 1 HRS, preventative measures can sometimes obviate its occurrence. For example, the incidence of renal impairment is most significant among patients with spontaneous bacterial peritonitis and a serum bilirubin level >4 mg/dL (68 μmol/L) and a serum creatinine level >1 mg/dL (88 μmol/L) [31], and prophylactic use of albumin in this scenario has been shown to reduce the incidence of renal failure [31]. Likewise, the use of prophylactic antibiotics in patients who have an episode of gastrointestinal bleeding has been shown to reduce the incidence of bacterial infections and therefore the likelihood of developing type 1 HRS [32].

Vasoconstrictor therapy

Given that one of the major pathophysiologic factors for the development of type 1 HRS is systemic arterial vasodilatation, leading to paradoxical renal vasoconstriction, it stands to reason to treat type 1 HRS by counteracting the systemic arterial vasodilatation. The resultant improvement in the effective arterial blood volume should lead to a dampening of the activities of the various systemic vasoconstrictors, thereby decreasing the renal vasoconstriction, with overall improvement in renal blood flow and glomerular filtration.

Terlipressin

The most widely used agent outside North America for the treatment of type 1 HRS is terlipressin, which is a vasopressin analog. Terlipressin binds to the V_1 receptors of the vascular smooth muscle cells to cause vasoconstriction in both the systemic and the splanchnic circulations [33]. It therefore reduces the extent of splanchnic and systemic vasodilatation. In addition, terlipressin has been shown to dilate intrahepatic vessels, thereby reducing intrahepatic resistance to portal inflow [34]. The overall result is a reduction in portal pressure, which also has a direct effect on improving renal function [35].

To date, there have been two randomized controlled trials comparing terlipressin and albumin with albumin alone [36], or terlipressin and albumin with placebo [37]. Both studies have shown efficacy in reversing type 1 HRS in approximately 34–43% of patients, but survival was not improved. Recurrence of HRS was not common after discontinuation of treatment, and any recurrence could be retreated with terlipressin with similar response as the initial course. Sub-analyses showed that patients with severe liver or renal dysfunction, as indicated by a serum bilirubin of >10 mg/dL (170 μmol/L) and a serum creatinine of >5.6 mg/dL (493 μmol/L) [24] were not likely to respond. In addition, those patients who did not have an increase in mean arterial pressure of >5 mmHg on day 3 were also likely to not respond to treatment [38]. The corollary from these observations is that patients who are very ill with severe liver and renal dysfunction should not be treated with terlipressin, and, for those who receive terlipressin, a lack of hemodynamic response on day 3 should also indicate that an alternative therapy should be given.

More recently, there are reports that a continuous infusion is superior to bolus doses of terlipressin, which were used in the randomized controlled trials in the management of type 1 HRS [39,40]. Equal efficacy was achieved with a lower total daily dose and with fewer side effects, due to a more sustained portal pressure lowering effect of a continuous infusion than with bolus injections. There are now also case reports documenting the efficacy of repeated courses of continuous infusions of terlipressin with albumin 20–40 g/day as a bridge therapy to liver transplantation for repeated recurrences of HRS [41,42]. All patients who were treated in this manner remained alive at 46 days to 8 months and ultimately received a liver transplant as definitive therapy. Therefore, long-term use of terlipressin is a plausible option, preventing irreversible renal failure and the need for dialysis while waiting for liver transplantation.

Midodrine

Midodrine is an α-agonist. It acts by binding to the α_1-adrenergic receptors on the vascular smooth muscle cells, which in turn leads to an increase in the intracellular calcium, thereby causing smooth muscle cell contraction and vasoconstriction. It therefore increases mean arterial pressure, and hence renal perfusion pressure. Its use in type 1 HRS has been propelled by two pilot studies [43,44], which showed improvement but not normalization of renal function. Because terlipressin is not available in North America except in the context of a clinical trial, the use of midodrine is popular. To date, there are no randomized controlled trials comparing midodrine with placebo as a treatment for type 1 HRS, but a few retrospective studies suggest that it is effective in approximately 30% of patients, especially when combined with octreotide [45,46]. One of the retrospective studies found that when midodrine was given at 15 mg three times daily, 88% patients had type 1 HRS reversal compared with 33% of those receiving <12.5 mg three times daily [45]. The most recent data suggest that terlipressin is superior to the midodrine–octreotide combination in reversing type 1 HRS [47]. With clinical trials of terlipressin for type 1 HRS just completed in North America, the use of the midodrine–octreotide combination may be phased out in the near future. Of note, the use of octreotide alone has not been shown to be effective in the treatment of type 1 HRS [48].

Norepinephrine

Like midodrine, norepinephrine is an α-agonist. To date, there are three randomized controlled trials comparing the safety and efficacy of norepinephrine with terlipressin in reversing type 1 HRS. A similar number of patients responded to norepinephrine with an improvement in mean arterial pressure and renal function when compared with the terlipressin groups [49–51]. Side-effect profiles and cumulative survival were also comparable between the two drugs. A meta-analysis comparing the use of terlipressin with norepinephrine also confirmed equal efficacy of the two drugs in the reversal of type 1 HRS [52]. The cost of norepinephrine is significantly lower than that of terlipressin. However, the use of norepinephrine requires cardiac monitoring in an intensive care unit, whereas terlipressin can be administered in a nonmonitored setting. Therefore, the cost-effectiveness argument for the use of norepinephrine for type 1 HRS may not be valid. However, it is a good alternative in situations where terlipressin is not available. There have been no randomized controlled trials comparing norepinephrine with the midodrine–octreotide combination.

Therefore, the choice of vasoconstrictor for the treatment of type 1 HRS depends on local drug availability and the access for cardiac monitoring. A meta-analysis comparing all randomized trials on vasoconstrictors with or without albumin versus no intervention or albumin alone for type 1 HRS reported a beneficial effect of vasoconstrictors on renal function, and a reduction in all-cause mortality favoring the vasoconstrictors (Figure 16.2a) [53]. A sub-analysis assessing only the terlipressin trials confirmed that terlipressin plus albumin was more efficacious than albumin alone in terms of improving renal function or reversal of HRS (Figure 16.2b) [53]. Since then, two further meta-analyses corroborated the same findings [52,54]. Thus, the available data suggest that terlipressin, where available, should be given for type 1 HRS.

Albumin

Albumin is a plasma protein that has ligand-binding, antioxidant, anti-inflammatory, and metabolic properties in addition to being a very effective volume expander [55]. It is given to patients with AKI to rule out prerenal failure. Albumin has not been established as a stand-alone treatment for type 1 HRS, especially as recent studies have not shown albumin alone to be able to reverse type 1 HRS, nor to improve survival when compared with the combination of albumin and vasoconstrictors [36,37,55]. It is not clear whether albumin has any additional beneficial effects on renal function when added to vasoconstrictors in the treatment of HRS.

In the largest retrospective study on the use of terlipressin for HRS, there was no difference in the outcome of patients irrespective of whether albumin was added to terlipressin [56]. Yet, in another prospective nonrandomized study, the use of albumin significantly improved renal function and survival [57]. Given the fact that there is no evidence that albumin actually does some harm, it seems prudent to use albumin in the treatment of HRS. The International Ascites Club recommends the use of 20–40 g/day albumin in combination with vasoconstrictors, after the initial dose of 1 g/kg of body weight on initial 2 days [13].

Figure 16.3 describes the pharmacologic approach to the management of type 1 HRS.

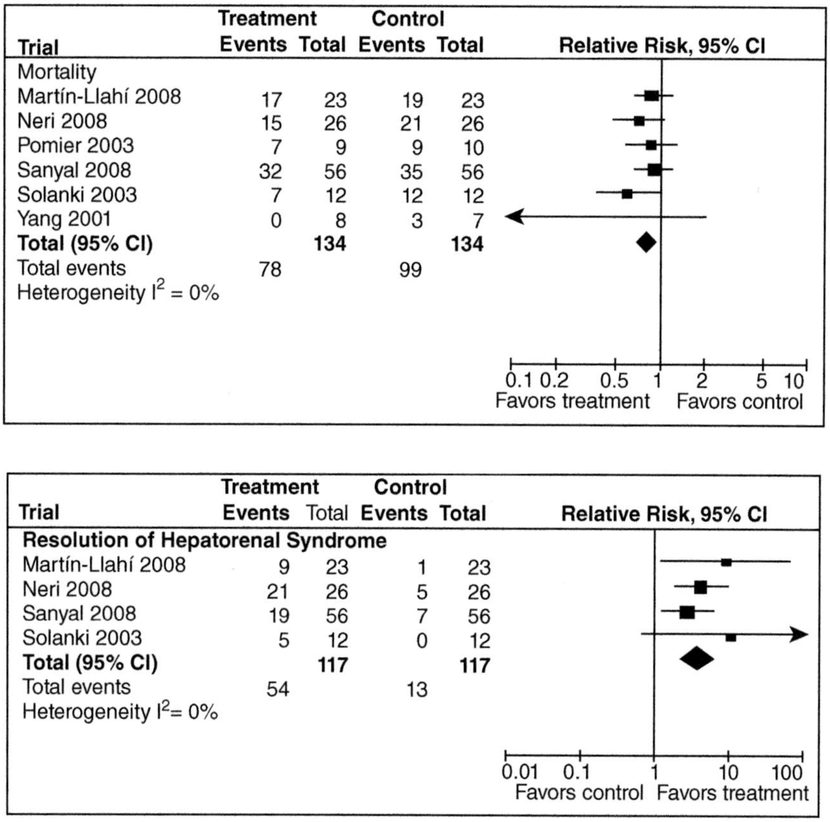

Figure 16.2 (A) Meta-analysis of all randomized controlled trials assessing the effects of terlipressin on all-cause mortality, and (B) meta-analysis of all randomized controlled trials assessing the effects of vasoconstrictors on renal function. *Source:* Gluud et al., 2010 [53]. Reproduced with permission of John Wiley & Sons.

Nonpharmacologic treatments of type 1 hepatorenal syndrome

Transjugular intrahepatic portosystemic shunt

Transjugular intrahepatic portosystemic shunt (TIPS) was first used as a treatment for HRS almost 20 years ago [58]. The rationale for using TIPS was because it is a very effective means of reducing sinusoidal portal hypertension, which is the initiator of the hemodynamic changes that lead to relative renal ischemia and hence decreased renal function. In addition, TIPS returns a significant portion of the splanchnic volume into the systemic circulation, leading to suppression of various vasoactive neurohormones, resulting in better renal perfusion. Indeed, several studies have demonstrated the efficacy of TIPS in improving renal function in patients with type 1 HRS [59–61]. In those patients who responded, ascites was also reported to decrease significantly. In addition, TIPS appears to confer a survival advantage over conventional medical treatment, with one study reporting an 18-month survival of 35% [60]. However, in that particular study, those who received medical therapy had more severe liver dysfunction with a significantly higher Child–Pugh score; that is, those who received TIPS might have had a survival advantage for the simple reason that they were less ill. The fact that there has not been any report on the use of TIPS as a treatment for type 1 HRS in the past decade suggests this may be a treatment option that is falling out of favor, as other treatment modalities such as terlipressin may have supplanted the use of TIPS as a treatment for type 1 HRS, especially as TIPS is associated with its own set of complications [62], and it is not uniformly associated with total reversal of HRS [59–61]. In the latest review on the clinical applications for TIPS [62], it has

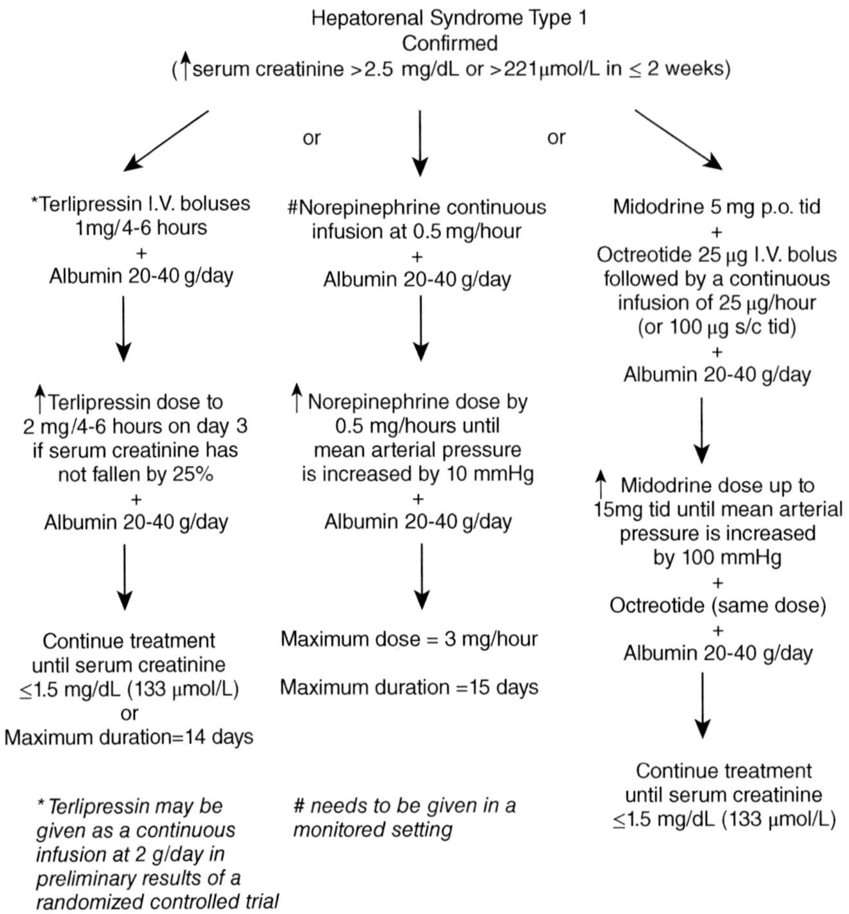

Figure 16.3 Pharmacologic treatments for type 1 hepatorenal syndrome. (Data from references 36,37,39,43,44,49,51.)

been suggested that TIPS should be considered as a treatment for HRS in those patients whose liver function is relatively preserved such as abstinent alcoholics, and/or patients who are possible candidates for liver transplantation. One study showed that TIPS could significantly improve post-transplant graft and patient survival in such candidates, possibly due to an improved pretransplant renal function and portal blood supply of the graft by reducing collateral flow. Long-term survival, however, was not affected [63].

Extracorporeal albumin dialysis

In patients with acute-on-chronic liver failure, many with renal failure, the use of extracorporeal albumin dialysis system as a means of filtering out various substances including vasodilators was thought to be beneficial to patients with HRS, as this process could help to improve the hemodynamic derangements of patients with type 1 HRS. Indeed, the use of one such system was able to reduce serum bilirubin and serum creatinine [64,65], and in one randomized controlled trial, survival also improved [66]. However, when treatment was stopped, serum creatinine returned to pretreatment high levels, suggesting that no real change in renal function was achieved with extracorporeal albumin dialysis, as confirmed by measurement of renal function using clearance techniques [67]. Rather, the bilirubin and creatinine were being filtered out by the dialysis. Therefore, extracorporeal albumin dialysis cannot be recommended as a treatment for type 1 HRS.

Treatment of type 2 hepatorenal syndrome

Patients with type 2 HRS usually present with refractory ascites and mild renal dysfunction. Treatment is usually directed towards the management of refractory ascites, and the options include repeat large-volume paracentesis or TIPS. For those patients with concomitant severe liver dysfunction, liver transplant is the appropriate definitive treatment.

Large-volume paracentesis is often the first line therapy for patients with refractory ascites [68]. There is always the concern for the development of post-paracentesis circulatory dysfunction even with the administration of albumin post-paracentesis [69]. The use of vasoconstrictors for type 2 HRS has been assessed in a few small studies. In total, 43 patients with type 2 HRS treated with terlipressin have been reported in the literature with similar response rates to patients with type 1 HRS [57,70–72]. The recurrence rate was high, making it impractical to use terlipressin in this population of patients [57,71].

The use of TIPS as a treatment for type 2 HRS has been specifically addressed in one study [73]. The insertion of TIPS was associated with a significant reduction of serum creatinine back to the normal range, associated with improved survival in 12 of the 18 patients. When the insertion of TIPS was preceded by the use of terlipressin, the reversal of HRS was maintained [70]. Given the fact that TIPS insertion alone was able to normalize renal function, it is not clear whether the use of terlipressin pre-TIPS would add any benefit to patient outcome.

Liver transplantation for hepatorenal syndrome

Liver transplantation is the definitive treatment for HRS, especially for patients with type 1 HRS who do not respond to vasoconstrictor therapy. Renal replacement therapy may need to be instituted in patients as a bridging therapy until liver transplantation [74]. Although HRS is usually reversible after liver transplantation [75], up to 40% of patients can remain dependent on dialysis for a period of time post-liver transplant [76], possibly related to the persistence of abnormal hemodynamics post-transplant [77]. There are several controversies surrounding the issue of liver transplantation for HRS. For example, in patients with type 1 HRS who have achieved HRS reversal, whether their priority for liver transplant as indicated by the model for end-stage liver disease (MELD) score should be calculated with the post-treatment serum creatinine, as their prognosis post-liver transplant is similar to patients without HRS [78]. Opponents to such a strategy argue that the clinical outcome of patients with type 1 HRS remains poor despite reversal of HRS, and therefore they should retain their priority for liver transplant [79] using their pretreatment serum creatinine to compute the MELD score. The other area of contention concerns the use of combined liver kidney transplant (CLKT) for patients with type 1 HRS. There are now data suggesting that patient and graft survivals are inferior for CLKT when compared with liver transplant alone [80], therefore many transplant centers are now starting to adopt a wait-and-see approach with respect to simultaneous kidney transplant in patients with cirrhosis and type 1 HRS. However, patients who have bad prognostic indicators for renal recovery such as the presence of alcoholic hepatitis, need for pretransplant dialysis [76], as well as the duration of dialysis of >8 weeks pretransplant [81], should be considered for CKLT. Finally, patients with type 2 HRS tend to have much lower priority for liver transplant, as their MELD score is usually lower, especially if their liver dysfunction is not too severe. However, their clinical course is not particularly benign, especially if the patient also has hyponatremia [82]. The mortality for patients with ascites on the liver transplant waiting list remains high (>20% at 180 days) despite a lower MELD score of <21 [83]. The controversy then becomes whether patients with type 2 HRS should also be given priority for liver transplantation, especially if hyponatremia is a recurring issue. To settle this issue, efforts are now being made to modify the criteria for allocation of donor organs such as assigning points for persistent ascites and low serum sodium in calculating the final score for organ allocation.

Acute kidney injury

HRS is a well-defined entity with rigid diagnostic criteria. However, there are cases of acute rises in serum creatinine that reach a level of >1.5 mg/dL (133 μmol/L) in decompensated cirrhosis that do not really fit into the diagnostic criteria for HRS. As mentioned in the section under differential diagnoses for type 1 HRS, some cases of acute renal failure in these patients are related to organic renal disease such as ATN. However, the majority of cases of AKI are related to prerenal azotemia [1,84]. In a retrospective study assessing the outcome of 152 hospitalized patients with a serum creatinine >1.5 mg/dL (133 μmol/L) [84], 70% of patients had stage 1 AKI as defined by the Acute Kidney Injury Network (AKIN) for other patient populations (an absolute increase of serum creatinine by 0.3 mg/dL (26.4 μmol/L) or a 50% increase from baseline within 48 hours) [85], 69% had prerenal azotemia that was responsive to volume replacement. HRS type 1, which was not volume responsive, only made up of 9% of AKI patients. Intrinsic renal disease including ATN and post-renal causes were the other differential diagnoses of AKI in these patients (Table 16.3). The International Ascites Club requires all patients who present with AKI to undergo volume challenge in order to exclude prerenal azotemia before diagnosing HRS. Likewise, intrinsic renal disease has to be excluded by a bland urinalysis, normal urine microscopy, and normal kidney sizes on abdominal ultrasound before a diagnosis of HRS can be accepted [13].

Table 16.3 Differential diagnosis of acute kidney injury in cirrhosis.

Prerenal azotemia
Over-diuresis
Large-volume paracentesis without adequate intravascular volume replacement
Gastrointestinal blood loss
Sepsis
Excessive vomiting
Intrinsic renal diseases
Acute glomerulonephritis
Acute tubular necrosis:
aminoglycosides
heme-pigment related
Interstitial nephritis:
penicilins
cephalosporins
ciprofloxacin
thiazide diuretics
Nephrotoxic drugs:
radiocontrast agents
methotrexate
cyclosporine
tacrolimus
Ischemia:
nonsteroidal anti-inflammatory drugs
Hemolytic uremic syndrome
Hepatorenal syndrome
Type 1
Post-renal causes
Ureteric obstruction
Bladder neck obstruction

Note: hepatorenal syndrome type 1 is a specific form of prerenal azotemia that is not responsive to volume replacement.

In a prospective study by Belcher et al. [6] that followed strictly the AKIN diagnostic criteria for AKI [85], patients with decompensated cirrhosis and AKI admitted into hospital were followed for their clinical outcome. Almost half of the patients had stage 1 AKI on admission, 30% had stage 2 AKI (doubling of serum creatinine from baseline), and the remainder of the patients had stage 3 AKI (trebling of serum creatinine from baseline). Progression of the renal dysfunction to the next AKIN stage was noted in 44% of patients, associated with more medical events, the development of more cirrhotic complications, and higher mortality [6]. In those patients who had AKIN stage 3 renal failure whose renal dysfunction progressed, those needing dialysis had a mortality rate of >70%. Of note, the lowest serum creatinine in this study cohort was 1.0 g/dL (88 μmol/L), not sufficient for the diagnosis of HRS, and yet this patient was amongst the nonsurvivors. High mortality rates were also reported in critically ill cirrhotic patients in intensive care units who developed AKI according to the AKIN criteria. Such patients were 6.9 times more likely to die than patients who were otherwise ill but who did not develop AKI [86].

The study by Belcher et al. [6] illustrates that it is the change in serum creatinine rather than the absolute serum creatinine value that is important in determining patient outcome. This is because serum creatinine is a poor indicator of the glomerular filtration rate [16], especially in decompensated cirrhosis due to reduced production of creatinine from creatine because of significant muscle wasting. For example, a serum creatinine of 1 mg/dL (88 μmol/L) in such a patient, which is still within the laboratory's normal range, is associated with a glomerular filtration rate of 50 mL/min, which represents substantial reduction in renal function [7]. Therefore, such a patient will not be able to withstand further renal insults with this diminished renal reserve. In a population of post-cardiac surgery patients, small increments of serum creatinine have been shown to have a negative impact on prognosis [87]. Similarly, in a population of ambulatory cirrhotic patients with ascites, whose baseline serum creatinine was within the normal

Table 16.4 Proposed diagnostic criteria of kidney dysfunction in cirrhosis.

Diagnosis	Definition
Acute kidney injury	• A rise in serum creatinine of ≥50% from baseline, or a rise of serum creatinine by ≥26.4 μmol/L (≥0.3 mg/dL) in <48 hours • HRS type I is a specific form of acute kidney injury
Chronic kidney disease	• Glomerular filtration rate of <60 mL/min for >3 months calculated using MDRD6 formula • HRS type II is a specific form of chronic kidney disease
Acute on chronic kidney disease	• Rise in serum creatinine of ≥50% from baseline or a rise of serum creatinine by ≥26.4 μmol/L (≥0.3 mg/dL) in <48 hours in a patient with cirrhosis whose glomerular filtration rate is <60 mL/min for >3 months calculated using MDRD6 formula

Source: Adapted from Wong et al., 2011 [88]. Reproduced with permission of BMJ Group.
Both the acute deterioration in renal function and the background chronic renal dysfunction can be functional or structural in nature.
MDRD6, Modification of Diet in Renal Disease formula calculated using six variables of serum creatinine, age, gender, albumin, blood urea nitrogen, and whether the patient is African-American.

laboratory range, small increases of serum creatinine of either 0.3 mg/dL (26.4 μmol/L) within 48 hours or a 50% rise in serum creatinine from a baseline value within the previous 6 months, irrespective of the final serum creatinine, which might still be within the laboratory's normal range, was associated with a decreased survival when followed-up for 1 year [5]. In addition, these episodes of AKI appear to be precipitated by the same events that lead to the development of type 1 HRS, suggesting that it may be the same pathophysiologic process that underlies the development of milder cases of AKI, perhaps to a less degree of intensity.

The recognition that acute trivial rises in serum creatinine could have a significant impact on the natural history of decompensated cirrhosis has led several groups of experts together to define the entity of "acute kidney injury" in cirrhosis modified from the AKIN criteria (Table 16.4) [88]. These new diagnostic criteria also acknowledge the entity of acute-on-chronic renal failure, suggesting that changes in hemodynamics can also occur in patients with structural renal disease, leading to further insults to renal function. This new concept of combined functional and structural damage in the kidneys of cirrhotic patients is quite innovative, but may be the reality of the future, as more cirrhotic patients develop structural renal disease from causes such as diabetes. A recent prospective study using these new diagnostic criteria of AKI in infected cirrhotic patients admitted into hospital found that they accurately predicted 30-day survival in these patients [89]. Further validation of these new diagnostic criteria in large cohorts of cirrhotic patients will be needed before they can be brought into daily practice.

Conclusions

The development of renal dysfunction still remains a common and dreaded complication of cirrhosis. Great strides have been made in the past decade in the understanding of the pathophysiology and in the development of effective treatment of renal dysfunction in cirrhosis, resulting in improved patient outcomes. The recognition that milder degrees of renal dysfunction could also be potentially deleterious to the prognosis of these patients has rekindled the enthusiasm in the search for newer knowledge, and thence new therapies for this once fatal complication of cirrhosis.

References

1 Garcia-Tsao G, Parikh CR, Viola A. Acute kidney injury in cirrhosis. Hepatology 2008;48:2064–77.
2 Warner NS, Cuthbert JA, Bhore R, et al. Acute kidney injury and chronic kidney disease in hospitalized patients with cirrhosis. J Investig Med 2011;59:1244–51.
3 Schrier R, Arroyo V, Bernardi M, et al. Peripheral arterial vasodilatation hypothesis: a proposal for the initiation of renal sodium and water retention in cirrhosis. Hepatology 1988;8:1151–7.
4 Montoliu S, Ballesté B, Planas R, et al. Incidence and prognosis of different types of functional renal failure in cirrhotic

patients with ascites. Clin Gastroenterol Hepatol 2010;8: 616–22.
5 Tsien CD, Rabie R, Wong F. Acute kidney injury in decompensated cirrhosis. Gut 2013;62:131–7.
6 Belcher JM, Garcia-Tsao G, Sanyal AJ, et al. Association of AKI with mortality and complications in hospitalized patients with cirrhosis. Hepatology 2013;57:753–62.
7 Gines P, Guevara M, Arroyo V, et al. Hepatorenal syndrome. Lancet 2003;362:1819–27.
8 Martin PY, Ginès P, Schrier RW. Nitric oxide as a mediator of hemodynamic abnormalities and sodium and water retention in cirrhosis. N Engl J Med 1998;339:533–41.
9 Bosch J, Abraldes JG, Fernández M, et al. Hepatic endothelial dysfunction and abnormal angiogenesis: new targets in the treatment of portal hypertension. J Hepatol 2010;53:558–67.
10 Castro A, Ros J, Jiménez W, et al. Intracellular calcium concentration in vascular smooth muscle cells of rats with cirrhosis. J Hepatol 1994;21:521–6.
11 Ruiz-del-Arbol L, Urman J, Fernandez J, et al. Systemic, renal, and hepatic hemodynamic derangement in cirrhotic patients with spontaneous bacterial peritonitis. Hepatology 2003;38:1210–8.
12 Stadlbauer V, Wright GA, Banaji M, et al. Relationship between activation of the sympathetic nervous system and renal blood flow autoregulation in cirrhosis. Gastroenterology 2008;134:111–9.
13 Salerno F, Gerbes A, Gines P, et al. Diagnosis, prevention and treatment of hepatorenal syndrome in cirrhosis. Gut 2007;56:1310–8.
14 Krag A, Bendtsen F, Henriksen JH, et al. Low cardiac output predicts development of hepatorenal syndrome and survival in patients with cirrhosis and ascites. Gut 2010;59:105–10.
15 Krag A, Bendtsen F, Burroughs AK, et al. The cardiorenal link in advanced cirrhosis. Med Hypotheses 2012;79:53–5.
16 Caregaro L, Menon F, Angeli P, et al. Limitations of serum creatinine level and creatinine clearance as filtration markers in cirrhosis. Arch Intern Med 1994;154:201–5.
17 Francoz C, Glotz D, Moreau R, et al. The evaluation of renal function and disease in patients with cirrhosis. J Hepatol 2010;52:605–13.
18 Belcher JM, Sanyal AJ, Peixoto AJ, et al. Kidney biomarkers and differential diagnosis of patients with cirrhosis and acute kidney injury. Hepatology 2014;60:622–32.
19 Salerno F, Cazzaniga M, Merli M, et al. Diagnosis, treatment and survival of patients with hepatorenal syndrome: a survey on daily medical practice. J Hepatol 2011;55:1241–8.
20 Mandal AK, Lansing M, Fahmy A. Acute tubular necrosis in hepatorenal syndrome: an electron microscopy study. Am J Kidney Dis 1982;2:363–74.
21 Guevara M, Arroyo V. Hepatorenal syndrome. Expert Opin Pharmacother 2011;12:1405–17.
22 Trawalé JM, Paradis V, Rautou PE, et al. The spectrum of renal lesions in patients with cirrhosis: a clinicopathological study. Liver Int 2010;30:725–32.
23 Wong F, Murray P. Kidney damage biomarkers: novel tools for the diagnostic assessment of acute kidney injury in cirrhosis. Hepatology 2014;60:455–7.
24 Boyer TD, Sanyal AJ, Garcia-Tsao G, et al. Predictors of response to terlipressin plus albumin in hepatorenal syndrome (HRS) type 1: relationship of serum creatinine to hemodynamics. J Hepatol 2011;55:315–21.
25 Olsen JC, Kamath PS. Acute-on-chronic liver failure: concept, natural history, and prognosis. Curr Opin Crit Care 2011;17:165–9.
26 Fasolato S, Angeli P, Dallagnese L, et al. Renal failure and bacterial infections in patients with cirrhosis: epidemiology and clinical features. Hepatology 2007;45:223–9.
27 Gustot T, Durand F, Lebrec D, et al. Severe sepsis in cirrhosis. Hepatology 2009;50:2022–33.
28 Perdomo Coral G, Alves de Mattos A. Renal impairment after spontaneous bacterial peritonitis: incidence and prognosis. Can J Gastroenterol 2003;17:187–90.
29 Terra C, Guevara M, Torre A, et al. Renal failure in patients with cirrhosis and sepsis unrelated to spontaneous bacterial peritonitis: value of MELD score. Gastroenterology 2005; 129:1944–53.
30 European Association for the Study of the Liver. EASL clinical practice guidelines on the management of ascites, spontaneous bacterial peritonitis, and hepatorenal syndrome in cirrhosis. J Hepatol 2010;53:397–417.
31 Sort P, Navasa M, Arroyo V, et al. Effect of intravenous albumin on renal impairment and mortality in patients with cirrhosis and spontaneous bacterial peritonitis. N Engl J Med 1999;341:403–9.
32 Chavez-Tapia NC, Barrientos-Gutierrez T, Tellez-Avila F, et al. Meta-analysis: antibiotic prophylaxis for cirrhotic patients with upper gastrointestinal bleeding – an updated Cochrane review. Aliment Pharmacol Ther 2011;34: 509–18.
33 Saner FH, Canbay A, Gerken G, et al. Pharmacology, clinical efficacy and safety of terlipressin in esophageal varices bleeding, septic shock and hepatorenal syndrome. Expert Rev Gastroenterol Hepatol 2007;1:207–17.
34 Kiszka-Kanewitz M, Henricksen JH, Hansen EF, et al. Effect of terlipressin on blood volume distribution in patients with cirrhosis. Scand J Gastroenterol 2004;39:486–92.
35 Jalan R, Forrest EH, Redhead DN, et al. Reduction in renal blood flow following acute increase in the portal pressure: evidence for the existence of a hepatorenal reflex in man? Gut 1997;40:664–70.
36 Sanyal AJ, Boyer T, Garcia-Tsao G, et al. A randomized, prospective, double-blind, placebo-controlled trial of terlipressin for type 1 hepatorenal syndrome. Gastroenterology 2008;134:1360–8.
37 Martín-Llahí M, Pépin MN, Guevara M, et al. Terlipressin and albumin vs albumin in patients with cirrhosis and hepatorenal syndrome: a randomized study. Gastroenterology 2008;134:1352–9.

38 Nazar A, Pereira GH, Guevara M, et al. Predictors of response to therapy with terlipressin and albumin in patients with cirrhosis and type 1 hepatorenal syndrome. Hepatology 2010;51:219–26.
39 Angeli P, Fasolato S, Cavallin M, et al. Terlipressin given as continuous intravenous infusion is the more suitable schedule for the treatment of type 1 hepatorenal syndrome (HRS) in patients with cirrhosis: results of a controlled clinical trial. Hepatology 2008;48 (Suppl): 378A.
40 Gerbes AL, Huber E, Gülberg V. Terlipressin for hepatorenal syndrome: continuous infusion as an alternative to i.v. bolus administration. Gastroenterology 2009;137: 1179–81.
41 Piano S, Morando F, Fasolato S, et al. Continuous recurrence of type 1 hepatorenal syndrome and long-term treatment with terlipressin and albumin: a new exception to MELD score in the allocation system to liver transplantation? J Hepatol 2011;55:491–6.
42 Caraceni P, Santi L, Mirici F, et al. Long-term treatment of hepatorenal syndrome as a bridge to liver transplantation. Dig Liver Dis 2011;43:242–5.
43 Angeli P, Volpin R, Gerunda G, et al. Reversal of type 1 hepatorenal syndrome with the administration of midodrine and octreotide. Hepatology 1999;29:1690–7.
44 Wong F, Pantea L, Sniderman K. The use of midodrine, octreotide and transjugular intrahepatic portosystemic stent shunt in the treatment of cirrhotic patients with ascites and renal dysfunction including hepatorenal syndrome. Hepatology 2004;40:55–64.
45 Esrailian E, Pantangco ER, Kyulo NL, et al. Octreotide/midodrine therapy significantly improves renal function and 30-day survival in patients with type 1 hepatorenal syndrome. Dig Dis Sci 2007;52:742–8.
46 Skagen C, Einstein M, Lucey MR, et al. Combination treatment with octreotide, midodrine, and albumin improves survival in patients with type 1 and type 2 hepatorenal syndrome. J Clin Gastroenterol 2009;43:680–5.
47 Cavallin M, Merli M, Fasolato S, et al. Terlipressin and albumin vs. midodrine plus octreotide and albumin in the treatment of hepatorenal syndrome in patients with cirrhosis: results of a controlled clinical trial by the Italian Association for the Study of the Liver. Hepatology 2011;54 (Suppl 1): 1426A.
48 Pomier-Layrargues G, Paquin SC, Hassoun Z, et al. Octreotide in hepatorenal syndrome: a randomized, double-blind, placebo-controlled, crossover study. Hepatology 2003;38: 238–43.
49 Sharma P, Kumar A, Shrama BC, et al. An open label, pilot, randomized controlled trial of noradrenaline versus terlipressin in the treatment of type 1 hepatorenal syndrome and predictors of response. Am J Gastroenterol 2008;103: 1689–97.
50 Alessandria C, Ottobrelli A, Debernardi-Venon W, et al. Noradrenalin vs terlipressin in patients with hepatorenal syndrome: a prospective, randomized, unblinded, pilot study. J Hepatol 2007;47:499–505.
51 Singh V, Ghosh S, Singh B, et al. Noradrenaline versus terlipressin in the treatment of hepatorenal syndrome: a randomized study. J Hepatol 2012;56:1293–8.
52 Dobre M, Demirjian S, Sehgal AR, et al. Terlipressin in hepatorenal syndrome: a systematic review and meta-analysis. Int Urol Nephrol 2011;43:175–84.
53 Gluud LL, Christensen K, Christensen E, et al. Systematic review of randomized trials on vasoconstrictor drugs for hepatorenal syndrome. Hepatology 2010;51:576–84.
54 Sagi SV, Mittal S, Kasturi KS, et al. Terlipressin therapy for reversal of type 1 hepatorenal syndrome: a meta-analysis of randomized controlled trials. J Gastroenterol Hepatol 2010;25:880–5.
55 Neri S, Pulvirenti D, Malaguarnera M, et al. Terlipressin and albumin in patients with cirrhosis and type I hepatorenal syndrome. Dig Dis Sci 2008;53:830–5.
56 Moreau R, Durand F, Poynard T, et al. Terlipressin in patients with cirrhosis and type 1 hepatorenal syndrome: a retrospective multicenter study. Gastroenterology 2002; 122:923–30.
57 Ortega R, Ginès P, Uriz J, et al. Terlipressin therapy with and without albumin for patients with hepatorenal syndrome: results of a prospective, nonrandomized study. Hepatology 2002;36:941–8.
58 Lake JR, Ring E, LaBerge J, et al. Transjugular intrahepatic portacaval stent shunts in patients with renal insufficiency. Transplant Proc 1993;25:1766–7.
59 Brensing KA, Textor J, Strunk H, et al. Transjugular intrahepatic portosystemic stent-shunt for hepatorenal syndrome. Lancet 1997;349:697–8.
60 Brensing KA, Textor J, Perz J, et al. Long term outcome after transjugular intrahepatic portosystemic stent-shunt in non-transplant cirrhotics with hepatorenal syndrome: a phase II study. Gut 2000;47:288–95.
61 Guevara M, Gines P, Bandi JC, et al. Transjugular intrahepatic portosystemic shunt in hepatorenal syndrome: effects on renal function and vasoactive systems. Hepatology 1998;28:416–22.
62 Rössle M, Gerbes AL. TIPS for the treatment of refractory ascites, hepatorenal syndrome and hepatic hydrothorax: a critical update. Gut 2010;59:988–1000.
63 Guerrini GP, Pleguezuelo M, Maimone S, et al. Impact of TIPS pre-liver transplantation for the outcome post transplantation. Am J Transplant 2009;9:192–200.
64 Jalan R, Sen S, Steiner C, et al. Extracorporeal liver support with molecular adsorbents recirculating system in patients with severe acute alcoholic hepatitis. J Hepatol 2003;38: 24–31.
65 Di Campli C, Santoro MC, Gaspari R, et al. Catholic university experience with molecular adsorbent recycling system in patients with severe liver failure. Transplant Proc 2005;37: 2547–50.

66 Mitzner SR, Stange J, Klammt S, et al. Improvement of hepatorenal syndrome with extracorporeal albumin dialysis MARS: results of a prospective, randomized, controlled clinical trial. Liver Transpl 2000;6:277–86.
67 Wong F, Raina N, Richardson R. Molecular adsorbent recirculating system is ineffective in the management of type 1 hepatorenal syndrome in patients with cirrhosis with ascites who have failed vasoconstrictor treatment. Gut 2010;59:381–6.
68 Wong F. Management of ascites in cirrhosis. J Gastroenterol Hepatol 2012;27:11–20.
69 Ruiz-del-Arbol L, Monescillo A, Jimenéz W, et al. Paracentesis-induced circulatory dysfunction: mechanism and effect on hepatic hemodynamics in cirrhosis. Gastroenterology 1997;113:579–86.
70 Alessandria C, Venon WD, Marzano A, et al. Renal failure in cirrhotic patients: Role of terlipressin in clinical approach to hepatorenal syndrome type 2. Eur J Gastroenterol Hepatol 2002;14:1363–8.
71 Alessandria C, Ottobrelli A, Debernardi-Venon W, et al. Noradrenalin vs. terlipressin in patients with hepatorenal syndrome: a prospective, randomized, unblinded, pilot study. J Hepatol 2007;47:499–505.
72 Testro AG, Wongseelashote S, Angus PW, et al. Long-term outcome of patients treated with terlipressin for types 1 and 2 hepatorenal syndrome. J Gastroenterol Hepatol 2008;23: 1535–40.
73 Testino G, Ferro C, Sumberaz A, et al. Type-2 hepatorenal syndrome and refractory ascites: role of transjugular intrahepatic portosystemic stent-shunt in eighteen patients with advanced cirrhosis awaiting orthotopic liver transplantation. Hepatogastroenterology 2003;50:1753–5.
74 Wong LP, Blackley MP, Andreoni KA, et al. Survival of liver transplant candidates with acute renal failure receiving renal replacement therapy. Kidney Int 2005;68:362–70.
75 Leung W, Al Beshir M, Marquez M, et al. Is type 1 hepatorenal syndrome reversible after liver transplantation? J Hepatol 2012;56 (Suppl 2): S258–9.
76 Marik PE, Wood K, Starzl TE. The course of type 1 hepatorenal syndrome post liver transplantation. Nephrol Dial Transplant 2006;21:478–82.
77 Hadengue A, Lebrec D, Moreau R, et al. Persistence of systemic and splanchnic hyperkinetic circulation in liver transplant patients. Hepatology 1993;17:175–8.
78 Restuccia T, Ortega R, Guevara M, et al. Effects of treatment of hepatorenal syndrome before transplantation on post-transplantation outcome: a case–control study. J Hepatol 2004;40:140–6.
79 Ginès P. Hepatorenal syndrome, pharmacological therapy, and liver transplantation. Liver Transpl 2011;17: 1244–6.
80 Locke JE, Warren DS, Singer AL, et al. Declining outcomes in simultaneous liver-kidney transplantation in the MELD era: ineffective usage of renal allografts. Transplantation 2008;85:935–42.
81 Davis CL, Feng S, Sung R, et al. Simultaneous liver–kidney transplantation: Evaluation to decision making. Am J Transplant 2007;7:1702–09.
82 Somsouk M, Guy J, Biggins SW, et al. Ascites improves upon serum sodium plus Model for End-Stage Liver Disease (MELD) for predicting mortality in patients with advanced liver disease. Aliment Pharmacol Ther 2009;30: 741–8.
83 Somsouk M, Kornfield, R, Vittinghoff E, et al. Moderate ascites identifies patients with low Model for End-Stage Liver Disease scores awaiting liver transplantation who have a high mortality risk. Liver Transpl 2011;17:129–36.
84 Warner NS, Cuthbert JA, Bhore R, et al. Acute kidney injury and chronic kidney disease in hospitalized patients with cirrhosis. J Investig Med 2011;59:1244–51.
85 Mehta RL, Kellum JA, Shah SV, et al. Acute Kidney Injury Network: report of an initiative to improve outcomes in acute kidney injury. Crit Care 2007;11:R31.
86 Lopes JA, Melo MJ, Costa AC, et al. Acute kidney injury and in-hospital mortality in critically ill patients with cirrhosis: a cohort study. Gut 2012;61:955–6.
87 Lassnigg A, Schmidlin D, Mouhieddine M, et al. Minimal changes of serum creatinine predict prognosis in patients after cardiothoracic surgery: a prospective cohort study. J Am Soc Nephrol 2004;15:1597–605.
88 Wong F, Nadim MK, Kellum JA, et al. Working Party proposal for a revised classification system of renal dysfunction in patients with cirrhosis. Gut 2011;60:702–9.
89 Wong F, O'Leary JG, Reddy KR, et al. New consensus definition of acute kidney injury accurately predicts 30-day mortality in patients with cirrhosis and infection. Gastroenterology 2013;145:1280–8.

CHAPTER 17

The hepatopulmonary syndrome

Moises Ilan Nevah Rubin and Michael B. Fallon
Division of Gastroenterology, Hepatology and Nutrition, Department of Internal Medicine, The University of Texas Health Science Center at Houston, Houston, TX, USA

Introduction

Cirrhosis and portal hypertension are associated with alterations in the vasculature in a number of organ systems that alter function in these organs and lead to increased mortality. Although the initial hemodynamic abnormality in cirrhosis is the development of an increased portosystemic gradient (the gradient between the portal vein and the systemic circulation) due to disrupted liver architecture and intrahepatic vasoconstriction, this is promptly followed by splanchnic vasodilatation which, in turn, is followed by systemic vasodilatation. Splanchnic and systemic vasodilatation lead to decreased effective blood volume that activates baroreceptors and neurohumoral systems and is followed by sodium and water retention, increased plasma volume expansion, and cardiac output and, hence, a hyperdynamic circulatory state. Although the development of portal hypertension and a hyperdynamic circulatory state underlie organ dysfunction in liver disease, the specific mechanisms involved appear to vary between organs and are incompletely characterized.

One recently recognized end-organ complication of cirrhosis is the hepatopulmonary syndrome (HPS), which results from vascular dilatation and/or angiogenesis in the pulmonary arteriolar circulation [1,2]. The major clinical manifestation is hypoxemia and the presence of HPS has a direct impact on pre- and post-liver transplant mortality [3–5]. The only known cure for the syndrome is liver transplantation.

Definition

HPS is defined as vascular alterations in pulmonary gas exchange regions, leading to a widened age-corrected alveolar–arterial oxygen gradient (AaPO2) on room air, with or without hypoxemia (AaPO2 $\geq$15 mmHg, or $\geq$20 mmHg, in patients $\geq$65 years old), in patients with underlying liver disease and/or portal hypertension [1].

The diagnosis of HPS requires the presence of a constellation of clinical and laboratory findings and a high index of suspicion. HPS can occur in patients with compensated or decompensated cirrhosis, and has been described in patients with prehepatic portal hypertension (minimal or no evidence of liver dysfunction) and acute liver injury [6–9].

The pulmonary vascular alterations in HPS result from microvascular dilatation and/or angiogenesis. Exclusion of cardiopulmonary diseases has been a key component of the diagnosis in prior definitions. Currently, it is well established that HPS may occur in patients with coexistent cardiac or pulmonary pathologies and be an important contributor to the degree of hypoxemia (Table 17.1) [1,10,11].

The severity of HPS can be stratified based on the degree of the patient's hypoxemia as: mild (PaO2 $\geq$80 mmHg), moderate (PaO2 $\geq$60 to <80 mmHg), severe (PaO2 $\geq$50 to <60 mmHg), or very severe (PaO2 <50 mmHg) (Table 17.1).

Epidemiology

HPS is relatively common in patients with cirrhosis being evaluated for liver transplantation and may occur across the spectrum of severity of liver disease [12–14]. Intrapulmonary vascular dilatation detected by contrast-enhanced echocardiography is present in 40–60% of patients being evaluated for liver transplantation and as many as 30% have sufficient vascular abnormalities to

Cirrhosis: A practical guide to management, First Edition. Edited by Samuel S. Lee and Richard Moreau.

Table 17.1 Diagnostic criteria and staging for hepatopulmonary syndrome (HPS).

Cirrhosis and/or portal hypertension
Age corrected alveolar–arterial oxygenation gradient ≥15 mmHg or PaO2 <70 mmHg
Intrapulmonary vasodilatation documented on contrast enhanced echocardiography
Absence of abnormalities that can explain hypoxemia (abnormal chest X-ray, pulmonary function tests or CT)
Mild HPS
Alveolar–arterial oxygenation gradient ≥15 mmHg and PaO_2 ≥80 mmHg
Moderate HPS
Alveolar-arterial oxygenation gradient ≥15 mmHg and PaO_2 <80 – ≥60 mmHg
Severe HPS
Alveolar-arterial oxygenation gradient ≥15 mmHg and PaO_2 <60 – ≥50 mmHg
Very severe HPS
Alveolar–arterial oxygenation gradient ≥15 mmHg and PaO_2 <50 mmHg

Adapted from the European Respiratory Society task force on PHD diagnostic criteria for HPS, Rodriguez-Roisin et al, 2004 [1]. CT, computed tomography; PaO_2, partial pressure of oxygen in the arterial blood.

impair gas exchange and cause a widened alveolar–arterial oxygen gradient [5,12,14,15]. Severe HPS, defined as a PaO2 <60 mmHg on room air, is found in 5–15% of patients evaluated for liver transplantation [1]. Although some studies find HPS to be more common in more advanced liver disease and in more severe portal hypertension, it clearly occurs in both compensated cirrhosis and in settings where portal hypertension is present in the absence of cirrhosis. In a prospective multicenter US study, the severity of liver disease was not different between patients with and without HPS [5].

HPS is commonly found in the setting of cirrhosis. It appears to occur less commonly in smokers and may be more common in Caucasians than in Hispanics or African-Americans. HPS has been described in portal hypertension without cirrhosis (prehepatic portal hypertension, nodular regenerative hyperplasia, congenital hepatic fibrosis, and hepatic venous outflow obstruction) [6,7,16] and hepatic dysfunction in the absence of established portal hypertension (acute and chronic hepatitis) [8,9,17]. Intrapulmonary shunting and hypoxemia have also been reported in metastatic carcinoid in the absence of portal hypertension [18] and in children with congenital cardiovascular abnormalities that result in reduced hepatic venous drainage to the lungs [19–21]. Together these observations suggest that factors normally produced or metabolized in the liver may influence the lung microvasculature in susceptible individuals when hepatic function or blood flow are altered.

Pathogenesis

HPS develops when pulmonary microvascular dilatation and/or angiogenesis develops in the setting of liver disease (Figure 17.1). The mechanisms that trigger these microvascular changes are incompletely characterized. In experimental HPS induced by common bile duct ligation (CBDL), both pulmonary microvascular dilatation and angiogenesis contribute to altered gas exchange [2,13]. Similar changes are not observed in other rodent models of cirrhosis and portal hypertension, suggesting that CBDL triggers unique molecular events that influence the pulmonary microvasculature [22–24]. The two most well-recognized events include increased microvascular endothelin signaling and accumulation of monocytes in the microvascular lumen. Upregulated endothelin-1 (ET-1) signaling occurs via increased circulating ET-1 levels, in part derived from cholangiocytes, and by increased lung endothelial endothelin B (ET_B) receptor expression in response to increased shear stress due to systemic vascular changes [25–27]. The result is enhanced ET_B receptor mediated endothelial-derived nitric oxide (NO) production. Monocyte accumulation within the microvasculature is enhanced by ET-1 alterations and also by tumor necrosis factor α (TNF-α) production from bacterial translocation of intestinal micro-organisms and possibly specific overexpression of monocyte chemotactic and angiogenic chemokines (i.e., fractalkine) [2,23–25,28–31]. Intravascular monocytes are an important source for local pulmonary production of NO, carbon monoxide (CO), and vascular endothelial growth factor (VEGF) which contribute to vascular and gas exchange abnormalities. Recently, *in vitro* studies have demonstrated that upregulation of the ERK signaling pathway and cholangiocyte VEGF overexpression may be associated with cholangiocyte ET-1 production [32]. Accordingly, in CBDL animals, inhibition of TNF-α, ET_B receptor signaling, CO production, tyroxine kinase receptor, or angiogenesis ameliorate HPS [2,23–25,28,29,33].

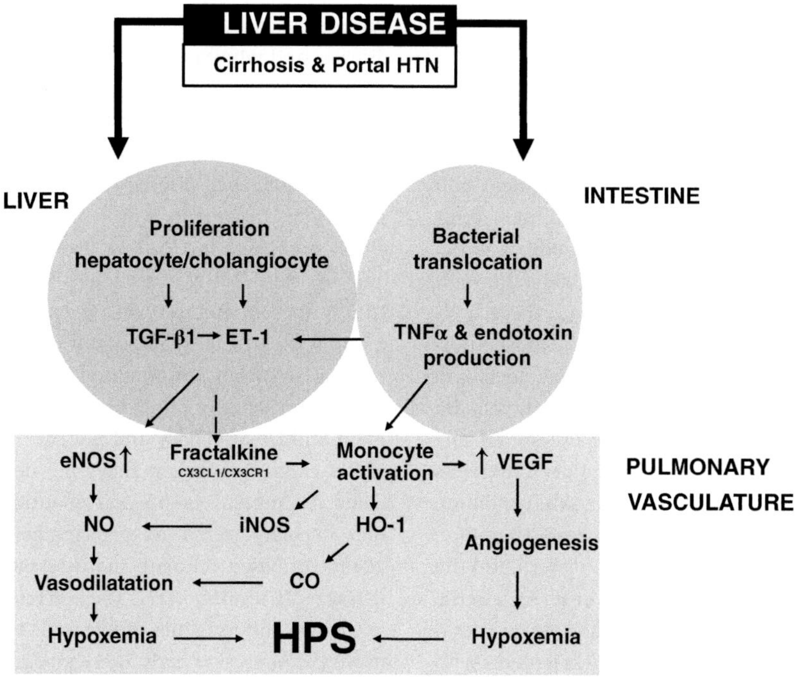

Figure 17.1 Pathogenesis of the hepatopulmonary syndrome. CO, carbon monoxide; eNOS, endothelial nitric oxide synthase; ET-1, endothelin-1; HO-1, heme oxygenase-1; HTN, hypertension; iNOS, inducible nitric oxide synthase; NO, nitric oxide; TGF-β1, transforming growth factor β1; TNFα, tumor necrosis factor α; VEGF, vascular endothelial growth factor.

Less is known about the pathogenesis of human HPS and how the mechanisms identified in the development of experimental HPS contribute to human disease. The fact that HPS occurs across a spectrum of etiologies and disease and portal hypertension severity and develops in less than 50% of cirrhotic patients, suggest that HPS develops in patients with an underlying predisposition. The recent finding that genetic variation in genes associated with vascular growth and development is associated with the risk of HPS raises the possibility that genetic susceptibility to angiogenesis might be a predisposing factor [34]. Systemic and pulmonary production of NO is increased in HPS, but is also increased in cirrhotic patients without HPS [35–38]. Inhibition of NO production does not reliably improve HPS despite improving systemic hemodynamics [35–38]. Therefore, the precise role of NO in human HPS is unknown. CO production does appear to be selectively increased in human HPS, although whether this derives from lung production or influences the vasculature is not known. Finally, whether monocytes adhere in the lung vasculature in human HPS, via increased circulating levels of adhesion molecules, and whether inhibition of TNF-α or bacterial translocation across the gastrointestinal tract alter the severity of HPS are not well defined [28,33,39,40].

The pathogenesis of altered oxygenation in HPS derives from the changes in the pulmonary microvascular bed. In humans, capillary dilatation and pleural arteriovenous malformations have been described in a limited number of cases [6,7,19,20,41]. In experimental HPS, both pulmonary vascular dilatation and angiogenesis occur [2,42]. Three mechanisms of hypoxemia have been described in human HPS: anatomic arteriovenous shunting, ventilation–perfusion mismatch (increased capillary blood flow), and diffusion–perfusion mismatching (impaired passage of oxygen from the alveolus into the vasculature). The relative contribution of these mechanisms to gas exchange abnormalities appear to vary based on the severity of HPS [43].

Clinical features

The majority of patients with HPS are either asymptomatic, particularly if discovered during evaluation for liver transplantation (LT), or develop the insidious onset of dyspnea [44]. Classically, dyspnea (platypnea) and hypoxemia (orthodeoxia) increase in the upright position in HPS due to the predominance of vasodilatation in the lung bases and the increased blood flow through these regions when upright [45]. However, these findings are uncommon and are of limited diagnostic utility [46,47]. Several other clinical features including spider angiomata, digital clubbing, and cyanosis, are also commonly described in HPS but are also not reliable diagnostic indicators. In addition, respiratory symptoms are common in cirrhosis due to poor physical condition, smoking, ascites, and/or intrinsic lung disease. Therefore, the presence of HPS may be difficult to discern and the diagnosis delayed and identified only after severe arterial hypoxemia has ensued. Finally, sleep-time oxygen desaturation also appears to occur commonly in patients with HPS and may worsen hypoxemia at night [48].

Chest radiography (CXR), chest computed tomography (CT), and/or pulmonary function tests (PFT) are often performed to evaluate dyspnea in cirrhosis and during LT evaluation. Commonly, CXR is normal in HPS even when hypoxemia is severe. However, lower lobe interstitial markings resulting from dilated vessels may be present and are often confused with pulmonary fibrosis [12,49]. Dilated vessels as well as parenchymal fibrosis may be visible on high resolution chest CT, but its role in the diagnosis of HPS has not been established. PFTs typically demonstrate well-preserved spirometry and lung volumes. However, the diffusing capacity for carbon monoxide (DLCO) is often reduced and may suggest the diagnosis. However, a decrease in DLCO commonly occurs in cirrhosis in the absence of HPS, limiting diagnostic utility [50,51].

Diagnosis

The diagnosis of HPS requires a high degree of clinical suspicion and rests on documentation of the presence of arterial gas exchange abnormalities resulting from intrapulmonary vasodilatation in the appropriate clinical setting. The threshold for pursuing the diagnosis is influenced by the presence of specific signs and symptoms, risk factors for intrinsic cardiopulmonary disease, and whether LT is being considered. In patients with risk factors for intrinsic cardiopulmonary disease (smoking and other cardiovascular risk factors, occupational exposure, liver diseases associated with intrinsic lung disease) such diseases are appropriate initial considerations. In patients with clubbing or dyspnea in the absence of risks for intrinsic cardiopulmonary disease and in those being considered for LT, screening for HPS is appropriate and cost-effective [52]. In the latter group it is particularly important to diagnose and differentiate HPS from portopulmonary hypertension, given that the presence of these disorders may influence treatment and LT candidacy and priority.

Gas exchange abnormalities are detected by arterial blood gas measurements and quantified by calculating the alveolar–arterial oxygen gradient (AaPO2 >15–20 mmHg based on age) and assessing for hypoxemia (PaO2 <70 mmHg) [1]. The inclusion of mild gas exchange abnormalities (increased AaPO2, PaO2 <70 mmHg, described as early HPS) appears to be important; based on recent findings, mortality is increased even in this subset of HPS patients relative to non-HPS cirrhotics [53,54]. Obtaining arterial blood gases in the sitting position may enhance the detection of arterial deoxygenation in HPS. Pulse oximetry is an established screening modality for detecting hypoxemia and HPS in patients being evaluated for LT. Using a threshold SpO2 value of <96% provides a sensitivity of 100% and specificity of 88% for detecting HPS patients with a PaO2 of <70 mmHg [55,56]. This technique can target the use of tests for HPS to those with a higher risk of disease. Those patients with a pulse oximetry of <96% should undergo further testing with room arterial blood gases and contrast echocardiography to exclude or confirm the diagnosis of HPS. Based on the utility of pulse oximetry for detecting hypoxemia in a wide range of disorders, this technique may also be useful for HPS screening in the general cirrhotic population (Figure 17.2).

In adults, contrast echocardiography using a transthoracic approach is the most sensitive and commonly employed screening technique for detecting intrapulmonary vascular dilatation. It is the preferred modality for the diagnosis of intrapulmonary shunting. Lung perfusion scanning, pulmonary angiography, and high resolution chest CT scanning are additional studies that may be useful as adjunctive tests. Typically, agitated saline is used to generate microbubbles during echocardiography.

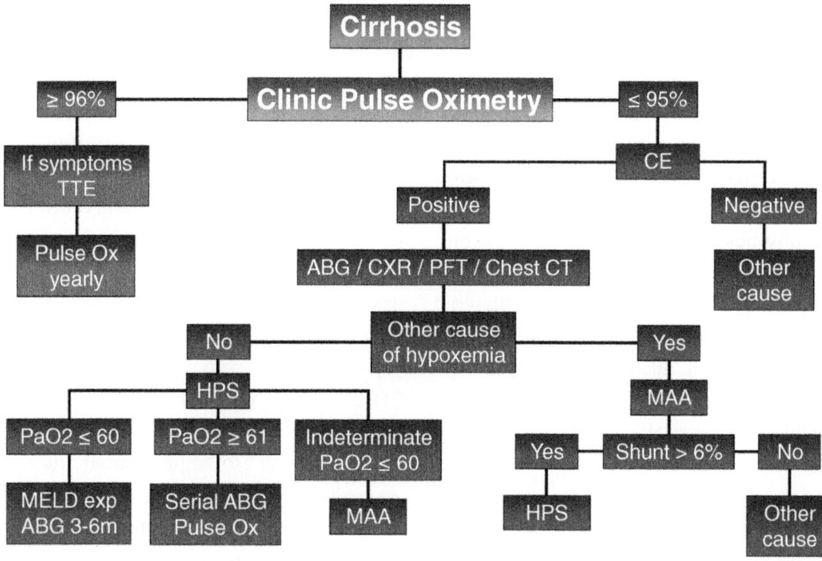

Figure 17.2 Evaluation of hypoxemia (based on pulse oximetry) in patients with cirrhosis. ABG, arterial blood gas; CE, contrast echocardiography; CT, computed tomography; CXR, chest X-ray; HPS, hepatopulmonary syndrome; MAA, macroaggregated albumin scan; MELD, model for end-stage liver disease; PaO2, partial pressure of oxygen; PFT, pulmonary function test; Pulse Ox, pulse oximetry; TTE, transthoracic echocardiography.

Intrapulmonary shunting and vasodilatation are considered when microbubbles are observed in the left cardiac chambers three cardiac cycles after intravenous injection [57–59]. Immediate visualization of injected contrast (microbubbles) in the left heart indicates intracardiac shunting. Transesophageal contrast echocardiography may increase the sensitivity of detecting intrapulmonary vasodilatation compared to transthoracic echocardiography, but is invasive and more expensive [57–59]. Echocardiography also assesses cardiac function and estimates pulmonary arterial systolic pressure, and is useful for screening for cardiac dysfunction and portopulmonary hypertension. As many as 40–60% of patients with cirrhosis and normal arterial blood gases may have a positive contrast echocardiogram, suggesting that mild intrapulmonary vasodilatation insufficient to alter gas exchange is common in cirrhotics [54,59,60]. Also, a positive result on contrast echocardiography in a hypoxemic patient with concomitant pulmonary dysfunction (pleural effusion, chronic obstructive pulmonary disease) does not establish HPS as a cause of gas exchange abnormalities, because either intrapulmonary vasodilatation or the underlying pulmonary process could be responsible. In these patients, additional testing with radionuclide lung perfusion scanning may be useful.

Radionuclide lung perfusion scanning using 20 μm technetium-labeled macroaggregated albumin particles (^{99m}TcMAA scan) may be used to quantify intrapulmonary shunting in HPS. Normally, all particles are trapped in the lung microvasculature, but in HPS, some particles escape through abnormal capillaries and lodge downstream. Quantitative imaging of the lung and brain using a standardized methodology has been validated as a means to calculate a shunt fraction [42,59,61]. Using this methodology, a positive ^{99m}TcMAA scan (shunt fraction >6%) is found only in HPS patients with a PaO2 <60 mmHg and not in those with intrinsic lung disease alone [59,61]. Therefore, a positive scan supports the presence of advanced HPS even in the setting of coexistent intrinsic lung disease. However, as a screening test in adults, ^{99m}TcMAA scanning is less sensitive than contrast echocardiography in detecting intrapulmonary vasodilatation in adults, and cannot evaluate cardiac function, intracardiac shunting, or pulmonary artery pressures.

Pulmonary angiography is an invasive and insensitive diagnostic modality for detecting intrapulmonary vasodilatation in HPS and is not useful as a screening test. Two types of angiographic findings have been reported: type 1, a diffuse "spongiform" appearance of pulmonary vessels during the arterial phase; and type 2, small discrete arteriovenous communications. The great majority of patients with HPS have either normal angiograms or type 1 findings even when hypoxemia is severe. Therefore, angiography has a very limited diagnostic or therapeutic role in HPS [62,63]. High-resolution chest CT may be a less invasive radiologic method to detect dilated pulmonary vessels and intrapulmonary shunting in HPS [18,64,65]. The degree of dilatation observed on CT has been found to correlate with the severity of gas exchange abnormalities in several studies, suggesting that CT may be useful in assessing the presence and severity of HPS.

Natural history and treatment

The natural history of HPS is incompletely characterized, although quality of life and survival are adversely affected by its presence [53]. Over time, the majority of patients appear to develop progressive intrapulmonary vasodilatation and worsening gas exchange, and spontaneous improvement, though reported, is rare [66]. Mortality in pretransplant patients with HPS is increased twofold relative to unaffected cirrhotic patients [3,4,53], although recent data suggest that pretransplantation HPS, regardless of severity, may not affect post-transplant mortality [67,68]. In addition, many patients with moderate to severe HPS have comparatively well-preserved hepatic synthetic function, making it likely that the presence of HPS will contribute to poor outcomes [4,53,69].

Currently, LT is the only effective treatment for patients with HPS and complete resolution of gas exchange abnormalities is reported in more than 80% of such patients [42,70]. However, an early prospective study found that those with severe HPS (preoperative PaO2 $\leq$50 mmHg and ^{99m}TcMAA shunt fraction $\geq$20%) had a marked increase in postoperative mortality, in part due to the development of unique postoperative complications recognized in these patients [71]. These findings support the current practice of providing model for end-stage liver disease (MELD) exception points to cirrhotic patients with HPS and a PaO2 <60 mmHg listed for LT. Since this initial study, a number of additional small studies and an analysis of Scientific Registry of Transplant Recipients data have found 1–3 year mortality after LT in HPS to range widely from 5% to 42% [3,4,15,67,68,71–74]. These studies highlight the need to define more precisely the influence of HPS on LT outcomes to guide MELD exception policy [75].

There is no effective or approved medical therapy for HPS. Somatostatin, almitrine, indomethacin, inhaled (nebulized) L-NAME, aspirin, and plasma exchange have all been tried without clear benefit [12,42].

In experimental HPS, inhibition of heme oxygenase-1 (by Tin protoporphyrin and Quercetin) has decreased CO-mediated vascular dilatation and improved gas exchange and intrapulmonary shunting [23,76]; human studies have yet to be performed and more information is needed.

A small open labeled clinical trial, several case reports, and a recent prospective trial using garlic have shown some benefit in HPS [77–81]. In this last trial, garlic was administered in a dosage of 1–2 mg/m^2/day. After 9 months of therapy, there was a statistically significant improvement in oxygen levels and decrease in AaPO2. This trial also documented reversal of HPS and survival benefits in a subset of treated patients. Further studies are required to validate these findings.

Recent case reports describe spontaneous resolution of HPS after complete withdrawal of methadone in two separate cirrhotic patients. Both patients had hepatitis C as the cause for their underlying liver disease; one of them achieved sustained virologic response after interferon and ribavirin therapy, 3 years prior to the resolution of the syndrome. Dyspnea and exercise tolerance improved after a few months of methadone withdrawal and, objectively, there was a significant decrease in the shunt fraction in the macroaggregated albumin scan. The authors hypothesize a role for opiate receptors in modulating NO signaling and release as the pathophysiologic mechanism for the effects [82,83].

Norfloxacin has been described in rat models to improve HPS by presumed decrease in bacterial translocation and endotoxemia which in turn reduces NO-mediated pulmonary vascular dilatation [29]. A published case report supported this hypothesis in a patient with hepatitis C cirrhosis, HPS, and brain abscess that experienced resolution of hypoxemia after successful treatment of the infectious process with the antibiotic [84]. The only randomized controlled trial of norfloxacin in humans failed to demonstrate improvement in oxygenation and AaPO2 [85].

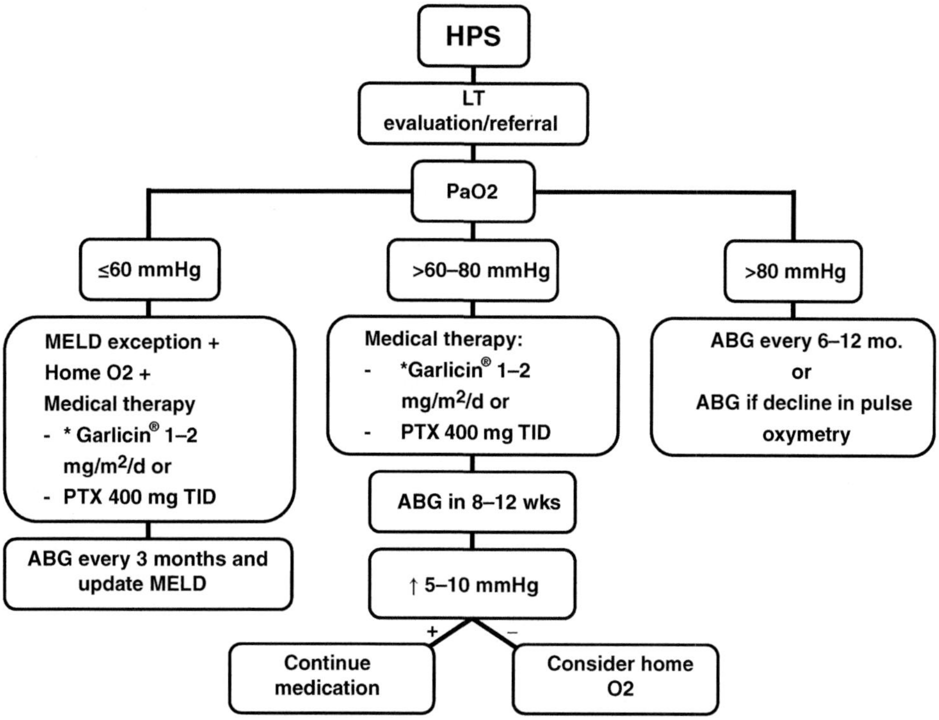

Figure 17.3 Proposed treatment algorithm for hepatopulmonary syndrome. ABG, arterial blood gas; HPS, hepatopulmonary syndrome; LT, liver transplantation; MELD, model for end-stage liver disease; mmHg, millimeters of mercury; PaO2, partial pressure of oxygen; PTX, pentoxifylline; TID, three times daily.

Recently, pentoxifylline (PTX), a phosphodiesterase inhibitor with known mild TNF-α and NO inhibitory properties, has been linked to improved oxygenation in experimental HPS [86–88]. However, in human HPS results with PTX are conflicting. In one study, tolerability of the drug was poor and no oxygenation benefit was observed after 6 weeks of therapy [87]. In a second study, tolerability to PTX was not a limiting factor and there was an overall improvement in PaO2 of more than 10 mmHg after 3 months of treatment [88]. The dose of PTX used in both trials was 400 mg three times daily. No studies have explored whether endothelin receptor antagonists or angiogenesis inhibitors, which have benefit in experimental HPS, are effective in human disease [2,25].

A number of case reports have evaluated the effects of lowering portal pressure with transjugular intrahepatic portosystemic shunt (TIPS) on HPS. Although several have reported significant improvement, no benefit has been found in others, making assessments of utility difficult [89–93]. These reports highlight the need to identify and target likely pathogenetic mechanisms and undertake randomized multicenter trials of sufficient size to determine efficacy. A recommended therapeutic algorithm is outlined in Figure 17.3.

Conclusions

The HPS is a common vascular complication of cirrhosis, and its presence increases mortality in cirrhotic patients. Identification of this syndrome requires thorough clinical evaluation, basic laboratory tests, exclusion of other disorders, and a high index of suspicion. The pathophysiology is distinct and yet to be fully characterized, but there is a key role of vasoactive mediators as initial triggers for vasodilatation and vascular remodeling. Direct actions of these substances in the gas-exchange capillaries, appear to result in pulmonary vasodilatation and angiogenesis in susceptible individuals leading to hypoxemia. Medical treatment for HPS is suboptimal and definitive therapy currently requires LT.

References

1 Rodriguez-Roisin R, Krowka MJ, Hervé P, Fallon MB; ERS Task Force Pulmonary-Hepatic Vascular Disorders (PHD) Scientific Committee. Pulmonary-hepatic vascular disorders (PHD). Eur Respir J 2004;24:861–80

2 Zhang J, Luo B, Tang L, et al. Pulmonary angiogenesis in a rat model of hepatopulmonary syndrome. Gastroenterology 2009;136:1070–80.

3 Schenk P, Schöniger-Hekele M, Fuhrmann V, Madl C, Silberhumer G, Müller C. Prognostic significance of the hepatopulmonary syndrome in patients with cirrhosis. Gastroenterology 2003;125:1042–52.

4 Swanson K, Wiesner R, Krowka M. Natural history of hepatopulmonary syndrome: impact of liver transplantation. Hepatology 2005;41:1122–9.

5 Fallon MB, Krowka MJ, Brown RS, et al. Impact of hepatopulmonary syndrome on quality of life and survival in liver transplant candidates. Gastroenterology 2008;135: 1168–75.

6 Binay K, Sen S, Biswas PK, Sanyal R, Majumdar D, Biswas J. Hepatopulmonary syndrome in inferior vena cava obstruction responding to cavoplasty. Gastroenterology 2000;118: 192–6.

7 Gupta D, Vijaya DR, Gupta R, et al. Prevalence of hepatopulmonary syndrome in cirrhosis and extrahepatic portal venous obstruction. Am J Gastroenterol 2001;96:3395–9.

8 Fuhrmann V, Madl C, Mueller C, et al. Hepatopulmonary syndrome in patients with hypoxic hepatitis. Gastroenterology 2006;131:69–75.

9 Regev A, Yeshurun M, Rodriguez M, et al. Transient hepatopulmonary syndrome in a patient with acute hepatitis A. J Viral Hep 2001;8:83–6.

10 Martinez G, Barberà JA, Navasa M, Roca J, Visa J, Rodriguez-Roisin R. Hepatopulmonary syndrome associated with cardiorespiratory disease. J Hepatol 1999;30:882–9.

11 Rodríguez-Roisin R, Agusti A, Roca J. The hepatopulmonary syndrome: new name, old complexities. Thorax 1992;47: 897–902.

12 Fallon M, Abrams G. Pulmonary dysfunction in chronic liver disease. Hepatology 2000;32:859–65.

13 Budhiraja R, Hassoun PM. Portopulmonary hypertension. Chest 2003;123:562–76.

14 Ferreira PP, Camara EJ, Paula RL, Zollinger CC, Cavalcanti AR, Bittencourt PL. Prevalence of hepatopulmonary syndrome in patients with decompensated chronic liver disease and its impact on short-term survival. Arq Gastroenterol 2008;45:34–7.

15 Pascasio JM, Grilo I, López-Pardo FJ, et al. Prevalence and severity of hepatopulmonary syndrome and its influence on survival in cirrhotic patients evaluated for liver transplantation. Am J Transplant 2014;14:1391–9.

16 Abrams G, Fallon M. The hepatopulmonary syndrome. Clin Liver Dis 1997;1:185–200.

17 Teuber G, Teupe C, Dietrich CF, Caspary WF, Buhl R, Zeuzem S. Pulmonary dysfunction in non-cirrhotic patients with chronic viral hepatitis. Eur J Intern Med 2002;13:311–8.

18 Lee D, Lepler L. Severe intrapulmonary shunting associated with metastatic carcinoid. Chest 1999;115:1203–7.

19 McFaul R, Tajik AJ, Mair DD, Danielson GK, Seward JB. Development of pulmonary arteriovenous shunt after superior vena cava-right pulmonary artery (Glenn) anastamosis: report of four cases. Circulation 1977;55:212–6.

20 Srivastava D, Preminger T, Lock JE, et al. Hepatic venous blood and the development of pulmonary arteriovenous malformations in congenital heart disease. Circulation 1995; 92:1217–22.

21 Duncan BW, Desai S. Pulmonary arteriovenous malformations after cavopulmonary anastomosis. Ann Thorac Surg 2003;76:1759–66.

22 Luo B, Abrams GA, Fallon MB. Endothelin-1 in the rat bile duct ligation model of hepatopulmonary syndrome: correlation with pulmonary dysfunction. J Hepatol 1998;29:571–8.

23 Zhang J, Ling Y, Luo B, et al. Analysis of pulmonary heme oxygenase-1 and nitric oxide synthase alterations in experimental hepatopulmonary syndrome. Gastroenterology 2003;125:1441–51.

24 Nunes H, Lebrec D, Mazmanian M, et al. Role of nitric oxide in hepatopulmonary syndrome in cirrhotic rats. Am J Respir Criti Care Med 2001;164:879–85.

25 Ling Y, Zhang J, Luo B, et al. The role of endothelin-1 and the endothelin B receptor in the pathogenesis of experimental hepatopulmonary syndrome. Hepatology 2004;39:1593–602.

26 Luo B, Liu L, Tang L, et al. Increased pulmonary vascular endothelin B receptor expression and responsiveness to endothelin-1 in cirrhotic and portal hypertensive rats: a potential mechanism in experimental hepatopulmonary syndrome. J Hepatol 2003;38:556–63.

27 Zhang M, Luo B, Chen SJ, Abrams GA, Fallon MB. Endothelin-1 stimulation of endothelial nitric oxide synthase in the pathogenesis of hepatopulmonary syndrome. Am J Physiol 1999;277:G944–52.

28 Zhang J, Ling Y, Tang L, et al. Pentoxifylline attenuation of experimental hepatopulmonary syndrome. J Appl Physiol 2007;102:949–55.

29 Rabiller A, Nunes H, Lebrec D, et al. Prevention of gram-negative translocation reduces the severity of hepatopulmonary syndrome. Am J Respir Crit Care Med 2002;166: 514–7.

30 Zhang J, Yang W, Luo B, Hu B, Maheshwari A, Fallon MB. The role of CX3CL1/CX3CR1 in pulmonary angiogenesis and intravascular monocyte accumulation in rat experimental hepatopulmonary syndrome. J Hepatol 2012;57:752–8.

31 Zhang J, Yang W, Hu B, Wu W, Fallon MB. Endothelin-1 activation of the endothelin B receptor modulates pulmonary endothelial CX3CL1 and contributes to pulmonary angiogenesis in experimental hepatopulmonary syndrome. Am J Pathol 2014;184:1706–14.

32 Yang W, Zhang J, Hu B, et al The role of receptor tyrosine kinase activation in cholangiocytes and pulmonary vascular endothelium in experimental hepatopulmonary syndrome. Am J Physiol Gastrointest Liver Physiol 2014;306:G72–80.
33 Sztrymf B, Rabiller A, Nunes H, et al. Prevention of hepatopulmonary syndrome by pentoxifylline in cirrhotic rats. Eur Respir J 2004;23:752–8.
34 Roberts KE, Kowut SM, Krowka MJ, et al. Genetic risk factors for hepatopulmonary syndrome in patients with advanced liver disease. Gastroenterology 2010;139:130–9.
35 Cremona G, Higenbottam TW, Mayoral V, et al. Elevated exhaled nitric oxide in patients with hepatopulmonary syndrome. Eur Respir J 1995;8:1883–5.
36 Degano B, Mittaine M, Hervé P, et al. Nitric oxide production by the alveolar compartment of the lungs in cirrhotic patients. Eur Respir J 2009;34:138–44.
37 Rolla G, Brussino L, Colagrande P, et al. Exhaled nitric oxide and oxygenation abnormalities in hepatic cirrhosis. Hepatology 1997;26:842–7.
38 Rolla G, Brussino L, Colagrande P. Exhaled nitric oxide and impaired oxygenation in cirrhotic patients before and after liver transplantation. Ann Intern Med 1998;129:375–8.
39 Sztrymf B, Libert JM, Mougeot C, et al. Cirrhotic rats with bacterial translocation have higher incidence and severity of hepatopulmonary syndrome. J Gastroenterol Hepatol 2005; 20:1538–44.
40 Raevens S, Coulon S, Van Steenkiste C, et al. Role of angiogenic factors/cell adhesion markers in serum of cirrhotic patients with hepatopulmonary syndrome. Liver Int 2014: in press.
41 Duncan BW, Desai S. Pulmonary arteriovenous malformations after cavopulmonary anastomosis. Ann Thorac Surg 2003;76:1759–66.
42 Rodriguez-Roisin R, Krowka MJ. Hepatopulmonary syndrome: a liver-induced lung vascular disorder. N Engl J Med 2008;358:2378–87.
43 Robert V, Chabot F, Vial B, Guiot P, Poussel JF, Polu JM. Hepatopulmonary syndrome: physiopathology of inpaired gas exchange. Rev Mal Respir 1999;16:769–79.
44 Sood G, Fallon MB, Niwas S, et al. Utility of a dyspnea-fatigue index for screening liver transplant candidates for hepatopulmonary syndrome. Hepatology 1998;28:2319 [abstract].
45 Robin ED, Laman D, Horn BR, Theodore J. Platypnea related to orthodeoxia caused by true vascular lung shunts. N Engl J Med 1976;294:941–3.
46 Gómez FP, Martínez-Pallí G, Barberà JA, Roca J, Navasa M, Rodríguez-Roisin R. Gas exchange mechanism of orthodeoxia in hepatopulmonary syndrome. Hepatology 2004;40:660–6.
47 Martinez GP, Barberà JA, Visa J, et al. Hepatopulmonary syndrome in candidates for liver transplantation. J Hepatol 2001;34:651–7.
48 Palma DT, Philips GM, Arguedas MR, Harding SM, Fallon MB. Oxygen desaturation during sleep in hepatopulmonary syndrome. Hepatology 2008;47:1257–63.
49 Malagari K, Nikita A, Alexopoulou E, et al. Cirrhosis-related intrathoracic disease. Imaging features in 1038 patients. Hepatogastroenterology 2005;52:558–62.
50 Lima B, França AV, Pazin-Filho A, et al. Frequency, clinical characteristics, and respiratory parameters of hepatopulmonary syndrome. Mayo Clin Proc 2004;79:42–8.
51 Møller S, Krag A, Madsen JL, Henriksen JH, Bendtsen F. Pulmonary dysfunction and hepatopulmonary syndrome in cirrhosis and portal hypertension. Liver Int 2009;29:1528–37.
52 Roberts DN, Arguedas MR, Fallon MB. Cost-effectiveness of screening for hepatopulmonary syndrome in liver transplant candidates. Liver Transpl 2007;13:206–14.
53 Fallon MB, Krowka MJ, Brown RS, et al. Impact of hepatopulmonary syndrome on quality of life and survival in liver transplant candidates. Gastroenterology 2008;135:1168–75.
54 Schenk P, Fuhrmann V, Madl C, et al. Hepatopulmonary syndrome: prevalence and predictive value of various cut offs for arterial oxygenation and their clinical consequences. Gut 2002;51:853–9.
55 Abrams GA, Sanders MK, Fallon MB. Utility of pulse oximetry in the detection of arterial hypoxemia in liver transplant candidates. Liver Transpl 2002;8:391–6.
56 Arguedas M, Singh H, Faulk DK, Fallon MB. Utility of pulse oximetry screening for hepatopulmonary syndrome. Clin Gastroenterol Hepatol 2007;5:749–54.
57 Aller R, Moya JL, Boixeda D, et al. Diagnosis of hepatopulmonary syndrome with contrast transesophageal echocardiography: advantages over contrast transthoracic echocardiography. Dig Dis Sci 1999;44:1243–48.
58 Vedrinne JM, Duperret S, Bizollon T, et al. Comparison of transesophageal and transthoracic contrast echocardiography for detection of an intrapulmonary shunt in liver disease. Chest 1997;111:1236–40.
59 Abrams GA, Jaffe CC, Hoffer PB, Binder HJ, Fallon MB. Diagnostic utility of contrast echocardiography and lung perfusion scan in patients with hepatopulmonary syndrome. Gastroenterology 1995;109:1283–8.
60 Martinez G, Barberà JA, Visa J, et al. Hepatopulmonary syndrome in candidates for liver transplantation. J Hepatol 2001;34:756–8.
61 Abrams G, Nanda NC, Dubovsky EV, Krowka MJ, Fallon MB. Use of macroaggregated albumin lung perfusion scan to diagnose hepatopulmonary syndrome:a new approach. Gastroenterology 1998;114:305–10.
62 Ryu JK, Oh JH. Hepatopulmonary syndrome: angiography and therapeutic embolization. Clin Imaging 2003;27:97–100.
63 Saad NEA, Lee DE, Waldman DL, Saad WE. Pulmonary arterial coil embolization for the management of persistent type I hepatopulmonary syndrome after liver transplantation. J Vasc Interv Radiol 2007;18:1576–80.
64 Koksal D, Kaçar S, Köksal AS, et al. Evaluation of intrapulmonary vascular dilatations with high-resolution computed thorax tomography in patients with hepatopulmonary syndrome. J Clin Gastroenterol 2006;40:77–83.

65 Suga K, Kawakami Y, Iwanaga H, Tokuda O, Matsunaga N. Findings of hepatopulmonary syndrome on breath-hold perfusion SPECT-CT fusion images. Ann Nucl Med 2009;23: 413–9.

66 Umeda A, Tagawa M, Kohsaka T, et al. Hepatopulmonary syndrome can show spontaneous resolution: possible mechanism of portopulmonary hypertension overlap? Respirology 2006;11:120–3.

67 Iyer VN, Swanson KL, Cartin-Ceba R, et al. Hepatopulmonary syndrome: favorable outcomes in the MELD exception era. Hepatology 2013;57:2427–35.

68 Gupta S, Castel H, Rao RV, et al. Improved survival after liver transplantation in patients with hepatopulmonary syndrome. Am J Transplant 2010;10:354–63.

69 Krowka M, Wiseman GA, Burnett OL, et al. Hepatopulmonary syndrome: a prospective study of relationships between severity of liver disease, Pao2 response to 100% oxygen, and brain uptake after 99mTc MAA lung scanning. Chest 2000; 118:615–24.

70 Krowka MJ, Mandell MS, Ramsay MA, et al. Hepatopulmonary syndrome and portopulmonary hypertension: a report of the multicenter liver transplant database. Liver Transpl 2004;10:174–82.

71 Arguedas M, Abrams GA, Krowka MJ, Fallon MB. Prospective evaluation of outcomes and predictors of mortality in patients with hepatopulmonary syndrome undergoing liver transplantation. Hepatology 2003;37:192–7.

72 Deberaldini M, Arcanjo AB, Melo E, et al. Hepatopulmonary syndrome: morbidity and survival after liver transplantation. Transplant Proc 2008;40:3512–6.

73 Schiffer E, Majno P, Mentha G, et al. Hepatopulmonary syndrome increases the postoperative mortality rate following liver transplantation: a prospective study in 90 patients. Am J Transplant 2006;6:1430–7.

74 Taille C, Cadranel J, Bellocq A, et al. Liver transplantation for hepatopulmonary syndrome: a ten-year experience in Paris, France. Transplantation 2003;79:1482–9.

75 Goldberg DS, Krok K, Batra S, Trotter JF, Kawut SM, Fallon MB. Impact of the hepatopulmonary syndrome MELD exception policy on outcomes of patients after liver transplantation: an analysis of the UNOS Database. Gastroenterology 2014;146:1256–65.

76 Tieppo J, Cuevas MJ, Vercelino R, et al. Quercetin administration ameliorates pulmonary complications of cirrhosis in rats. J Nutr 2009;139:1339–46.

77 Abrams GA, Fallon MB. Treatment of hepatopulmonary syndrome with allium sativum L. (garlic): a pilot trial. J Clin Gastroenterol 1998;27:232–5.

78 Akyüz F, Kaymakoğlu S, Demir K, Aksoy N, Adalet I, Okten A. Is there any medical therapeutic option in hepatopulmonary syndrome? A case report. Eur J Intern Med 2005;16: 126–8.

79 De B, Dutta D, Pal SK, Gangopadhyay S, Das Baksi S, Pani A. The role of garlic in hepatopulmonary syndrome: a randomized controlled trial. Can J Gastroenterol 2010;24:183–4.

80 Caldwell S, Jeffers LJ, Narula OS, Lang EA, Reddy KR, Schiff ER. Ancient remedies revisited: does *Allium sativum* (garlic) palliate the hepatopulmonary syndrome? J Clin Gastroenterol 1992;15:248–50.

81 Najafi Sani M, Kianifar HR, Kianee A, Khatami G. Effect of oral garlic on arterial oxygen pressure in children with hepatopulmonary syndrome. World J Gastroenterol 2006; 12:2427–31.

82 Lau EMT, McCaughan G, Torzillo PJ. Improvement in hepatopulmonary syndrome after methadone withdrawal: a case report with implications for disease mechanism. Liver Transpl 2010;16:870–3.

83 Kitzing B, Torzillo PJ, Allman KC. Resolution of hepatopulmonary syndrome after methadone withdrawal as demonstrated by right to left shunt study. Clin Nucl Med 2011;36:152–3.

84 Añel RML, Sheagren JN. Novel presentation and approach to management of hepatopulmonary syndrome with use of antimicrobial agents. Clin Infect Dis 2001;32:e131–6.

85 Gupta S, Faughnan ME, Lilly L, Hutchison S, Fowler R, Bayoumi AM. Norfloxacin therapy for hepatopulmonary syndrome: a pilot randomized controlled trial. Clin Gastroenterol Hepatol 2010;8:1095–8.

86 Zhang J, Ling Y, Tang L, et al. Pentoxifylline attenuation of experimental hepatopulmonary syndrome. J Appl Physiol 2007;102:949–55.

87 Tanikella R, Philips GM, Faulk DK, Kawut SM, Fallon MB. Pilot study of pentoxifylline in hepatopulmonary syndrome. Liver Transpl 2008;14:1199–203.

88 Gupta LB, Kumar A, Jaiswal AK, et al. Pentoxifylline therapy for hepatopulmonary syndrome: a pilot study. Arch Intern Med 2008;168:1820–3.

89 Reigler JL, Lang KA, Johnson SP, Westerman JH. Transjugular intrahepatic portosystemic shunt improves oxygenation in hepatopulmonary syndrome. Gastroenterology 1995;109:978–83.

90 Selim KM, Akriviadis EA, Zuckerman E, Chen D, Reynolds TB. Transjugular intrahepatic portosystemic shunt: a successful treatment for hepatopulmonary syndrome. Am J Gastroenterol 1998;93:455–8.

91 Allgaier HP, Haag K, Ochs A, et al. Hepatopulmonary syndrome: successful treatment by transjugular intrahepatic portosystemic stent-shunt (TIPS). J Hepatol 1995;23:102–5.

92 Paramesh A, Husain SZ, Shneider B, et al. Improvement of hepatopulmonary syndrome after transjugular intrahepatic portasystemic shunting: case report and review of literature. Pediatr Transplantation 2003;7:157–62.

93 Corley DA, Scharschmidt B, Bass N, Somberg K, Gold W. Lack of efficacy of TIPS for hepatopulmonary syndrome. Gastroenterol 1997;113:728–31.

CHAPTER 18

Hyponatremia and other electrolyte/ion disorders

Salvatore Piano,[1] Filippo Morando,[1] and Paolo Angeli[1,2]
[1]*Department of Medicine (DIMED), University of Padova, Padova, Italy*
[2]*Department of Medicine (DIMED), Unit of Hepatic Emergencies and Liver Transplantation, University of Padova, Padova, Italy*

Hyponatremia

Epidemiology and pathogenesis

Unlike hypernatremia, hyponatremia is very common in patients with cirrhosis and ascites. Its prevalence depends on the criteria used to define it. In a prospective study in patients with cirrhosis and ascites, the prevalence of hyponatremia, defined by a serum sodium concentration ≤135 mmol/L, was found to be 28%. Patients with cirrhosis develop two types of hyponatremia: (i) hypovolemic hyponatremia, or (ii) hypervolemic hyponatremia. Hypovolemic hyponatremia is characterized by low serum sodium associated with contraction of plasma volume, lack of edema, ascites, and prerenal renal failure. Hypervolemic or dilutional hyponatremia is due to a marked impairment of renal solute-free water excretion, resulting in a disproportionate renal retention of water with respect to sodium. As a consequence, the most stricking difference between these two conditions lies in the volume status which is reduced in hypovolemic hyponatremia and increased in hypervolemic hyponatremia. Hypervolemic hyponatremia is much more common than hypovolemic hyponatremia in patients with cirrhosis and ascites, thus, this chapter discusses to hypervolemic hyponatremia.

Clinically significant hyponatremia (serum sodium value ≤130 mmol/L) in patients with cirrhosis is associated with severe liver disease as reflected by a high Child–Pugh score, poor control of ascites, and serum creatinine value >108 μmol/L [1]. Its pathogenesis is related to a higher rate of renal retention of water in relation to sodium because of a reduction in solute-free water clearance [2–4]. The pathogenesis of water retention in cirrhosis is complex and involves several factors: increased plasma levels of vasopressin (AVP), reduced renal synthesis of prostaglandins, and reduced delivery of filtrate to the ascending limb of the loop of Henle, the diluting segment of the nephron. Patients with cirrhosis and ascites have increased plasma concentrations of AVP which are closely correlated with the reduction in solute-free water excretion [5–7]. Several studies have provided evidence that increased release [2–4] rather than reduced metabolism of AVP [8] is responsible for the increased plasma concentration of AVP in these patients. Taking into account that most patients with cirrhosis and ascites have a degree of hyponatremia and hypo-osmolality that would suppress AVP release in normal subjects [9], a nonosmotic stimulation of AVP release due to a reduction in effective circulating volume is considered the afferent factor leading to increased plasma concentration of AVP. In this context, it should be highlighted that AVP is part of the neurohumoral response to splanchnic arterial vasodilatation which also includes hyperactivation of antinatiuretic and vasopressor systems such as the renin-angiotensin-aldosterone axis and the sympathetic nervous system [9,10]. Bichet et al. [7] showed that the expansion of central blood volume by means of head-out water immersion suppressed plasma renin activity, and the plasma levels of aldosterone, norephineprine, and AVP, resulting in an improvement in both sodium and water excretion. These results were confirmed, almost 20 years later, by clinical studies that showed that in patients with hepatorenal syndrome (HRS) who responded to the prolonged administration

Cirrhosis: A practical guide to management, First Edition. Edited by Samuel S. Lee and Richard Moreau.

of vasoconstrictors and albumin there was a significant improvement in plasma levels of sodium associated with a decrease in the plasma level of AVP [11,12].

The first step in the action of AVP on water excretion is its binding to V2 receptors on the basolateral membrane of the principal cells of the collecting duct. The activation of the V2 receptors stimulates adenyl cyclase via the stimulatory G protein and promotes the formation of cyclic adenosine monophosphate (cAMP). The post-cAMP events that mediate the increase in water permeability are related to the presence of a number of the water channel family that are exclusively expressed in the principal cells of the collecting duct, aquaporin-2. AVP stimulates the translocation of aquaporin-2 from sub-apical multivescicular bodies to the apical membrane [13]. According to this pathogenetic interpretation of hyponatremia in cirrhosis, urinary excretion of aquaporin-2 would be expected to be increased and not reduced as was found by Esteva-Font et al. [14]. The authors found urinary aquaporin-2 excretion in patients with cirrhosis and hyponatremia lower than in patients without hyponatremia and did not find a correlation between plasma level of AVP and urinary aquaporin-2 excretion. Nevertheless, the reduced urinary excretion of aquaporin-2 in patients with cirrhosis and hyponatremia may represent the molecular basis of the phenomenon of escaping the effects of AVP similar to that found in healthy subjects [14]. In fact, if the AVP–aquaporin-2 system was persistently activated in cirrhosis, solute-free water reabsorption would be permanently increased relative to sodium retention, and serum sodium levels would decline steadily to levels incompatible with life. Fortunately, this does not happen in clinical practice as, in most patients with cirrhosis, hyponatremia, when developed, is stable for weeks or even for a few months. Therefore, in patients with cirrhosis who develop hyponatremia, a reduced availability of aquaporin-2 may be part of a protective mechanism that counteracts the AVP-induced increase in solute-free water reabsorption in the collecting ducts and the further fall in serum sodium concentration.

Two additional factors are thought to be relevant in the pathogenesis of hyponatremia in cirrhosis: a reduced production of solute-free water due to reduced sodium delivery to the distal tubule and increased release of renal prostaglandins [15]. The former may be the consequence of a reduction in glomerular filtration rate (GFR) or an increase in sodium reabsorption in the proximal tubule [16,17]. As a consequence of its complex pathogenic mechanisms, impaired water excretion in cirrhotic patients with ascites may be induced and/or worsened by several factors including diuretics, nonsteroidal anti-inflammatory drugs (NSAIDs) and other drugs [18–20], as well as by large-volume paracentesis if not followed by adequate plasma expansion [21], and bacterial infections. As far as diuretics are concerned, it should be stated that they can precipitate hypovolemic hyponatremia causing an excessive increase in sodium excretion and thus dehydration, as well as hypervolemic hyponatremia. With reference to the latter, it should be noted that loop diuretics may directly interfere with the urine diluting process by impairing free water generation through the inhibition of NaCl reabsorption in the thick ascending limb of the loop of Henle. On the other hand, any type of diuretic may stimulate a further release of AVP by means of a further reduction in the effective circulating volume [22]. Finally, among the drugs that can precipitate hyponatremia in cirrhosis, an acute reduction in serum sodium concentration is common during treatment with terlipressin, an AVP agonist, for severe portal-hypertensive bleeding. It develops rapidly after the start of therapy, may be severe in some patients, is associated with neurologic complications, and is usually reversible after terlipressin withdrawal [23].

Clinical consequences and prognostic implications

The symptoms of hyponatremia (anorexia, apathy, nausea, vomiting) associated with cirrhosis and ascites do not differ from those of hyponatremia in other diseases in which hyponatremia is coupled with an increase in extracellular fluid volume. Few data exist on the clinical consequences of hyponatremia in patients with cirrhosis because hyponatremia almost always occurs in the setting of advanced liver failure, which causes a wide array of clinical manifestations. Nevertheless, from a clinical point of view, hyponatremia was found to be associated with a greater likelihood of hepatic encephalopathy, hepatorenal syndrome (HRS), and spontaneous bacterial peritonitis (SBP) [1]. The relationship between hyponatremia and HRS and/or SBP should probably be viewed from a pathophysiologic perspective. HRS and SBP can precipitate hyponatremia in patients with cirrhosis [24] because they are characterized by a

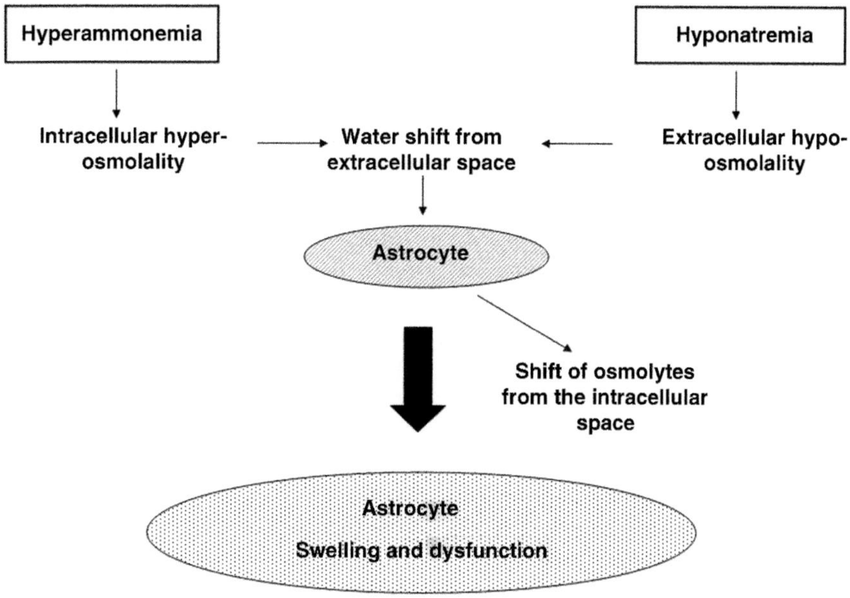

Figure 18.1 Pathogenesis of hepatic encephalopathy: role of hyponatremia.

further impairment of the effective circulating volume and, thus, to a maximal activation of all the factors that are involved in the physiopathology of hyponatremia. Nevertheless, it is also proven that hyponatremia represent a significant risk factor for the development of HRS in patients with cirrhosis [25]. Both these clinical conditions further impair the cardiocirculatory system and further increase the plasma levels of AVP, thus favoring the development of hyponatremia in patients with cirrhosis and ascites. However, the terms of the relationship must be reversed when considering encephalopathy [1], because hyponatremia appears to precipitate and aggravate hepatic encephalopathy in patients with cirrhosis. In our experience, serum levels of sodium and ammonia appear to be the major determinants of electroencephalographic abnormalities in patients with cirrhosis [26]. In addition, the existence of hyponatremia was found to be a major risk factor for the development of overt encephalopathy in all patients with cirrhosis and ascites [27], particularly in those with refractory ascites [28]. Finally, it has been observed that in patients with cirrhosis who were treated with transjugular intrahepatic portosystemic shunt, hyponatremia was a major risk factor for hepatic encephalopathy [29].

In order to explain these clinical observations it may be hypothesized, on the basis of experimental and human studies [30–33], that an increased ammonia level and reduced sodium concentration act synergistically to induce swelling of astrocytes (Figure 18.1). The consequent cerebral edema would not be sufficient to cause an increase in intracranial pressure, but astrocyte swelling would result in a number of alterations in neurologic function, which would facilitate the development of hepatic encephalopathy. Other neurologic manifestations such as headache, focal motor deficits, seizures, and cerebral herniation are very uncommon in patients with cirrhosis compared with other patients who develop hyponatremia. As it has been stated that the most important factor in determining the severity of neurologic symptoms is the rate of fall in serum sodium concentration, it is likely that the relatively low incidence of neurologic manifestations in patients with cirrhosis and hypervolemic hyponatremia is related to the fact that in most of these patients hyponatremia is chronic rather than acute, and this gives sufficient time for the brain to adjust to the reduced osmolality of the extracellular fluid.

For several years hyponatremia has been recognized as a powerful prognostic indicator in patients with cirrhosis and ascites [34]. The presence of hyponatremia is associated with a low probability of survival in patients with cirrhosis and ascites [35] as well as in patients with acute-on-chronic liver failure [36]. In addition, it has been shown that hyponatremia is an independent predictive factor of the impaired health-related quality of life in these patients [35]. Nevertheless, full recognition of the prognostic value of reduced serum sodium concentration in patients with advanced cirrhosis has occurred with the development of the Model of end-stage liver disease (MELD) as reliable indicator of 90-day survival in patients who are candidates for liver transplantation (LT). This scoring system utilizes three widely available laboratory values: total bilirubin (mg/dL), creatinine (mg/dL), and international normalized ratio (INR) of the prothrombin time [37,38]. Creatinine was initially thought to capture the prognostic implications of all the clinical complications associated with the circulatory derangements in cirrhosis: ascites, hyponatremia, and renal failure. However, it has been subsequently reported that hyponatremia, uncontrolled ascites [39], as well as type 1 HRS were predictive of short-term mortality independently of the MELD score [40]. From a speculative point of view it is relevant to note that the independent predictive value of serum sodium concentration disappears when GFR measured by means of insulin clearance was incorporated into the MELD score [41]. The independent prognostic significance of low serum sodium concentration was subsequently confirmed by several authors worldwide and a variety of prognostic models incorporating serum sodium and MELD have been proposed [42–44]. The most advanced is that of Kim et al. [45] which is based on the very simple concept that "the lower MELD the higher prognostic relevance of hyponatremia".

Patients with cirrhosis and hyponatremia are at increased risk of developing neurologic complications including central pontine myelinolysis after LT [46,47]. Although central pontine myelinolysis is thought to be brought about by a rapid change in serum sodium in the early postoperative period rather than by hyponatremia per se, it can be considered as a hyponatremia-related complication. Two recent studies have shown that the existence of hyponatremia before LT in patients with cirrhosis is associated not only with an increased risk of neurologic complications after LT, but also with an increased risk of renal failure and infectious complications, longer duration of hospital stay, and, more importantly, increased short-term mortality after LT [46,47]. More recently, however, the effect of pretransplant hyponatremia on short-term mortality after LT has not been confirmed [48].

Management

The first step in the management of hyponatremia in cirrhosis is to identify whether hyponatremia is hypovolemic or hypervolemic, because management differs markedly. The management of hypovolemic hyponatremia is essentially based upon the administration of sodium with the aim of normalizing the depleted body sodium stores, while the key to management of hypervolemic hyponatremia is to increase renal solute-free water excretion. The administration of hypertonic sodium chloride cannot be recommended, on a regular basis, for the management of hypervolemic hyponatremia because it has a partial and short-lived effect in increasing serum sodium concentration in cirrhosis and it further increases ascites and edema in these patients.

The treatment of hypervolemic hyponatremia has some ambitious aims. First, as hyponatremia has been shown to be a predisposing factor for hepatic encephalopathy in some studies [27,28], the improvement of serum sodium concentration may help to reduce the risk of this complication. Second, treatment of hyponatremia may improve survival and quality of life in patients with cirrhosis [35]. Third, in patients awaiting LT, the normalization of serum sodium concentration before transplantation may help to reduce the frequency and severity of neurologic complications after LT [46,47]. Unfortunately, because of the lack of pharmacologic agents, these potentially beneficial effects of treating hyponatremia in cirrhosis have not been evaluated in prospective randomized controlled trials (RCTs). The traditional options for treatment of hypervolemic hyponatremia in cirrhosis include: (i) fluid restriction with or without reduction of the doses/withdrawal of diuretics, and (ii) the administration of albumin. Fluid restriction alone or associated with a reduction of the doses/withdrawal of diuretics, in particular of loop diuretics, has been the standard of care for the management of hypervolemic hyponatremia in cirrhosis for many years. Nevertheless, its efficacy in improving serum sodium is modest and it is probably only helpful in preventing a further reduction in serum sodium concentration. In some prospective randomized studies comparing the efficacy of vaptans with placebo,

Table 18.1 Vaptans.

Compound	Conivaptan	Lixivaptan	Satavaptan	Tolvaptan
Phase	2	2	3	Approved by FDA
Receptor	$V1_a/V2$	V2	V2	V2
Route of administration	i.v.	oral	oral	oral
Urine volume	↑	↑	↑	↑
Urine osmolality	↓	↓	↓	↓
Sodium excretion/24 hours	↔	↔*	↔*	↔
Company	Astellas Pharma	Cardiokine	SanofiAventis	Otsuka

* = increase 24 hour sodium excretion at high dose.

in which patients from both groups were treated with fluid restriction, the efficacy of this intervention in improving serum sodium concentration (>5 mmol/L) ranged from 0% to less than 30% [49–51]. Some reports in a small series of patients and the preliminary results of a still unpublished RCT suggest that the administration of albumin (20–40 g/day) for a short period of time improves serum sodium concentration in patients with hypervolemic hyponatremia [52–54]. This beneficial effect of albumin is probably related to an improvement in the effective circulating volume with a consequent reduction in the activity of the sodium and water-retaining systems, including AVP.

A new family of drugs, known as vaptans (Table 18.1), which increase renal solute-free water excretion through the inhibition of the V2 receptors located in the principal cells of the collecting ducts, has recently been investigated in the management of hypervolemic hyponatremia associated with different conditions including cirrhosis [55–57]. Nevertheless, among the different compounds, only tolvaptan has been approved, limited to Japan and the United States, for the management of hyponatremia in cirrhosis. RCTs have demonstrated that the vaptans, including lixivaptan, tolvaptan, and satavaptan, are effective in improving serum sodium concentration in patients with hyponatremia [58–61]. In short-term studies, normalization of serum sodium concentration was observed in 27–54% of patients. In particular, the rate of normalization of serum sodium concentration in patients with cirrhosis was 33% by week 4 [59,62]. The most common side effect of the vaptans is thirst, which is related to the pharmacodynamic effect of these drugs. The long-term effects of tolvaptan on serum sodium concentration was evaluated in patients with cirrhosis, in patients with chronic heart failure (CHF), and in those with syndrome of inappropriate secretion of AVP (SIADH). More than 60% and 45% of patients in the mild and marked hyponatremia groups, respectively, exhibited normal serum sodium levels by week 4. Correction rates seemed to be generally similar among patients with CHF and SIADH/other but may have been somewhat lower among patients with cirrhosis (Figure 18.2). Mean dosage of tolvaptan was 30 mg/day [59]. Hyponatremia recurred in tolvaptan-treated patients after discontinuation [62].

The long-term effect of satavaptan has been evaluated in three randomized double-blind studies comparing satavaptan with placebo in patients with cirrhosis and uncomplicated ascites as well as in those with difficult-to-treat ascites. Satavaptan was more effective than placebo in improving the serum sodium concentration in patients with hyponatremia. Satavaptan was not more effective than placebo in the control of ascites in any of the populations studied but, overall, in one of the studies mortality was higher in patients treated with satavaptan than with placebo [63].

Thus, further studies are needed to determine the efficacy of vaptans in the long-term management of hyponatremia in cirrhosis including their impact on survival because concerns about the administration of vaptans in patients with cirrhosis include: (i) hypernatremia and dehydration, (ii) a too rapid increase in serum sodium concentration, which could lead to neurologic complications, particularly central pontine myelinolysis; and (iii) renal failure resulting from depletion of the intravascular volume. Central pontine myelinolyis has never been reported thus far in any of the studies with vaptans. Likewise, no significant impairment of renal function was found in vaptan-treated groups compared with placebo. However, all patients in the previous

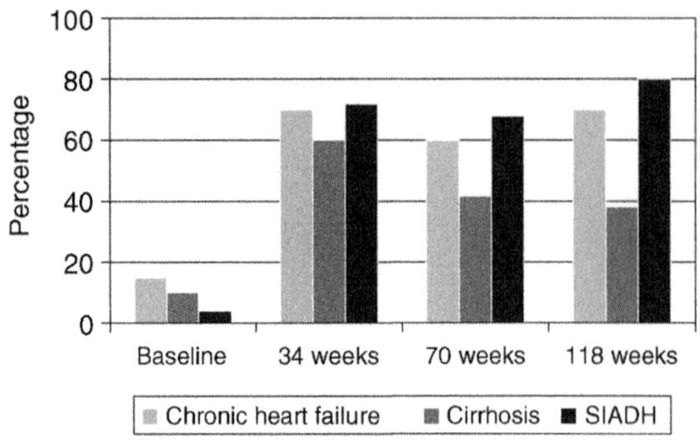

Figure 18.2 Rate of normalization of serum sodium concentration during long-term treatment with tolvaptan (adapted from ref. no 59).

mentioned studies were treated in a hospital for the first days of therapy, had free access to water, and followed strict investigation protocols with low doses of diuretics and with daily measurement of serum sodium and interruption of drug administration if serum sodium increased more than 8 mmol/day. Therefore, it is not known whether the rate of central pontine myelinolysis and renal impairment could be higher under different study conditions. Taken together, the available information on side effects of treatment with vaptans in patients with cirrhosis suggest that the drugs should be given under strict clinical and analytical surveillance, particularly at the initiation of therapy or when the dosage of the drug is increased [64].

Disorders of potassium homeostasis

Hypokalemia and hyperkalemia are frequently observed in patients with cirrhosis and ascites as a result of diuretic therapy. So it is important to differentiate between untreated and treated patients. Over 98% of the body's potassium (K^+) is intracellular. Because of this it is often difficult to make extrapolations regarding total potassium store from serum potassium concentration [64]. K^+ homeostasis is regulated by the kidney. Furthermore, aldosterone, serum pH, insulin, and catecholamines affect the movement of K^+ between the serum and intracellular compartments [64].

Hypokalemia

Epidemiology and pathogenesis

Secondary hyperaldosteronism, hyperactivity of sympathetic nervous system [65], hyperinsulinemia [66], and respiratory alkalosis [67] are common in patients with advanced cirrhosis. These are potential causes of hypokalemia in patients with cirrhosis not treated with diuretics (Table 18.2). Nevertheless, serum K^+ levels are usually normal in these patients [68]. Most K^+ is found within the intracellular compartment and the correlation between serum K^+ and total body K^+ is poor. The evaluation of total body potassium by the dilution of $^{42}K^+$ and the determination of body's total exchangeable pool has been shown total body potassium depletion in patients with decompensated cirrhosis [68]. Once could note that these studies do not take into account that patients with cirrhosis and ascites have an increase in total body water. Indeed, when the results were expressed in millimol per kilogram of dry body weight, no differences in total body K^+ between cirrhotic

Table 18.2 Main potential causes of hypokalemia in patients with cirrhosis.

Factors that affect cellular shift of potassium
Respiratory alkalosis
Hyperinsulinism
Hyperactivity of sympathetic nervous system
Hyperaldosteronism
Factors that affect potassium loss
Extrarenal causes
• Severe or chronic diarrhea
• Prolonged vomiting
Renal causes
• Hyperaldosteronism
• Diuretics (loop diuretics)
• Magnesium deficiency

patients and healthy subjects were shown [69]. In summary, the total body K^+ depletion in diuretic-free patients with liver cirrhosis may reflect an excess of total body water rather than a true deficit. Secondary hyperaldosteronism is not able to induce hypokalemia in patients with cirrhosis because these patients have a reduced distal tubular delivery of serum sodium resulting from increased proximal tubular reabsorption [17]. Hyperinsulinemia is not able to induce hypokalemia because patients with cirrhosis are frequently affected by insulin resistance [70]. Hypokalemia is common in patients treated with diuretics. Up to 30% of patients with cirrhosis and ascites treated with loop diuretics develop hypokalemia [71]. There are two main reasons for the high prevalence of hypokalemia in patients treated by loop diuretics: (i) loop diuretics reduce the reabsorption of potassiun in the loop of Henle; and (ii) loop diuretics increase the sodium delivery into the distal tubule where secondary hyperaldosteronism leads to an increased reabsorption of sodium and secretion of potassium. When aldosterone antagonist and loop diuretics are combined hypokalemia is less common [72].

Clinical consequences and diagnosis

Symptoms of hypokalemia include mild weakness, paralytic ileus, cardiac arrhythmias (atrial tachycardia, ventricular tachycardia, ventricular fibrillation), and rhabdomyolisis. Hypokalemia significantly increases renal ammonia production and excretion in the proximal tubule and may cause hepatic encephalopathy [73]. Electrocardiographic changes such as decreased T-wave amplitude, T-wave inversion, and prolongation of QT interval, are common. The presence of precipitating factors (loop diuretics, severe or chronic diarrhea, prolonged vomiting, malnutrition and/or low protein intake, magnesium deficiency, alkalosis) should be investigated before treatment.

Management

Loop diuretics should be discontinued if serum potassium concentration is less than 3.0 mmol/L [63]. Oral replacement using potassium chloride is the preferred method for patients with mild symptoms who are able to tolerate oral intake. One cautionary note about KCl tablets (which typically contain ~8 mmol potassium) is that they can irritate the gastrointestinal mucosa and cause bleeding and ulceration, especially if taken in large quantities. For patients with severe symptoms or with serum potassium less than 2.5 mmol/L, intravenous replacement is needed. It is safer not to exceed a dose of 20 mmol/L, as there is a danger of rebound hyperkalemia. The concentration of potassium in intravenous solutions should not exceed 60 mmol/L (40 mmol/L if infusing by peripheral line). Aldosterone antagonists could be useful in patients with ascites and without renal failure.

Hyperkalemia

Epidemiology and pathogenesis

Hyperkalemia can occur in patients with cirrhosis as a result of acute renal failure and/or diuretic treatment. Hyperkalemia is observed up to 18% of patients treated with antialdosterone antagonists or other potassium-sparing diuretics [72]. It has been stated that the association of antialdosterone antagonists and loop diuretics could reduce the onset of hyperkalemia [72]. The pathophysiology of hyperkalemia in patients with cirrhosis and HRS is not different from that found in acute oliguric renal failure of other etiologies. A reduced secretion of potassium in the nephron and the redistribution of potassium from cells into the extracellular fluid because of acidosis contribute to the development of hyperkalemia in this setting.

Clinical consequences and diagnosis

Symptoms of hyperkalemia are nonspecific and include fatigue, palpitation, paresthesias, and cardiac arrhythmias. Electrocardiographic changes such as "peaked" T-wave, PR prolongation, QRS widening, and atrioventricular block are common. Severe hyperkalemia is able to trigger life-threatening arrhythmias such as ventricular fibrillation and asystole. Acid–base status and renal function should be investigated to identify precipitating causes.

Management

Aldosterone antagonists should be discontinued if the serum potassium is higher than 6 mmol/L [63]. The goals of therapy are to stabilize membrane potential, move potassium intracellularly, and eliminate potassium from the body [74]. Patients with electrocardiographic changes or serum potassium concentrations higher than 7 mmol/L should receive an intravenous calcium infusion, which antagonizes the effect of potassium on cardiac membrane potential. Calcium gluconate 10 mL as 10% solution should be infused over 2–5 minutes and repeated in 10 minutes if there is no effect seen on the electrocardiogram. Intracellular shift of potassium can be achieved by insulin infusion. Ten units of regular insulin may be administered intravenously along with an intravenous bolus of dextrose (25 g as a 50% solution) [74]. Insulin should be used without dextrose in hyperglycemic patients. Direct elimination of potassium can be achieved by the administration of sodium polystyrene sulfonate, a cation exchange resin. In the lumen of intestine, it exchange sodium for secreted potassium. It may be given orally or by retention enema, although the oral route is considered to be more effective [74]. The resin causes constipation and, hence, should be administered with a cathartic. Loop diuretics should be used in hypervolemic patients. Dialysis should be considered in patients with severe hyperkalemia, renal failure, and no response to medical therapy. The administration of sodium bicarbonate could be useful in patients with metabolic acidosis.

Disorders of magnesium and phosphate homeostasis

Hypomagnesemia

Epidemiology and pathogenesis

Hypomagnesemia has been described in 9–11% of patients with cirrhosis [75,76] and 30% of patients with chronic alcohol abuse [77]. Approximately 99% of total body magnesium (Mg^{2+}) is intracellular, with only 1% present in the extracellular space. As Mg^{2+} is predominantly distributed intercellularly and in the bone, serum concentrations do not accurately reflect total body Mg^{2+} stores. Parenteral Mg^{2+} tolerance testing is more accurate that serum Mg^{2+} in the evaluation of total body Mg^{2+} but is not routinely used in clinical practice [75]. Nevertheless, when total body Mg^{2+} was evaluated with parenteral Mg^{2+} tolerance, Mg^{2+} deficiency was described in 73.7% of patients with cirrhosis [75]. The main factors that can cause hypomagnesemia in patients with cirrhosis are reported in Table 18.3.

Table 18.3 Main potential causes of hypomangesemia in patients with cirrhosis.

Inadeguate intake of magnesium
Malnutrition
Alcoholism
Magnesium loss
Gastrointestinal loss
• Severe or chronic diarrhea
• Malabsorption syndrome
• Proton pump inhibitors
• Vomiting
Renal loss
• Diuretics (loop diuretics)
• Hyperaldosteronism
• Chronic alcohol consumption

Hypomagnesemia may result from inadequate intake (malnutrition, alcoholism), increased gastrointestinal loss (chronic diarrhea, malabsorption syndrome, steatorrhea, vomiting), or, most commonly, increased losses in urine. Renal magnesium wasting can result from inhibition of magnesium reabsorption in the thick ascending loop of Henle or distal convoluted tubule following administration of loop diuretics. Hyperaldosteronism has been associated with hypomagnesemia [78]. Mechanisms whereby aldosterone causes Mg^{2+} depletion are unclear, but recently it has been suggested that altered Mg^{2+} metabolism in hyperaldosteronism may relate to transient receptor potential melastatin cation channels 7 (TRPM7) downregulation [79]. Furthermore, spironolactone is able to improve Mg^{2+} reabsorption in patients with secondary hyperaldosteronism [80]. Chronic alcohol abuse causes renal tubular dysfunction that leads to increased fractional excretion of Mg^{2+} [77]. The renal tubular dysfunction is reversible after 4 weeks of abstinence [77]. Recently, it has been reported that the chronic use of proton pump inhibitors can lead to severe hypomagnesemia due to decreased intestinal Mg^{2+} absorption [81]. Finally, hypomagnesemia has been associated with insulin resistance and nonalcoholic steatohepatitis [82].

Clinical consequences and diagnosis

Most patients with hypomagnesemia are asymptomatic. Hypomagnesemia often coexists with other metabolic disorders, such as hypocalcemia or hypokalemia. This co-presentation makes it difficult to distinguish the clinical manifestations related to the Mg^{2+} deficiency. Manifestations of severe hypomagnesemia include hyperreflexia, tetany, and generalized seizures. The most life-threatening cardiovascular effect of hypomagnesemia is ventricular arrhythmia. Although there are no electrocardiographic findings consistently associated with hypomagnesemia, both ventricular and supraventricular arrhythmias are associated with hypomagnesemia. Hypomagnesemia and hypokalemia could induce further prolongation of the QT interval in patients with cirrhosis triggering torsade de pointes [83]. The presence of precipitating factors (loop diuretics, alcohol consumption, proton pump inhibitor use, prolonged vomiting, malnutrition, K^+ deficiency, calcium deficiency) should be investigated before treatment.

Management

Patients with mild to moderate deficiency should be treated with diet or oral Mg^{2+} oxide (400 mg two or three times daily) for as long as the risk factors for Mg^{2+} deficiency exist. Oral Mg^{2+} gluconate (500 mg two or three times daily) can also be used [84]. Parenteral therapy is indicated for patients with symptomatic hypomagnesemia and tetany or in the presence of arrhythmias. Mg^{2+} repletion should be achieved by intravenous administration of 2 g Mg^{2+} sulfate in 100 mL 5% dextrose in water over 5–10 minutes and followed by a continuous infusion of 4–6 g/day for 3–5 days if renal function is relatively normal [84]. Patients with renal insufficiency should receive 25–50% of the initial dose recommended for patients with normal kidney function. Loop diuretics should be discontinued. Aldosterone antagonists could be used because they can increase Mg^{2+} reabsorption in the cortical collecting duct [80]. Hypokalemia and hypocalcemia should be treated.

Hypophosphatemia

Epidemiology and pathogenesis

Hypophosphatemia has been described in 40–50% of hospitalized alcoholics [85–87]. Thus, it may occur also in patients with alcohol-related liver disease who are still drinking [88]. More recently, hypophosphatemia has been described in 35% of alcoholics with alcohol-related liver disease and in 29% of those without alcohol-related liver disease [77]. However, cases of severe or even life-threatening hypophosphatemia have been described in patients with cirrhosis due to other etiologies such as primary biliary cirrhosis [89] or virus-related cirrhosis [90]. The main causes of hypophosphatemia in patients with cirrhosis are reported in Table 18.4.

Table 18.4 Main potential causes of hypophosphatemia in patients with cirrhosis.

Decreased intestinal absorption of phosphate
Vitamin D deficiency
Internal redistribution of phosphate
Respiratory alkalosis
• Alcohol withdrawal
• Hepatic coma
• Sepsis
Increased urinary excretion of phosphate
• Renal tubular defect (chronic alcoholism, jaundice, Fanconi's syndrome, drugs)
• Vitamin D deficiency

Hyperventilation with respiratory alkalosis, associated with alcohol withdrawal or hepatic coma, can causes a reduction of CO_2 tension in extracellular fluid as well as inside the cells. As a consequence of the increase in intracellular pH, phosphofructokinase, the rate-regulating enzyme of glycolysis, is activated, and the rate of phosphorylation of glucose and its metabolites increases, consuming phosphate ions [86]. Among the other causes of hypophosphatemia, reduced renal phosphate tubular reabsorption seems to be the major one. A reduced renal phosphate tubular reabsorptive capacity evaluated by means of maximum capacity for reabsorption of phosphate to GFR (TmPO4/GFR) has been found in 82% and 86% of alcoholics with hypophosphatemia with and without alcohol-related liver disease, respectively [88]. Although the reduced TmPO4/GFR may be related to hyperparathyroidism secondary to a deficit of vitamin D, whose prevalence is high in these patients, more recent data support the hypothesis that a proximal tubular dysfunction is responsible and that an impairment of liver function is not required for the development of this renal tubular defect [88]. Hypophosphatemia and renal tubular function disappeared after 4 weeks of abstinence in alcoholic patients [77]. A reduced renal phosphate tubular reabsorptive capacity, as part of a more complex proximal tubular defect, is thought to be also the major determinant of hypophosphatemia either in patients with biliary cirrhosis [89] or in those with virus-related cirrhosis with jaundice [90]. Nevertheless, hypophosphatemia may be precipitated in patients with cirrhosis of any etiology or by infusion of glucose or amino acid solution or by refeeding or hyperalimentation. All these situations in fact stimulate the uptake of phosphorus in the cells due to the stimulation of insulin release.

Finally, a number of case reports suggest that in patients with HIV infection, hypophosphatemia may develop during treatment with tenofovir disoproxil fumarate (TDF) as a result of a loss of kidney function including reduced renal phosphate tubular reabsorption [91]. This report was not confirmed by a recent systematic meta-analysis in HIV patients. Nevertheless, a renal tubular dysfunction has been recently described in 15% of patients treated with TDF or adefovir [92]. Thus, waiting for perspective clinical studies, patients with HBV-related chronic liver disease receiving long-term TDF should be monitored for serum creatinine, phosphate, and calcium levels and urinalysis [93].

Clinical consequences and diagnosis

Hypophosphatemia has been implicated in the development of several complications: myopathy, congestive cardiomyopathy, respiratory failure, neurologic dysfunction, and hemolysis [94–98]. To detect hypophosphatemia in the alcoholic patient with or without liver disease, serum phosphate levels should be evaluated at the time of admission and then every 24 hours for the first 3–5 days, because the early phase of alcoholic withdrawal is associated with a high rate of respiratory alkalosis which is one of the causes of hypophosphatemia.

Management

Specific information is not available on the beneficial effects of phosphorus administration in patients with cirrhosis. Nevertheless, oral phosphate salts with careful clinical monitoring could be used to normalize serum phosphate levels in these patients. Cow's milk is a good and easily accessible source of phosphate. It contains 1 mg (0.032 mmol) of elemental phosphate per milliliter. Alternatively, oral preparations in the form of sodium phosphate or potassium phosphate can be used. The phosphate distribution varies among patients, so there are no formulas to determine the magnitude of the phosphate deficit, but the average patient requires 1000–2000 mg (32–64 mmol) phosphate per day for 7–10 days to replenish body stores. An important side effect of oral phosphate supplementation is diarrhea [98]. Intravenous phosphate administration could be required for symptomatic patients. However, caution is needed because it can precipitate arterial hypotension, hypocalcemia, volume excess, hypernatremia, metabolic acidosis, and hyperphosphatemia [98].

References

1 Angeli P, Wong F, Watson H, Gines P, and the participants to CAPPS. Hyponatremia in cirrhosis: results of a survey. Hepatology 2006;44:1535–42.
2 Arroyo V, Rodes J, Gutierrez-Lizarraga MA. Prognostic value of spontaneous hyponatremia in cirrhosis with ascites. Dig Dis 1976;21:249–256.
3 Borroni G, Maggi A, Sangiovanni A, Cazzaniga M, Salerno F. Clinical relevance of hyponatraemia for the hospital outcome of cirrhotic patients. Dig Liver Dis 2000;32:605–10.
4 Porcel A, Diaz F, Rendom P, Macias M, Martin-Herrera L, Giron-Gonzalez J. Dilutional hyponatremia in patients with cirrhosis and ascites. Arch Intern Med 2002;162:323–8.
5 Bichet DG, Van Putten VJ, Schrier RW. Potential role of increased sympathetic activity in impaired sodium and water excretion in cirrhosis. N Engl J Med 1982;307:1552–7.
6 Salerno F, Del Bo A, Maggi A, et al. Vasopressin-release and water metabolism in patients with cirrhosis. J Hepatol 1994; 21:822–30.
7 Bichet D, Szatalowicz V, Chaimovitz C, Schrier RW. Role of vasopressin in abnormal water excretion in cirrhotic patients. Ann Intern Med 1982;96:423–7.
8 Solis-Herruzo JA, Gonzalez Gamarra A, Castellano G, et al. Metabolic clearance rate of arginine vasopressin in patients with cirrhosis. Hepatology 1992;16:974–9.
9 Gines P, Berl T, Bernardi M, et al. Hyponatremia in cirrhosis: from pathogenesis to treatment. Hepatology 1998;8:851–64.
10 Schrier RW, Arroyo V, Bernardi M, et al. Peripheral arteriolar vasodilation hypothesis: a proposal for the initiation of renal sodium and water retention in cirrhosis. Hepatology 1988;8: 1151–7.
11 Angeli P, Volpin R, Gerunda G, et al. Reversal of type 1 hepatorenal syndrome with the administration of midrine and octreotide. Hepatology 1999;29:1690–7.
12 Ortega R, Gines P, Uriz J, et al. Terlipressin therapy with and without albumin for patients with hepatorenal syndrome: results of a prospective, nonrandomized study. Hepatology 2002;36:941–8.
13 Nielsen S, Chou LC, Marples D, et al. Vasopressin increases water permeability of the kidney collecting duct by inducing translocation of AQP-CD water channels to plasma membrane. Proc Natl Acad Sci USA 1995;92:1013–7.
14 Esteva-Font C, Baccaro ME, Fernández-Llama P, et al. Aquaporin-1 and aquaporin-2 urinary excretion in cirrhosos: relationship with ascites and hepatorenal syndrome. Hepatology 2006;44:1555–63.
15 Epstein M. Derangements of renal water handling in liver disease. Gastroenterology 1985;89:1415–25.

16 Gatta A, Caregaro L, Angeli P, et al. Impaired renal water excretion in liver cirrhosis. Scand J Gastroenterol 1988;23: 523–8.

17 Angeli P, Gatta A, Caregaro L, et al. Tubular site of renal sodium retention in ascitic liver cirrhosis evaluated by lithium clearance. Eur J Clin Invest 1990;20:111–7.

18 Boyer TD, Zia P, Reynolds TB. Effect of indomethacin and prostaglandin A1 on renal function and plasma renin activity in alcoholic liver disease. Gastroenterology 1979; 77:215–22.

19 Quintero E, Ginés P, Arroyo V, et al. Sulindac reduces the urinary excretion of prostaglandins and impairs renal function in cirrhosis. Nephron 1986;41:298–303.

20 Miller M, Moses AM. Drug induced states of impaired water excretion. Kidney Int 1976;10:96–103.

21 Ginès P, Tito LL, Arroyo V, et al. Randomized comparative study of therapeutic paracentesis with and without intravenous albumin in cirrhosis. Gastroenterology 1988;94: 1493–502.

22 Ginès P, Jiménez W. Aquaretic agents: a new potential treatment of dilutional hyponatremia in cirrhosis. J Hepatol 1996;24:506–12.

23 Solà E, Lens S, Guevara M, et al. Hyponatremia in patients treated with terlipressin for severe gastrointestinal bleeding due to portal hypertension. Hepatology 2010;52: 124: 1783–90.

24 Follo A, Llovet JM, Navasa M, et al. Renal impairment after spontaneous bacterial peritonitis in cirrhosis: course, predictive factors and prognosis. Hepatology 1994;20:1495–501.

25 Peres G, Gines A, Escorsell A, et al. Incidence, predictive factors, and prognosis of hepatorenal syndrome in cirrhosis. Gastroenterology 1993;105:229–36.

26 Amodio P, Del Piccolo F, Petteno E, et al. Prevalence and prognostic value of quantified electroencephalogram (EEG) alterations in cirrhotic patients. J Hepatol 2001;35:37–45.

27 Guevara M, Baccaro ME, Torre A, et al. Hyponatremia is a risk factor of hepatic encephalophathy in patients with cirrhosis: a prospective study with time dependent analysis. Am J Gastroenterol 2009;1004:1382–9.

28 Guevara M, Baccaro ME, Rıos J, et al. Risk factors for hepatic encephalopathy in patients with cirrhosis and refractory ascites: relevance of serum sodium concentration. Liver Int 2010;30:1137–42.

29 Jalan R, Elton RA, Redhead DN, et al. Analysis of prognostic variables in the prediction of shunt failure, variceal rebleeding, early mortality and encephalopathy following the transjugular intrahepatic portosystemic stent-shunt (TIPSS). J Hepatol 1995;23:123–8.

30 Restuccia T, Gomez-Anson B, Guevara M, et al. Effects of dilutional hyponatremia on brain organic osmolytes and water content in patients with cirrhosis. Hepatology 2004;39: 1613–22.

31 Haussinger D. Low grade cerebral edema and the pathogenesis of hepatic encephalopathy in cirrhosis. Hepatology 2006;43:1187–90.

32 Cordoba J, Alonso J, Rovira A, et al. The development of low-grade cerebral edema in cirrhosis is supported by the evolution of (1)H-magnetic resonance abnormalities after liver transplantation. J Hepatol 2001;35:598–604.

33 Kale RA, Gupta RK, Saraswat VA, et al. Demonstration of interstitial cerebral edema with diffusion tensor MR imaging in type C hepatic encephalopathy. Hepatology 2006;43: 698–706.

34 Baldus WP, Feichter RN, Summerskill WH. The kidney in cirrhosis: clinical and biochemical features of azotemia in hepatic failure. Ann Intern Med 1964;560:353–65.

35 Planas R, Montoliu S, Ballesté B, et al. Natural history of patients hospitalized for management of cirrhotic ascites. Clin Gastroenterol Hepatol 2006;4:1385–94.

36 Krshna YR, Saraswat VA, Das K, et al. Clinical features and predictors of outcome in acute hepatitis A and hepatitis E virus hepatitis on cirrhosis. Liver Int 2009;29: 392–8.

37 Gines P, Wong F, Smajda Lew E, Diamand F. Hyponatremia is a major determinant of impaired health-related quality of life in cirrhosis with ascites [Abstract]. Hepatology 2007;46: 567A.

38 Kamath PS, Wiesner RH, Malinchoc M, et al. A model to predict survival in patients with end-stage liver disease. Hepatology 2001;33:464–70.

39 Freeman RB Jr, Weisner RH, Harper A, et al. The new liver allocation system: moving toward evidence-based transplaction policy. Liver Transpl 2002;8:851–8.

40 Heuman DM, Abou-Assi SG, Abib A, et al. Persistent ascites and low serum sodium identify patients with cirrhosis and low MELD scores who are at high risk for early death. Hepatology 2004;40 802–10.

41 Alessandria C, Ozdogan O, Guevara M, et al. MELD score and clinical type predict prognosis in hepatorenal syndrome: relevance to liver transplantation. Hepatology 2005;41: 1282–9.

42 Lim YS, Larson TS, Benson JT, et al. Serum sodium, renal function, and survival of patients with end-stage liver disease. J Hepatol 2010;52:523–8.

43 Luca A, Angermayr B, Bertolini G, et al. An integrated MELD model including serum sodium and age improves the prediction of early mortality in patients with cirrhosis. Liver Transpl 2007;13:1174–80.

44 Huo TI, Wang YW, Yang YY, et al. Model for end-stage liver disease score to serum sodium ratio index as a prognostic predictor and its correlation with portal pressure in patients with liver cirrhosis. Liver Int 2007;27:498–506.

45 Kim WR, Biggins SW, Kremers WK, et al. Hyponatremia and mortality among patients on the liver-transplant waiting list. N Engl J Med 2008;359:1018–26.

46 Londono MC, Guevara M, Rimola A, et al. Hyponatremia impairs early posttransplantation outcome in patients with cirrhosis undergoing liver transplantation. Gastroenterology 2006;130:1135–43.

47 Yun BC, Kim R, Benson JT, et al. Impact of pretransplant hyponatremia on outcome following liver transplantation. Hepatology 2009;49:1610–5.
48 Dawwas MF, Lewsey JD, Neuberger JM, et al. The impact of serum sodium concentration on mortality after liver transplantation: a cohort multicenter study. Liver Transpl 2007;13:1115–24.
49 Gerbes A, Gülberg V, Ginès P, et al; VPA Study Group. Therapy of hyponatremia in cirrhosis with a vasopressin receptor antagonist: a randomized double-blind multicenter trial. Gastroenterology 2003;124:933–9.
50 Wong F, Blei AT, Blendis LM, et al. A vasopressin receptor antagonist (VPA-985) improves serum sodium concentration in patients with hyponatremia: a multicenter, randomized, placebo-controlled trial. Hepatology 2003;37:182–91.
51 Ginès P, Wong F, Watson H, et al. Effects of satavaptan, a selective vasopressin V_2 receptor antagonist, on ascites and serum sodium in cirrhosis with hyponatremia: a randomized trial. Hepatology 2008;48:204–13.
52 McCormick PA, Mistry P, Kaye G, et al. Intravenous albumin infusion is an effective therapy for hyponatraemia in cirrhotic patients with ascites. Gut 1990;31:204–7.
53 Tulassay T, Tulassay Z, Rascher W. Effects of albumin infusion in cirrhotic patients. Gut 1990;31:1419–20.
54 Jalan R, Mookerjee R, Cheshire L, et al. Albumin infusion for severe hyponatremia in patients with refractory ascites: a randomized clinical trail. J Hepatol 2007;46:232A.
55 Quittnat F, Gross P. Vaptans and the treatment of water-retaining disorders. Semin Nephrol 2006;26:234–43.
56 Ginès P. The Vaptans: a promising therapy in the management of advanced cirrhosis. J Hepatol 2007;46; 1150–2.
57 Chen S, Jalandhara N, Batlle D. Evaluation and management of hyponatremia: an emerging role for vasopressin receptor antagonists. Nat Clin Pract Nephrol 2007;3:82–95.
58 Schrier RW, Gross P, Gheorghiade M, et al; for the SALT Investigators. Tolvaptan a selective oral vasopressin V_2-receptor antagonist, for hyponatremia. N Engl J Med 2006:355–20.
59 Berl T, Quittnat-Pelletier F, Verbalis JG, et al. Oral tolvaptan is safe and effective in chronic hyponatremia. J Am Soc Nephrol 2010;21:705–12.
60 Ginès P. Wong F, Watson H. Long-term improvement of serum sodium by the V2-receptor antagonist satavaptan in patients with cirrhosis and hyponatremia. J Hepatol 2007;46:90A.
61 Wong F. Watson H, Gerbes A. et al. Satavaptan for the management of ascites in cirrhosis: efficacy and safety across the spectrum of ascites severity. Gut 2012;61:108–16.
62 Cardenas A, Gines P, Marotta P, et al. Tolvaptan, an oral vasopressin antagonist, in the tretament of hyponatremia in cirrhosis. J Hepatol 2012;56:571–8.
63 European Association for the Study of the Liver, Ginès P, Angeli P, Lenz K, Møller S, Moore K, Moreau R, et al. EASL clinical practice guidelines on the management of ascites, spontaneous bacterial peritonitis, and hepatorenal syndrome in cirrhosis. J Hepatol 2010;53:347–417.
64 Clausen T. Hormonal and pharmacological modification of plasma potassium homeostasis. Fundam Clin Pharmacol 2010;24:595–605.
65 Solà E, Ginès P. Renal and circulatory dysfunction in cirrhosis: current management and future perspectives. J Hepatol 2010;53:1135–45.
66 Wong F, Logan A, Blendis L. Hyperinsulinemia in preascitic cirrhosis: effects on systemic and renal hemodynamics, sodium homeostasis, forearm blood flow, and sympathetic nervous activity. Hepatology 1996;23:414–22.
67 Funk GC, Doberer D, Osterreicher C, et al. Equilibrium of acidifying and alkalinizing metabolic acid–base disorders in cirrhosis. Liver Int 2005;25:505–12.
68 Casey TH, Summerskill WH, Orvis AL. Body and serum potassium in liver disease. I. relationship to hepatic function and associated factors. Gastroenterology 1965;48:198–207.
69 Mas A, Bosch J, Piera C, et al. Intracellular and exchangeable potassium in cirrhosis: evidence against the occurrence of potassium depletion in cirrhosis with ascites. Dig Dis Sci 1981;26:723–7.
70 García-Compeán D, Jáquez-Quintana JO, Lavalle-González FJ, et al. The prevalence and clinical characteristics of glucose metabolism disorders in patients with liver cirrhosis: a prospective study. Ann Hepatol 2012;11:240–8.
71 Sarin SK, Sachdev G, Mishra SP, et al. Bumetanide, spironolactone and a combination of the two, in the treatment of ascites due to liver disease: a prospective, controlled, randomized trial. Digestion 1988;41:101–7.
72 Angeli P, Fasolato S, Mazza E, et al. Combined versus sequential diuretic treatment of ascites in non-azotaemic patients with cirrhosis: results of an open randomised clinical trial. Gut 2010;59:98–104.
73 Artz SA, Paes IC, Faloon WW. Hypokalemia-induced hepatic coma in cirrhosis: occurrence despite neomycin therapy. Gastroenterology 1966;51:1046–53.
74 Weisberg LS. Management of severe hyperkalemia. Crit Care Med 2008;36:3246–51.
75 Angeli P, Albino G, Carraro P, et al. Cirrhosis and muscle cramps: evidence of a causal relationship. Hepatology 1996;23:264–73.
76 Madden AM, Bradbury W, Morgan MY. Taste perception in cirrhosis: its relationship to circulating micronutrients and food preferences. Hepatology 1997;26:40–8.
77 De Marchi S, Cecchin E, Basile A, et al. Renal tubular dysfunction in chronic alcohol abuse: effects of abstinence. N Engl J Med 1993;329:927–34.
78 Runyan AL, Sun Y, Bhattacharya SK, et al. Responses in extracellular and intracellular calcium and magnesium in aldosteronism. J Lab Clin Med 2005;146:76–84.

79 Sontia B, Montezano AC, Paravicini T, et al. Downregulation of renal TRPM7 and increased inflammation and fibrosis in aldosterone-infused mice: effects of magnesium. Hypertension 2008;51:915–21.
80 Gao X, Peng L, Adhikari CM, et al. Spironolactone reduced arrhythmia and maintained magnesium homeostasis in patients with congestive heart failure. J Card Fail 2007;13:170–7.
81 Regolisti G, Cabassi A, Parenti E, et al. Severe hypomagnesemia during long-term treatment with a proton pump inhibitor. Am J Kidney Dis 2010;56:168–74.
82 Rodríguez-Hernández H, Gonzalez JL, Rodríguez-Morán M, et al. Hypomagnesemia, insulin resistance, and non-alcoholic steatohepatitis in obese subjects. Arch Med Res 2005;36:362–6.
83 Faigel DO, Metz DC, Kochman ML. Torsade de pointes complicating the treatment of bleeding esophageal varices: association with neuroleptics, vasopressin, and electrolyte imbalance. Am J Gastroenterol 1995;90:822–4.
84 Martin KJ, González EA, Slatopolsky E. Clinical consequence and management of hypomagnesemia. J Am Soc Nephrol 2009;20:2291–5.
85 Stein JH, Smith WO, Ginne HE. Hypophosphatemia in acute alcoholism. Am J Med Sci 1966;252:78–83.
86 Knochel JP, Derangements of phosphate, magnesium and calcium homeostasis in shronic alcoholism. In Epstein M. (ed.) The Kidney in Liver Diseases. New York: Elsevier Biomedical, 1983: pp. 203–27.
87 Ryback RS, Eckardt MJ, Pautler CP. Clinical relationship between serum phosphorous and other blood chemistry values in alcoholics. Arch Intern Med 1980;140:673–7.
88 Angeli P, Gatta A, Caregaro L, et al. Hypophosphatemia and renal tubular dysfunction in alcoholics: are they related to liver function impiarment? Gastroenterology 1991;100:502–12.
89 Bando H, Hashimoto N, Hirota Y, et al. Severe hypophosphatemic osteomalacia with Fanconi syndrome, renal tubular acidosis, vitamin D deficiency and primary biliary cirrhosis. Intern Med 2009;48:353–8.
90 Moutzouri E, Liberapoulus N, Elisaf M. Life-threatening hypophosphatemia in a cirrhotic patient with jaundice. Arch Med Sci 2011;7:736–9.
91 Cooper RD, Wiebe N, Smith N, et al. Systematic review and meta-analysis: renal safety of tenofovir disoproxil fumarate in HIV-infected patients. Clin Infect Dis 2010;51: 496–505.
92 Fontana RJ. Side effects of long-term oral antiviral therapy for hepatitis B. Hepatology 2009;49(Suppl. 5):185–95.
93 Gara N, Zhao X, Collins MT, et al. Renal tubular dysfunction during long-term adefovir or tenofovir therapy in chronic hepatitis B. Aliment Pharmacol Ther 2012;35: 1317–25.
94 Lotz M, Zisman E, Bartter FC. Evidence for a phosphorous-depletion syndrome in man. N Engl J Med 1968;278:409–15.
95 Darsee JR, Nutter DO. Reversible severe congestive cardiomyopathy in three cases of hypophosphatemia. Ann Intern Med 1978;89:867–70.
96 Newman JH, Neff TA, Ziporin P. Acute respiratory failure associated with hypophosphatemia. N Engl J Med 1977; 296:1101–3.
97 Silvis SE, Paragas PD. Paresthesias, weakness, seizures and hypophosphatemia in patients receiving hyperalimentation. Gastroenterology 1972;62:513–20.
98 Gaasbeek A, Meinders E. Hypophosphatemia: an update on its etiology and treatment. Am J Med 2005;118:1094–101.

CHAPTER 19

Portopulmonary hypertension[1]

Rodrigo Cartin-Ceba and Michael J. Krowka
Division of Pulmonary and Critical Care Medicine, Mayo Clinic, Rochester, MN, USA

Introduction

Portopulmonary hypertension (PPH) is the well-recognized relationship of pulmonary arterial hypertension (PAH) that evolves as a consequence of portal hypertension [1]. PPH is included within Group I of the 5th World symposium on pulmonary hypertension [2]. The first clinical and pathologic report of what we now know as PPH was provided by Mantz and Craige in 1951 [3]. These authors described necropsy results of a 53-year-old female with spontaneous portocaval shunt (due to a probable congenital portal vein narrowing) that originated at the confluence of the portal, splenic, and mesenteric veins, coursed through to mediastinum and was lined by varying amounts of thrombus thought to have embolized via the innominate vein into the right heart and pulmonary arteries. In addition to embolized small pulmonary arteries, an extreme endothelial proliferation and recanalization process was documented [3]. Since the 1980s, enhanced recognition and renewed importance of PPH has evolved with the evolution of liver transplantation (LT) and potential outcomes associated with PPH. Specific screening recommendations and diagnostic criteria are now clearly defined for this syndrome. Despite the lack of randomized controlled trials for its medical treatment, extrapolation of the therapeutic advances in treating pulmonary artery hypertension with specific effects in PPH has stimulated ongoing interest and importance in this syndrome. This chapter summarizes the most recent advances in the comprehensive management of patients with PPH.

Definition

PPH is only one of the various pulmonary hemodynamic patterns that complicate advanced liver disease [4,5] and therefore the importance of accurate interpretation of hemodynamics obtained by right heart catheterization (RHC) is vital in order to provide appropriate management. The vascular pathology that characterizes PPH includes obstruction to arterial flow due to vasoconstriction, endothelial and smooth muscle proliferation, *in situ* thrombosis, and plexogenic arteriopathy [6,7]; these changes increase the resistance to pulmonary arterial blood flow which is the main mechanism of the disease. PPH is defined as a mean pulmonary artery pressure (MPAP) $\geq$25 mmHg associated with pulmonary vascular resistance (PVR) $\geq$240 dyn/s/cm^{-5} and pulmonary artery wedge pressure (PAWP) <15 mmHg based upon RHC. A summary of the diagnostic criteria and severity classification of PPH is presented in Table 19.1. It is also very important to recognize the three main abnormal hemodynamic patterns that can be present during RHC in patients with portal hypertension (Figure 19.1):

1 Hyperdynamic circulatory state induced by liver dysfunction;

Cirrhosis: A practical guide to management, First Edition. Edited by Samuel S. Lee and Richard Moreau.

Table 19.1 Diagnostic and severity criteria for portopulmonary hypertension.

Variable	Criterion
Portal hypertension	Clinical diagnosis (ascites, varices, splenomegaly)
Mean pulmonary artery pressure (MPAP)	≥25 mmHg; and
Pulmonary vascular resistance (PVR)[a]	>240 dyn/s/cm^{-5}
Pulmonary artery wedge pressure (PAWP)	<15 mmHg
Transpulmonary gradient[b] (TPG)	>12 mmHg
Degree of severity	
Mild	25 < MPAP < 35 mmHg
Moderate	35 ≤ MPAP ≤ 45 mmHg
Severe	45 mmHg ≤ MPAP

TPG (MPAP–PAWP) distinguishes between simple volume excess causing increased MPAP and the pulmonary artery vasculopathy that characterizes PPH.

[a] PVR = (MPAP–PCWP) × 80/cardiac output.

[b] In the case where PAWP is >15 mmHg (abnormal), an abnormal.

2 Excess pulmonary venous volume due to diastolic dysfunction and/or renal insufficiency (pulmonary venous hypertension); and
3 Pulmonary artery hypertension due to vascular obstruction [6].

Distinguishing these patterns is of paramount important for adequate management and treatment.

Screening

Transthoracic echocardiography (TTE) has been the most practical screening method to detect PPH [8–10]. By assessing the tricuspid regurgitant peak velocity (TR), estimating the right atrial pressure by inferior vena cava changes with inspiration and using the modified Bernoulli equation, an estimate of right ventricle systolic pressure (RVSP) can be determined in ~80% of patients with portal hypertension [8]. This quantitative approach allows one to decide which patients should proceed to RHC for the definitive characterization of pulmonary hemodynamics. The presence of RVSP >50 mmHg has been the cutoff criterion to proceed to RHC in the current Mayo Clinic algorithm followed since 1996 [5]; rarely, immeasurable TR with abnormal qualitative right ventricular size or function results in RHC. TTE was noted to have a 97% sensitivity and 77% specificity to detect moderate to severe PAH prior to LT [8].

Identifying which patients indeed have PPH, deciding who needs PAH-specific therapy based on severity, and determining the risks and timing for potential LT are clinical issues based upon RHC results and are summarized in Figure 19.2. Those PPH patients with MPAP >35 mmHg are particularly vulnerable to poor outcomes with attempted LT, especially if there is no attempt to treat the PPH with current PAH-specific therapy [11]. With current treatments, PPH outcomes are variable, yet in highly selected PPH patients, with aggressive treatment and successful LT, pulmonary hemodynamics may completely normalize. Right ventricular size and

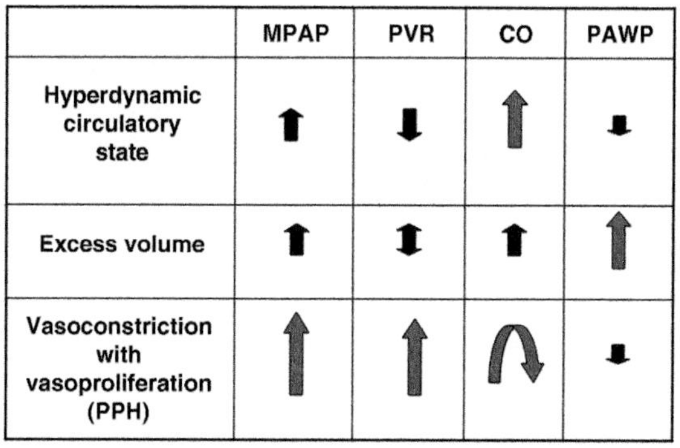

Figure 19.1 Pulmonary hemodynamic patterns documented by right heart catheterization in advanced liver disease. CO, cardiac output; MPAP, mean pulmonary artery pressure; PAWP, pulmonary artery wedge pressure; PPH, portopulmonary hypertension; PVR, pulmonary vascular resistance.

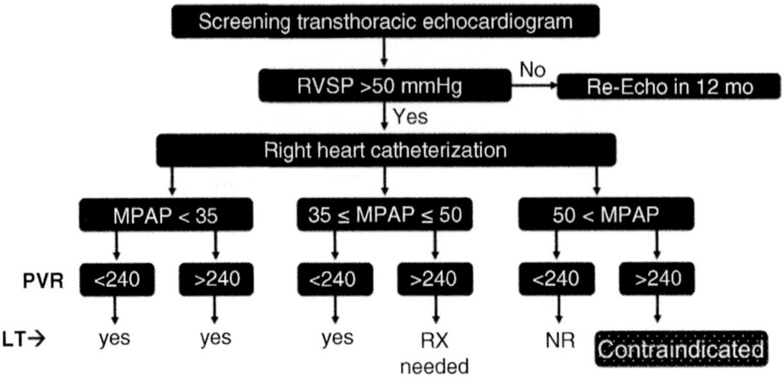

Figure 19.2 Current PPH screening evaluation and treatment algorithm used at the Mayo Clinic. Contraindicated, high risk of intraoperative event at graft reperfusion; LT, liver transplantation; MPAP, mean pulmonary artery pressure (normal <25 mmHg); NR, never reported; PVR, pulmonary vascular resistance [normal <240 dyn/s/cm^{-5} (or 3 Wood units)]; RVSP, right ventricular systolic pressure estimated by transthoracic echocardiography; RX, vasomodulating treatment advised prior to LT; Yes, risk to proceed with liver transplant is minimal.

function normalizes and liberation from PAH-specific therapy may be allowed.

Importantly, PPH should be distinguished from the other major pulmonary vascular consequence of liver disease, hepatopulmonary syndrome (HPS) [4,11]. In HPS, arterial hypoxemia is caused by intrapulmonary vascular dilatations (exactly opposite to the vascular obstructions documented in PPH) that form as a remodeling process due to factors yet to be identified. In addition, the pulmonary hemodynamics associated with HPS reflect a normal pulmonary vascular resistance and usually a high flow state characterized by an increased cardiac output (CO). The distinction between these two syndromes is summarized in Table 19.2 and is quite important especially if LT is to be considered because of the differences in risk and outcomes between these two syndromes [11].

Epidemiology and natural history

It is unclear as to who coined the term "portopulmonary hypertension", but Yoshida et al. [12] appear to be the first authors to use the term in 1993 as they described the first successful case of PPH to undergo successful LT (39-year-old male with long-standing chronic active hepatitis). Subsequently, several small series and case reports with autopsy results have described pulmonary arterial obstruction and pulmonary plexogenic arteriopathy with and *without* thromboemboli [7,13–16]. Two distinct pulmonary vascular obstructive patterns causing PAH in association with portal hypertension are well described:

1 Chronic pulmonary emboli from spontaneous or surgical portocaval shunts and/or *in situ* thrombus; and
2 A vasoconstrictive, proliferative endothelial/smooth muscle process due to circulating mediators that bypassed normal hepatic metabolism due to flow patterns of portal hypertension.

Large series have confirmed the coexistence of these portal and pulmonary vascular abnormalities and have shown that they are not coincidental. An unselected series of 17 901 patients documented PAH associated with cirrhosis more than five times more frequently than PAH without cirrhosis [17]. Within the 1981–1987 NIH national registry of "primary" pulmonary hypertension from 32 centers reported by Rich et al. [18], additional analyses by Groves et al. [19] concluded that 8.3% likely had PPH (17/204; 187 had primary pulmonary hypertension). Hadengue et al. [20] reported the largest prospective study of patients with portal hypertension (n = 507) in which portopulmonary hemodynamic measurements concluded that 2% had PPH.

With the era of PAH-specific therapy and LT, prospective studies have focused on the frequency of PPH in clinical settings, national registries, and individual transplant center experiences. Humbert et al. [21] reported a 10.4% frequency of PPH (70/674) from 17 French university hospitals pulmonary hypertension registry

Table 19.2 Distinctions between portopulmonary hypertension (PPH) and hepatopulmonary syndrome (HPS).

Variable	PPH	HPS
Presentation onset		
Pediatric	Rare	Yes
Adult	Most common	Yes
Symptoms	Exertional dyspnea Chest pain/syncope	Exertional dyspnea
Clinical exam	↑Second heart sound Systolic murmur	Clubbing/cyanosis Systolic murmur
Genetic predisposition	Yes	Unknown
Liver diseases	Autoimmune (common)	No relation
Portocaval shunts	Spontaneous (common)	No relation
Child–Turcotte–Pugh classes	No relation	No relation
MELD scores	No relation	No relation
Lung biopsies	Not indicated	Not indicated
Chest radiograph	Cardiomegaly Enlarged central arteries	Normal
Electrocardiogram	RBBB T wave inversion V1–V4	Normal
Transthoracic echo	↑ RV size; ↓ RV function + shunt	Normal RV ++++ shunt
Arterial hypoxemia	Mild	May be severe
Abnormal overnight oximetry	Common	Common
Pulmonary hemodynamics	↑MPAP; ↑PVR	↑MPAP; normal PVR
Pulmonary angiography	Enlarged central arteries Distal pruning	Spongy appearance Discrete AV communications (uncommon)
Liver transplant	MELD exception if MPAP, PVR improved	MELD exception if $PaO_2 < 60$ mmHg
Causes of death	Right heart failure GI complications	GI complications

GI, gastrointestinal; MELD, Model end-stage liver disease; MPAP, mean pulmonary artery pressure; PVR, pulmonary vascular resistance; RBBB, right bundle branch block; RV, right ventricle.

clinic experiences over a 12-month period (2002–2003). The US-based REVEAL Registry documented a 5.3% PPH frequency (174/3; 525) in which there were 68% prevalent and 32% incident cases satisfying the criteria that MPAP >25 mmHg and PVR >240 dyn/s/cm^{-5} with PAWP <15 mmHg [22]. Of interest were the additional 29 patients that satisfied MPAP and PVR criteria, but in whom the PAWP was >15 mmHg; each of those patients had a transpulmonary gradient >12 mmHg (abnormal). Following slightly different PVR diagnostic criteria as part of outpatient RHC diagnostic assessments, the largest PPH-liver transplant center experiences reported to date are as follows: 8.5% (Baylor 102/1205; PVR >120 dyn/s/cm^{-5}), 6.1% (Clichy, France 10/165; PVR >120 dyn/s/cm^{-5}), and 5.3% (Mayo Clinic 66/1235; PVR >240 dyn/s/cm^{-5}) [5,23,24].

The natural history of PPH has been difficult to characterize and has also been confounded by small series from eras in which none of the current PAH-specific therapies were available versus the current era with the evolving PAH-specific therapies and LT experiences. Robalino and Moodie [25] reported a dismal 5-year survival rate of 4% (n = 78) in an era prior to the availability of continuous IV prostacyclin infusion. Swanson et al. [26] reported a 14% 5-year survival rate in PPH patients (n = 19) denied LT and not treated with any of the current PAH-specific therapies. From the French National Center for PAH (n = 154 over a 20-year span until 2004), Le Pavec et al. [27] described 1, 3, and 5-year survival rates of 88%, 75%, and 68%, respectively, PPH patients (but mainly Child A and alcoholic cirrhotics). Only one-third had been treated

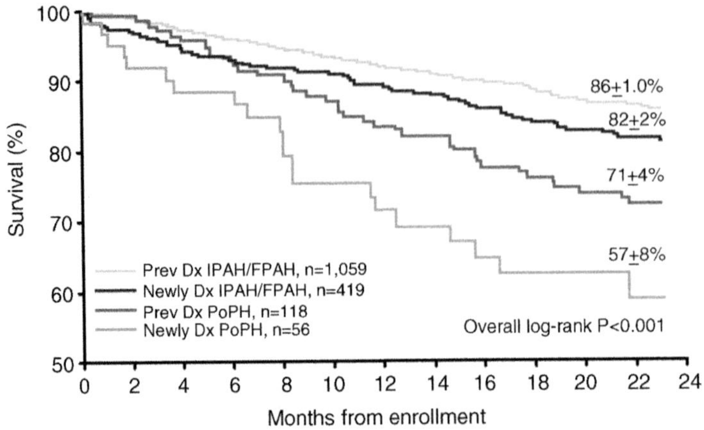

Figure 19.3 Two-year survival patterns for portopulmonary hypertension (PPH) and idiopathic pulmonary artery hypertension (IPAH) categorized by previous versus newly diagnosed at the time of entry into the registry. FPAH, familial pulmonary arterial hypertension. (Krowka et al., 2012 [22]. Reproduced with permission of Chest.) (See colour plate section.)

with PAH-specific therapies with severity of cirrhosis and reduced CO poor prognostic factors. Causes of death in all series mentioned herein were equally distributed between right heart failure due to PPH and direct complications of liver disease (bleeding, sepsis, hepatocellular carcinoma).

From the REVEAL registry (Registry to Evaluate Early And Long-term pulmonary arterial hypertension disease management) two important PPH observations were reported [22]. First, PPH treatment patterns reported in the REVEAL registry demonstrated that the use of any PAH-specific therapy for PPH was delayed compared with patients diagnosed with idiopathic pulmonary artery hypertension (IPAH). Specifically, at the time of entry into the registry only 25% were on PAH-specific therapy; by the end of 12 months' follow-up 74% of those alive were on treatment. Second, although baseline hemodynamics in PPH (MPAP and PVR) were significantly better than those with IPAH, the 1 and 3-year survival rates were worse (Figure 19.3); the 5-year survival rate for all PPH patients was 40% versus 64% for IPAH. Liver disease etiologies and causes of death were not determined in the registry and survival was not analyzed by the type of PAH-specific therapy.

Two caveats are important in characterizing the natural history of PPH. First, aside from one study evaluating the effect of riociguat (a soluble guanylate cyclase stimulator) in PAH [28], controlled randomized studies evaluating PAH-specific therapies have excluded PPH patients. This universal exclusion in the United States further complicated the understanding of PPH outcomes compared to other PAH disorders. Second, beginning in 2002, a higher priority for LT was an option for highly selected patients with PPH in the United States [29]. Formalization of higher priority pulmonary hemodynamic criteria were put forth in 2006 and standardized in 2010. Only patients with moderate to severe PPH (MPAP >35 mmHg) who attained significant hemodynamic improvement with PAH-specific therapy (MPAP <35 mmHg and PVR <400 dyn/s/cm^{-5}) were granted higher priority for LT. From 2002 through 2010, 155 PPH patients were granted such priority and transplanted by regional review boards [30].

Etiology and pathogenetic mechanisms

It is not clear why only 6–8% of patients with portal hypertension develop PPH, which is indistinguishable from the histopathology of other PAH phenotypes [6,7]. Based upon autopsy and lung explant studies, PPH is characterized by a spectrum of obstructive and remodeling changes in the pulmonary arterial bed. Initially, medial hypertrophy with smooth muscle proliferation and a transition to myofibroblasts has been documented. Intuitively, this vasoconstrictive process could be responsive to pulmonary arterial vasodilator therapy. As this proliferative pathologic process advances, platelet aggregates, *in situ* thrombosis, intimal fibrosis, and finally, taking a sporadic, web-like shape involving the entire pulmonary arterial wall with recanalization for the passage of pulmonary arterial blood [6,7]. This web-like pathology is termed plexogenic arteriopathy and it is unknown whether such structures are irreversible [7].

The factors leading to such pulmonary vascular obstruction in the setting of liver disease are complex, but originate from the development of portal hypertension. The pulmonary vascular pathology occurs within the context of a hyperdynamic state caused by extrahepatic (splanchnic) vasodilatation [31]. It is unknown if this persistent high flow state initiates (by shear stress) or exacerbates (in combination with circulating mediators) the pulmonary vascular proliferative process. Genetic predisposition may also have a role because not all patients with portal hypertension due to cirrhosis develop PPH [32]. It has been demonstrated that the pulmonary endothelial cells lack prostacyclin synthase in PPH patients (hence a lack of prostacyclin vasodilatation) [33], the pulmonary vascular bed is exposed to increased levels of circulating endothlin-1 in the setting of cirrhosis (a potent vasoconstrictor and facilitator of smooth muscle proliferation) [34,35], and may be deficient in local nitric oxide effect (for vasodilatation) [36]. The role of other circulating and receptor factors that may affect the pulmonary endothelium is speculative. These factors include vasoconstrictive/proliferative mediators such as serotonin, thromboxane, vasoactive intestinal peptide, and vascular endothelial growth factor (VEGF); as well as the possible imbalance of endothelin receptors (ET_A - mediating vasoconstriction; ET_B (mediating vasodilatation) in the pulmonary arterial bed [36]. The mechanistic link between estrogen signaling, serum estradiol levels, circulating endothelial progenitor cells, and the development of PPH is a current research hypothesis of interest [37,38].

It is also hypothesized that, initially, the intrahepatic injury leads to an intrahepatic increased resistance to flow. Such injury evokes mediators that cause splanchnic vasodilatation via enhanced local nitric oxide effect and presumed angiogenesis effect [31,39]. The splanchnic bed becomes hyporesponsive to vasoconstrictors; excess volume occurs due to renal retention and a hyperdynamic state is generated. This high flow exacerbates the existing portal hypertension due to increased intrahepatic resistance to flow, leading to the creation of alternative flow pathways: portocaval shunts and esophagogastric varices. Presumably, such aberrant pathways allow other mediators to reach the pulmonary arterial bed and, in the setting of high flow, "trigger" the pulmonary arterial proliferative process.

Therefore, in PPH, the resulting pulmonary hemodynamics have been well-described: increased MPAP, high CO, normal PCWP, but an increased calculated PVR to the proliferative, obstructive process in the pulmonary arterial bed. Note that if the pulmonary vascular pathologic proliferative process does not occur, only a high flow states exists with no obstruction to flow with resultant normal calculated PVR. Marked excess volume due to fluid retention may occur and be reflected by increased PAWP. Depending upon the existence of proliferation and the degree of such fluid retention, an increase in *both* PVR and PAWP can be seen, confusing the interpretation of pulmonary hemodynamics [5]. In that scenario, which may occur in up to 25% of PPH patients [31], the existence of obstruction to pulmonary arterial flow is manifested by an increased transpulmonary gradient (MPAP–PAWP >12 mmHg). These patients should not be excluded from the diagnosis of PPH due to high PAWP alone.

As the pulmonary vasoproliferative process progresses, the increasing resistance to flow will at some point begin to restrict the degree of cardiac output flowing through the pulmonary vascular bed. Strain on the right ventricle will be seen with dilatation of the right ventricle and reduction in systolic function (as measured by reduced longitudinal contractility). Progressive reduction in cardiac output will then evolve with right heart failure leading to hepatic venous engorgement and worsening portal hypertension. Death from either right heart failure or portal hypertension complications will occur if no PAH-specific therapeutic intervention is attempted [31].

Clinical manifestations

The predominant presenting symptom of PPH is dyspnea on exertion or at rest. The presence of chest pain and syncope are symptoms suggestive of severe PPH [31]. As other reasons for dyspnea include ascites, anemia, fluid retention, and muscle wasting – all manifestations of advanced liver disease – the consideration of PPH as a diagnosis may be overlooked. Physical findings in PPH may be absent or subtle and non-specific; however, some important findings may be noted such as the presence of hyperdynamic precordium, an accentuated second heart sound (best heard at the apex) reflecting forceful closure of the pulmonic valve due to high pulmonary artery pressures, and a systolic murmur during right ventricular systolic function due to tricuspid valve regurgitation. With severe PPH there may be marked distension of the jugular veins, peripheral edema, ascites, and a right ventricular third heart sound (S3). The lung examination is usually normal and it is quite uncommon to have clubbing or cyanosis (as seen in HPS). Mild hypoxemia is common and often associated with abnormal overnight pulse oximetry. Rarely is severe hypoxemia documented, as opposed to being commonly seen in HPS [31].

The chest radiograph usually demonstrates cardiomegaly and enlargement of the central pulmonary arteries as the duration and severity of PPH progresses (usually over many months) [31]. The electrocardiogram may show right ward electrical axis, right bundle branch block pattern and, when PPH is severe, the presence of inverted T-waves in the precordial V1–V4 leads can be seen which suggests severe effect on the right ventricle. Although rare, it is important to rule out chronic pulmonary emboli as a cause of pulmonary artery hypertension even in the setting of liver disease, especially in the setting of portal vein and hepatic vein thromboses. Pulmonary function tests are usually not helpful in the diagnosis or management because a common abnormality seen in PAH, a reduced single breath diffusing capacity, is frequently seen in most patients with advanced liver disease.

At least one study has suggested that autoimmune liver disorders (primary biliary cirrhosis, and cirrhosis from autoimmune hepatitis) and female gender are more frequently associated with PPH [40]. Mainly affecting adults, PPH has been reported in the pediatric age group [31]. The presence of spontaneous portocaval shunts is more frequent in those with PPH; patients with previous surgical portocaval shunts have a high frequency of PPH years after that surgery [41–43]. Splenectomy accomplished during portocaval shunt surgery may also be a risk factor for PPH [44]. Other disorders that affect the liver may cause pulmonary hypertension. Of particular concern is the Rendu–Osler–Weber syndrome, also called hereditary hemorrhagic telangiectasia [45]. In this syndrome there can be numerous intrahepatic arteriovenous communications within the liver causing a high flow state (with normal PVR and leading to right heart failure). Liver transplant can ameliorate the right heart failure, as well as reduce the frequency and severity of epistaxis [45]. Finally, there appears to be no relationship to the existence or severity of PPH with the severity of liver dysfunction as characterized by the Child–Turcotte–Pugh or Model for end-stage liver disease (MELD) scores [20,31].

Important similarities and differences between PPH and other phenotypes of PAH exist. Compared with IPAH, PPH is characterized by higher CO and generally less degrees of severity as measured by MPAP and PVR [22,46]. In addition, PPH patients not infrequently have a history of splenectomy which may be an independent factor to develop PAH [44]. Finally, it is not uncommon for patients to have an initial diagnosis of IPAH, to later determine because of thrombocytopenia and other imaging (even in the setting of normal liver function tests) that portal hypertension exists and PPH is the correct diagnosis.

Medical treatment

The management of PPH includes an emergent number of different therapeutic agents. The immediate goal of PAH-specific treatment for PPH is to improve pulmonary hemodynamics by reducing the obstruction to pulmonary arterial flow. This can be accomplished by medications that selectively or in combination result in vasodilatation, antiplatelet aggregation, and antiproliferative effects [31]. These goals may be attained by augmenting the lack of pulmonary endothelial prostacyclin synthase deficiency (prostacyclin infusion), blocking circulating endothelin-1 effects (endothelin receptor antagonists), and enhancing local nitric oxide vasodilatation effects (phosphodiesterase inhibitors) [31]. The ultimate goal, in addition to favorably affecting pulmonary hemodynamics (↓ MPAP, ↓ PVR, and ↑ CO), is to stabilize, improve, or normalize right ventricular function.

Uncontrolled, small series and recent case reports have demonstrated that PAH-specific therapies used for other types of PAH could be beneficial for patients with PPH (Table 19.3) [47–63]. It is important to stress that improvements in both MPAP and PVR are the ideal goals in treating PPH. However, MPAP may not decrease as much as desired as increases in CO associated

Table 19.3 Pulmonary vasodilator use in portopulmonary hypertension.

Study first author (medication)	Number of patients	Comments
Endothelin receptor antagonists		
Hoeper [55] (bosentan)	18	1- and 3-year survival rates 94% and 89%, respectively
Cartin-Ceba [48] (ambrisentan)	13	At 1 year, MPAP and PVR improved in 8/8; PVR normalized in 5
Savale [64] (bosentan)	34	Event free survival estimates were 82%, 63%, and 47% at 1, 2, and 3 years, respectively
Phosphodiesterase inhibitors		
Reichenberger [61] (sildenafil)	12	Improvement at 3 months; not sustained at 1 year
Gough [51] (sildenafil)	11	PVR decreased in all at first RHC follow-up
Hemnes [53] (sildenafil)	10	At 1-year MPAP and PVR decreased in 3/5 patients
Prostacyclins		
Kuo [59] (IV epoprostenol)	4	MPAP and PVR improved
Krowka [58] (IV epoprostenol)	15	15 MPAP and PVR improved
Ashfaq [47] (IV epoprostenol)	16	Successful LT in 11 patients; 5-year survival 67%
Fix [50] (IV epoprostenol)	19	PVR improved in 14/14; MPAP improved in 11/14
Sussman [63] (IV epoprostenol)	8	MPAP and PVR improved in 7/8
Sakai [62] (IV treprostinil)	3	Successful LT in two patients (moderate portopulmonary hypertension)
Hoeper [55] (inhaled iloprost)	13	1- and 3-year survival rates 77% and 46%, respectively
Melgosa [60] (inhaled iloprost)	21	Acute, but no long-term hemodynamic improvement
Combination therapy		
Hollatz [56] (sildenafil and protacyclins)	11	MPAP and PVR improved in all patients, all underwent LT and 7/11 are off PAH-specific therapy
Raevens [83] (sildenafil and bosentan combined in 6 patients, 1 patient only on prostacyclins)	7	MPAP and PVR improved in the 5/6 patients treated with combination of sildenafil and bosentan, 2 underwent LT

IV, intravenous; LT, liver transplantation; MPAP, mean pulmonary artery pressure; PVR, pulmonary vascular resistance.

with reduced obstruction to flow (measured by decreased PVR) will result in higher flow (and subsequent pressure).

Prostacyclins

The most dramatic PAH-specific therapy effects in PPH have been with the use of continuous prostacyclin infusion via a central catheter and oral endothelin receptor antagonists. In a summary of 48 patients treated with intravenous epoprostenol from five studies, MPAP decreased by 25% (48 → 36 mmHg, PVR decreased by 52% (550 → 262 dyn/s/cm^{-5}) and CO increased by 38% (6.3 → 8.7 L/min; $P<0.01$)) [13,46–50]. Other prostacyclins (intravenous treprostinil and inhaled iloprost) have resulted in significant pulmonary hemodynamic improvement in PPH [56,60,62].

Endothelin receptor antagonists

Regarding the use of endothelin receptor antagonists, Hoeper et al. [55] documented 1 and 3-year survival rates of 94% and 89% in 18 patients with PPH and Child A severity liver disease using the nonselective endothelin antagonist bosentan. No liver toxicity was noted. However, Eriksson et al. [49] have correctly warned about potential liver toxicity with the use of bosentan, occurring in up to 10% of patients without documented PPH. Although Kahler et al. [57] have reported success in PPH with the use of a selective endothelin receptor antagonist (ET_A) sitaxsentan, this medication was never approved in the United States, has been associated with fatal hepatic failure, and was withdrawn from the market in late 2010. Cartin-Ceba et al. [48] reported 13 PPH patients using the ET_A receptor antagonist ambrisentan (10 mg/day) and documented at 1 year improvement in each of eight PPH patients (MPAP 58 → 41 mmHg and PVR 445 → 174 dyn/s/cm^{-5}; $P=0.004$); of note was that five of eight patients normalized their PVR. In further support of ambrisentan in PPH, Halank et al. [52] described significant improvement in both exercise capacity and symptoms in 14 PPH patients. Importantly, neither of the uncontrolled ambrisentan studies was associated with hepatic toxicity. This may be due to the differences in chemical structure (ambrisentan–propionic acid; bosentan and sitaxsentan–sulfa base) and distinct hepatic metabolic pathways [54]. More recently, Savale et al. [64] described 34 patients with PPH treated with bosentan documenting significant hemodynamic improvement and event-free survival estimates were 82%, 63%, and 47% at 1, 2, and 3 years, respectively.

Phosphodiesterase-5 inhibitors

PDE-5 inhibitors prevent the breakdown of cyclic guanosine monophosphate, the mediator of nitric oxide-induced vasodilatation. The use of PDE inhibition (sildenafil) to enhance nitric oxide vasodilating effect either alone or in combination with other PAH-specific therapies has successfully improved PPH pulmonary hemodynamics and facilitated successful LT, with most experiences being in those with less severe PPH [51,53,61].

Other therapies

The dramatic hemodynamic improvement with the 6-week addition of imatinib 400 mg/day (a tyrosine kinase inhibitor) to pre-LT IV epoprostenol and post-LT bosentan therapy, resulted in liberation of all PAH-specific medications and normalization of right ventricular function 1 year post-LT. This observation suggests a possible fourth pathway of PAH-specific therapies effectiveness (blocking platelet-derived growth factor receptors) in treating PPH [65].

The use of beta-blockers or transjugular intrahepatic portosystemic shunting (TIPS) in the setting PPH may be problematic. The former, used to prevent gastrointestinal bleeding by reducing the degree of portal hypertension, may impair needed right ventricular function. In moderate to severe PPH (n = 10; mean MPAP 52 mmHg), withdrawal of beta-blockade increased CO by 28%, decreased PVR by 19%, with no change in MPAP, and increased 6-minute walk test results by 79 m [66]. TIPS, as a treatment for uncontrollable gastrointestinal bleeding or refractory ascites, can temporarily increase MPAP, CO, and PVR. In a study of 16 cirrhotic patients without pulmonary hypertension, the increase in MPAP was greater than that noted in CO, suggesting an increase in the PVR after TIPS [67]. Such changes remained for at least 30 days post-TIPS and reflected neurohumoral effects as opposed to increased preload. A significant increase in right ventricular work was documented and the potential effect on right ventricular function could be deleterious in patients with pre-existing PPH [68].

Liver transplantation

The majority of patients with PPH have cirrhosis and LT is a potentially curative intervention. Over 6000 LTs were accomplished in the United States in 2013; as of mid-2014, there were approximately 16 000 patients on the wait list in over 120 US liver transplant centers (www.unos.org and http://optn.transplant.hrsa.gov/). Assuming up to 8.5% of LT candidates have PPH, at any point in time there may be ~1300 PPH-LT candidates [27]. The outcome of PPH following LT remains unpredictable despite screening, careful patient selection, higher priority for LT, and advances in single and combination PAH-specific therapies (Table 19.4) [69–78]. Current policy adopted by the American Association for the Study of Liver Diseases (AASLD) calls for screening TTE to detect pulmonary hypertension in every patient considered for LT in the United States [79]. This policy originated from documentation that PPH was first diagnosed in the operating room in 65% of patients (n = 43; 18 peer-reviewed studies) reported in a literature review with a 35% mortality rate in patients subsequently transplanted; pre-LT MPAP >35 mmHg (untreated) was associated with higher mortality [80]. Studies by Castro et al. [71], Starkel et al. [77], and Saner et al. [75] reported first diagnosing PPH in the operating room after anesthesia induction (in eras prior to current PAH-specific therapies), noting that mild to moderate PPH patients (MPAP <35 mmHg) do quite well without pre-LT PAH-specific therapy intervention. The goal of screening is to identify and pre-LT treat those who have the highest risk of cardiopulmonary adversity during and after LT. Pulmonary hemodynamics in LT candidates may change over time, therefore repetitive screening (every 12 months) is highly appropriate [23].

Effective PAH-specific therapy has resulted in successful LT and liberation from pre-LT PAH-specific therapy (Table 19.4). Importantly, it is to be stressed that a key moment during the LT procedure is with reperfusion when preload can increase, cytokines may be released,

Table 19.4 Liver transplant outcomes in the setting of portopulmonary hypertension.

Outcome	References
PPH Wait-list mortality	[23,50,51,63]
PPH MELD exception pre-LT	[30,63]
Case canceled in operating room	[24,59,72,80]
Intraoperative death	[24,26,27,30,74,80]
Transplant hospitalization death	[24,30,47,73–75,77,78,80]
PPH Post-LT	
resolved; PAH-specific discontinued	[30,47,48,50,51,56,62,63,65,70]
resolved/stable without PAH-specific therapy	[12,23,47,71,77]
improved/stabilized/PAH-specific therapy continued	[30,50,53,56,61–63,69]
progressive despite PAH-specific therapy	[24]
Late death not due to PPH	[24,26,47]
Late death due to PPH	[24,27]
Multiorgan (H-Lu-Lv; Lu-Lv transplant)[a]	[76]
De novo PAH post-LT[b]	[82]

[a]H-Lu-Lv, heart, double lung, liver; Lu-Lv, double lung, liver transplants. It is noted that multiorgan transplants have been reported in the literature cystic fibrosis, alpha-1 antitrypsin deficiency and sarcoidosis, but these entities also affect lung parenchyma and many cases were accomplished in the era prior to current PAH-specific medications, therefore were not included herein.
[b]PAH, pulmonary artery hypertension; a literature review of 13 such cases.

thrombi may migrate into the pulmonary circulation, and intraoperative death follows from acute right heart failure [81].

Table 19.5 Model end-stage liver disease exception criteria for portopulmonary hypertension.

1. Moderate to severe PPH diagnosis confirmed by right heart catheterization
   (a) MPAP $\geq$35 mmHg
   (b) PVR $\geq$240 dyn/s/cm^{-5}
   (c) PAWP $\leq$15 mmHg
2. PAH-specific therapy initiated; improvement documented
   (a) MPAP <35 mmHg
   (b) PVR <400 dyn/s/cm^{-5} [a]
   (c) Satisfactory right ventricular function by transthoracic echocardiography
3. MELD exception updated every 3 months
   (a) Give additional MELD exception if RHC data satisfies criteria 2

MELD, Model end-stage liver disease; MPAP, mean pulmonary artery pressure; PAH, pulmonary arterial hypertension; PAWP, pulmonary artery wedge pressure; PPH, portopulmonary hypertension; PVR, pulmonary vascular resistance; RHC, right heart catheterization.
[a] If PVR is normal, higher MPAP may be allowed and reconsidered due to physiology that is now high flow rather than obstruction to flow due to the therapy.

Although supporting data are limited, LT programs in the United States now allow higher priority to conduct LT if pulmonary hemodynamics can be significantly improved and meet standardized MELD exception guidelines. Current treatment targets for PPH MELD exception in the United States are shown in Table 19.5. The intention and results of such recent policy in the US transplant programs has been the hope not only to interrupt the natural history of PPH (reduce waitlist death), but also improve post-LT survival and liberate patients from PAH-specific therapy after successful LT if pulmonary hemodynamics have normalized (Table 19.4).

Although the role of LT in the setting of PPH is evolving with experience, the recognition that severe PPH (measured hemodynamically and qualitatively by echocardiography) can resolve post-LT with aggressive pre-LT PAH-specific therapy is quite remarkable. Although preliminary observations are encouraging, the normalization of pulmonary hemodynamics post-LT does not necessarily equate to pulmonary vascular pathology resolution or long-term stability. Finally, it should be noted that clinically significant PAH could develop *de novo* following LT (i.e., normal pulmonary hemodynamics are noted at the time of LT) for reasons that are clearly not understood [82].

Conclusions

PPH is an uncommon and serious yet treatable pulmonary vascular consequence of portal hypertension. Presenting as exertional dyspnea, PPH may lead to right heart failure and death if untreated. There is no relationship between the existence and degree of PPH and the severity of advanced liver disease. Due to the spectrum of pulmonary hemodynamic changes associated with hepatic dysfunction, screening by transthoracic echocardiography and confirmation by RHC is necessary for accurate diagnosis and therapeutic considerations. Despite the lack of controlled studies, PAH-specific therapies in PPH can significantly improve pulmonary hemodynamics and right ventricular function. The potential to "cure" PPH, at least hemodynamically, with a combination of PAH-specific therapy and LT appears to be an attainable goal in a cohort of PPH patients yet to be optimally characterized. Controlled multicenter studies and long-term follow-up post-LT are needed.

References

1 Simonneau G, Robbins IM, Beghetti M, et al. Updated clinical classification of pulmonary hypertension. J Am Coll Cardiol 2009;54(Suppl):S43–54.

2 Simonneau G, Gatzoulis MA, Adatia I, et al. Updated clinical classification of pulmonary hypertension. J Am Coll Cardiol 2013;62(Suppl):D34–41.

3 Mantz FA Jr, Craige E. Portal axis thrombosis with spontaneous portacaval shunt and resultant cor pulmonale. AMA Arch Pathol 1951;52:91–7.

4 Rodriguez-Roisin R, Krowka MJ, Herve P, Fallon MB. Pulmonary-hepatic vascular disorders (PHD). Eur Respir J 2004;24:861–80.

5 Krowka MJ, Swanson KL, Frantz RP, McGoon MD, Wiesner RH. Portopulmonary hypertension: results from a 10-year screening algorithm. Hepatology 2006;44:1502–10.

6 Krowka MJ, Edwards WD. A spectrum of pulmonary vascular pathology in portopulmonary hypertension. Liver Transpl 2000;6:241–2.

7 Edwards BS, Weir EK, Edwards WD, Ludwig J, Dykoski RK, Edwards JE. Coexistent pulmonary and portal hypertension: morphologic and clinical features. J Am Coll Cardiol 1987;10:1233–8.

8 Kim WR, Krowka MJ, Plevak DJ, et al. Accuracy of Doppler echocardiography in the assessment of pulmonary hypertension in liver transplant candidates. Liver Transpl 2000;6: 453–8.

9 Donovan CL, Marcovitz PA, Punch JD, et al. Two-dimensional and dobutamine stress echocardiography in the preoperative assessment of patients with end-stage liver disease prior to orthotopic liver transplantation. Transplantation 1996;61:1180–8.

10 Cotton CL, Gandhi S, Vaitkus PT, et al. Role of echocardiography in detecting portopulmonary hypertension in liver transplant candidates. Liver Transpl 2002;8:1051–4.

11 Rodriguez-Roisin R, Krowka MJ. Hepatopulmonary syndrome: a liver-induced lung vascular disorder. N Engl J Med 2008;358:2378–87.

12 Yoshida EM, Erb SR, Pflugfelder PW, et al. Single-lung versus liver transplantation for the treatment of portopulmonary hypertension: a comparison of two patients. Transplantation 1993;55:688–90.

13 Lebrec D, Capron JP, Dhumeaux D, Benhamou JP. Pulmonary hypertension complicating portal hypertension [Case Reports]. Am Rev Respir Dis 1979;120:849–56.

14 Matsubara O, Nakamura T, Uehara T, Kasuga T. Histometrical investigation of the pulmonary artery in severe hepatic disease. J Pathol 1984;143:31–7.

15 Naeye RL. "Primary" pulmonary hypertension with coexisting portal hypertension: a retrospective study of six cases. Circulation 1960;22:376–84.

16 Sankey EA, Crow J, Mallett SV, et al. Pulmonary platelet aggregates: possible cause of sudden peroperative death in adults undergoing liver transplantation. J Clin Pathol 1993;46:222–7.

17 McDonnell PJ, Toye PA, Hutchins GM. Primary pulmonary hypertension and cirrhosis: are they related? Am Rev Respir Dis 1983;127:437–41.

18 Rich S, Dantzker DR, Ayres SM, et al. Primary pulmonary hypertension: a national prospective study. Ann Intern Med 1987;107:216–23.

19 Groves BM, Brundage BH, Elliot CG, et al. Pulmonary hypertension associated with hepatic cirrhosis. In: Fishman AP (ed.) The Pulmonary Circulation: Normal and Abnormal. Philadelphia: University of Pennsylvania Press, 1990. pp. 359–69.

20 Hadengue A, Benhayoun MK, Lebrec D, Benhamou JP. Pulmonary hypertension complicating portal hypertension: prevalence and relation to splanchnic hemodynamics. Gastroenterology 1991;100:520–8.

21 Humbert M, Sitbon O, Chaouat A, et al. Pulmonary arterial hypertension in France: results from a national registry. Am J Respir Crit Care Med 2006;173:1023–30.

22 Krowka MJ, Miller DP, Barst RJ, et al. Portopulmonary hypertension: a report from the US-based REVEAL Registry. Chest 2012;141:906–15.

23 Colle IO, Moreau R, Godinho E, et al. Diagnosis of portopulmonary hypertension in candidates for liver transplantation: a prospective study. Hepatology 2003;37:401–9.

24 Ramsay MA, Simpson BR, Nguyen AT, Ramsay KJ, East C, Klintmalm GB. Severe pulmonary hypertension in liver transplant candidates. Liver Transpl Surg 1997;3:494–500.

25 Robalino BD, Moodie DS. Association between primary pulmonary hypertension and portal hypertension: analysis of its pathophysiology and clinical, laboratory and hemodynamic manifestations [Case Reports Review]. J Am Coll Cardiol 1991;17:492–8.
26 Swanson KL, Wiesner RH, Nyberg SL, Rosen CB, Krowka MJ. Survival in portopulmonary hypertension: Mayo Clinic experience categorized by treatment subgroups. Am J Transplant 2008;8:2445–53.
27 Le Pavec J, Souza R, Herve P, et al. Portopulmonary hypertension: survival and prognostic factors. Am J Respir Crit Care Med 2008;178:637–43.
28 Ghofrani HA, Galie N, Grimminger F, et al. Riociguat for the treatment of pulmonary arterial hypertension. N Engl J Med 2013;369:330–40.
29 Krowka MJ, Fallon MB, Mulligan DC, Gish RG. Model for end-stage liver disease (MELD) exception for portopulmonary hypertension. Liver Transpl 2006;12(Suppl 3):S114–6.
30 Krowka MJ, Wiesner RH, Rosen CB, Nyberg SL, Heimbach JK. Portopulmonary hypertension outcomes in the era of MELD exception. Liver Transpl 2012;18:S259.
31 Krowka MJ. Portopulmonary hypertension. Semin Respir Crit Care Med 2012;33:17–25.
32 Roberts KE, Fallon MB, Krowka MJ, et al. Genetic risk factors for portopulmonary hypertension in patients with advanced liver disease. Am J Respir Crit Care Med 2009;179:835–42.
33 Tuder RM, Cool CD, Geraci MW, et al. Prostacyclin synthase expression is decreased in lungs from patients with severe pulmonary hypertension. Am J Respir Crit Care Med 1999; 159:1925–32.
34 Kamath PS, Carpenter HA, Lloyd RV, et al. Hepatic localization of endothelin-1 in patients with idiopathic portal hypertension and cirrhosis of the liver. Liver Transpl 2000;6: 596–602.
35 Benjaminov FS, Prentice M, Sniderman KW, Siu S, Liu P, Wong F. Portopulmonary hypertension in decompensated cirrhosis with refractory ascites. Gut 2003;52:1355–62.
36 Pellicelli AM, Barbaro G, Puoti C, et al. Plasma cytokines and portopulmonary hypertension in patients with cirrhosis waiting for orthotopic liver transplantation. Angiology 2010; 61:802–6.
37 Yeager ME, Frid MG, Stenmark KR. Progenitor cells in pulmonary vascular remodeling. Pulm Circ 2011;1:3–16.
38 Arnal JF, Fontaine C, Billon-Gales A, et al. Estrogen receptors and endothelium: arteriosclerosis, thrombosis, and vascular biology. 2010;30:1506–12.
39 Iwakiri Y, Groszmann RJ. The hyperdynamic circulation of chronic liver diseases: from the patient to the molecule. Hepatology 2006;43(Suppl 1):S121–31.
40 Kawut SM, Krowka MJ, Trotter JF, et al. Clinical risk factors for portopulmonary hypertension. Hepatology 2008;48: 196–203.
41 Lockhart A. Pulmonary arterial hypertension in portal hypertension. Clin Gastroenterol 1985;14:123–38.
42 Senior RM, Britton RC, Turino GM, Wood JA, Langer GA, Fishman AP. Pulmonary hypertension associated with cirrhosis of the liver and with portacaval shunts. Circulation 1968;37:88–96.
43 Talwalkar JA, Swanson KL, Krowka MJ, Andrews JC, Kamath PS. Prevalence of spontaneous portosystemic shunts in patients with portopulmonary hypertension and effect on treatment. Gastroenterology 2011;141:1673–9.
44 Peacock AJ. Pulmonary hypertension after splenectomy: a consequence of loss of the splenic filter or is there something more? Thorax 2005;60:983–4.
45 Dupuis-Girod S, Chesnais AL, Ginon I, et al. Long-term outcome of patients with hereditary hemorrhagic telangiectasia and severe hepatic involvement after orthotopic liver transplantation: a single-center study. Liver Transpl 2010;16: 340–7.
46 Kuo PC, Plotkin JS, Johnson LB, et al. Distinctive clinical features of portopulmonary hypertension. Chest 1997;112: 980–6.
47 Ashfaq M, Chinnakotla S, Rogers L, et al. The impact of treatment of portopulmonary hypertension on survival following liver transplantation. Am J Transplant 2007;7: 1258–64.
48 Cartin-Ceba R, Swanson K, Iyer V, Wiesner RH, Krowka MJ. Safety and efficacy of ambrisentan for the treatment of portopulmonary hypertension. Chest 2011;139:109–14.
49 Eriksson C, Gustavsson A, Kronvall T, Tysk C. Hepatotoxicity by bosentan in a patient with portopulmonary hypertension: a case-report and review of the literature. J Gastrointest Liver Dis 2011;20:77–80.
50 Fix OK, Bass NM, De Marco T, Merriman RB. Long-term follow-up of portopulmonary hypertension: effect of treatment with epoprostenol. Liver Transpl 2007;13:875–85.
51 Gough MS, White RJ. Sildenafil therapy is associated with improved hemodynamics in liver transplantation candidates with pulmonary arterial hypertension. Liver Transpl 2009;15:30–6.
52 Halank M, Knudsen L, Seyfarth HJ, et al. Ambrisentan improves exercise capacity and symptoms in patients with portopulmonary hypertension. Z Gastroenterol 2011;49: 1258–62.
53 Hemnes AR, Robbins IM. Sildenafil monotherapy in portopulmonary hypertension can facilitate liver transplantation. Liver Transpl 2009;15:15–9.
54 Hoeper MM. Liver toxicity: the Achilles' heel of endothelin receptor antagonist therapy? Eur Respir J 2009;34: 529–30.
55 Hoeper MM, Seyfarth HJ, Hoeffken G, et al. Experience with inhaled iloprost and bosentan in portopulmonary hypertension. Eur Respir J 2007;30:1096–102.
56 Hollatz TJ, Musat A, Westphal S, et al. Treatment with sildenafil and treprostinil allows successful liver transplantation of patients with moderate to severe portopulmonary hypertension. Liver Transpl 2012;18:686–95.

57 Kahler CM, Graziadei I, Vogelsinger H, Desole S, Cima K, Vogel W. Successful treatment of portopulmonary hypertension with the selective endothelin receptor antagonist Sitaxentan. Wien Klin Wochenschr 2011;123: 248–52.
58 Krowka MJ, Frantz RP, McGoon MD, Severson C, Plevak DJ, Wiesner RH. Improvement in pulmonary hemodynamics during intravenous epoprostenol (prostacyclin): a study of 15 patients with moderate to severe portopulmonary hypertension. Hepatology 1999;30:641–8.
59 Kuo PC, Johnson LB, Plotkin JS, Howell CD, Bartlett ST, Rubin LJ. Continuous intravenous infusion of epoprostenol for the treatment of portopulmonary hypertension. Transplantation 1997;63:604–6.
60 Melgosa MT, Ricci GL, Garcia-Pagan JC, et al. Acute and long-term effects of inhaled iloprost in portopulmonary hypertension. Liver Transpl 2010;16:348–56.
61 Reichenberger F, Voswinckel R, Steveling E, et al. Sildenafil treatment for portopulmonary hypertension. Eur Respir J 2006;28:563–7.
62 Sakai T, Planinsic RM, Mathier MA, de Vera ME, Venkataramanan R. Initial experience using continuous intravenous treprostinil to manage pulmonary arterial hypertension in patients with end-stage liver disease. Transpl Int 2009;22: 554–61.
63 Sussman N, Kaza V, Barshes N, et al. Successful liver transplantation following medical management of portopulmonary hypertension: a single-center series. Am J Transplant 2006;6:2177–82.
64 Savale L, Magnier R, Le Pavec J, et al. Efficacy, safety, and pharmacokinetics of bosentan in portopulmonary hypertension. Eur Respir J 2013;41:96–103.
65 Tapper EB, Knowles D, Heffron T, Lawrence EC, Csete M. Portopulmonary hypertension: imatinib as a novel treatment and the Emory experience with this condition. Transplant Proc 2009;41:1969–71.
66 Provencher S, Herve P, Jais X, et al. Deleterious effects of beta-blockers on exercise capacity and hemodynamics in patients with portopulmonary hypertension. Gastroenterology 2006;130:120–6.
67 Van der Linden P, Le Moine O, Ghysels M, Ortinez M, Deviere J. Pulmonary hypertension after transjugular intrahepatic portosystemic shunt: effects on right ventricular function. Hepatology 1996;23:982–7.
68 van der Heijde RM, Lameris JS, van den Berg B, Wagenvoort CA, Hilvering C, van Buuren HR. Pulmonary hypertension after transjugular intrahepatic portosystemic shunt (TIPS). Eur Respir J 1996;9:1562–4.
69 Austin MJ, McDougall NI, Wendon JA, et al. Safety and efficacy of combined use of sildenafil, bosentan, and iloprost before and after liver transplantation in severe portopulmonary hypertension. Liver Transpl 2008;14:287–91.
70 Bandara M, Gordon FD, Sarwar A, et al. Successful outcomes following living donor liver transplantation for portopulmonary hypertension. Liver Transpl 2010;16:983–9.
71 Castro M, Krowka MJ, Schroeder DR, et al. Frequency and clinical implications of increased pulmonary artery pressures in liver transplant patients. Mayo Clin Proc 1996;71:543–51.
72 Fukazawa K, Pretto EA Jr. Poor outcome following aborted orthotopic liver transplantation due to severe portopulmonary hypertension. J Hepatobilary Pancreat Sci 2010; 17:505–8.
73 Kawut SM, Taichman DB, Ahya VN, et al. Hemodynamics and survival of patients with portopulmonary hypertension. Liver Transpl 2005;11:1107–11.
74 Krowka MJ, Mandell MS, Ramsay MA, et al. Hepatopulmonary syndrome and portopulmonary hypertension: a report of the multicenter liver transplant database. Liver Transpl 2004;10:174–82.
75 Saner FH, Nadalin S, Pavlakovic G, et al. Portopulmonary hypertension in the early phase following liver transplantation. Transplantation 2006;82:887–91.
76 Scouras NE, Matsusaki T, Boucek CD, et al. Portopulmonary hypertension as an indication for combined heart, lung, and liver or lung and liver transplantation: literature review and case presentation. Liver Transpl 2011;17:137–43.
77 Starkel P, Vera A, Gunson B, Mutimer D. Outcome of liver transplantation for patients with pulmonary hypertension. Liver Transpl 2002;8:382–8.
78 Taura P, Garcia-Valdecasas JC, Beltran J, et al. Moderate primary pulmonary hypertension in patients undergoing liver transplantation. Anesth Analg 1996;83:675–80.
79 Murray KF, Carithers RL Jr. AASLD practice guidelines: evaluation of the patient for liver transplantation. Hepatology 2005;41:1407–32.
80 Krowka MJ, Plevak DJ, Findlay JY, Rosen CB, Wiesner RH, Krom RA. Pulmonary hemodynamics and perioperative cardiopulmonary-related mortality in patients with portopulmonary hypertension undergoing liver transplantation. Liver Transpl 2000;6:443–50.
81 Ramsay M. Portopulmonary hypertension and right heart failure in patients with cirrhosis. Curr Opin Anaesthesiol 2010;23:145–50.
82 Koch DG, Caplan M, Reuben A. Pulmonary hypertension after liver transplantation: case presentation and review of the literature. Liver Transpl 2009;15:407–12.
83 Raevens S, De Pauw M, Reyntjens K, et al. Oral vasodilator therapy in patients with moderate to severe portopulmonary hypertension as a bridge to liver transplantation. Eur J Gastroenterol Hepatol 2013;25:495–502.

CHAPTER 20

Cirrhotic cardiomyopathy

Hongqun Liu and Samuel S. Lee
University of Calgary Cumming School of Medicine, Calgary, Canada

Introduction

Scientists and clinicians have gradually come to realize the importance of the abnormalities in the cardiovascular system in patients with cirrhosis or portal hypertension. Although the circulation becomes hyperdynamic when stressed, characterized by increased cardiac output and decreased peripheral vascular resistance and arterial pressure, the ventricular response is blunted, manifested by depressed contractile responsiveness and altered diastolic relaxation. The blunted response plus electrophysiologic abnormalities are termed "cirrhotic cardiomyopathy." Cirrhotic cardiomyopathy is generally latent and overt heart failure is rare because in cirrhosis the characteristic vasculature is systemic vasodilatation that reduces cardiac afterload thus "autotreating" the ventricle. However, major stresses on the cardiovascular system such as hemorrhage [1], infections [2], insertion of transjugular intrahepatic portosystemic shunt (TIPS) [3], and liver transplantation [4] can further damage the heart and unmask the presence of cirrhotic cardiomyopathy and thereby convert latent to overt heart failure [5]. Taking liver transplantation for example, 25–70% of patients develop cardiovascular complications after orthotopic liver transplantation [6]. Up to 56% of transplant recipients have pulmonary edema following surgery [7]. Moreover, cardiac causes are one of the leading causes of death post-transplantation (23%) [6]. The importance of cirrhotic cardiomyopathy has eventually been recognized. This chapter briefly elucidates the whole picture of cirrhotic cardiomyopathy.

Pathology

The abnormalities of the heart in cirrhosis were first described in autopsies 6 decades ago [8] and later confirmed by other studies [9,10]. The gross change includes myocardial hypertrophy, histologic abnormalities include cardiomyocytes, edema, fibrosis, exudation, nuclear vascuolation, and pigmentation. Lunseth et al. [11] documented a subgroup of 12 of 108 autopsied patients in whom they found idiopathic ventricular hypertrophy and vascular dilatation. Interestingly, cardiac hypertrophy seems to occur in the early and moderate stages of cirrhosis; patients with advanced cirrhosis mitigated the cardiac mass increase [11]. This phenomenon was further confirmed by Pozzi et al. [12] with echocardiography and color echo Doppler. They found that left ventricle wall thickness was increased to peak value and decreased in cirrhosis with tense ascites, both right and left atria and right ventricle diameters were significantly greater than controls.

Pathophysiology

Mechanistic changes

The mechanistic changes in cirrhotic cardiomyopathy include decreased density of β-adrenergic receptors, changes in membrane lipid content and membrane fluidity, and membrane ion channels such as calcium and potassium channels. Collagen shifts from type III to I (from compliant to a less compliant isoform) also impact diastolic function in the cirrhotic heart [13].

Cirrhosis: A practical guide to management, First Edition. Edited by Samuel S. Lee and Richard Moreau.

Early investigators noticed that patients with cirrhosis have attenuated cardiovascular responses to endogenous and exogenous catecholamines [14]. Since the β-adrenergic receptor system is the main determinant of ventricular contractility, investigators suspected that the β-adrenergic receptor system of the heart may be abnormal in cirrhosis.

Because of the difficulties in obtaining human heart tissue, Gerbes et al. [15] evaluated β-adrenoceptors on human lymphocytes to reflect the status of cardiac β-adrenoceptors. They found that lymphocyte β-adrenoceptor density was significantly lower in patients with cirrhosis and ascites. Later, using the bile duct ligated (BDL) cirrhotic rat model, it was found that cardiomyocyte sarcolemmal plasma membrane β-adrenoceptor density was significantly decreased [16], while the binding affinity of β-adrenoceptor to isoproterenol was unchanged [16,17]. Moreover, it was found that the β-adrenoceptor signal transduction pathway was impaired at different levels, including membrane content and function of the stimulatory G-protein [18], uncoupling of the receptor–ligand complex from G-protein [17], and impaired activity of the adenyl cyclase enzyme [18,19]. Using microarray, Ceolotto et al. [20] found that the β-adrenergic signaling pathway is impaired in the post-receptor cascades which included a significant overexpression of G-protein alpha-inhibiting subunit 2 (Gαi2), cyclic nucleotide phosphodiesterase (PDE2a), regulator of G-protein signaling 2 (RGS2), and downexpression of adenylate cyclase (Adcy3). These post-receptor cascade alterations favor cardiac contractile inhibition and therefore have an important role in cirrhotic cardiomyopathy.

The membrane lipid composition is changed in the cirrhotic heart. The increased cholesterol elevated the cholesterol: phospholipid ratio, which determined the membrane lipid biophysical characteristics. The more rigid membrane in cirrhotic heart limited the movement of the protein receptors embedded in the plasma membrane and, thus, hampered the coupling process between G-proteins and the β-adrenergic-receptor–ligand complex which results in abnormal cardiac contractility [17].

Another mechanistic change is in the ion channels in the membrane. Using bile duct-ligated rats, Ward et al. [21] found reduced expression and density of L-type Ca^{2+} channels in cirrhotic cardiomyocytes and the inward cellular calcium current in these cardiomyocytes was decreased. As is well known, intracellular calcium handling is the key factor to determining the contraction of cardiomyocytes, therefore the reduced L-type Ca^{2+} channel and inward cellular calcium current contribute to the depressed cardiac contractility in cirrhotic heart. Interestingly, in a model of portal vein-ligated (PVL) rats, Zavecz et al. [22] found a similar phenomenon; the density of L-type Ca^{2+} channels in heart from PVL was significantly decreased and L-type Ca^{2+} channels together with the sarcoplasmic reticulum Ca^{2+} pool were the cause of changed excitation–contraction coupling. The decreased density of potassium currents in ventricular myocytes mainly contribute to prolonging the QT interval [23].

Contractile inhibitory factors

There are many contractile inhibitory factors in cirrhotic cardiomyopathy such as tumor necrosis factor α (TNFα) [24], endocannabinoid [25], nitric oxide (NO) [26], carbon monoxide [27], and oxidative stress. These inhibitors have an important role in the depressed contractility of cirrhotic heart.

TNFα is increased in serum [24] and heart (unpublished data) in cirrhosis. Using gene knockout or antibody to eliminate TNFα, Yang et al. [24] demonstrated the improved cardiomyocyte contractility in cirrhotic heart. Furthermore, when incubated cardiomyocytes isolated from sham operated mice with TNFα, the cell contraction and relaxation velocities were significantly depressed. These results clearly demonstrated the inhibitory effects of TNFα on cardiac contractility. Endocannabinoid was significantly increased in cirrhotic rats [28] not only systematically, but also locally in the heart [29]. Western blot analysis showed that the quantity of cannabinoid receptor-1 (CB-1) has no change in cirrhotic heart [25,29], the local increase of endocannabinoid results in the cardiac contractile inhibition in cirrhotic heart. CB-1 receptor antagonist significantly improved cardiac contractility both *in vivo* and *in vitro* [25,29], while endocannabinoid uptake blockers inhibited cardiac contractility [25]. The negative inotropic effect of NO on cardiac contractility in cirrhosis is via guanosine 3,5′-cyclic monophosphate, NO inhibitor nitro-L-arginine methyl ester significantly improved the inhibited cardiac contractility in cirrhotic heart [26]. Another gas molecule, carbon monoxide, also has a significant role in contractile abnormality in cirrhotic cardiomyopathy [27]. Oxidative stress has been confirmed to have an important role in heart failure [30], Fernando et al. [31] verified that oxidative stress was significantly increased in the rat model of portal hypertension. We found not that only the oxidative stress was significantly increased in cirrhotic heart, but also the antioxidant gene was downregulated. Erythropoietin not only significantly decreased oxidative related DNP-derivatized protein but also activated antioxidant gene, nuclear factor (erythroid-derived 2)-like 2(Nrf2). Erythropoietin thus exerts cardioprotective effects [32].

Clinical features

For clinical features see Table 20.1.

Systolic dysfunction

The circulation of cirrhotic patients is hyperdynamic which includes lower mean arterial pressure (MAP), lower systemic vascular resistance (SVR), and higher cardiac output. It is well accepted that cardiac function is normal in most patients at rest due to peripheral vasodilatation [39,40], However, when challenged, the systolic dysfunction is revealed. Wong et al. [41] found that under the challenge of peak physical exercise, the heart rate, ejection fraction, and cardiac index were significantly decreased in cirrhotic patients compared with control subjects; these decreases are more pronounced in decompensated patients and were not related to the etiology of the cirrhosis. Limas et al. [42] infused angiotensin to correct the decreased peripheral

Table 20.1 Clinical feature and prognosis of cirrhotic cardiomyopathy.

Clinical feature	Prognosis	Evidence	Comments	Reference
Diastolic dysfunction	High mortality after TIPS insertion	E/A <1 at day 28 post-TIPS predicted 1-year survival (60% mortality)	E/A ratio might be a useful predictor in patients who receive TIPS	Cazzaniga et al. (2007) [33]
	Mortality after TIPS insertion	E/A <1 at baseline predicted 5-year survival (60% mortality)	Large two-center study; day-28 post-TIPS E/A not available	Rabie et al. (2009) [34]
	Poor diuresis after TIPS insertion	E/A ≤1 at baseline associated with slow/poor diuresis post-TIPS	Diastolic dysfunction impedes the increase of CO after TIPS, "underfilling" vascular slows clearance of the ascites	Rabie et al. (2009) [34]
Low cardiac output or systolic dysfunction	Patients with low CI have high mortality	The one year mortality was 63% in patients with CI <1.5 l/min/m^2	Of 24 patients, the group with the lowest CO had highest mortality at all time points examined	Krag et al. (2010) [35]
	Lower CO precipitates or aggravates HRS post-SBP	Six out of eight patients (75%) with low CO and HRS died after infection resolution	Of 23 patients, 8 developed HRS; this group had lower CO which declined further after infection resolution	Ruiz del Arbol et al. (2003) [36]
	Lower CO Precipitates hepatorenal syndrome	Of 66 patients, 27 who went on to develop HRS during follow-up had lower CO	Decreased CO and MAP were more pronounced in the HRS group	Ruiz del Arbol et al. (2005) [37]
Overt left ventricular failure	Poor outcomes post-liver transplantation?	Reversible LVF occurred in 7/754 patients post-transplant	True prevalence of LVF may be higher than 1% reported in this retrospective series	Sampathkumar et al. (1998) [38]
QTc prolongation	Unclear; risk of torsade de pointes arrhythmia?	Found in 30–60% of patients with advanced cirrhosis	Probably subclinical but no large prospective study to date	(Many studies)

CI, cardiac index; CO, cardiac output; E/A, ratio of early- to late-diastolic filling wave velocity; HRS, hepatorenal syndrome; LVF, left ventricular failure; MAP, mean arterial pressure; QTc, corrected QT interval; SBP, spontaneous bacterial peritonitis; TIPS, transjugular intrahepatic portosystemic shunt.

vascular resistance back to within a normal range, and found that the pulmonary wedge pressure was increased tremendously but the cardiac output did not change. Using ouabain, a short-acting cardiac glycoside, the same group demonstrated that this significantly shortened the total electromechanical systole, pre-ejection period, and left ventricular ejection time in normal volunteers. Ouabain has no effect on systolic time intervals and cardiac output in cirrhotic patients [42]. Mikulic et al. [43] showed that the infusion of dobutamine, a β_1-adrenergic receptor agonist, did not change cardiac stroke volume significantly in cirrhotic patients. Isoproterenol, a β-adrenergic receptor agonist, required a higher dose to increase 25 beats/minute in cirrhotic patients compared with control volunteers [44]. Lee et al. [16] infused isoprenaline to test the cardiac response and found that compared with sham-operated controls, cirrhotic rats needed a significantly higher dose (four times) of isoprenaline to raise basal heart rate by 50 beats/min and that the maximal chronotropic response in cirrhotic rats was 30% lower than that in controls. Krag et al. [45] investigated the effects of terlipressin on the cardiovascular system in cirrhotic patients. They found that terlipressin increased end diastolic and end systolic volumes, MAP and SVR, but there were no increases in stroke volume or ejection fraction. The total effects on heart were to decrease cardiac output and cardiac index. The reduction in wall motion and wall thickening is related to the severity of the liver disease. Krag et al. concluded that the suppression of cardiac systolic function is related to the degree of hepatic decompensation [45]. The TIPS procedure leads to a sudden increase in cardiac preload. The exact risk of precipitating acute congestive heart failure after TIPS insertion remains inconclusive. Huonker et al. [3] found that TIPS increased right atrial pressure, mean pulmonary artery pressure, pulmonary capillary wedge pressure, left atrial diameter, and left ventricular end diastolic volume. Braverman et al. [46] reported that TIPS caused high-output congestive heart failure; Gines et al. [47] showed that 12% of the patients with TIPS developed heart failure. A recent study by Pimenta et al. [48] showed that systolic function was impaired in those whose brain natriuretic peptide (BNP) was elevated even at rest.

As techniques improve, the conception of "normal cardiac function" in cirrhotic patients at rest is challenged. Unlike conventional two-dimensional echocardiography, which detects fluid movement, tissue Doppler perceives tissue dynamics. Using tissue Doppler, a newer echocardiographic modality, Kazankov et al. [49] demonstrated that myocardial dysfunction is present even at rest. They found that both systolic and diastolic myocardial functions were compromised in cirrhotic patients at rest. Left ventricular ejection fraction (LVEF), mean peak systolic tissue velocity, and mean systolic strain rate were all reduced in cirrhotic patients.

Diastolic dysfunction

Unlike systolic function, which is considered to be "normal" at rest, diastolic function is abnormal even without cardiac stress. Challenges such as TIPS aggravate diastolic function. Finucci et al. [50] evaluated the left ventricular diastolic function in cirrhotic patients and found impaired left ventricular relaxation, decreased ratio of early- to late-diastolic filling wave velocity (E/A), and delayed early diastolic transmittal filling in patients with cirrhosis compared with controls. A study by Wong et al. [41] demonstrated similar findings. They found an increased isovolumic relaxation time, reduced E/A ratio, and a dilated left atrium in cirrhotic patients. The E/A ratio is more pronounced in ascitic cirrhosis than in pre-ascitic patients. Furthermore, high sodium diet exacerbated myocardial diastolic dysfunction in cirrhosis [51]. Pozzi et al. [12] showed that in cirrhotic patients with tense ascites the A wave velocity is significantly increased, the E/A ratio is markedly reduced, and the deceleration time of the E wave is markedly increased. Furthermore, the removal of the ascitic fluid (paracentesis) reduced the A wave velocity and increased the E/A ratio to values similar to those of cirrhotic patients without ascites. This implies that ascites has an important role in cardiac diastolic dysfunction.

More evidence of diastolic dysfunction can be found in the increased atrial natriuretic peptide (ANP) in cirrhosis. The stretch of atrial fibers stimulates ANP release [52]. It is the relaxation dysfunction that causes the volume accumulation in the cardiac atria that elicits the atria to secret ANP. BNP is secreted by ventricles and therefore reflects the ventricle functions. Wong et al. [53] demonstrated that BNP is correlated with cardiac septal thickness, ventricle inflow deceleration time, and left ventricular mass. Under challenges such as TIPS, diastolic dysfunction is further aggravated. Huonker et al. [3] compared the cardiac diastolic function before and after TIPS and found that 9 hours after TIPS, the left atrial diameter and left ventricular end diastolic volume were significantly increased; right atrial, MAP, and pulmonary capillary wedge pressures were doubled. The total pulmonary resistance increased by about 35%.

Prolongation of the QT interval

The ECG QT interval is a measure of the time between the start of the Q wave and the end of the T wave in the heart's electrical cycle. Its prolongation is essentially caused by a delayed repolarization which is initiated by the outward potassium currents. Ward et al. [23] demonstrated that two types of potassium channels in ventricular myocytes were functionally abnormal in experimental cirrhosis induced in rats by bile duct ligation. Day et al. [54] first reported QT interval prolongation in patients with alcoholic liver diseases in 1993. This phenomenon was later confirmed by other researchers and QT abnormalities were shown to be independent from the eitiology of cirrhosis. Ytting et al. [55] found that QT prolongation is more frequent in cirrhotic patients (50%).

Since QT interval length varies with heart rate, the correct interpretation of the QT interval requires correction by heart rate. There are different formulas: the Bazett formula, $QT_c = Q - T/(RR)^{1/2}$, over-corrects at high heart rates and under-corrects at low heart rates. Fridericia has published an alternative correction formula using the cube-root of RR: $QT_c = Q - T/(RR)^{1/3}$. Bazett and Fridericia assumed that the relationship between QT and RR is exponential. Sagie et al. ($QT_c = QT + 0.154(1-RR)$) and Hodges ($QTc = QT = 105\ (1/RR - 1)$) believed it to be a linear relationship. Zambruni et al. [56] recently generated a new formula: $QT = 453.65 \times RR^{1/3.02}$. They pointed out that their formula and the Fridericia correction are better suited to cirrhotic patients.

Using the Bazett formula, Henriksen et al. [57] defined that $QT_c > 0.440\ s^{1/2}$ as prolonged QT_c interval.

QT prolongation had no connection with gender, etiology, or current alcohol consumption but with the severity of cirrhosis. The QT length is positively correlated with Child–Pugh score system ($r = 0.53$; $P < 0.01$). Interestingly, the follow-up showed that those whose Child–Pugh score was worse, their QT length was further prolonged [58]. Besides liver function, portosystemic shunt is also associated with QT prolongation. First, the QT interval is longer in cirrhotic patients with portal hypertension than those without [55], and those with noncirrhotic portal hypertension and preserved liver function; second, TIPS, a procedure artificially decreasing portal hypertension and increasing portosystemic shunting, worsens this abnormality [59]. All of these events imply that it is the portosystemic shunt that causes QT prolongation. Besides the prolonged QT interval, there is a compromised relation between the electrical and mechanical functions of the heart in cirrhotic patients. The difference between electrical and mechanical systole time is significantly more dispersed in patients with cirrhosis [60]. However, the clinical significance of this electromechanical dyssynergy is unclear.

Diagnosis

There is no solidly established criteria for diagnosis and therefore judgment is based on high clinical suspicion (Figure 20.1). An expert working party created the diagnostic criteria shown in Table 20.2.

Management

Since the systemic vasodilatation that reduces cardiac afterload and thus, "autotreating" the ventricle, the overt ventricular failure is usually absent. However, if overt heart failure occurs in any circumstance, such as TIPS or other portosystemic shunting procedures, infection and liver transplantation, and so on, the treatment should be as for other noncirrhotic forms of congestive heart failure. These measures include bed-rest, administration of oxygen, salt and water restriction, and diuretic therapy.

There is no long-term comprehensive management protocol. The reagents used for noncirrhotic congestive heart failure may not suitable for cirrhotic cardiomyopathy. Angiotensin-converting enzyme inhibitors dilate systemic vascular and decrease cardiac afterload and therefore have therapeutic effects on heart failure. However, the vasculature has already been dilated in cirrhosis and therefore vasodilators, especially angiotensin converting enzyme inhibitors, precipitate profound

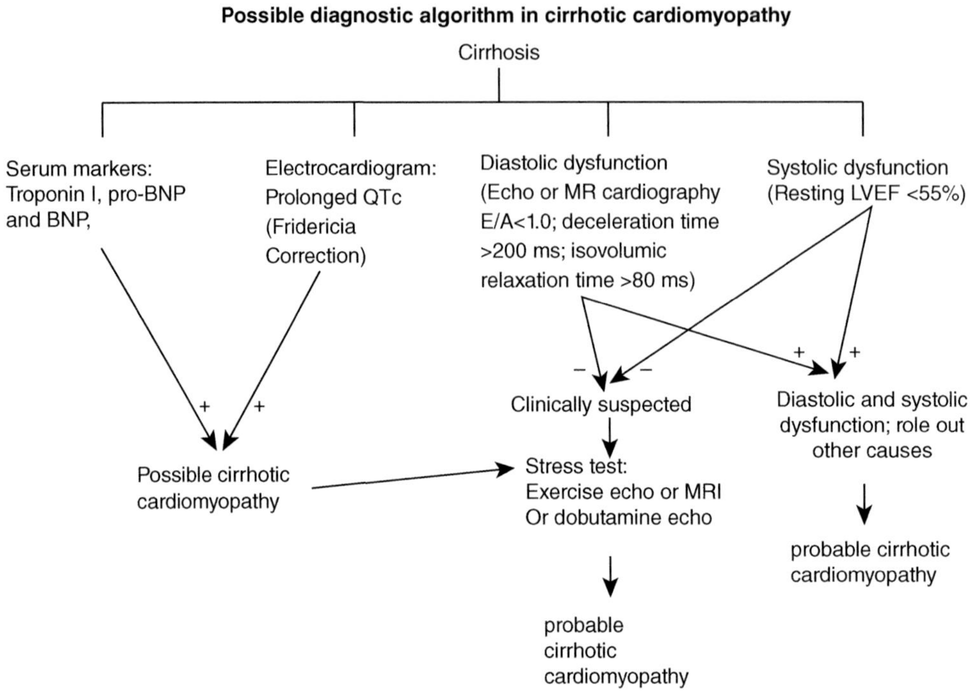

Figure 20.1 Diagnostic algorithm for cirrhotic cardiomyopathy. BNP, brain natriuretic peptide; LVEF, left ventricular ejection fraction; MR, magnetic resonance; MRI, magnetic resonance imaging.

arterial hypotension in cirrhotic patients. The cardiac glycosides given to boost systolic contractility in non-cirrhotic congestive heart failure might not be effective in cirrhotic cardiomyopathy. Limas et al. [42] found that ouabain caused significant shortening of total electromechanical systole, pre-ejection period, and left ventricular ejection time in normal volunteers; ouabain neither improved left ventricular function nor altered systolic time intervals. It is well known that the density of cardiac β-adrenergic receptors is downregulated in cirrhosis, so β-adrenergic receptors agonists, such as dobutamine, are likely not useful. Mikulic et al. [43] found that dobutamine did not change cardiac stroke volume significantly in cirrhotic patients.

Pozzi et al. [62] demonstrated that K-canrenoate, an aldosterone antagonist, significantly decreased left ventricular hypertrophy and wall thickness and left ventricular end-diastolic volume in Child A cirrhotic patients. K-canrenoate had a trend towards improved diastolic function indices in the E/A ratio. Since aldosterone promotes myocardial fibrosis, the aldosterone antagonist, spironolactone, reduces myocardial collagen turnover [63], Pozzi et al. [62] speculated that the effects of K-canrenoate on cirrhotic cardiomyopathy is via the blockage of the fibrogenic effects of the aldosterone system.

Another possibility for long-term treatment is beta-blockers. The overactivity of the sympathetic system overdrives the heart, so long-term stimulation might cause decreased density of β-adrenergic receptors. The density of β-adrenergic receptors are decreased in non-cirrhotic heart failure [64] and yet beta-blockers are a fundamental treatment in chronic heart failure [65]. Beta-blockers have cardioprotective effects. In cirrhotic patients, beta-blockers improve the prolonged QT interval in cirrhotic patients [57]. However, a recent study showed that beta-blockers cause paracentesis-induced circulatory dysfunction in patients with cirrhosis and refractory ascites [66]. The long-term effect of beta-blockers on cardiac morphology, contractile and electrophysiologic abnormalities in patients with cirrhotic cardiomyopathy needs further investigation.

Our laboratory recently demonstrated the protective effect of erythropoietin on the rat model of cirrhotic cardiomyopathy [32]. Erythropoietin is a hypoxia-induced hormone, the major regulator of erythropoiesis.

Table 20.2 Proposal for diagnostic and supportive criteria for cirrhotic cardiomyopathy agreed upon at a working party held at the 2005 World Congress of Gastroenterology in Montreal.

Definition of cirrhotic cardiomyopathy

General definition:

Cirrhotic cardiomyopathy is defined as chronic cardiac dysfunction in patients with cirrhosis, characterized by blunted contractile responsiveness to stress, and/or altered diastolic relaxation with electrophysiological abnormalities, in the absence of known cardiac disease

Diagnostic criteria:

1 Abnormal systolic contractile responses to stress
2 Diastolic dysfunction at rest
3 Absence of clinically significant cardiopulmonary disease

Systolic dysfunction (at least one of the following):

1 Blunted increase in cardiac output with exercise, volume challenge or pharmacologic stimuli
2 Resting LVEF <55%

Diastolic dysfunction (at least one of the following):

1 E/A ratio (age corrected) <1.0
2 Prolonged deceleration time (>200 ms)
3 Prolonged isovolumic relaxation time (>80 ms)

Supportive criteria:

1 Electrophysiologic abnormalities including the following:
- Abnormal chronotropic response to stress
- Electromechanical uncoupling/dyssynchrony
- Prolonged QTc interval

2 Heart chamber alterations: enlarged LA, increased LVWT
3 Increased pro-BNP and BNP
4 Increased troponin I

BNP, brain natriuretic peptide; LA, left atrium; LVEF, left ventricular ejection fraction; LVWT, left ventricular wall thickness.

Source: Yang et al., 2012 [61]. Reproduced with permission of Elsevier.

Many studies have demonstrated that erythropoietin has anti-inflammatory and antioxidant properties [67]. Erythropoietin alleviates left ventricular hypertrophy in patients with congestive heart failure and enhances exercise performance, increases ejection fraction, decreases mortality, improves cardiac function, and shortens hospitalization [68,69]. Erythropoietin is protective in many types of heart diseases including congestive heart failure [68], myocarditis [70], cardiomyopathy [71], and ischemic injury [72]. Erythropoietin protects cardiomyocytes from ischemic injury, decreases oxidative stress, attenuates myocardial inflammation by suppression of TNFα, and improves cardiac contractile function.

We found that erythropoietin has pleiotropic effects on cirrhotic heart: antioxidative stress, enhancing antioxidant gene expression, and inhibiting TNFα. Erythropoietin improves cardiac contractility in cirrhotic hearts in the rat model [32]. Whether this study is applicable to cirrhotic cardiomyopathy in patients needs further investigation.

Prognosis

Since vasodilatation that reduces cardiac afterload and thus, "autotreating" the ventricle, overt heart failure is rare in cirrhotic patients and therefore cirrhotic cardiomyopathy is often overlooked. However, when stressed, heart failure has a significant role in mobility and mortality; 7–21% of deaths in the post-transplant period are due to cirrhotic cardiomyopathy. How to predict the outcome is critically important. First of all, because "cirrhotic cardiomyopathy" is based on chronic liver disease, the Model for end-stage liver disease (MELD) score should be considered as predictive factor in liver transplantation outcome. Cirrhotic patients with MELD scores greater than 14 are generally not considered for surgical intervention. Patients with MELD scores of 8–14 are at greater perioperative risk [73]. However, the predictive value of MELD on the survival of liver transplantation is inconclusive [6,74,75].

BNP is thought to reflect cardiac dysfunction [74]. BNP concentrations correlate with cardiac function and hypertrophy [76] and seems to be the most sensitive index to identify subclinical asymptomatic left ventricular dysfunction [73]. There are cardiac abnormalities in cirrhotic patients, so plasma BNP is an excellent indicator of cardiac function in these patients. Furthermore, BNP plasma levels correlate with MELD scores in cirrhotic patients. Multivariate analysis showed that BNP predicts the cardiac ejection fraction: patients whose baseline BNP concentrations were more than 70 pg/mL had an ejection fraction of around 45% [73]. Pimenta et al. [48] found that BNP levels are not only related to cardiac systolic function, but also associated with medium-term survival, suggesting its potential utility as a prognostic marker in cirrhosis. Besides cardiac function, renal function also affects BNP levels. Ruiz-del-Arbol et al. [36] demonstrated that decreased cardiac output is related to the development of hepatorenal syndrome which also impacts patients' survival rates. Bernal et al. [77] demonstrated that pretransplant NT-proBNP levels were significantly associated with risk for cardiovascular events after the procedure.

Troponin, a marker of cardiac injury, might be an indicator reflecting heart damage in cirrhotic cardiomyopathy. Pateron et al. [78] found that 31% of patients with cirrhosis had an increase in serum cardiac troponin I concentrations. These patients had no cardiac ischemia on clinical or ECG examination. The elevated troponin levels in patients with cirrhosis were correlated with a decrease in the stroke volume index and an increase in left ventricular mass. Coss et al. [79] confirmed Pateron et al.'s study and found that pretransplant troponin I levels were increased in approximately one-quarter of their patients and correlated with markers of cardiac dysfunction/disease such as left ventricular wall thickness and a low ejection fraction. Moreover, an abnormal pretransplant troponin I level (>0.07 ng/mL) was one of the independent predictors for the cardiovascular complications after liver transplantation. Because of the predictive value, Liu and Lee [80] speculated that troponin I is perhaps a marker of cirrhotic cardiomyopathy with latent cardiac dysfunction that is not recognized by conventional screening methods.

References

1 Wu IC, Yu FJ, Chou JJ, et al. Predictive risk factors for upper gastrointestinal bleeding with simultaneous myocardial injury. Kaohsiung J Med Sci 2007;23:8–16.

2 Lee SS. Cardiac dysfunction in spontaneous bacterial peritonitis: a manifestation of cirrhotic cardiomyopathy? Hepatology 2003;38:1089–91.

3 Huonker M, Schumacher YO, Ochs A, Sorichter S, Keul J, Rossle M. Cardiac function and haemodynamics in alcoholic cirrhosis and effects of the transjugular intrahepatic portosystemic stent shunt. Gut 1999;44:743–8.

4 Therapondos G, Flapan AD, Plevris JN, Hayes PC. Cardiac morbidity and mortality related to orthotopic liver transplantation. Liver Transpl 2004;10:1441–53.

5 Baik SK, Fouad TR, Lee SS. Cirrhotic cardiomyopathy. Orphanet J Rare Dis 2007;2:15.

6 Fouad TR, Abdel-Razek WM, Burak KW, Bain VG, Lee SS. Prediction of cardiac complications after liver transplantation. Transplantation 2009;87:763–70.

7 Lossnitzer D, Steen H, Zahn A, et al. Myocardial late gadolinium enhancement cardiovascular magnetic resonance in patients with cirrhosis. J Cardiovasc Magn Reson 2010;12:47.

8 Spatt SD, Rosenblatt P. The incidence of hypertension in portal cirrhosis; a study of 80 necropsied cases of portal cirrhosis. Ann Intern Med 1949;31:479–83.

9 Hall EM, Olsen AY, Davis FE. Portal cirrhosis; clinical and pathologic review of 782 cases from 16, 600 necropsies. Am J Pathol 1953;29:993–1027.

10 Loyke HF. The relationship of cirrhosis of the liver to hypertension: a study of 504 cases of cirrhosis of the liver. Am J Med Sci 1955;230:627–32.

11 Lunseth JH, Olmstead EG, Abboud F. A study of heart disease in one hundred eight hospitalized patients dying with portal cirrhosis. AMA Arch Intern Med 1958;102:405–13.

12 Pozzi M, Carugo S, Boari G, et al. Evidence of functional and structural cardiac abnormalities in cirrhotic patients with and without ascites. Hepatology 1997;26:1131–7.

13 Glenn TK, Honar H, Liu H, ter Keurs HE, Lee SS. Role of cardiac myofilament proteins titin and collagen in the pathogenesis of diastolic dysfunction in cirrhotic rats. J Hepatol 2011;55:1249–55.

14 Abelmann WH, Kowalski HJ, Mc NW. The hemodynamic response to exercise in patients with Laennec's cirrhosis. J Clin Invest 1955;34:690–5.

15 Gerbes AL, Remien J, Jungst D, Sauerbruch T, Paumgartner G. Evidence for down-regulation of beta-2-adrenoceptors in

cirrhotic patients with severe ascites. Lancet 1986;1: 1409–11.
16 Lee SS, Marty J, Mantz J, Samain E, Braillon A, Lebrec D. Desensitization of myocardial beta-adrenergic receptors in cirrhotic rats. Hepatology 1990;12:481–5.
17 Ma Z, Meddings JB, Lee SS. Membrane physical properties determine cardiac beta-adrenergic receptor function in cirrhotic rats. Am J Physiol 1994;267:G87–93.
18 Ma Z, Miyamoto A, Lee SS. Role of altered beta-adrenoceptor signal transduction in the pathogenesis of cirrhotic cardiomyopathy in rats. Gastroenterology 1996;110:1191–8.
19 Ma Z, Lee SS, Meddings JB. Effects of altered cardiac membrane fluidity on beta-adrenergic receptor signalling in rats with cirrhotic cardiomyopathy. J Hepatol 1997;26:904–12.
20 Ceolotto G, Papparella I, Sticca A, et al. An abnormal gene expression of the beta-adrenergic system contributes to the pathogenesis of cardiomyopathy in cirrhotic rats. Hepatology 2008;48:1913–23.
21 Ward CA, Liu H, Lee SS. Altered cellular calcium regulatory systems in a rat model of cirrhotic cardiomyopathy. Gastroenterology 2001;121:1209–18.
22 Zavecz JH, Bueno O, Maloney RE, O'Donnell JM, Roerig SC, Battarbee HD. Cardiac excitation-contraction coupling in the portal hypertensive rat. Am J Physiol Gastrointest Liver Physiol 2000;279:G28–39.
23 Ward CA, Ma Z, Lee SS, Giles WR. Potassium currents in atrial and ventricular myocytes from a rat model of cirrhosis. Am J Physiol 1997;273:G537–44.
24 Yang YY, Liu H, Nam SW, Kunos G, Lee SS. Mechanisms of TNFalpha-induced cardiac dysfunction in cholestatic bile duct-ligated mice: interaction between TNFalpha and endocannabinoids. J Hepatol 2010;53:298–306.
25 Gaskari SA, Liu H, Moezi L, Li Y, Baik SK, Lee SS. Role of endocannabinoids in the pathogenesis of cirrhotic cardiomyopathy in bile duct-ligated rats. Br J Pharmacol 2005;146:315–23.
26 Liu H, Ma Z, Lee SS. Contribution of nitric oxide to the pathogenesis of cirrhotic cardiomyopathy in bile duct-ligated rats. Gastroenterology 2000;118:937–44.
27 Liu H, Song D, Lee SS. Role of heme oxygenase-carbon monoxide pathway in pathogenesis of cirrhotic cardiomyopathy in the rat. Am J Physiol Gastrointest Liver Physiol 2001;280:G68–74.
28 Tam J, Liu J, Mukhopadhyay B, Cinar R, Godlewski G, Kunos G. Endocannabinoids in liver disease. Hepatology 2011;53:346–55.
29 Batkai S, Mukhopadhyay P, Harvey-White J, Kechrid R, Pacher P, Kunos G. Endocannabinoids acting at CB1 receptors mediate the cardiac contractile dysfunction in vivo in cirrhotic rats. Am J Physiol Heart Circ Physiol 2007;293: H1689–95.
30 Ahmed Z, Tang WH. Pharmacologic strategies to target oxidative stress in heart failure. Curr Heart Fail Rep 2012;9: 14–22.
31 Fernando B, Marley R, Holt S, et al. N-acetylcysteine prevents development of the hyperdynamic circulation in the portal hypertensive rat. Hepatology 1998;28: 689–94.
32 Liu L, Liu H, Nam SW, Lee SS. Protective effects of erythropoietin on cirrhotic cardiomyopathy in rats. Dig Liver Dis 2012;44:1012–7.
33 Cazzaniga M, Salerno F, Pagnozzi G, et al. Diastolic dysfunction is associated with poor survival in patients with cirrhosis with transjugular intrahepatic portosystemic shunt. Gut 2007;56:869–75.
34 Rabie RN, Cazzaniga M, Salerno F, Wong F. The use of E/A ratio as a predictor of outcome in cirrhotic patients treated with transjugular intrahepatic portosystemic shunt. Am J Gastroenterol 2009;104:2458–66.
35 Krag A, Bendtsen F, Henriksen JH, Moller S. Low cardiac output predicts development of hepatorenal syndrome and survival in patients with cirrhosis and ascites. Gut 2010;59: 105–10.
36 Ruiz-del-Arbol L, Urman J, Fernandez J, et al. Systemic, renal, and hepatic hemodynamic derangement in cirrhotic patients with spontaneous bacterial peritonitis. Hepatology 2003;38:1210–8.
37 Ruiz-del-Arbol L, Monescillo A, Arocena C, et al. Circulatory function and hepatorenal syndrome in cirrhosis. Hepatology 2005;42:439–47.
38 Sampathkumar P, Lerman A, Kim BY, et al. Post-liver transplantation myocardial dysfunction. Liver Transpl Surg 1998;4:399–403.
39 Keller H, Bezjak V, Stegaru B, Buss J, Holm E, Heene DL. Ventricular function in cirrhosis and portasystemic shunt: a two-dimensional echocardiographic study. Hepatology 1988;8:658–62.
40 Ahmed SS, Howard M, ten Hove W, Leevy CM, Regan TJ. Cardiac function in alcoholics with cirrhosis: absence of overt cardiomyopathy: myth or fact? J Am Coll Cardiol 1984; 3:696–702.
41 Wong F, Girgrah N, Graba J, Allidina Y, Liu P, Blendis L. The cardiac response to exercise in cirrhosis. Gut 2001;49: 268–75.
42 Limas CJ, Guiha NH, Lekagul O, Cohn JN. Impaired left ventricular function in alcoholic cirrhosis with ascites: ineffectiveness of ouabain. Circulation 1974;49:754–60.
43 Mikulic E, Munoz C, Puntoni LE, Lebrec D. Hemodynamic effects of dobutamine in patients with alcoholic cirrhosis. Clin Pharmacol Ther 1983;34:56–9.
44 Ramond MJ, Comoy E, Lebrec D. Alterations in isoprenaline sensitivity in patients with cirrhosis: evidence of abnormality of the sympathetic nervous activity. Br J Clin Pharmacol 1986;21:191–6.
45 Krag A, Bendtsen F, Mortensen C, Henriksen JH, Moller S. Effects of a single terlipressin administration on cardiac function and perfusion in cirrhosis. Eur J Gastroenterol Hepatol 2010;22:1085–92.

46 Braverman AC, Steiner MA, Picus D, White H. High-output congestive heart failure following transjugular intrahepatic portal-systemic shunting. Chest 1995;107:1467–9.
47 Gines P, Uriz J, Calahorra B, et al. Transjugular intrahepatic portosystemic shunting versus paracentesis plus albumin for refractory ascites in cirrhosis. Gastroenterology 2002;123: 1839–47.
48 Pimenta J, Paulo C, Gomes A, Silva S, Rocha-Goncalves F, Bettencourt P. B-type natriuretic peptide is related to cardiac function and prognosis in hospitalized patients with decompensated cirrhosis. Liver Int 2010;30:1059–66.
49 Kazankov K, Holland-Fischer P, Andersen NH, et al. Resting myocardial dysfunction in cirrhosis quantified by tissue Doppler imaging. Liver Int 2011;31:534–40.
50 Finucci G, Desideri A, Sacerdoti D, et al. Left ventricular diastolic function in liver cirrhosis. Scand J Gastroenterol 1996;31:279–84.
51 Wong F, Liu P, Lilly L, Bomzon A, Blendis L. Role of cardiac structural and functional abnormalities in the pathogenesis of hyperdynamic circulation and renal sodium retention in cirrhosis. Clin Sci (Lond) 1999;97:259–67.
52 Potter LR, Yoder AR, Flora DR, Antos LK, Dickey DM. Natriuretic peptides: their structures, receptors, physiologic functions and therapeutic applications. Handb Exp Pharmacol 2009:341–66.
53 Wong F, Siu S, Liu P, Blendis LM. Brain natriuretic peptide: is it a predictor of cardiomyopathy in cirrhosis? Clin Sci (Lond) 2001;101:621–8.
54 Day CP, James OF, Butler TJ, Campbell RW. QT prolongation and sudden cardiac death in patients with alcoholic liver disease. Lancet 1993;341:1423–8.
55 Ytting H, Henriksen JH, Fuglsang S, Bendtsen F, Moller S. Prolonged Q-T(c) interval in mild portal hypertensive cirrhosis. J Hepatol 2005;43:637–44.
56 Zambruni A, Di Micoli A, Lubisco A, Domenicali M, Trevisani F, Bernardi M. QT interval correction in patients with cirrhosis. J Cardiovasc Electrophysiol 2007;18: 77–82.
57 Henriksen JH, Bendtsen F, Hansen EF, Moller S. Acute nonselective beta-adrenergic blockade reduces prolonged frequency-adjusted Q-T interval (QTc) in patients with cirrhosis. J Hepatol 2004;40:239–46.
58 Bernardi M, Calandra S, Colantoni A, et al. Q-T interval prolongation in cirrhosis: prevalence, relationship with severity, and etiology of the disease and possible pathogenetic factors. Hepatology 1998;27:28–34.
59 Trevisani F, Merli M, Savelli F, et al. QT interval in patients with non-cirrhotic portal hypertension and in cirrhotic patients treated with transjugular intrahepatic porto-systemic shunt. J Hepatol 2003;38:461–7.
60 Henriksen JH, Fuglsang S, Bendtsen F, Christensen E, Moller S. Dyssynchronous electrical and mechanical systole in patients with cirrhosis. J Hepatol 2002;36:513–20.
61 Yang YY, Lin HC. The heart: pathophysiology and clinical implications of cirrhotic cardiomyopathy. J Chin Med Assoc 2012;75:619–23.
62 Pozzi M, Grassi G, Ratti L, et al. Cardiac, neuroadrenergic, and portal hemodynamic effects of prolonged aldosterone blockade in postviral child A cirrhosis. Am J Gastroenterol 2005;100:1110–6.
63 MacFadyen RJ, Barr CS, Struthers AD. Aldosterone blockade reduces vascular collagen turnover, improves heart rate variability and reduces early morning rise in heart rate in heart failure patients. Cardiovasc Res 1997;35:30–4.
64 Gaemperli O, Liga R, Spyrou N, et al. Myocardial beta-adrenoceptor down-regulation early after infarction is associated with long-term incidence of congestive heart failure. Eur Heart J 2010;31:1722–9.
65 Fonarow GC. When to initiate beta-blockers in heart failure: is it ever too early? Curr Heart Fail Rep 2005;2:94–9.
66 Serste T, Francoz C, Durand F, et al. Beta-blockers cause paracentesis-induced circulatory dysfunction in patients with cirrhosis and refractory ascites: a cross-over study. J Hepatol 2011;55:794–9.
67 Xanthos T, Vasileiou PV, Kakavas S, Syggelou A, Iacovidou N. the potential role of erythropoietin as a pleiotropic agent in post-cardiac arrest syndrome. Curr Pharm Des 2011; 17:1517–29.
68 Mancini DM, Katz SD, Lang CC, LaManca J, Hudaihed A, Androne AS. Effect of erythropoietin on exercise capacity in patients with moderate to severe chronic heart failure. Circulation 2003;107:294–9.
69 Silverberg DS, Wexler D, Sheps D, et al. The effect of correction of mild anemia in severe, resistant congestive heart failure using subcutaneous erythropoietin and intravenous iron: a randomized controlled study. J Am Coll Cardiol 2001;37:1775–80.
70 Hirose S, Takahashi M, Ogawa R, et al. Erythropoietin attenuates the development of experimental autoimmune myocarditis. Cardiovasc Drugs Ther 2007;21:17–27.
71 Hamed S, Barshack I, Luboshits G, et al. Erythropoietin improves myocardial performance in doxorubicin-induced cardiomyopathy. Eur Heart J 2006;27:1876–83.
72 Lipsic E, Schoemaker RG, van der Meer P, Voors AA, van Veldhuisen DJ, van Gilst WH. Protective effects of erythropoietin in cardiac ischemia: from bench to bedside. J Am Coll Cardiol 2006;48:2161–7.
73 Padillo J, Rioja P, Munoz-Villanueva MC, et al. BNP as marker of heart dysfunction in patients with liver cirrhosis. Eur J Gastroenterol Hepatol 2010;22:1331–6.
74 Kim YK, Shin WJ, Song JG, et al. Evaluation of intraoperative brain natriuretic peptide as a predictor of 1-year mortality after liver transplantation. Transplant Proc 2011;43: 1684–90.
75 Narayanan Menon KV, Nyberg SL, Harmsen WS, et al. MELD and other factors associated with survival after liver transplantation. Am J Transplant 2004;4:819–25.

76 Waku S, Iida N, Ishihara T. Significance of brain natriuretic peptide measurement as a diagnostic indicator of cardiac function. Methods Inf Med 2000;39:249–53.

77 Bernal V, Pascual I, Lanas A, et al. Cardiac function and amino-terminal pro-brain natriuretic peptide levels in liver-transplanted cirrhotic patients. Clin Transplant 2012;26:111–6.

78 Pateron D, Beyne P, Laperche T, et al. Elevated circulating cardiac troponin I in patients with cirrhosis. Hepatology 1999;29:640–3.

79 Coss E, Watt KD, Pedersen R, Dierkhising R, Heimbach JK, Charlton MR. Predictors of cardiovascular events after liver transplantation: a role for pretransplant serum troponin levels. Liver Transpl 2011;17:23–31.

80 Liu H, Lee SS. Predicting cardiovascular complications after liver transplantation: 007 to the rescue? Liver Transpl 2011; 17:7–9.

CHAPTER 21
Adrenal insufficiency

Emily Dannhorn and James O'Beirne
Sheila Sherlock Liver Centre, Royal Free Hospital, London, UK

Introduction

The concept of inadequate cortisol production during critical illness such as in septic shock has been termed relative adrenal insufficiency (RAI) and, more recently, critical illness-related corticosteroid insufficiency (CIRCI). Both these conditions have been described in critically ill patients where cortisol production and/or utilization by peripheral tissues is insufficient, leading to adverse outcomes such as increased levels of shock and mortality [1].

Due to similarities between liver failure and septic shock numerous investigators have studied the prevalence and impact of adrenal insufficiency (AI) in liver disease of various etiologies and severities. Initial results are intriguing; AI appears to be common not only in critically ill patients with liver disease, but also in patients with stable cirrhosis and post-liver transplantation. In addition, emerging evidence appears to show that AI is more prevalent in patients developing complications of cirrhosis and its presence may affect the efficacy of treatment of those complications.

Currently, there is no randomized trial evidence to support the routine administration of supplemental steroids to patients with AI and complications of cirrhosis. This is partly due to difficulties encountered in the accurate measurement of cortisol in patients with cirrhosis but initial data would suggest that the presence of AI may worsen outcomes and therefore in appropriate settings the presence of AI should be considered and treated, especially if patients are not responding to conventional treatment.

Background

The hypothalamic–pituitary–adrenal axis (HPA) is instrumental in the body's ability to deal with stress, particularly in the context of critical illness, during which cortisol has many vital roles. These include, but are not limited to, preserving vascular tone and permeability, increasing myocardial contractility, stimulating anti-inflammatory cytokine production, and initiation of lipolysis and protein catabolism [2]. Animal studies have clearly demonstrated that adrenalectomized subjects succumb rapidly to shock and corticosteroid replacement in these situations is protective [3]. In septic shock, supplemental corticosteroids have been shown to lead to faster shock reversal and low levels of serum cortisol are associated with increased mortality [4,5]. Further studies showed that some patients with septic shock had inappropriately low levels of cortisol, subnormal responses to adrenocortical stimulation, and blunted pressor responses to norepinephrine that could be restored by the administration of corticosteroids. The finding of inappropriately low cortisol levels in critically unwell patients led to the new term of relative adrenal insufficiency (RAI) [6]. More recently, the term CIRCI (critical illness-related corticosteroid insufficiency) has been used to describe a clinical picture caused by inadequate cortisol activity either by inadequate production and/or peripheral corticosteroid resistance, which is characterized by a much amplified and prolonged systemic inflammatory response [7].

Septic shock and liver failure share the same hemodynamic features (i.e., systemic vasodilatation, low mean

Cirrhosis: A practical guide to management, First Edition. Edited by Samuel S. Lee and Richard Moreau.

arterial pressure, and raised cardiac output), therefore the prevalence of AI has also been studied in patients with liver disease. RAI appears to be prevalent in patients with cirrhosis and septic shock and is associated with increased mortality [8]. RAI has also been identified in patients with stable cirrhosis, nonseptic complications of cirrhosis (bleeding, ascites), and in patients post-liver transplantation [9]. The presence of AI even in the absence of critical illness in patients with cirrhosis suggests that adrenal dysfunction may be a complication of liver disease per se, leading to the term hepato-adrenal syndrome [10]. This chapter discusses the importance of AI in cirrhosis and its complications, methods of diagnosis in the correct clinical context, and treatment options. Areas where evidence is currently limited are highlighted.

Physiology of the hypothalamic–pituitary–adrenal axis

The body's ability to respond appropriately to situations of stress is dependent on cortisol production by the adrenal gland regulated by the HPA axis. Under normal nonstressed conditions, cortisol secretion is pulsatile in fashion, and demonstrates marked diurnal variation. Peak levels are seen between 6 and 8 a.m. (6–23 μg/dL), with the lowest levels noted at midnight.

During conditions of stress, corticotropin-releasing hormone (CRH) is released from the hypothalamus in response to inflammatory cytokines and other stimuli. CRH stimulates release of adrenocorticotropic hormone (ACTH) from the anterior pituitary, which in turn promotes the release of cortisol from the adrenal cortex. This process is tightly regulated by a series of negative feedback loops such that the release of cortisol is extremely sensitive to changes in levels of ACTH.

Following its secretion, 90% of cortisol circulates in plasma bound to cortisol binding globulin (CBG), and to a lesser extent albumin. Less than 10% of cortisol circulates in the biologically active free form. Cortisol is able to diffuse rapidly across cell membranes, where it undergoes binding to glucocorticoid receptors. The glucocorticoid receptor is responsible for downstream signaling within the cell, and has several different isoforms that can be expressed differentially within various tissues, signaling different pathways [11]. Following binding to glucocorticoid receptors, the complex is translocated into the nucleus of the cell, where the effects of cortisol are exerted.

Cortisol is not stored within the adrenal gland and therefore needs to be produced rapidly on demand from its precursors during times of stress. The main substrate for cortisol synthesis is cholesterol, particularly high-density lipoprotein (HDL) cholesterol. More than 80% of cortisol is produced from cholesterol at times of stress, and this is of particular relevance in conditions where cholesterol levels are low (including liver disease), where inadequate levels of substrate may limit adequate synthesis [10,12].

Relative adrenal insufficiency and critical illness-related corticosteroid insufficiency

RAI is insufficient glucocorticoid activity relative to the severity of the patient's illness. RAI is usually seen in critically ill patients with low levels of serum cortisol and/or subnormal responses to adrenal stimulation. The definition of RAI does not encompass the subset of patients with apparently normal adrenal responses who appear to benefit from glucocorticoid supplementation. Therefore, a better definition is that of CIRCI. CIRCI is defined as a circulating level of cortisol inadequate for the severity of the patient's illness and comprises both suppression of the HPA axis and also tissue resistance to the actions of cortisol [7].

Pathophysiology

During critical illness, inflammatory cytokines activate the HPA axis, resulting in a rise in serum cortisol. Annane et al. [13] demonstrated clearly that extremes in cortisol levels in this context, either low or high, are associated with poor prognosis. In addition, it appeared that patients with a subnormal response to challenge with synthetic ACTH also had a worse prognosis. These two findings suggest that, in a subset of critically ill patients, cortisol levels are inadequate relative to the severity of the systemic disease, or the adrenal glands are unable to respond adequately to the correct level of stimulus resulting in RAI.

RAI/CIRCI arises from combined effects of both suppression of the HPA axis and resistance of tissue to circulating cortisol levels. Dysregulation of the HPA axis is multifactorial in critical illness, and causes include decreased ACTH response to CRH, inhibition of cortisol synthesis, and adrenal hypoperfusion. Although incompletely understood, the pro-inflammatory cytokine milieu has a central role in the process. Elevated levels of the pro-inflammatory cytokines tumor necrosis factor α (TNF-α) and interkeukin 1 (IL-1) have been shown to cause decreased ACTH response to CRH, and high levels of TNF-α can cause a reduction in cortisol synthesis by direct inhibition of the action of ACTH on the adrenal gland [14,15]. Furthermore, it has been shown that patients who demonstrate abnormal responses to exogenous ACTH also have higher levels of TNF-α [16]. Tissue resistance to glucocorticoids is thought to be due to downregulation of glucocorticoid receptor function and decreased transmission of activated receptors due to chronic exposure to pro-inflammatory cytokines such as TNF-α, IL-6, lipopolysaccharide (LPS), and macrophage migratory inhibitory factor [17–19]. This results in a picture consistent with adrenal failure, although levels of cortisol may be normal or even supranormal.

Although widely documented in the literature, there is significant variation in reported incidence of RAI/CIRCI. This can be attributed to inconsistencies within patient populations studied, differences in diagnostic methods used to assess cortisol levels (serum total cortisol, serum free cortisol or other, including salivary cortisol levels), and a lack of concrete diagnostic criteria. Standardized methods of diagnosis have not been designed, and there is as yet no consensus regarding the optimal diagnostic tests or criteria required to determine the presence of RAI.

Adrenal insufficiency and liver disease

Clinically, patients with cirrhosis have a hyperdynamic circulation, associated with decreased vascular resistance, hypotension, and increased cardiac output – a similar picture to that seen in patients with septic shock. Even in stable conditions, patients with cirrhosis demonstrate raised circulating levels of pro-inflammatory cytokines (TNF-α, IL-1, and IL-6) and endotoxin, which can have dysregulating effects on the HPA. Additionally, normal circadian rhythms within this population are disrupted by the effects of ammonia, which could affect the ability of the HPA axis to respond appropriately to stress [20,21].

Substrate depletion is an important contributor to adrenal dysfunction in liver disease. At times of stress most cortisol is synthesized from HDL cholesterol in the Apo-1 form, which is synthesized in the liver. The adrenal gland is therefore reliant on adequate substrate in order to produce levels of cortisol appropriate to the stress situation. Patients with cirrhosis have low levels of HDL cholesterol compared to controls – a finding that is proportional to disease severity as measured by Child–Pugh score [12]. The impact of this finding is observed in critically ill liver patients where adrenal responses correlate with baseline HDL levels and adrenal dysfunction can be seen to develop in patients with previously normal adrenal function and low HDL levels during prolonged critical illness – the adrenal exhaustion syndrome [10,22]. Another possible cause of AI in patients with cirrhosis is adrenal hemorrhage secondary to coagulopathy. In the study by Harry et al. [23], out of 12 patients that died, 8 had a postmortem and 1 patient was shown to have sustained adrenal hemorrhage (Figure 21.1).

Prevalence and clinical relevance of adrenal insufficiency in liver disease

The true prevalence of RAI/CIRCI in cirrhosis is controversial as varying definitions have been used and there are inherent difficulties in measurement of cortisol in patients with liver disease. What is clear is that whichever definition is used the prevalence of the syndrome appears to correlate with disease severity and also carries prognostic significance.

RAI/CIRCI in critically ill patients with liver disease

In patients with acute liver injury and liver failure, Harry et al. [23] found that the prevalence of AI was increased in line with the severity of liver disease and the degree of organ failure. In this study of 45 patients with either acute liver injury or acute liver failure, patients underwent adrenal function testing with the short Synacthen test (SST). An impaired response to adrenal stimulation was seen in 37% of patients with subnormal responses to

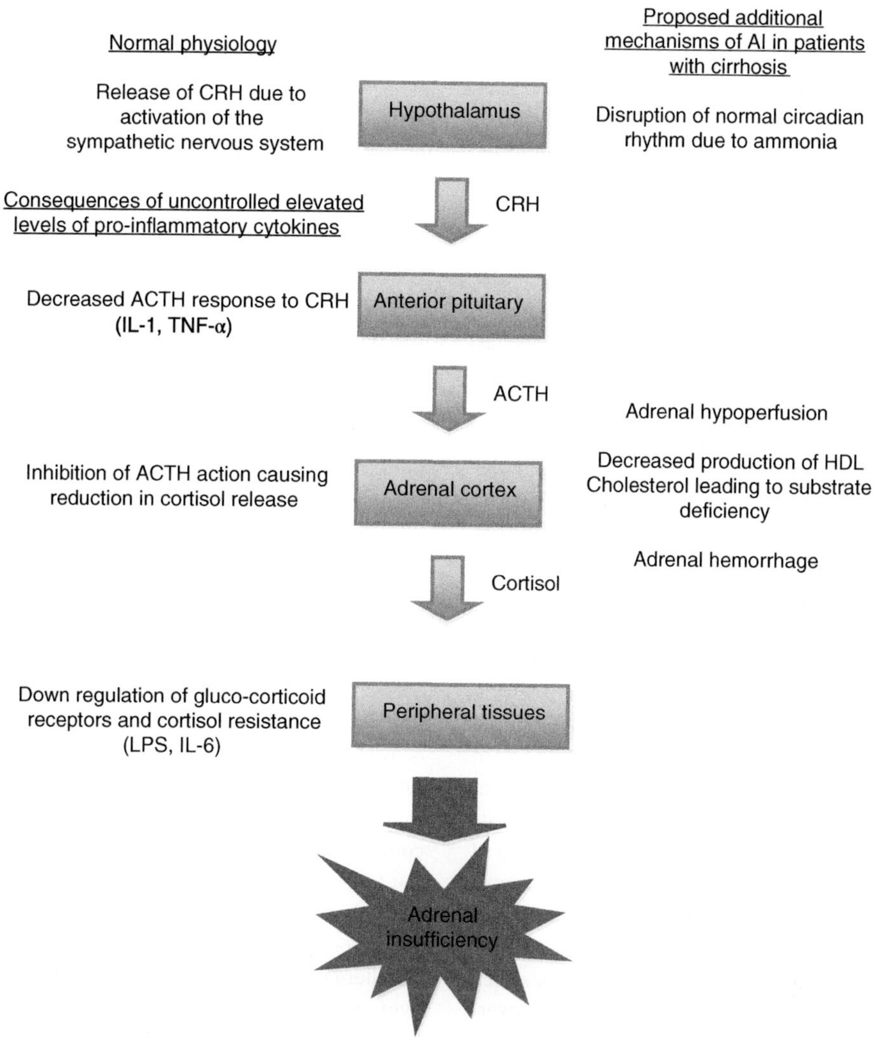

Figure 21.1 Pathophysiology of adrenal dysfunction in liver disease – The normal events leading to activation of the HPA and consequences of uncontrolled elevated levels of proinflammatory cytokines on the left of the figure. Factors that may be more relevant in patients with liver disease outlined on the right of the figure. ACTH, adrenocorticotropic hormone; CRH, corticotropin-releasing hormone; IL, interleukin; LPS, lipopolysaccharide; TNF, tumor necrosis factor.

adrenal stimulation seen more frequently in patients with more severe organ failure, need for emergency transplantation, and nonsurvivors.

In patients with cirrhosis and septic shock. Tsai et al. [8] studied 101 septic cirrhotic patients, who underwent adrenal function testing. The results demonstrated that 51% of patients fulfilled their criteria for AI (baseline cortisol <9 μg/dL or an increment of <9 μg/dL after stimulation with 250 μg Synacthen). Patients with AI had lower mean arterial pressure and were more likely to need vasopressor support. Of note, a correlation was demonstrated between the degree of adrenal dysfunction and severity of disease, as per Child–Pugh, MELD, and Apache III scores. The response to adrenal stimulation was also an independent predictor of mortality, which was increased in the AI group.

Using an alternative definition of AI, Marik et al. [10] reported the prevalence of AI within 340 patients admitted to a liver intensive care unit. The incidence of AI was found to be 66% in critically ill cirrhotic patients, with a prevalence of 33% in acute liver failure patients. In this study, the mortality rate of patients with AI was 39% overall. Patients who were subsequently treated with steroids had a mortality rate of 26% compared with 46% in those not treated with steroids, although this was not assessed in a randomized fashion. The use of hydrocortisone in cirrhotic patients with septic shock has now been assessed in a retrospective cohort study and a randomized controlled clinical trial [24,25]. In the first study, the effect of treating patients with cirrhosis and septic shock with low dose hydrocortisone was evaluated in a prospective fashion. Critically ill cirrhotic patients (n=25) with either an inappropriately low random cortisol (<15 g/dL) or a subnormal (<9 g/dL) response to SST received 50 mg hydrocortisone four times daily. The patients treated with steroids were compared with a group of patients treated on the same intensive treatment unit prior to the introduction of adrenal function testing in septic shock. AI was diagnosed in 18/25 (68%). In the treated group of patients there was quicker resolution of shock and an increase in hospital survival compared to the 50 historical controls that had not undergone adrenal function testing (64% vs. 32%). In a randomized trial of patients with cirrhosis and septic shock, 75 patients underwent adrenal function testing and were randomized to receive intravenous 50 mg hydrocortisone four times daily or placebo within 48 hours of shock onset. Hydrocortisone therapy was continued until shock reversal (cessation of vasopressors) and the primary outcome was all cause 28-day mortality. The overall incidence of AI in the study population was 76% and was not significantly different between treated patients and controls. There was no difference in survival between the two groups although hydrocortisone-treated patients had a faster resolution of shock. However, in hydrocortisone-treated patients there was a higher incidence of shock relapse and gastrointestinal bleeding. The incidence of shock relapse in this study was much higher than in other studies using low dose hydrocortisone suggesting that one factor leading to the overall negative result may have been the abrupt cessation of steroid supplementation rather than tapering. This could be important in patients with cirrhosis if one considers that AI may be a pre-existing condition rather than a result of the sepsis per se.

Prevalence of adrenal insufficiency in stable cirrhosis

AI has been documented in patients with stable liver disease in a number of studies. In the majority of these studies, the prevalence of AI appears to increase with increasing disease severity, as per MELD or Child score. A number of studies have shown that there does not appear to be a significant proven association with prognosis, although this conclusion has been limited by short follow-up or indeed no follow-up reported. Within these studies, a range of prevalence of AI has been demonstrated, from 6.3% to 58% depending on the adrenal function assay used (Table 21.1). More recently, AI has been associated with the incidence of complications and death in a large cohort of patients with cirrhosis [26].

Galbois et al. [27] studied 88 stable inpatients, admitted for complications of cirrhosis but without hemorrhage or hemodynamic compromise. All patients had measurement of levels of CBG, total serum cortisol, and salivary cortisol before and after stimulation with 250 μg Synacthen. The definitions used to define AI were baseline serum total cortisol <9 μg/dL, or a concentration 60 minutes after Synacthen <18 μg/dL, or an increment following stimulation of <9 μg/dL (i.e., Δ cortisol). Using salivary cortisol assays, a basal value of <1.8 ng/mL, or a concentration 1 hour after Synacthen <12.7 ng/mL, or Δ <3 ng/mL was used to diagnose AI. Serum free cortisol was calculated using serum total cortisol and CBG levels with Coolens' equation. Salivary cortisol showed an excellent correlation with calculated free cortisol; however, it correlated less well with serum total cortisol levels – this led to significant differences in the frequency of the diagnosis of AI depending on the test used. Using serum total cortisol levels, 33% of the patients were considered to have AI, compared to the use of salivary cortisol levels, where only 9.1% of patients fulfilled the definition of AI. Of the patients diagnosed with AI using serum total cortisol levels, 21 had normal adrenal function according to salivary cortisol measurements.

In a further study by Tan et al. [28], the relationship between serum total cortisol, serum free cortisol, and calculated free cortisol was investigated within a cohort of 43 stable cirrhotic patients, compared with a healthy control group. Patients underwent testing before and after adrenal stimulation with 250 μg Synacthen. Baseline (T_0) serum total cortisol levels were similar between the patient and control groups, but peak and incremental

Table 21.1 Prevalence of adrenal insufficiency (AI) in patients with stable cirrhosis.

Author	No of patients	Type of liver disease	Definition of adrenal insufficiency	Patients fulfilling definition (%)	Outcome in adrenally insufficient patients
Galbois [27]	88	Stable cirrhosis	Short Synacthen test Peak <18 μg/dL Any part 9 μg/dL	33	Not reported
Tan [28]	43	Stable cirrhosis	Short Synacthen test Increment <9 μg/dL	58	AI not associated with outcome
Thevenot [34]	85	Stable cirrhosis	Short Synacthen test Peak <18 μg/dL	6.3	No association of AI with outcome
Fede [9]	101	Stable cirrhosis	Low dose short Synacthen test Peak <18 μg/dL	38	Not reported
Zietz [52]	52	Stable cirrhosis	CRH test Peak <18 μg/dL	57	Not reported
McDonald [53]	27	Stable cirrhosis	Short Synacthen test No definition of AI used	39% reduction in cortisol increment compared with controls	Not reported

levels were significantly lower. However, using plasma free cortisol levels, there was no difference found between patients and healthy controls, suggesting that measured serum total cortisol levels were spuriously low in the cirrhotic patient group. A total of 58% of patients fulfilled criteria for AI with Δcortisol <9 μg/dL following adrenal stimulation. Comparatively, using serum free cortisol levels, only 12% of patients had AI.

Adrenal function testing in cirrhosis – which test?

It is clear from the studies outlined above that the prevalence of AI in cirrhosis depends on which test is used. At the present time this area is not settled as the more accurate tests for cortisol are not available outside of a research setting and normal ranges have not been defined. Current guidelines for critically unwell patients propose a definition of Δ serum total cortisol of <9 μg/dL following SST, or a random serum total cortisol of <10 μg/dL in order to diagnose AI. However, this definition pertains to a general patient population, and is not specific for liver disease. In the majority of published literature in this area, the same cutoff values for diagnosing AI have been applied to patients regardless of whether they are critically ill or stable. This may not be correct and traditional assays based on serum total cortisol levels may be inaccurate due to patients with cirrhosis having subnormal CBG or albumin levels leading to a spuriously low total cortisol level and hence overestimation of the prevalence of AI. Differences also exist in the stimulation tests used: some studies have used the low dose (1 μg) Synacthen test, as opposed to the standard dose of 250 μg [9]. This renders studies difficult to compare, and provides challenges with regards to collating data from multiple studies [29].

Assessment of adrenocortical function is usually based on the short ACTH stimulation test (SST), with measurement of serum total cortisol before and after administration of a synthetic ACTH (cosyntropin). The standard high dose test involves administration of 250-μg cosyntropin. A normal response after 30 or 60 minutes is a peak of 18–20 μg/dL and an increment of >9 μg/dL. Most studies have used the 250-μg dose to stimulate adrenal function. However, this dose results in an elevation of ACTH levels of up to 100 times higher than expected physiologically in severe stress situations. An alternative low-dose stimulation test (1-μg dose of cosyntropin) has therefore been proposed in an attempt to elicit a more physiologic assessment of adrenal reserve [30].

There is no consensus regarding whether the low-dose test is superior to the high-dose ACTH stimulation test although the low-dose SST may be more sensitive and detect partial AI that may be missed by the standard high-dose test [30,31].

Comparision of studies is made more complicated when accounting for the fact that assessing adrenal function in cirrhotic patients appears to be inaccurate due to changes in the plasma levels of cortisol binding globulin and albumin. Ninety percent of serum cortisol circulates bound to CBG and albumin; only 10% exists in the biologically active free form. Traditional laboratory assays have only measured serum total cortisol. Therefore, in conditions associated with lower plasma levels of CBG and albumin, including cirrhosis, liver failure, and sepsis, there is potential for overdiagnosing AI. Measurement of serum free cortisol would therefore seem to be the ideal assay; however, this is difficult outside of a research setting and is time consuming, expensive, and therefore impractical within routine clinical practice. Other methods of estimating the serum free cortisol level include salivary cortisol levels, free cortisol index, and calculation using Coolens' equation [27,32,33].

In patients with cirrhosis (95 nonseptic and 30 septic), Thevenot et al. [34] measured levels pre and post administration of 250 µg Synacthen of serum total cortisol, serum free cortisol, and salivary cortisol. They demonstrated that serum total cortisol levels overestimated AI in patients with end-stage liver disease. Of note, they showed that salivary cortisol levels correlated well with free cortisol levels, indicating that salivary cortisol may well provide a good surrogate marker for serum free cortisol.

However, in current clinical practice, measurement of serum total cortisol remains the most readily available test and in patients with cirrhosis and a serum albumin >25 g/dL serum total cortisol appears to give results comparable with serum free cortisol. For the purposes of standardization the 250 µg standard dose SST should be used, as this is the most widely available test within current clinical settings. A result demonstrating Δ cortisol <9 µg/dL can be used to diagnose AI within this population [35].

Adrenal function and the complications of cirrhosis – who should be tested and who should be treated?

Cirrhosis and septic shock

Current guidance recommends that patients with septic shock who are poorly responsive to fluid resuscitation and vasopressors are treated with supplemental corticosteroids. There is no consensus regarding the optimal steroid dose regimen, or indeed regarding duration of treatment; however, doses greater than 300 mg/day hydrocortisone are not recommended and steroid tapering after shock resolution is recommended [36]. Of note, the guidelines also suggest that, for patients with septic shock, ACTH testing should not be used to select patients for treatment with corticosteroids, due to potentially unreliable laboratory assays of plasma cortisol concentration in critically ill patients. In this regard the recent CORTICUS study [37] has shown that supplemental corticosteroids in a general population of patients with septic shock is not associated with any significant benefit other than faster shock reversal and this benefit was independent of the presence or absence of AI. However, these results may not be applicable to patients with cirrhosis and sepsis who may already have pre-existing AI associated with cirrhosis. In early uncontrolled studies of cirrhosis and septic shock the presence of AI was associated with a worse outcome and more use of vasopressors. Moreover, the use of supplemental corticosteroids was associated with improved hemodynamic responses and better survival than historical controls, suggesting a role for supplemental steroids in septic patients with liver disease [8,10,24,38]. These findings are in contrast to the recent report by Arabi et al. [25], which found no benefit of hydrocortisone in cirrhotic patients with septic shock. As mentioned previously, one reason for this apparent lack of benefit may have been the rather abrupt taper of steroids after resolution of shock. Previous studies have demonstrated that abrupt cessation of steroids, as opposed to a gradual dose tapering, is associated with rebound of hemodynamic collapse and increased inflammatory markers [39]. It is conceivable that this effect may be even more pronounced in those who already have baseline AI such as patients with cirrhosis, which may account for the high rate of shock relapse in the Arabi study. Further studies addressing the role of supplemental hydrocortisone, duration of treatment and impact of AI in septic patients with cirrhosis are needed. For the moment our current practice is to treat patients with cirrhosis and septic shock fulfilling the surviving sepsis guidance with hydrocortisone (100 mg intravenous bolus followed by 10 mg/hour) until shock resolution. Following shock resolution, steroids are tapered according to the presence or absence of AI on a baseline SST (Figure 21.2).

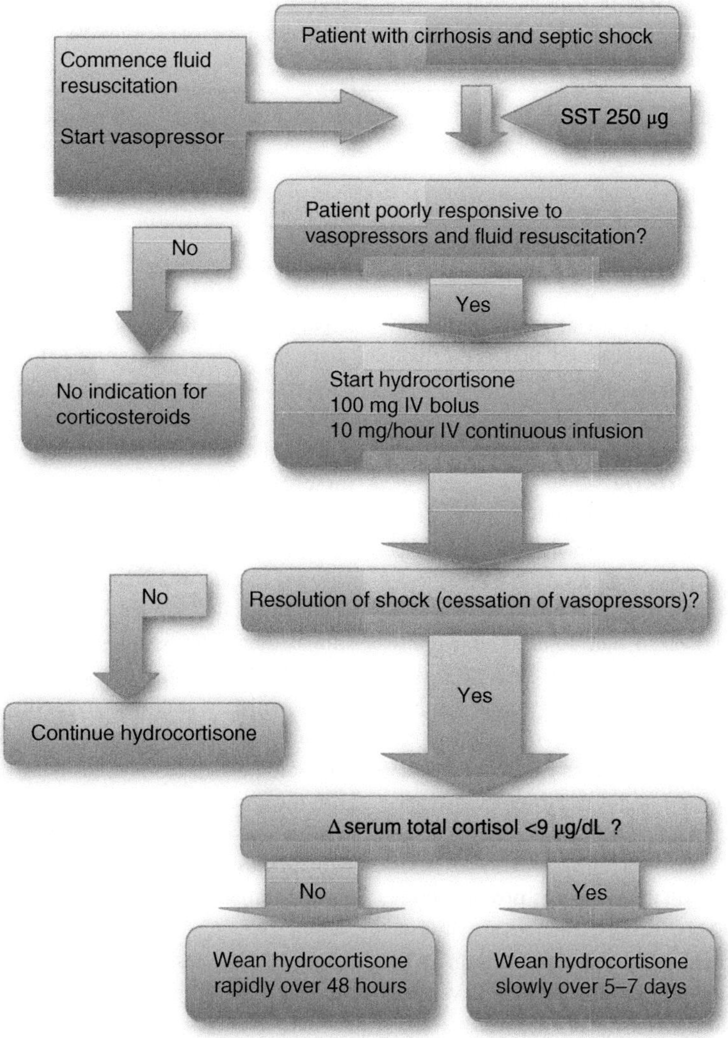

Figure 21.2 Suggested algorithm for the diagnosis and management of adrenal insufficiency (AI) in septic shock and cirrhosis. SST, short Synacthen test.

Complications of cirrhosis

The prevalence of AI increases with increasing severity of liver disease. Recent data have shown that the presence of AI is also more frequent in patients with complications of cirrhosis. Acevedo et al. [40] performed a prospective study of 160 patients admitted to a single center with complications of cirrhosis but without septic shock. All patients underwent an SST and AI was defined as a Δ serum total cortisol <9 μg/dL. AI was found in 26% of the admissions and compared with patients without AI these patients exhibited more circulatory dysfunction, hyponatremia, and more frequently exhibited markers of systemic inflammation respose syndrome (SIRS) (Table 21.2). Interestingly, patients with AI more frequently developed infections and septic shock than non-AI patients. Mortality was also significantly higher in the AI group than the non-AI group (19% vs. 7%; $P = 0.04$).

The association of AI with markers of circulatory dysfunction raises the possibility that treatment of cirrhotic patients with supplemental corticosteroids may

Table 21.2 Serum sodium and markers of circulatory dysfunction in cirrhotic patients with adrenal insufficiency (AI) (n = 43) compared with cirrhotic patients without AI on admission to hospital (n = 123). MAP, mean arterial pressure; Na, sodium; PRA, plasma rennin activity; SIRS, systemic inflammatory response syndrome.

	MAP (mmHg)	PRA (ng/mL/hour)	Noradrenaline (pg/mL)	Serum Na <130 (%)	SIRS (%)
AI	77	6.7	548	44	51
No AI	82	4.0	448	21	27

lead to improved outcomes. There are as yet no randomized trials in this area; however, recent data suggest that this may be a fruitful area of research.

Adrenal insufficiency, refractory ascites, and hepatorenal syndrome

The development of ascites and ultimately hepatorenal syndrome is defined by a progressive alteration in systemic hemodynamics such as low mean arterial pressure, decreased systemic vascular resistance, and a raised cardiac output [41]. It is now clear that despite the overall increase in cardiac output, some patients with cirrhosis have a "latent" cardiomyopathy that results in an inability to maintain organ perfusion in the face of progressive systemic vasodilatation or an acute insult such as bleeding or infection [42,43]. This cirrhotic cardiomyopathy is characterized by chronotropic and inotropic incompetence, diastolic dysfunction, and electrocardiographic abnormalities such as prolongation of the QT interval [44]. Many of these changes are similar to those found in patients with acute and chronic AI, raising the possibility that AI contributes to the development of cirrhotic cardiomyopathy. This is an important concept as the cardiomyopathy associated with AI is reversible with treatment and therefore in patients with cirrhosis at risk of complications, AI may be an important therapeutic target [45]. As yet, the link between adrenal function and cirrhotic cardiomyopathy is yet to be proven and as yet there are no randomized clinical trials that show benefit of supplemental steroids in patients with complications of cirrhosis. However, emerging evidence points to a potential therapeutic role for supplemental hydrocortisone in certain clinical settings. One such area is refractory ascites.

In a pilot study, Alessandria et al. [46] examined adrenal responses in 25 patients with ascites. Of the patients, 16 had refractory ascites and of these 50% had AI. Patients with refractory ascites or type 2 hepatorenal syndrome underwent treatment with 50 mg hydrocortisone 6-hourly for 7 days. In the treated patients there was significant improvement noted in mean arterial pressure, plasma renin activity, natriuresis, and renal function. Although this was a small pilot study these data suggest that addressing AI in patients with circulatory dysfunction can result in an amelioration of the hyperdynamic circulatory state and provides a rationale for considering treatment. In contrast, however, a recent study of AI in patients with variceal bleeding has shown that although the prevalence of AI in patients with bleeding was significantly higher than stable cirrhotic patients and healthy controls (60% vs. 48%), the presence of AI was not associated with a worse outcome [47].

In the absence of controlled clinical trial data, concrete recommendations for testing and treating AI in patients with cirrhosis and complications cannot be made. However, AI appears to be common and carries prognostic significance. Therefore, in certain clinical situations (Figure 21.3), testing for and treating AI in patients without other therapeutic options or where prognosis is likely to be poor appears reasonable [48].

Adrenal insufficiency and liver transplantation

Liver transplantation (LT) is the treatment for many of the complications of chronic liver disease. The high prevalence of adrenal dysfunction in stable cirrhotic patients would suggest that AI would also be prevalent in the perioperative stage. Postoperatively, however, AI may not be clinically apparent as the use of corticosteroids both intra- and postoperatively is common and may effectively "mask" AI. Increasingly, transplant centers are using steroid-free immunosuppressant regimens in order to minimize the known risks of steroids

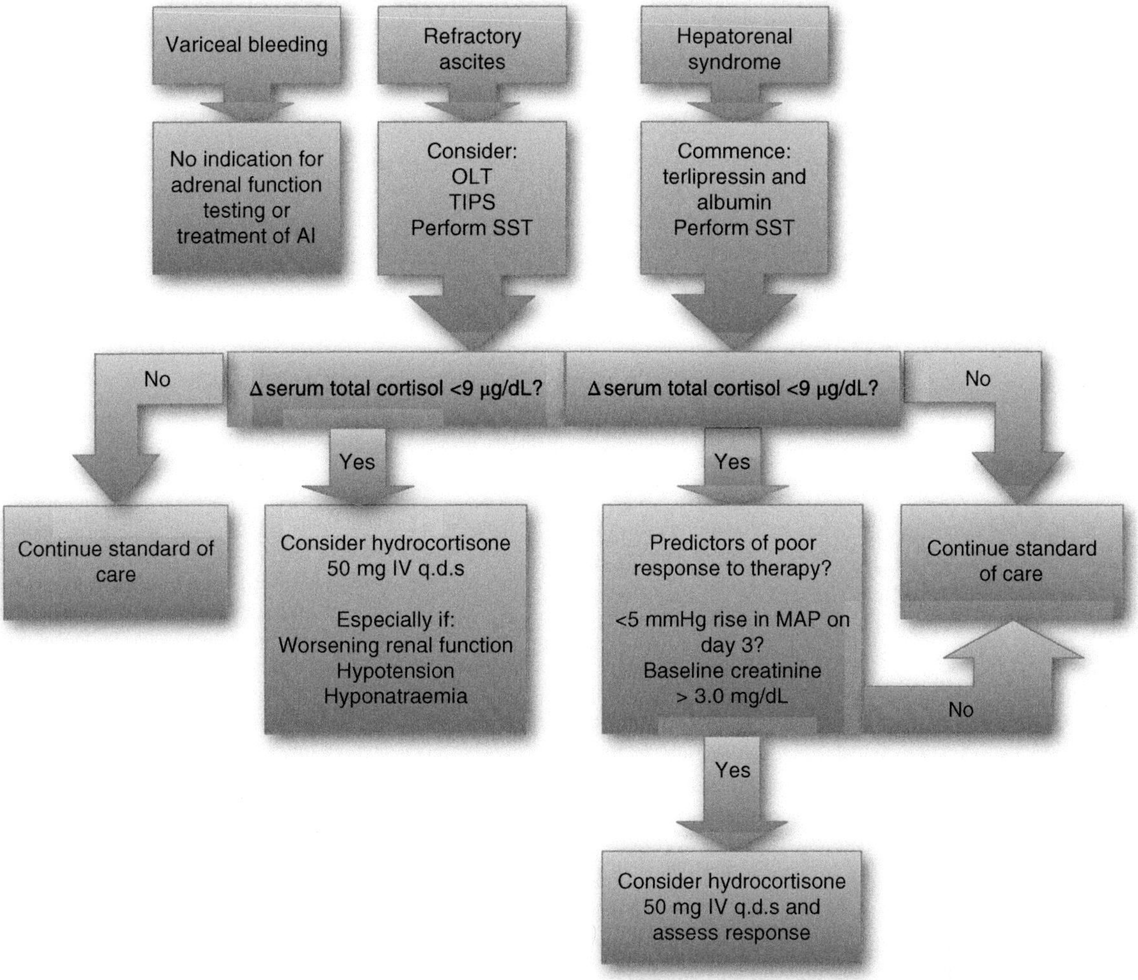

Figure 21.3 Suggested algorithm for adrenal function testing and treatment of adrenal insufficiency (AI) in patients with complications of cirrhosis. MAP, mean arterial pressure; OLT, orthotopic liver transplantation; q.d.s., four times daily; SST, short Synacthen test; TIPS, transjugular intrahepatic portosystemic shunt.

such as new onset diabetes, wound infections, and concerns about the risk of recurrent hepatitis C infection in the graft. Therefore, the identification and treatment of AI in the postoperative phase of LT may become increasingly important [49].

In centers using a steroid-free immunosuppressant regiment, the prevalence of AI has been demonstrated to be as high as 92%; however, this was using the low-dose SST [10]. Therefore, AI may be common in post-LT patients and has the potential to cause significant morbidity if not recognized. The effect of perioperative corticosteroid administration has been shown by Patel et al. [50] who studied 90 patients undergoing first elective LT: 45 before and 45 after the protocolized intraoperative intravenous administration of 1 g methylprednisolone. Patients receiving corticosteroids had significantly reduced requirements for fluid administration, vasopressors, renal replacement therapy, invasive ventilation, and intensive care stay compared with patients not receiving steroids. These data suggest that the use of steroids in this context may have addressed a "latent" tendency towards AI although none of the patients underwent formal adrenal function testing. Corticosteroid use postoperatively prevents transplant patients developing AI; however, their prolonged use can suppress the HPA axis, and cause functional adrenal gland atrophy (FAGA), potentially leading to AI late post-transplant after steroid withdrawal [51]. SST was used to assess 87 transplant recipients postoperatively before complete steroid cessation. FAGA was apparent in 27%, and was associated with length and cumulative steroid dose, as well as total cholesterol and ACTH concentrations. Therefore, attention should be paid to the rapidity of withdrawal of steroids post-LT and consideration should be given to adrenal function testing in those patients who are at high risk of FAGA.

Conclusions

Dysfunction of the HPA axis in patients with liver disease is not uncommon, occurring both in times of acute illness and in patients with stable cirrhosis. Indeed, liver disease per se may affect the HPA axis. As yet, there are no concrete definitions available, resulting in discrepancies within prevalence across published studies. In addition, agreement needs to be reached regarding the optimal diagnostic investigation, which must be practical in clinical settings. Allowing for the limitations associated with measuring adrenal function using serum total cortisol, more data on adrenal function using standard adrenal stimulation testing are required. Currently, there are no guidelines regarding the use of supplemental steroids in patients with complications or at risk of complications of cirrhosis. Studies to determine the role of corticosteroid supplementation will be carried out but at the present time the practical approach is to consider AI in patients with cirrhosis where the prognosis is poor, especially where response to therapy is suboptimal.

References

1 Marik PE, Pastores SM, Annane D, et al. Recommendations for the diagnosis and management of corticosteroid insufficiency in critically ill adult patients: consensus statements from an international task force by the American College of Critical Care Medicine. Crit Care Med 2008;36:1937–49.

2 Streeten DH, Anderson GH, Dalakos TG, et al. Normal and abnormal function of the hypothalamic-pituitary-adrenocortical system in man. Endocr Rev 1984;5:371–94.

3 Hinshaw LB, Beller BK, Chang AC, et al. Corticosteroid/antibiotic treatment of adrenalectomized dogs challenged with lethal *E. coli*. Circ Shock 1985;16:265–77.

4 Sprung CL, Caralis PV, Marcial EH, et al. The effects of high-dose corticosteroids in patients with septic shock: a prospective, controlled study. N Engl J Med 1984;311:1137–43.

5 Annane D, Sébille V, Troché G, Raphaël JC, Gajdos P, Bellissant E. A 3-level prognostic classification in septic shock based on cortisol levels and cortisol response to corticotropin. J Am Med Assoc 2000;283:1038–45.

6 Gonzalez H, Nardi O, Annane D. Relative adrenal failure in the ICU: an identifiable problem requiring treatment. Crit Care Clin 2006;22:105–18 –vii.

7 Marik PE. Critical illness-related corticosteroid insufficiency. Chest 2009;135:181–93.

8 Tsai M-H, Peng Y-S, Chen Y-C, et al. Adrenal insufficiency in patients with cirrhosis, severe sepsis and septic shock. Hepatology 2006;43:673–81.

9 Fede G, Spadaro L, Tomaselli T, et al. Assessment of adrenocortical reserve in stable patients with cirrhosis. J Hepatol 2011;54:243–50.

10 Marik PE, Gayowski T, Starzl TE, Hepatic Cortisol Research and Adrenal Pathophysiology Study Group. The hepatoadrenal syndrome: a common yet unrecognized clinical condition. Crit Care Med 2005;33:1254–9.

11 Duma D, Jewell CM, Cidlowski JA. Multiple glucocorticoid receptor isoforms and mechanisms of post-translational modification. J Steroid Biochem Mol Biol 2006;102:11–21.

12 Atogo-Asse F-E, Vincent RP, Hughes SA, et al. High density lipoprotein in patients with liver failure; relation to sepsis, adrenal function and outcome of illness. Liver International 2011;32:128–36.

13 Annane D, Sébille V, Troché G. A 3-level prognostic classification in septic shock based on cortisol levels and cortisol response to corticotropin. J Am Med Assoc 2000;23:1038–45.

14 Kwon YS, Suh GY, Jeon K, et al. Serum cytokines and critical illness-related corticosteroid insufficiency. Intensive Care Med 2010;36:1845–51.

15 Gaillard RC, Turnill D, Sappino P, Muller AF. Tumor necrosis factor alpha inhibits the hormonal response of the pituitary gland to hypothalamic releasing factors. Endocrinology 1990;127:101–6.

16 Jäättelä M, Ilvesmäki V, Voutilainen R, Stenman UH, Saksela E. Tumor necrosis factor as a potent inhibitor of adrenocorticotropin-induced cortisol production and steroidogenic P450 enzyme gene expression in cultured human fetal adrenal cells. Endocrinology 1991;128:623–9.

17 Yang N, Ray DW, Matthews LC. Current concepts in glucocorticoid resistance. Steroids 2012;77:1041–9.

18 Ishiguro Y, Yamagata K, Sakuraba H, et al. Macrophage migration inhibitory factor and activator protein-1 in ulcerative colitis. Ann N Y Acad Sci 2004;1029:348–9.

19 Flaster H, Bernhagen J, Calandra T, Bucala R. The macrophage migration inhibitory factor-glucocorticoid dyad:

regulation of inflammation and immunity. Mol Endocrinol 2007;21:1267–80.
20 Ahabrach H, Piedrafita B, Ayad A, et al. Chronic hyperammonemia alters the circadian rhythms of corticosteroid hormone levels and of motor activity in rats. J Neurosci Res 2010;88:1605–14.
21 Montagnese S, Middleton B, Mani AR, Skene DJ, Morgan MY. On the origin and the consequences of circadian abnormalities in patients with cirrhosis. Am J Gastroenterol 2010;105:1773–81.
22 Marik PE. Adrenal-exhaustion syndrome in patients with liver disease. Intensive Care Med 2006;32:275–80.
23 Harry R, Auzinger G, Wendon J. The clinical importance of adrenal insufficiency in acute hepatic dysfunction. Hepatology 2002;36:395–402.
24 Fernández J, Escorsell A, Zabalza M, et al. Adrenal insufficiency in patients with cirrhosis and septic shock: effect of treatment with hydrocortisone on survival. Hepatology 2006;44:1288–95.
25 Arabi YM, Aljumah A, Dabbagh O, et al. Low-dose hydrocortisone in patients with cirrhosis and septic shock: a randomized controlled trial. Cmaj 2010;182:1971–7.
26 Acevedo J, Fernández J, Prado V, et al. Relative adrenal insufficiency in decompensated cirrhosis: relationship to short-term risk of severe sepsis, hepatorenal syndrome, and death. Hepatology 2013;58:1757–65.
27 Galbois A, Rudler M, Massard J, et al. Assessment of adrenal function in cirrhotic patients: salivary cortisol should be preferred. J Hepatol 2010;52:839–45.
28 Tan T, Chang L, Woodward A, et al. Characterising adrenal function using directly measured plasma free cortisol in stable severe liver disease. J Hepatol 2010;53:841–8.
29 Fede G, Spadaro L, Tomaselli T, et al. Adrenocortical dysfunction in liver disease: a systematic review. Hepatology 2012;55:1282–91.
30 Thaler LM, Blevins LS. The low dose (1-microg) adrenocorticotropin stimulation test in the evaluation of patients with suspected central adrenal insufficiency. J Clin Endocrinol Metab 1998;83:2726–9.
31 Abdu TA, Elhadd TA, Neary R, Clayton RN. Comparison of the low dose short synacthen test (1 microg), the conventional dose short synacthen test (250 microg), and the insulin tolerance test for assessment of the hypothalamo-pituitary-adrenal axis in patients with pituitary disease. Jo Clin Endocrinol Metab 1999;84:838–43.
32 le Roux CW, Sivakumaran S, Alaghband-Zadeh J, Dhillo W, Kong WM, Wheeler MJ. Free cortisol index as a surrogate marker for serum free cortisol. Ann Clin Biochem 2002;39: 406–8.
33 Coolens JL, Van Baelen H, Heyns W. Clinical use of unbound plasma cortisol as calculated from total cortisol and corticosteroid-binding globulin. J Steroid Biochem 1987;26: 197–202.
34 Thevenot T, Borot S, Remy-Martin A, et al. Assessment of adrenal function in cirrhotic patients using concentration of serum-free and salivary cortisol. Liver Int 2011;31:425–33.
35 Fede G, Spadaro L, Tomaselli T, et al. Comparison of total cortisol, free cortisol, and surrogate markers of free cortisol in diagnosis of adrenal insufficiency in patients with stable cirrhosis. Clin Gastroenterol Hepatol 2014;12:504–12, e8; quiz 23–4.
36 Surviving Sepsis Campaign. International guidelines for management of severe sepsis and septic shock: 2008. 2007;34:17–60.
37 Sprung CL, Annane D, Keh D, et al. Hydrocortisone therapy for patients with septic shock. N Engl J Med 2008;358:111–24.
38 Harry R, Auzinger G, Wendon J. The effects of supraphysiological doses of corticosteroids in hypotensive liver failure. Liver Int 2003;23:71–7.
39 Keh D, Boehnke T, Weber-Cartens S, et al. Immunologic and hemodynamic effects of "low-dose" hydrocortisone in septic shock. Am J Respir Crit Care Med 2003;167:512–20.
40 Acevedo J, Fernández J, Castro M, Roca D, Ginès P, Arroyo V. Impact of relative adrenal insufficiency on circulatory function and mortality in advanced cirrhosis. J Hepatol 2011;54:S61.
41 Braillon A, Cales P, Valla D, Gaudy D, Geoffroy P, Lebrec D. Influence of the degree of liver failure on systemic and splanchnic haemodynamics and on response to propranolol in patients with cirrhosis. Gut 1986;27:1204–9.
42 Krag A, Bendtsen F, Henriksen JH, Møller S. Low cardiac output predicts development of hepatorenal syndrome and survival in patients with cirrhosis and ascites. Gut 2010;59: 105–10.
43 Ruiz-del-Arbol L, Urman J, Fernández J, et al. Systemic, renal, and hepatic hemodynamic derangement in cirrhotic patients with spontaneous bacterial peritonitis. Hepatology 2003;38:1210–8.
44 Møller S, Henriksen JH. Cirrhotic cardiomyopathy. J Hepatol 2010;53:179–90.
45 Theocharidou E, Krag A, Bendtsen F, Møller S, Burroughs AK. Cardiac dysfunction in cirrhosis: does adrenal function play a role? A hypothesis. Liver Int 2012;32:1327–32.
46 Alessandria C, Mezzabotta L, Carello M, et al. Relative adrenal insufficiency in cirrhosis: relevance in patients with ascites and treatment with hydrocortisone in refractory ascites. Dig Liver Dis 2009;41:A13.
47 Triantos CK, Marzigie M, Fede G, et al. Critical illness-related corticosteroid insufficiency in patients with cirrhosis and variceal bleeding. Clin Gastroenterol Hepatol 2011;9:595–601.
48 Boyer TD, Sanyal AJ, Garcia-Tsao G, et al. Predictors of response to terlipressin plus albumin in hepatorenal syndrome (HRS) type 1: relationship of serum creatinine to hemodynamics. J Hepatol 2011;55:315–21.
49 Pulitanò C, Guzzetti E, Arru M, Ferla G, Aldrighetti L. In defense of the administration of perioperative steroids in liver transplantation. Liver Transpl 2008;14:124–5.

50 Patel S, Broomhead R, Burroughs AK, Mallett SV, O'Beirne J. Effect of intra-operative methylprednisolone on post liver transplant (LT) intensive care unit (ITU) course: further evidence for the existence of hepato-adrenal syndrome? J Hepatol 2010;52:S197.

51 Toniutto P, Fabris C, Fumolo E, et al. Prevalence and risk factors for delayed adrenal insufficiency after liver transplantation. Liver Transpl 2008;14:1014–9.

52 Zietz B, Lock G, Plach B, et al. Dysfunction of the hypothalamic-pituitary-glandular axes and relation to Child–Pugh classification in male patients with alcoholic and virus-related cirrhosis. Eur J Gastroenterol Hepatol 2003;15:495–501.

53 McDonald JA, Handelsman DJ, Dilworth P, Conway AJ, McCaughan GW. Hypothalamic-pituitary adrenal function in end-stage non-alcoholic liver disease. J Gastroenterol Hepatol 1993;8:247–53.

CHAPTER 22
Coagulopathy and clotting disorders

Marco Senzolo[1] and A.K. Burroughs[2]

[1]*Multivisceral Transplant Unit, Gastroenterology, Department of Surgical and Gastroenterological Sciences, University Hospital of Padua, Padua, Italy*
[2]*The Royal Free Sheila Sherlock Liver Centre and University Department of Surgery, Department of Intensive Care, Royal Free Hospital, London, UK*

Introduction

The liver has a key role in blood coagulation being involved in both primary and secondary hemostasis [1]. It is the site of synthesis of most coagulation factors and their inhibitors except for von Willebrand factor (vWf) [2]. Liver failure is accompanied by multiple changes in the hemostatic system, because of reduced plasma levels of procoagulative and anticoagulative clotting factors synthesized by the intact liver [3]. Therefore, the hemostatic system is in a delicate balance between prothrombotic and antithrombotic processes, aiming to prevent excessive blood loss from injured vessels and prevent spontaneous thrombosis. Moreover, during liver failure, there is a reduced capacity to clear activated hemostatic proteins and protein inhibitor complexes from the circulation. Thus, the global effect of liver disease with regard to hemostasis is complex, so that patients with advanced liver disease can experience severe bleeding or even thrombotic complications. Finally, when marked portal hypertension develops with secondary splenomegaly, thrombocytopenia develops due to splenic sequestration, but thrombocytopenia may also be due to decreased hepatic thrombopoietin synthesis. Demonstrated decreased platelet function could be balanced by the concomitant increase in vWf. This delicate hemostatic balance can be easily be tipped towards bleeding or thrombosis by superimposed conditions such as infections.

Hemostatic factors

Procoagulant factors

The liver is the site of synthesis of fibrinogen and factors II, V, VII, IX, X, XI, and XII [4]; vWf is synthesized by the endothelium [5]. Factor VIII is synthesized mainly by the hepatic sinusoidal endothelial cells [6,7], but also by endothelial and nonparenchymal cells in the kidney, spleen, lungs, and brain [8]. Thus, the plasma concentration of factor VIII, which is one of the most procoagulant factors, is not decreased with liver disease, but it has been shown to be increased [9]. This occurs possibly because of increased endothelial synthesis and reduced clearance via low density lipoprotein receptor-related protein [5] and increased vWf [10]. However, the biologic activity of the synthesized molecule is lower than the plasma concentration [11].

Vitamin K is an essential cofactor for the production of biologically active forms of the coagulation factors II, VII, IX, and X. It promotes hepatic post-ribosomal conversion of certain glutamic acid residues in the protein precursors, to gamma-carboxyglutamic acid (Gla). These active forms of the clotting factors chelate calcium at the Gla site resulting in effective hemostatic function. In chronic liver disease, the gamma-carboxylation is impaired due to deficiency or antagonism of vitamin K, and inert precursors are synthesized (known as proteins induced by vitamin K absence, PIVKA) and released into the bloodstream [12]. The clinical significance of these precursors is not clear. In cholestasis, reduction of vitamin K absorption from the small intestine due to decreased bile salt production can be compensated by parenteral administration of 10 mg/day vitamin K for 24–48 hours, but in parenchymal liver disease, decreased levels of coagulation factors are dependent on a decreased synthesis, so that there is no improvement with vitamin K administration [13]. This therapeutic trial can be used to assess the eventual vitamin K deficit. Nevertheless, 25% of patients with acute liver injury have a subclinical deficit of vitamin K that may benefit from parenteral administration with corresponding improvement of the

Cirrhosis: A practical guide to management, First Edition. Edited by Samuel S. Lee and Richard Moreau.

international normalized ratio (INR) [14]. However, this approach is not recommendend due to alterations in prognostic scores in liver failure and possible changes in indications to liver transplantation. In acute liver failure, the first factors whose plasma concentrations fall are those with the shortest half-life, factors V and VII (12 hours and 4–6 hours, respectively), and factors II, VII, and X will subsequently also be found to be low [15]. Factor VIII, together with vWf, is usually elevated, whereas there is only a slight reduction of factors IX and X. The differential effects on clotting factor levels during acute liver failure occur because high levels of cytokines increase levels of tissue factor which activate factors II, V, VII, X, whereas any thrombin generated is inhibited by antithrombin III, preventing activation of factors VIII, XI, and consequently XI, thus preserving their plasma levels [9].

Higher plasma des-gamma-carboxy (PIVKA) prothrombin concentrations are found in patients with hepatocellular carcinoma, due to local production by tumor cells. This abnormal prothrombin is thought to be a growth factor for this tumor and to be associated with poor prognosis [16].

Von Willebrand factor

Plasma concentration of vWf is substantially increased in patients with acute liver failure, due to its increased synthesis as an acute phase protein in response to tissue injury [17–19]. With liver injury this may also be secondary to endotoxemia associated with endothelial dysfunction [5]. In chronic liver disease, endothelial shear stress related to portal hypertension may also contribute to the high plasma levels of vWf via a nitric oxide (NO) stimulus [20]. Elevated levels of vWf seem to support platelet adhesion despite their reduced functional capacity [21]. Moreover, increased levels of high molecular weight vWf multimers have been found to be increased in end-stage liver disease, due to the concomitant decrease in ADAMTS13 (a disintegrin-like and metalloproteinase with thrombospondin type-1 motifs 13) which specifically cleaves multimeric vWf between Tyr1605 and Met 1606 [22]. These high molecular weight multimeric forms may be responsible for microthrombi formation in the terminal branches of portal venules, further aggravating cirrhosis.

A correlation between severity of liver disease, hepatic venous pressure gradient (HVPG) and vWf plasma antigen levels has been documented and vWf higher than 315% has been shown to be a good predictor of liver decompensation and death in a cohort of 286 patients [23].

Fibrinogen

Plasma fibrinogen is an acute-phase reactant, and remains normal or increased in patients with liver disease [24]. Lower levels due to decreased synthesis, yet above 100 mg/dL, have been reported only in patients with very severe liver disease [25]. However, this synthesized form is a nonfunctional fibrinogen. About 60–70% of patients with liver disease have nonfunctional forms of fibrinogen due to an increased activity of sialyltransferase expressed by immature hepatocytes generated during hepatic injury. This leads to a low molecular weight fibrinogen with abnormal α chains and higher sialic acid content [26]. This counterbalances the high fibrinogen concentrations found in patients with chronic hepatitis, cholestatic jaundice, and hepatocellular carcinoma, which does not result in increased clotting ability. Clinically, this results in an abnormal thrombin time (TT), despite almost normal prothrombin time (PT) and partial thromboplastin time (PTT), with an apparently normal concentration of fibrinogen. This abnormality is reversed following recovery of liver function and after liver transplantation [27].

Platelets

Abnormalities in both number and function of platelets are common in patients with liver disease and contribute to the impaired hemostasis seen in these patients.

About 70% of patients with chronic liver disease develop thrombocytopenia, which is usually mild to moderate ($70–90 \times 10^9$/L), and worsens with disease progression and increased hypersplenism which increases platelet sequestration [28–30]. Severe thrombocytopenia defined as platelet count less than 20×10^9/L occurs in only 1% of patients [31].

Thrombocytopenia has not been associated with an increased risk of bleeding from esophageal varices (i.e., structural bleeding) or other sources, although there are only few studies evaluating this, but it has been shown to be correlated with blood loss during surgery (i.e., hemostatic bleeding) [32]. A higher spleen diameter : platelet count ratio has been shown to have a high predictive value for the presence of esophageal varices in patients with cirrhosis [31].

The issue of sequestration versus other causes of thrombocytopenia in cirrhosis has been evaluated recently by comparing platelet number in extrahepatic portal hypertension, with that of cirrhotic patients having a similar-sized spleen. This has shown less severe thrombocytopenia in the noncirrhotic patients [33]. Synthetic function of the liver is essential for platelet production via thrombopoietin, which regulates platelet production in the bone marrow [34]. Although thrombopoietin is increased in patients with thrombocytopenia due to a homeostatic response [35], this occurs to a lesser degree with severe or chronic liver diseases than in those subjects with a normal liver [36]. Lower thrombopoietin mRNA levels in cirrhotic liver tissue [37] have been shown, confirming impaired thrombopoietin synthesis. In addition, a low platelet production from the bone marrow in cirrhotic patients has been shown [38].

Hepatitis C virus (HCV) infection [39], acute viral infection, alcohol abuse, and folate deficiency can result in myelosuppression [40], further lowering platelet counts. Consumption coagulopathy is not common in cirrhosis and even if disseminated intravascular coagulation (DIC) is present at a chronic low level, it does not influence platelet count [41,42]. Thrombocytopenia may also be contributed to by immune-mediated mechanisms due to an increase in production from B cells of antibodies binding platelet surface antigen GPIIb-IIIa and GPIb/I, which has been shown in viral-related cirrhosis B and C [43] and cholestatic liver diseases (primary biliary cirrhosis, PBC; primary sclerosing cholangitis, PSC) [44]. Among 368 patients with viral-induced cirrhosis, elevated titers of platelet-associated immunoglobulin G were observed in 88% with HCV and 47% with hepatitis B virus (HBV) infection [39].

Platelet function, as well as decreased platelet number, has been shown to be impaired in patients with liver disease with several laboratory activation tests [45]. Platelet aggregation in response to ADP, arachidonic acid, collagen, and thrombin is subnormal, probably due to a defective signal transduction mechanism [46]. Intrinsic defects [47] and abnormal plasma factors [48] have also been shown to contribute to platelet function abnormalities. An abnormal content of arachidonic acid in platelet membranes is found in liver disease and induces less aggregation ability mediated by thromboxane A2 [49]. In plasma from cirrhotic patients, the presence of an abnormal high-density lipoprotein (HDL) may alter NO content in the cell, leading to abnormal aggregability [50].

However, more recent data have questioned this hypothesis. Urinary excretion of 11-deydro-thromboxane (tx) B_2, a stable metabolite of TxA_2, was increased in cirrhosis suggesting activation of platelets [51]. Moreover, recent flow cytometry analysis of platelet activation, as well as platelet-monocyte aggregates, is consistent with hyperactivation of platelets in cirrhosis [52]. These recent findings could be explained by the activation of platelet adhesion by thrombin which is increased in cirrhosis and elevated levels of vWf, especially its high molecular multimeric forms.

Cholestatic liver diseases that can demonstrate a normal or hypercoagulable state by thromboelastography [53] have normal or hyperactive platelet function when assessed by platelet function assay (PFA-100) closure time and flow cytometric study of receptors [54]. When the platelet number is too low, cytometry or aggregation studies may be difficult to interpret; thromboelastography, which is a global test of clot formation and dissolution, measures both platelet function and number by maximum amplitude parameter [55], and can be used to assess platelet function.

Splenectomy is generally contraindicated in patients with cirrhosis, because of the high mortality rate and risk of secondary portal vein thrombosis, leading to increased risk of bleeding from esophageal-gastric varices and more difficult surgery during subsequent liver transplant [56]. Splenic embolization with 30–50% reduction in flow can normalize or significantly improve platelet number in some patients with cirrhosis [57] and may be helpful if invasive procedures such as embolization of hepatocellular carcinoma or interferon therapy for viral hepatitis are required. Insertion of transjugular intrahepatic portosystemic shunt (TIPS) has been shown to increase, but not to normalize, platelet number in some cases [58,59].

Anticoagulant factors

Antithrombin III

Antithrombin III is a non-vitamin-K-dependent glycoprotein synthesized by the liver but also by the endothelium [60]. Its plasma concentration decreases in patients with liver disease, in parallel with the severity of liver dysfunction, probably due to reduced synthesis and/or increased consumption due to hyperfibrinolysis [61]. Usually, the antithrombin III deficit is mild and thrombosis as a complication is very rare, reported only sporadically [62]. The decrease in antithrombin III may be responsible for the demonstrated low plasma levels of anti-Xa activity found in patients with cirrhosis undergoing therapy with low molecular weight heparin [63]. However, the decreased level of anti-Xa activity does not correspond to a reduced anticoagulation response in patients with liver disease compared with control subjects [64].

Proteins C and S

Proteins C and S are vitamin-K-dependent glycoproteins synthesized mainly by hepatocytes [65]. Therefore, during acute or chronic liver disease, their concentrations can be decreased, but usually not below 20% of normal values [66]. In patients with liver disease who also have genetic deficiency, plasma concentration is often lower than 20%. When there is severe liver disease, it can be difficult to exclude coexistent genetic deficiency as levels may be very low, due to very depressed synthesis [67]. In this situation a concomitant finding of a normal level of factor II and protein C: factor VII ratio can help to confirm a coexistent genetic deficit [68]. In acquired deficiency of vitamin K, a defective protein C lacking gamma-carboxyl (PIVKA) is produced [1].

In cirrhotic patients, the decreased level of protein C causes resistance to thrombomodulin activation which increases thrombin generation compared with control subjects, especially in Child C patients in whom the imbalance between factor VIII and C is greater.

Protein C deficiency is not associated with extrahepatic portal vein thrombosis [69]. Genetic deficiency of protein S is extremely rare, yet accounts up to 7% of patients with Budd–Chiari syndrome (BCS) or portal vein thrombosis, especially in series from Asia [70].

Disorders of the fibrinolytic system

All the proteins involved in fibrinolysis, except for tissue plasminogen activator (tPA) and plasminogen activator inhibitor-1 (PAI-1), are synthesized in the liver, and indeed reduced plasma levels of plasminogen [71], α2-antiplasmin, histidine-rich glycoprotein [72], factor XIII [73], and thrombin-activable fibrinolysis inhibitor (TAFI) [71] are documented in patients with cirrhosis. Conversely, tPA levels are increased in liver disease, due to decreased clearance, whereas its inhibitor PAI-1 is normal or only slightly increased in plasma. Therefore, the insufficient inhibitor concentrations accounts for net increased fibrinolysis [74].

Hyperfibrinolysis is correlated with the severity of liver dysfunction in cirrhosis as assessed by Child–Pugh score [75]. Ascitic patients show a greater degree of fibrinoslyis, because ascitic fluid has increased fibrinolytic activity: up to 20 L is reabsorbed daily, with fibrinolysis being correlated with endotoxin levels [76]. Increased levels of D-dimers, prothrombin fragments 1+2 (F1+2) fibrin degradation products and plasmin–α2-antiplasmin complexes are found [77]. Many studies using different methodologies demonstrate hyperfibrinolysis (thromboelastography [78], diluted whole blood clot lysis assay [79], and euglobin clot lysis time [80]). Recently, TAFI has been evaluated: it is decreased by an average of 26% in cirrhosis and by 50% in acute liver failure [81,82]. However, there is some controversy regarding hyperfibrinolytic activity in cirrhotic patients, as not all studies have confirmed this. This may due to the particular *in vitro* assay used. In contrast, *in vivo* correlation between hyperfibrinolysis and an increased risk of variceal bleeding, compatible with the circadian rhythm of hyperfibrinolytic activity has been shown [83]. In addition, increased fibrinolytic activity during liver transplantation and hepatic resection correlates with blood loss [84].

Interestingly, patients with cholestatic liver disease are characterized by a normal or hypercoagulable state: higher PAI-1 concentrations are seen than with other etiologies, balancing the increased tPA activity. This results in less hyperfibrinolysis in the reperfusion phase during liver transplantation, and antifibrinolytic therapy is not usually administered [85]. Thus, the clinical issue is whether cirrhotic patients when under "stress" (e.g., during infection, surgery, or bleeding) exhibit increased fibrinolysis, resulting in an increased bleeding tendency, which is not manifest when patients are stable.

Disseminated intravascular coagulation and accelerated intravascular coagulation

DIC is characterized by intravascular fibrin deposition due to activation of the clotting cascade, which overwhelms the anticoagulation pathway. DIC causes consumption of coagulation factors and platelets, and secondary fibrinolysis occurs, causing an increased bleeding tendency [86].

Hemostatic abnormalities that are present in cirrhotic patients share common laboratory features with DIC (i.e., an prolonged PT and PTT, low fibrinogen level, elevated fibrin-degradation product and D-dimer, and thrombocytopenia) [87–89]. However, despite DIC-like laboratory abnormalities (so-called pseudo-DIC) being observed, autopsy studies in cirrhotics have shown little evidence for fibrin deposition and clinically manifest DIC is very rare [87].

More sensitive tests, quantifying proteolytic cleavage products of the coagulation reaction (i.e., fibrinopeptide A, F1+2, and fibrinolysis reactions (fibrin D-dimer, high molecular weight fibrin–fibrinogen complexes or soluble fibrin)), demonstrate an abnormal profile called the accelerated intravascular coagulation and fibrinolysis phenomenon (AICF) in about 30% of cirrhotic patients [78,90].

However, Ben Ari et al. [78] analyzed 52 patients with stable liver disease showing that despite normal F1+2 thrombin–antithrombin III complex and D-dimer levels, thromboelastographic studies were able to detect hyperfibrinolysis. AICF may be important in the portal venous system, as this phenomenon is more pronounced there than in systemic blood. This could be related to higher levels of endotoxemia in portal blood, which can trigger release of interleukin 6 (IL-6) and tumor necrosis factor α (TNF-α), thus activating intravascular coagulation [91].

Assessment of the risk of thrombosis and anticoagulation

Thrombotic complications can paradoxically occur in cirrhotic patients even if clinically they are regarded as having hemorrhagic tendencies. Despite prolonged coagulation tests, these patients cannot be viewed as being "anticoagulated," due to the demonstratated normal thrombin generation due to the contemporary decrease in synthesis of both pro- and anticoagulant factors [3].

Wanless et al. [92] contend that portal vein and hepatic vein microthrombi cause disease progression in cirrhotic patients. Hepatic vein and portal vein thrombosis was found in at least 70% and 36%, respectively, of explanted livers and were associated with regions of confluent fibrosis (focal parenchymal extinction).

The formation of microthrombi could be due to the increased platelet aggregation due to increased high weight multimeric forms of vWf [21] or a combination of increased blood flow and imbalance between pro- and anticoagulation factors in patients with advanced cirrhosis, which results in increased thrombin generation [93]. Moreover, increased thrombin generation due to factor V Leiden mutation was associated with a 3.28-fold increased risk of rapid fibrosis progression in a Caucasian hepatitis C cohort [94].

The proposed pathogenic mechanism lies in thrombin's wide range of biologic activity, which includes amplification of Par-1 signaling leading to activation of stellate cells [95].

Portal vein thrombosis complicates cirrhosis in 0.6–15% of cases, possibly leading to worsening of liver function, and mesenteric infarction if the mesenteric vein is involved [96]. Moreover, in these patients early anticoagulation is indicated as it has been shown to repermeate portal vein in about 46–75% of cases and prevent the extension of the thrombus without causing complications [97–99]. A proposed algorithm is represented in Figure 22.1.

In BCS, even if a prothrombotic cause is not identified, anticoagulation should be started immediately after this diagnosis, because many genetic prothrombotic defects remain yet to be discovered and acquired disorders common in BCS may be elusive such as polycythemia vera or paroxysmal nocturnal hemoglobinuria. Early anticoagulation ameliorates prognosis. Anticoagulation therapy should continue even after liver transplantation because of the high rate of recurrence and thrombotic complications after orthotopic liver transplantation, and also because multiple prothrombotic disorders not limited to protein deficiencies may exist [67].

Aside from organ-specific thrombosis, patients with cirrhosis have been shown to be at greater risk of venous thromboembolism and pulmonary embolism than non-cirrhotic patients. In hospitalized cirrhotic patients, the incidence of deep venous thrombosis ranges from 0.5% to 8%, with only 1 in 4 receiving thromboprophylaxis [98,100]. Patients with cholestatic disease such as PBC and PSC often exhibit a procoagulant state demonstrated by thromboelastography, and may be prone to thrombosis, but this has not yet been confirmed [53]. No guidelines are available regarding management of thrombotic complications or prevention of emboli in cirrhotic patients with atrial fibrillation. Thus, each

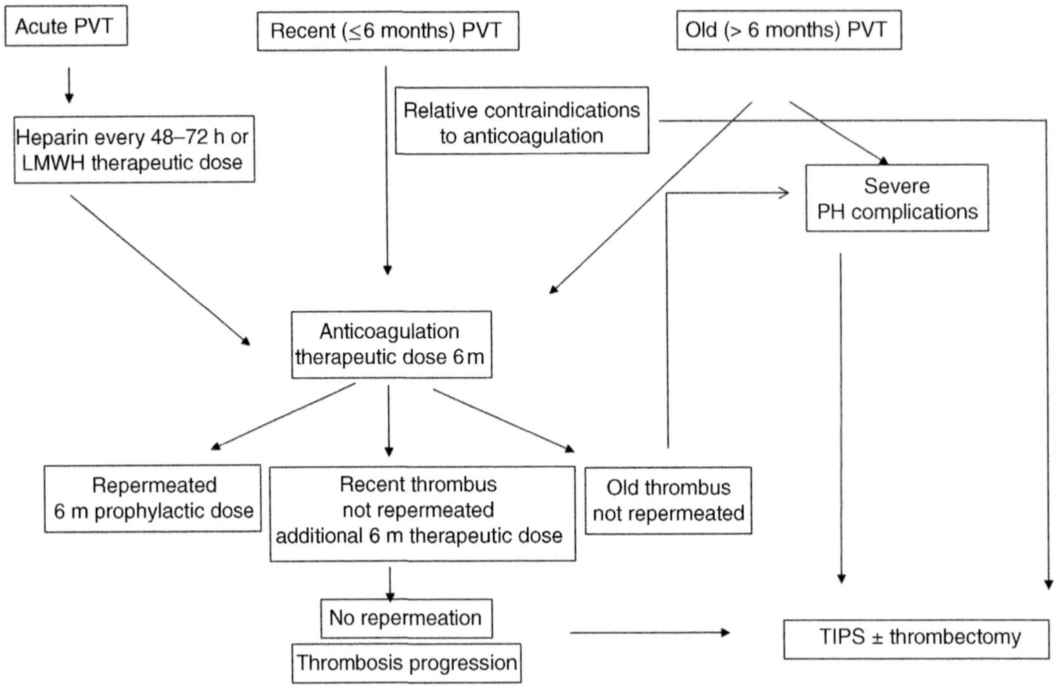

Figure 22.1 Proposed treatment algorithm to treat portal vein thrombosis (PVT) in cirrhosis. LMWH, low molecular weight heparin; PH, portal hypertension; TIPS, transjugular intrahepatic portosystemic shunt.

patient must be assessed individually. An endoscopic screen for varices must be performed and appropriate prophylaxis against variceal bleeding should be instituted particularly if there has been recent bleeding. Antiplatelet drugs and nonsteroidal anti-inflammatory drugs (NSAIDs) should be avoided as they may precipitate bleeding and increase fluid retention and risk of renal failure.

Assessment of the risk of bleeding

The role played by coagulation defects in the occurrence of bleeding in cirrhosis is still unclear. This is particularly because of the difficulty (and cost) in measuring static procoagulant and anticoagulant activities, and assessing the balance between the two. In addition, there are very few tests that reflect or predict coagulation *in vivo*; PT and INR are poorly correlated with the risk of bleeding during interventional procedures in patients with cirrhosis [101]. Recently, generation of thrombin has been explored *in vitro* in patients with cirrhosis and found to be normal. In this study, a resetting of the coagulation and anticoagulation systems at a lower level was postulated, because during liver disease both procoagulant and anticoagulant pathways are affected in a parallel manner. However, the *in vitro* technique has some drawbacks, the major one being that platelets are substituted by phospholipids [3]. Recently, the same authors have shown that when platelets were adjusted to correspond to whole-blood counts, patients with cirrhosis generated significantly less thrombin than control subjects when platelet count was less than 60×10^9/L [102].

Clinical signs of coagulopathy in liver disease depend on the degree of impairment of the hemostatic system. Commonly, minor signs of bleeding tendency such as gum bleeding and epistaxis are present, but major bleeding can also be encountered. The role of hemostatic abnormalities in the risk of variceal bleeding is not clear. Impaired laboratory studies may indicate worse hepatic synthesis serving more as a co-marker of disease rather than as a cause of hemorrhage. Hyperfibrinolysis has been shown to be associated but does not necessarily cause increased risk of variceal bleeding, in a cohort of 61 cirrhotics. Higher levels of fibrinogen degradation products were associated with a greater risk of variceal bleeding compared to patients without (odds ratio 8), but Child–Pugh score and endoscopic characteristics of varices remain the most important prognostic factors [103]. Recently, the role of infection and endogenous heparin-like substances demonstrated by thromboelastography has been evaluated in variceal bleeding. Infection may be a trigger factor for bleeding [104] and both infection and heparin-like substances may be mechanisms responsible for the persistence of bleeding in some [105]. Thromboelastography, which is a quick and reliable method to assess clot formation and lysis [55], also allows detection of heparin-like substances. Studies from our group have shown worsening coagulation detected by thromboelastography during infection, due to low molecular weight heparin-like substances [106].

Invasive procedures

Historically, PT and platelet count have been used to assess the risk of bleeding prior to invasive procedures. Cirrhotic patients have increased mortality and morbidity during surgery [107], mainly due to increased bleeding in 60% of cases [108,109]. Early studies linked PT to this risk during surgery (PT prolongation >1.5 and >2.5 seconds associated with 47% and 87% mortality, respectively) [110], hence platelet count $<50\times10^9$/L and PT >3 s have been considered relative contraindications to elective surgery [109]. In addition, portal hypertension and collateral veins increase the risk of bleeding during surgical dissection. Recently, severity of liver disease has been shown to be correlated with the risk of bleeding complications during brain surgery with mortality up to 63% in Child C patients [111] and mortality after cardiac surgery [112]. Recently, a paper by Giannini et al. [113] demonstrated an increased risk of bleeding following invasive procedures in patients with platelet counts of less than 75×10^9/L (10/32 versus 0/18; $P=0.008$).

Hyperfibrinolysis [114] and clotting activation, due to increased tPA levels, have been described in patients undergoing liver resection [115]. However, another study performed in patients undergoing laparoscopic liver biopsy failed to demonstrate any correlation between the risk of bleeding evaluated at the hepatic puncture site and coagulation tests, so that the degree of injury may be the important factor [116].

Liver biopsy is widely used diagnostically and to grade the severity of liver disease or fibrosis. Moreover, it is an essential tool used after liver transplantation to diagnose rejection and other causes of graft dysfunction. Bleeding complications occur in 0.35–0.5%, leading to mortality in 0.1% [117]. Despite the evidence that there were no threshold abnormalities of clotting tests associated with risk of bleeding during laparoscopic liver biopsy, INR and platelet count are considered essential to evaluate the bleeding risk for percutaneous liver biopsy [118]. An audit from the British Society of Gastroenterology (BSG) [119] performed in 1991 showed a doubling of the risk of bleeding in patients with INR ≥1.5, but that only 7.1% of the bleeding occurred with INR >1.5, and 90% occurred with a INR ≤1.3. Thus, having a normal INR no more excludes the risk of bleeding than an elevated INR suggests it. A cutoff for platelet count is difficult to justify from the literature. Most textbooks in the UK, and BSG guidelines, require platelet counts above 80×10^9/L [13], whereas a survey from the Mayo Clinic suggested 50×10^9/L as a cutoff [120]. Current recommendations state that a percutaneous liver biopsy can be performed safely without support when platelet counts are above 60×10^9/L [118]; however, all the guidelines have set the platelet thresholds based on "expert" suggestions rather than any firm evidence.

Blake et al. [121] advocated evaluating the use of bleeding time to assess the risk of bleeding for percutaneous liver biopsy, but this is not carried out in clinical practice. If clotting parameters are outside stipulated ranges, a transjugular liver biopsy can be more safely performed, without plasma or platelet therapy [122]. A plugged liver biopsy is also said to be safer, but it may cause greater risk of bleeding in hypocoagulable patients [117].

Risk of bleeding from variceal ulcers after variceal band ligation correlates only with severity of liver disease, but not with conventional coagulation tests nor thromboelastography parameters [123].

During minor procedures such as thoracentesis, paracentesis, or lumbar puncture performed in patients with liver disease, there are no firm guidelines as to the hemostatic threshold for performing these tests. The largest review on 608 patients who underwent paracentesis or thoracentesis with mild coagulation abnormalities showed 0.2% having excessive bleeding requiring transfusion and 0.02% mortality. There was no correlation with PT, PTT, platelet count, and the risk of bleeding [124]. In another study performed in 200 cirrhotic patients with INR ≥3 and platelet count ≤19 000/mm^3 who underwent paracentesis, no complications were seen, regardless of baseline INR and platelet count [125].

Bleeding occurs after dental extraction in about 3% of procedures even with INR >3 and platelet count <30 000/mm^3 [126]. Local use of tranexanic acid could be beneficial, because the oral and uterine cavities are areas of excessive fibrinolysis. Therefore, local antifibrinolytic agents can be useful in the general population, but clearly in those patients with other coagulation defects.

A contraindication to the procedure is clinically evident in DIC or fibrinolysis [127]. Whereas it is impossible using the evidence-based techniques currently available to establish "safe" coagulation tests for these procedures, equally, if not more important, is to limit such procedures to circumstances in which the perceived benefit of the procedure is clearly greater than the risk.

Coagulation during infection and sepsis

The overall cumulative incidence of infection in cirrhotic patients is estimated to be at least 30% [128], and is possibly associated with increased risk of variceal bleeding [104]. Infection is associated with early rebleeding and increased mortality [129,130]. Prophylactic antibiotic therapy led to less early rebleeding and better control of bleeding in a randomized study [131].

Using thromboelastography, 20 cirrhotic patients who experienced early rebleeding were found to have worsening thromboelastographyparameters the day before rebleeding [105]. Moreover, patients with bacterial infection have worse thromboelastography-parameters, which can be corrected *in vitro* by heparinase I, which can cleave heparin-like substances [106]. The presence of heparin-like substances is associated in some with increased anti-Xa activity [132]. Heparin-like substances have been detected hours after variceal bleeding [133]. Based on this evidence, the hypothesis has been postulated that endotoxins and inflammation due to infection can release heparinoids from the endothelium and mast cells [106]. One study, not yet replicated, showed increased heparan sulfate concentrations in patients with variceal bleeding compared to patients without [134]. Moreover, sepsis can cause impairment of platelet function, decreasing platelet number and aggregability, due to increased NO production [135].

Cytokines, in particular IL-6 and TNF-α released during infection, can trigger DIC with hyperfibrinolysis [136]. One study showed a strong association between both fragment F1+2 and D-dimer with endotoxemia. These markers interestingly returned to normal after antibiotic therapy [88]. Another report recently showed decreased platelet count and levels of factors VII, X, V, and II, in cirrhotic patients and severe sepsis, suggesting consumptive coagulopathy [137], whereas a further study found decreased activity of protein C, which is associated with increased fibrinolysis [138].

References

1 Lisman T, Leebeek FW, de Groot PG. Haemostatic abnormalities in patients with liver disease. J Hepatol 2002;37: 280–7.
2 Rapaport SI. Coagulation problems in liver disease. Blood Coagul Fibrinolysis 2000;11 (Suppl 1): S69–S74.
3 Tripodi A, Salerno F, Chantarangkul V, et al. Evidence of normal thrombin generation in cirrhosis despite abnormal conventional coagulation tests. Hepatology 2005;41:553–8.
4 Kelly DA, Summerfield JA. Hemostasis in liver disease. Semin Liver Dis 1987;7:182–91.
5 Ferro D, Quintarelli C, Lattuada A, et al. High plasma levels of von Willebrand factor as a marker of endothelial perturbation in cirrhosis: relationship to endotoxemia. Hepatology 1996;23:1377–83.
6 Wion KL, Kelly D, Summerfield JA, Tuddenham EG, Lawn RM. Distribution of factor VIII mRNA and antigen in human liver and other tissues. Nature 1985;317:726–9.
7 Hollestelle MJ, Geertzen HG, Straatsburg IH, van Gulik TM, van Mourik JA. Factor VIII expression in liver disease. Thromb Haemost 2004;91:267–75.
8 Hollestelle MJ, Thinnes T, Crain K, et al. Tissue distribution of factor VIII gene expression in vivo--a closer look. Thromb Haemost 2001;86:855–61.
9 Kerr R. New insights into haemostasis in liver failure. Blood Coagul Fibrinolysis 2003;14 (Suppl 1): S43–5.

10 Hollestelle MJ, Geertzen HG, Straatsburg IH, van Gulik TM, van Mourik JA. Factor VIII expression in liver disease. Thromb Haemost 2004;91:267–75.

11 Maisonneuve P, Sultan Y. Modification of factor VIII complex properties in patients with liver disease. J Clin Pathol 1977;30:221–7.

12 Blanchard RA, Furie BC, Jorgensen M, Kruger SF, Furie B. Acquired vitamin K-dependent carboxylation deficiency in liver disease. N Engl J Med 1981;305:242–8.

13 Sherlock S, Dooley J. Diseases of the Liver and Biliary System, 11th edn. Oxford: Blackwell Publishing, 2002. pp. 47–64.

14 Pereira SP, Rowbotham D, Fitt S, Shearer MJ, Wendon J, Williams R. Pharmacokinetics and efficacy of oral versus intravenous mixed-micellar phylloquinone (vitamin K1) in severe acute liver disease. J Hepatol 2005;42:365–70.

15 Kerr R, Newsome P, Germain L, et al. Effects of acute liver injury on blood coagulation. J Thromb Haemost 2003;1: 754–9.

16 Weitz IC, Liebman HA. Des-gamma-carboxy (abnormal) prothrombin and hepatocellular carcinoma: a critical review. Hepatology 1993;18:990–7.

17 Baruch Y, Neubauer K, Ritzel A, Wilfling T, Lorf T, Ramadori G. Von Willebrand gene expression in damaged human liver. Hepatogastroenterology 2004;51:684–8.

18 Escolar G, Cases A, Vinas M, et al. Evaluation of acquired platelet dysfunctions in uremic and cirrhotic patients using the platelet function analyzer (PFA-100): influence of hematocrit elevation. Haematologica 1999;84:614–9.

19 Kelly DA, Tuddenham EG. Haemostatic problems in liver disease. Gut 1986;27:339–49.

20 Albornoz L, Alvarez D, Otaso JC, et al. Von Willebrand factor could be an index of endothelial dysfunction in patients with cirrhosis: relationship to degree of liver failure and nitric oxide levels. J Hepatol 1999;30:451–5.

21 Lisman T, Bongers TN, Adelmeijer J, et al. Elevated levels of von Willebrand factor in cirrhosis support platelet adhesion despite reduced functional capacity. Hepatology 2006;44: 53–61.

22 Uemura M, Fujimura Y, Matsumoto M, et al. Comprehensive analysis of ADAMTS13 in patients with liver cirrhosis. Thromb Haemost 2008;99:1019–29.

23 Ferlitsch M, Reiberger T, Hoke M, et al. Von Willebrand factor as new non-invasive predictor of portal hypertension, decompensation and mortality in patients with liver cirrhosis. Hepatology 2012;56:1439–47.

24 Lechner K, Niessner H, Thaler E. Coagulation abnormalities in liver disease. Semin Thromb Hemost 1977;4:40–56.

25 Dymock IW, Tucker JS, Woolf IL, Poller L, Thomson JM. Coagulation studies as a prognostic index in acute liver failure. Br J Haematol 1975;29:385–95.

26 Francis JL, Armstrong DJ. Fibrinogen-bound sialic acid levels in the dysfibrinogenaemia of liver disease. Haemostasis 1982;11:215–22.

27 Barr RD, Allardyce M, Brunt PW, McPhie JL. Dysfibrinogenaemia and liver cell growth. J Clin Pathol 1978;31: 89–92.

28 Noguchi H, Hirai K, Aoki Y, Sakata K, Tanikawa K. Changes in platelet kinetics after a partial splenic arterial embolization in cirrhotic patients with hypersplenism. Hepatology 1995;22:1682–8.

29 Sohma Y, Akahori H, Seki N, et al. Molecular cloning and chromosomal localization of the human thrombopoietin gene. FEBS Lett 1994;353:57–61.

30 Yanaga K, Tzakis AG, Shimada M, et al. Reversal of hypersplenism following orthotopic liver transplantation. Ann Surg 1989;210:180–3.

31 Giannini E. Platelet count/spleen diameter ratio: proposal and validation of a non-invasive parameter to predict the presence of oesophageal varices in patients with liver cirrhosis. Gut 2003;52:1200–5.

32 Clavien PA, Camargo CA Jr, Croxford R, Langer B, Levy GA, Greig PD. Definition and classification of negative outcomes in solid organ transplantation: application in liver transplantation. Ann Surg 1994;220:109–20.

33 Robson SC, Kahn D, Kruskal J, Bird AR, Kirsch RE. Disordered hemostasis in extrahepatic portal hypertension. Hepatology 1993;18:853–7.

34 Panasiuk A, Prokopowicz D, Zak J, Panasiuk B. Reticulated platelets as a marker of megakaryopoiesis in liver cirrhosis; relation to thrombopoietin and hepatocyte growth factor serum concentration. Hepatogastroenterology 2004;51: 1124–8.

35 Jelkmann W. The role of the liver in the production of thrombopoietin compared with erythropoietin. Eur J Gastroenterol Hepatol 2001;13:791–801.

36 Kitano K, Shimodaira S, Ito T, et al. Liver cirrhosis with marked thrombocytopenia and highly elevated serum thrombopoietin levels. Int J Hematol 1999;70:52–5.

37 Martin T.G III, Somberg KA, Meng YG, et al. Thrombopoietin levels in patients with cirrhosis before and after orthotopic liver transplantation. Ann Intern Med 1997;127:285–8.

38 Wang GL, Jiang BH, Rue EA, Semenza GL. Hypoxia-inducible factor 1 is a basic-helix-loop-helix-PAS heterodimer regulated by cellular O2 tension. Proc Natl Acad Sci U S A 1995;92:5510–4.

39 Nagamine T, Ohtuka T, Takehara K, Arai T, Takagi H, Mori M. Thrombocytopenia associated with hepatitis C viral infection. J Hepatol 1996;24:135–40.

40 Peck-Radosavljevic M. Thrombocytopenia in liver disease. Can J Gastroenterol 2000;14:60D–6D.

41 Violi F, Leo R, Basili S, Ferro D, Cordova C, Balsano F. Association between prolonged bleeding time and gastrointestinal hemorrhage in 102 patients with liver cirrhosis: results of a retrospective study. Haematologica 1994;79:61–5.

42 Violi F, Ferro D, Basili S, et al. Hyperfibrinolysis increases the risk of gastrointestinal hemorrhage in patients with advanced cirrhosis. Hepatology 1992;15:672–6.

43 Kajihara M, Kato S, Okazaki Y, et al. A role of autoantibody-mediated platelet destruction in thrombocytopenia in patients with cirrhosis. Hepatology 2003;37:1267–76.
44 Feistauer SM, Penner E, Mayr WR, Panzer S. Target platelet antigens of autoantibodies in patients with primary biliary cirrhosis. Hepatology 1997;25:1343–5.
45 Violi F, Basili S, Raparelli V, Chowdary P, Gatt A, Burroughs AK. Patients with liver cirrhosis suffer from primary haemostatic defects? Fact or fiction? J Hepatol 2011;55: 1415–27.
46 Escolar G, Cases A, Vinas M, et al. Evaluation of acquired platelet dysfunctions in uremic and cirrhotic patients using the platelet function analyzer (PFA-100): influence of hematocrit elevation. Haematologica 1999;84:614–9.
47 Laffi G, Marra F, Gresele P, et al. Evidence for a storage pool defect in platelets from cirrhotic patients with defective aggregation. Gastroenterology 1992;103:641–6.
48 Younger HM, Hadoke PW, Dillon JF, Hayes PC. Platelet function in cirrhosis and the role of humoral factors. Eur J Gastroenterol Hepatol 1997;9:989–92.
49 Owen JS, Hutton RA, Day RC, Bruckdorfer KR, McIntyre N. Platelet lipid composition and platelet aggregation in human liver disease. J Lipid Res 1981;22:423–30.
50 Riddell DR, Owen JS. Nitric oxide and platelet aggregation. Vitam Horm 1999;57:25–48.
51 Davi G, Ferro D, Basili S, et al. Increased thromboxane metabolites excretion in liver cirrhosis. Thromb Haemost 1998;79:747–51.
52 Lisman T, Adelmeijer J, de Groot PG, Janssen HL, Leebeek FW. No evidence for an intrinsic platelet defect in patients with liver cirrhosis: studies under flow conditions. J Thromb Haemost 2006;4:2070–2.
53 Ben Ari Z, Panagou M, Patch D, et al. Hypercoagulability in patients with primary biliary cirrhosis and primary sclerosing cholangitis evaluated by thrombelastography. J Hepatol 1997;26:554–9.
54 Pihusch R, Rank A, Gohring P, Pihusch M, Hiller E, Beuers U. Platelet function rather than plasmatic coagulation explains hypercoagulable state in cholestatic liver disease. J Hepatol 2002;37:548–55.
55 Salooja N, Perry DJ. Thrombelastography. Blood Coagul Fibrinolysis 2001;12:327–37.
56 Bolognesi M, Merkel C, Sacerdoti D, Nava V, Gatta A. Role of spleen enlargement in cirrhosis with portal hypertension. Dig Liver Dis 2002;34:144–50.
57 N'Kontchou G, Seror O, Bourcier V, et al. Partial splenic embolization in patients with cirrhosis: efficacy, tolerance and long-term outcome in 32 patients. Eur J Gastroenterol Hepatol 2005;17:179–84.
58 Jabbour N, Zajko A, Orons P, Irish W, Fung JJ, Selby RR. Does transjugular intrahepatic portosystemic shunt (TIPS) resolve thrombocytopenia associated with cirrhosis? Dig Dis Sci 1998;43:2459–62.
59 Karasu Z, Gurakar A, Kerwin B, et al. Effect of transjugular intrahepatic portosystemic shunt on thrombocytopenia associated with cirrhosis. Dig Dis Sci 2000;45:1971–6.
60 Schipper HG, ten Cate JW. Antithrombin III transfusion in patients with hepatic cirrhosis. Br J Haematol 1982;52: 25–33.
61 Liebman HA, McGehee WG, Patch MJ, Feinstein DI. Severe depression of antithrombin III associated with disseminated intravascular coagulation in women with fatty liver of pregnancy. Ann Intern Med 1983;98:330–3.
62 Carmassi F, Morale M, De Negri F, Carrai M. Modulation of hemostatic balance with antithrombin III replacement therapy in a case of liver cirrhosis associated with recurrent venous thrombosis. J Mol Med 1995;73:89–93.
63 Bechmann LP, Sichau M, Wichert M, Gerken G, Kroger K, Hilgard P. Low-molecular-weight heparin in patients with advanced cirrhosis. Liver Int 2011;31:75–82.
64 Marco S, Isabel RK, Valeria R, et al. Increased anticoagulant response to low molecular weight heparin in plasma from patients with advanced cirrhosis. J Thromb Haemost 2012;10:1823–9.
65 Fair DS, Marlar RA. Biosynthesis and secretion of factor VII, protein C, protein S, and the protein C inhibitor from a human hepatoma cell line. Blood 1986;67:64–70.
66 Mannucci PM, Vigano S. Deficiencies of protein C, an inhibitor of blood coagulation. Lancet 1982;2:463–7.
67 Senzolo M, Cholongitas CE, Patch D, Burroughs AK. Update on the classification, assessment of prognosis and therapy of Budd–Chiari syndrome. Nat Clin Pract Gastroenterol Hepatol 2005;2:182–90.
68 Minnema MC, Janssen HL, Niermeijer P, de Man RA. Budd–Chiari syndrome: combination of genetic defects and the use of oral contraceptives leading to hypercoagulability. J Hepatol 2000;33:509–12.
69 Primignani M, Martinelli I, Bucciarelli P, et al. Risk factors for thrombophilia in extrahepatic portal vein obstruction. Hepatology 2005;41:603–8.
70 Bhattacharyya M, Makharia G, Kannan M, Ahmed RP, Gupta PK, Saxena R. Inherited prothrombotic defects in Budd–Chiari syndrome and portal vein thrombosis: a study from North India. Am J Clin Pathol 2004;121: 844–7.
71 Stein SF, Harker LA. Kinetic and functional studies of platelets, fibrinogen, and plasminogen in patients with hepatic cirrhosis. J Lab Clin Med 1982;99:217–30.
72 Leebeek FW, Kluft C, Knot EA, De Maat MP. Histidine-rich glycoprotein is elevated in mild liver cirrhosis and decreased in moderate and severe liver cirrhosis. J Lab Clin Med 1989;113:493–7.
73 Biland L, Duckert F, Prisender S, Nyman D. Quantitative estimation of coagulation factors in liver disease: the diagnostic and prognostic value of factor XIII, factor V and plasminogen. Thromb Haemost 1978;39:646–56.

74 Hersch SL, Kunelis T, Francis RB Jr. The pathogenesis of accelerated fibrinolysis in liver cirrhosis: a critical role for tissue plasminogen activator inhibitor. Blood 1987;69: 1315–9.
75 Hu KQ, Yu AS, Tiyyagura L, Redeker AG, Reynolds TB. Hyperfibrinolytic activity in hospitalized cirrhotic patients in a referral liver unit. Am J Gastroenterol 2001;96:1581–6.
76 Agarwal S, Joyner KA Jr, Swaim MW. Ascites fluid as a possible origin for hyperfibrinolysis in advanced liver disease. Am J Gastroenterol 2000;95:3218–24.
77 Paramo JA, Rocha E. Hemostasis in advanced liver disease. Semin Thromb Hemost 1993;19:184–90.
78 Ben Ari Z, Osman E, Hutton RA, Burroughs AK. Disseminated intravascular coagulation in liver cirrhosis: fact or fiction? Am J Gastroenterol 1999;94:2977–82.
79 Comp PC, Jacocks RM, Rubenstein C, Radcliffe R. A lysine-absorbable plasminogen activator is elevated in conditions associated with increased fibrinolytic activity. J Lab Clin Med 1981;97:637–45.
80 Francis RB Jr, Feinstein DI. Clinical significance of accelerated fibrinolysis in liver disease. Haemostasis 1984;14: 460–5.
81 Lisman T, Leebeek FW, Mosnier LO, et al. Thrombin-activatable fibrinolysis inhibitor deficiency in cirrhosis is not associated with increased plasma fibrinolysis. Gastroenterology 2001;121:131–9.
82 Colucci M, Binetti BM, Branca MG, et al. Deficiency of thrombin activatable fibrinolysis inhibitor in cirrhosis is associated with increased plasma fibrinolysis. Hepatology 2003;38:230–7.
83 Piscaglia F, Siringo S, Hermida RC, et al. Diurnal changes of fibrinolysis in patients with liver cirrhosis and esophageal varices. Hepatology 2000;31:349–57.
84 Lewis JH, Bontempo FA, Awad SA, et al. Liver transplantation: intraoperative changes in coagulation factors in 100 first transplants. Hepatology 1989;9:710–4.
85 Segal H, Cottam S, Potter D, Hunt BJ. Coagulation and fibrinolysis in primary biliary cirrhosis compared with other liver disease and during orthotopic liver transplantation. Hepatology 1997;25:683–8.
86 Amitrano L, Guardascione MA, Brancaccio V, Balzano A. Coagulation disorders in liver disease. Semin Liver Dis 2002;22:83–96.
87 Carr JM. Disseminated intravascular coagulation in cirrhosis. Hepatology 1989;10:103–10.
88 Violi F, Ferro D, Basili S, et al. Association between low-grade disseminated intravascular coagulation and endotoxemia in patients with liver cirrhosis. Gastroenterology 1995;109:531–9.
89 Kemkes-Matthes B, Bleyl H, Matthes KJ. Coagulation activation in liver diseases. Thromb Res 1991;64:253–61.
90 Joist JH. AICF and DIC in liver cirrhosis: expressions of a hypercoagulable state. Am J Gastroenterol 1999;94:2801–3.
91 Basili S, Ferro D, Violi F. Endotoxaemia, hyperfibrinolysis, and bleeding in cirrhosis. Lancet 1999;353:1102
92 Wanless IR, Wong F, Blendis LM, Greig P, Heathcote EJ, Levy G. Hepatic and portal vein thrombosis in cirrhosis: possible role in development of parenchymal extinction and portal hypertension. Hepatology 1995;21:1238–47.
93 Tripodi A, Primignani M, Chantarangkul V, et al. An imbalance of pro- vs anti-coagulation factors in plasma from patients with cirrhosis. Gastroenterology 2009;137: 2105–11.
94 Papatheodoridis GV, Papakonstantinou E, Andrioti E, et al. Thrombotic risk factors and extent of liver fibrosis in chronic viral hepatitis. Gut 2003;52:404–9.
95 Anstee QM, Dhar A, Thursz MR. The role of hypercoagulability in liver fibrogenesis. Clin Res Hepatol Gastroenterol 2011;35:526–33.
96 Amitrano L, Guardascione MA, Brancaccio V, et al. Risk factors and clinical presentation of portal vein thrombosis in patients with liver cirrhosis. J Hepatol 2004;40:736–41.
97 Francoz C, Belghiti J, Vilgrain V, et al. Splanchnic vein thrombosis in candidates for liver transplantation: usefulness of screening and anticoagulation. Gut 2005;54:691–7.
98 Rodriguez-Castro KI, Simioni P, Burra P, Senzolo M. Anticoagulation for the treatment of thrombotic complications in patients with cirrhosis. Liver Int 2012;32:1465–76.
99 Senzolo M, Sartori M, Rossetto V, et al. Prospective evaluation of anticoagulation and transjugular intrahepatic portosistemic shunt for the management of portal vein thrombosis in cirrhosis. Liver Int 2012;32:919–27.
100 Espiritu JD. Pulmonary embolism in a patient with coagulopathy from end-stage liver disease. Chest 2000;117:924–5.
101 Caldwell SH, Hoffman M, Lisman T, et al. Coagulation disorders and hemostasis in liver disease: pathophysiology and critical assessment of current management. Hepatology 2006;44:1039–46.
102 Tripodi A, Primignani M, Chantarangkul V, et al. Thrombin generation in patients with cirrhosis: the role of platelets. Hepatology 2006;44:440–5.
103 Violl F, Basili S, Ferro D, Quintarelli C, Alessandril C, Cordova C. Association between high values of D-dimer and tissue-plasminogen activator activity and first gastrointestinal bleeding in cirrhotic patients. CALC Group. Thromb Haemost 1996;76:177–83.
104 Goulis J, Patch D, Burroughs AK. Bacterial infection in the pathogenesis of variceal bleeding. Lancet 1999;353:139–42.
105 Chau TN, Chan YW, Patch D, Tokunaga S, Greenslade L, Burroughs AK. Thrombelastographic changes and early rebleeding in cirrhotic patients with variceal bleeding. Gut 1998;43:267–71.
106 Montalto P, Vlachogiannakos J, Cox DJ, Pastacaldi S, Patch D, Burroughs AK. Bacterial infection in cirrhosis impairs coagulation by a heparin effect: a prospective study. J Hepatol 2002;37:463–70.

107 Perkins L, Jeffries M, Patel T. Utility of preoperative scores for predicting morbidity after cholecystectomy in patients with cirrhosis. Clin Gastroenterol Hepatol 2004;2:1123–8.
108 Patel T. Surgery in the patient with liver disease. Mayo Clin Proc 1999;74:593–9.
109 Friedman LS. The risk of surgery in patients with liver disease. Hepatology 1999;29:1617–23.
110 Garrison RN, Cryer HM, Howard DA, Polk HC Jr. Clarification of risk factors for abdominal operations in patients with hepatic cirrhosis. Ann Surg 1984;199:648–55.
111 Chen CC, Hsu PW, Lee ST, et al. Brain surgery in patients with liver cirrhosis. J Neurosurg 2012;117:348–53.
112 Lopez-Delgado JC, Esteve F, Javierre C, et al. Predictors of long-term mortality in patients with cirrhosis undergoing cardiac surgery. J Cardiovasc Surg (Torino) 2014; in press.
113 Giannini EG, Greco A, Marenco S, Andorno E, Valente U, Savarino V. Incidence of bleeding following invasive procedures in patients with thrombocytopenia and advanced liver disease. Clin Gastroenterol Hepatol 2010;8:899–902.
114 Tsuji K, Eguchi Y, Kodama M. Postoperative hypercoagulable state followed by hyperfibrinolysis related to wound healing after hepatic resection. J Am Coll Surg 1996;183: 230–8.
115 Meijer C, Wiezer MJ, Hack CE, et al. Coagulopathy following major liver resection: the effect of rBPI21 and the role of decreased synthesis of regulating proteins by the liver. Shock 2001;15:261–71.
116 Ewe K. Bleeding after liver biopsy does not correlate with indices of peripheral coagulation. Dig Dis Sci 1981;26: 388–93.
117 Burroughs AK, Dagher L. Gastroenterological Endoscopy. New York: Thieme; 2002. pp. 252–9.
118 Grant A, Neuberger J. Guidelines on the use of liver biopsy in clinical practice. British Society of Gastroenterology. Gut 1999 Oct;45 (Suppl 4): 1–11.
119 Gilmore IT, Burroughs A, Murray-Lyon IM, Williams R, Jenkins D, Hopkins A. Indications, methods, and outcomes of percutaneous liver biopsy in England and Wales: an audit by the British Society of Gastroenterology and the Royal College of Physicians of London. Gut 1995;36:437–41.
120 McGill DB, Rakela J, Zinsmeister AR, Ott BJ. A 21-year experience with major hemorrhage after percutaneous liver biopsy. Gastroenterology 1990;99:1396–400.
121 Blake JC, Sprengers D, Grech P, McCormick PA, McIntyre N, Burroughs AK. Bleeding time in patients with hepatic cirrhosis. BMJ 1990;301:12–5.
122 Papatheodoridis GV, Patch D, Watkinson A, Tibballs J, Burroughs AK. Transjugular liver biopsy in the 1990s: a 2-year audit. Aliment Pharmacol Ther 1999;13:603–8.
123 Vieira da Rocha EC, D'Amico EA, Caldwell SH, et al. A prospective study of conventional and expanded coagulation indices in predicting ulcer bleeding after variceal band ligation. Clin Gastroenterol Hepatol 2009;7: 988–93.
124 Pache I, Bilodeau M. Severe haemorrhage following abdominal paracentesis for ascites in patients with liver disease. Aliment Pharmacol Ther 2005;21:525–9.
125 Lin CH, Chen SC, Ko PC. Preprocedure coagulation tests are unnecessary before abdominal paracentesis in emergency departments. Hepatology 2005;41:402–3.
126 Perdigao JP, de Almeida PC, Rocha TD, et al. Postoperative bleeding after dental extraction in liver pretransplant patients. J Oral Maxillofac Surg 2012;70:e177–84.
127 Runyon BA. Paracentesis of ascitic fluid: a safe procedure. Arch Intern Med 1986;146:2259–61.
128 Bernard B, Grange JD, Khac EN, Amiot X, Opolon P, Poynard T. Antibiotic prophylaxis for the prevention of bacterial infections in cirrhotic patients with gastrointestinal bleeding: a meta-analysis. Hepatology 1999;29:1655–61.
129 Goulis J, Armonis A, Patch D, Sabin C, Greenslade L, Burroughs AK. Bacterial infection is independently associated with failure to control bleeding in cirrhotic patients with gastrointestinal hemorrhage. Hepatology 1998;27: 1207–12.
130 Bernard B, Cadranel JF, Valla D, Escolano S, Jarlier V, Opolon P. Prognostic significance of bacterial infection in bleeding cirrhotic patients: a prospective study. Gastroenterology 1995;108:1828–34.
131 Hou MC, Lin HC, Liu TT, et al. Antibiotic prophylaxis after endoscopic therapy prevents rebleeding in acute variceal hemorrhage: a randomized trial. Hepatology 2004;39:746–53.
132 Zambruni A, Thalheimer U, Coppell J, et al. Endogenous heparin-like activity detected by anti-Xa assay in infected cirrhotic and non-cirrhotic patients. Scand J Gastroenterol 2004;39:830–6.
133 Thalheimer U, Triantos C, Samonakis D, et al. Endogenous heparinoids in acute variceal bleeding. Gut 2005;54: 310–1.
134 McKee RF, Hodson S, Dawes J, Garden OJ, Carter DC. Plasma concentrations of endogenous heparinoids in portal hypertension. Gut 1992;33:1549–52.
135 Thalheimer U, Triantos CK, Samonakis DN, Patch D, Burroughs AK. Infection, coagulation, and variceal bleeding in cirrhosis. Gut 2005;54:556–63.
136 Grignani G, Maiolo A. Cytokines and hemostasis. Haematologica 2000;85:967–72.
137 Plessier A, Denninger MH, Consigny Y, et al. Coagulation disorders in patients with cirrhosis and severe sepsis. Liver Int 2003;23:440–8.
138 Wong F, Bernardi M, Balk R, et al. Sepsis in cirrhosis: report on the 7th meeting of the International Ascites Club. Gut 2005;54:718–25.

CHAPTER 23

Agents and drugs: precautions in patients with cirrhosis

Felix Stickel
Department of Gastroenterology and Hepatology, University Hospital Zürich, Switzerland

Introduction

Administering drugs to patients with acute or chronic liver diseases – either for the underlying liver disease, or to treat nonhepatic conditions – is everyday routine in medical practice. Concerns of physicians that many of the functions that the liver harbors to handle foreign substances could be impaired due to the underlying liver disease are understandable bearing in mind that the liver has a central role in the absorption, distribution, and elimination kinetics of most drugs and many active or inactive drug metabolites [1]. Moreover, the liver is not only the primary site of biotransformation of xenobiotics, but also affects drug distribution, bioavailability, and biliary excretion. In addition, patients with hepatic dysfunction may also be more sensitive to the effects, both desired and adverse, of several drugs, and tolerate an event of drug-induced liver injury (DILI) less well than individuals without pre-existing liver diseases. However, only few methods are available for the assessment of the metabolic function of the liver, and among those that are established, all capture only a proportion of the liver's function [2]. Avoiding known hepatotoxins and adjustment of dosage of drugs without intrinsic hepatotoxicity in patients with liver dysfunction may therefore be required to avoid excessive accumulation of the drug, active drug metabolite(s) thereof, and subsequent adverse effects, either hepatic or extrahepatic. As no surrogate parameter is currently available to reliably reflect the patency of hepatic metabolism of drugs, their pharmacokinetic characteristics and interactions with other drugs must be considered to avoid therapeutic misadventures in patients with impaired liver function. While this is true for certain substances that are primarily metabolized by the liver, a common misconception prevails that subjects with pre-existing liver diseases are more susceptible to develop DILI than those without. In fact, clinical data supporting this general attitude of caution are limited to only a few drugs, while the majority of prescription and over-the-counter drugs can be used safely.

Impaired liver function and drug biotransformation

Any foreign compound that enters the human body undergoes metabolism and elimination via exhalation, urinary clearance, or biliary/fecal excretion. Anatomically and functionally, the liver is located between the gastrointestinal tract and the systemic circulation. Drugs (and multiple other molecules contained in the gut) are absorbed predominantly in the small bowel and transported to the liver via the portal vein. Together, the intestinal epithelium and the liver are responsible for the presystemic elimination, the so-called first-pass metabolism of drugs and other xenobiotics before these reach the post-hepatic circulation. Drug-metabolizing enzyme systems are present in many tissues of the body, including the gut epithelia, but their magnitude is expressed in liver tissue. Here, biotransformation takes place by the action of multiple drug-metabolizing enzymes including microsomal cytochrome P450 isoenzymes, mixed-function monooxygenases, glutathione-S-transferases, and UDP-glucuronosyltransferases, to name but a few. Some of these can be induced through variable mechanisms which may lead to large interindividual variability in

Cirrhosis: A practical guide to management, First Edition. Edited by Samuel S. Lee and Richard Moreau.

Table 23.1 Drugs to avoid or to be used with special precautions in patients with liver diseases.

Drug name/group	Liver disease	Remarks/precautions
Paracetamol/acetaminophen >2 g/day	Alcoholic liver disease/cirrhosis	Can be safely used up to 4 g/day in noncirrhotic patients
"Biologicals" (infliximab, etanercept, adalimumab, certolizumab)	Untreated hepatitis B virus infection	Co-treatment with antiviral agent required (e.g., lamivudine, tenofovir)
"Disease modifiers" (sulfasalazine, chloroquine, gold, methotrexate, azathioprine)	Untreated hepatitis B virus infection	Co-treatment with antiviral agent required (e.g., lamivudine, tenofovir) Add folate to methotrexate
Isoniazide-containing antituberculosis treatment regimens	Alcoholic liver disease, chronic viral hepatitis B/C, particularly when coinfected with HIV	Regular liver enzyme level monitoring, switch to isoniazide – sparing regimens according to guidelines [37]
HAART	HIV–HCV coinfected subjects	Increased incidence of DILI related to nearly all classes of HAART agents; regular laboratory testing including lactate (lactic acidosis)
Antidepressants	All causes of advanced liver diseases	Avoid MAO inhibitors, tricyclic antidepressants, and nefazodone
Hormonal agents Tamoxifen Antiandrogens (flutamide, cyproterone acetate)	Nonalcoholic fatty liver disease/insulin resistance Chronic viral hepatitis	Regular liver laboratory testing; restriction of use to clear indications
Herbal preparations	All liver diseases	Lack of efficacy and safety data; restrict use to clinical trials

DILI, drug-induced liver injury; HAART, highly active antiretroviral therapy; HCV, hepatitis C virus; MAO, monoamine oxidase inhibitor.

pharmacokinetics and susceptibility for drug-related liver damage [2]. Obviously, the capacity to handle drugs can be hampered with a reduced compartment of metabolically active liver cells such as in severe acute or chronic liver injury. Accounting for this impairment of liver function, pharmacotherapy in clinical hepatology requires the assessment of liver function beyond the determination of routine laboratory biomarkers such as liver-related serum transaminases (alanine aminotransferase, ALT; aspartate aminotransferase, AST) or markers of synthetic (coagulation factors, albumin) or excretory (conjugated bilirubin) function. However, available methods reflecting the metabolic function of the liver are neither satisfactory nor routinely used in clinical practice [3]. Thus, decision making in clinical practice to date relies on data from clinical population-based studies, case reports, spontaneous reporting of adverse events to pharmacovigilance authorities, safety data of registrations trials, and the few randomized trials in which the incidence of DILI in specific cohorts was deliberately sought. In addition to scientific data, information on safety, applicability, and contraindications of certain drugs are provided in the manufacturers' package inserts of drugs to guide prescribers and users. However, the most important factor in this context is that acting physicians are aware of the true limitations and risks of several drugs in the context of hepatic insufficiency, keep in mind the possibility of DILI even with drugs generally considered safe, and are able to translate this knowledge into clinical judgment [4].

In the following sections, individual drugs associated with a risk of causing DILI are described with a special focus on the context of prescribing them to patients with coexisting liver diseases. Among these, the use of only a few is associated with an increased risk of DILI when administered to patients with pre-existing liver diseases (Table 23.1).

Acetaminophen/paracetamol

Paracetamol is among the most widely used antipyretic analgesics in the world, and a common cause of fulminant hepatic failure [5], but differs from most other drugs resulting in DILI in that its hepatotoxicity is dose related and thus predictable once the threshold of toxicity has been exceeded. Hepatotoxicity of paracetamol is due to biotransformation of the drug to a toxic metabolite that requires conjugation with glutathione via activity of glutathione transferase to be inactivated [6]. Once glutathione is depleted, the toxic metabolite, *N*-acetyl-*p*-benzoquinone imine (NAPQI), binds to other nucleophilic groups in the cell. Cell death ensues, especially in zone III hepatocytes around the terminal hepatic vein, but also in nonliver cells that are able to activate the parent compound such as renal tubular cells, which can lead also to kidney failure. NAPQI formation is enhanced with induction of cytochrome-P450 2E1 (CYP2E1), an isoenzyme responsible for the oxidative degradation of ethanol and other chemicals (Figure 23.1). CYP2E1 can be induced, and thus capable of increased NAPQI production, by excessive alcohol consumption, obesity, and fasting, thereby exhausting glutathione stores required for NAPQI detoxification [7].

Awareness of paracetamol as a potential cause of liver injury is relatively high, but this often leads to its avoidance in patients with liver disease. However, contrary to common belief, paracetamol can be safely used even in patients with cirrhosis, although a maximum safe dose has not yet been established.

Data from a randomized trial indicate an increased incidence of liver enzyme elevations up to 20-fold the upper limit of normal in healthy subjects taking 4 g/day paracetamol [8], and an earlier study in regular and excessive alcohol drinkers showed massive elevations of transaminases and fulminant liver failure in 20% of subjects who ingested paracetamol at doses of 4–6 g/day [9]. However, another more recent study in which

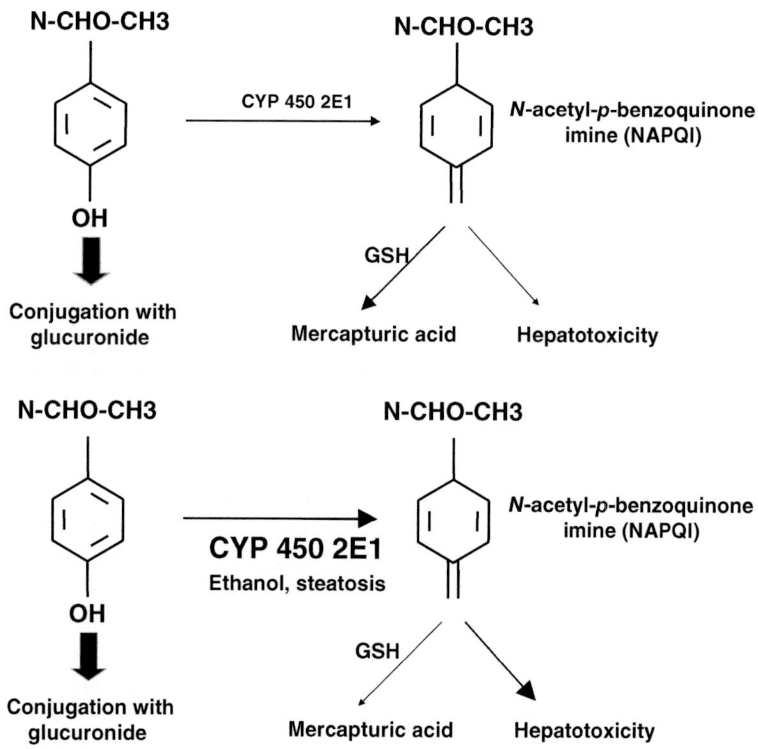

Figure 23.1 Under normal therapeutic circumstances, the magnitude of a therapeutic dose (>90%) of paracetamol is glucuronidated (or sulfated) and then excreted. A small percentage is metabolized by cytochrome P450 enzymes (CYP) to the reactive intermediate *N*-acetyl-*p*-benzoquinone imine (NAPQI), which is readily detoxified by conjugation with glutathione (GSH) (A). In situations of overdose and/or induced CYP enzymes, as in chronic drinkers or the heavily obese, detoxification mechanisms are exhausted and excessive formation of NAPQI occurs. In addition, glutathione stores may be depleted prior to paracetamol ingestion (malnutrition) aggravating the heaptic insufficiency to detoxify NAPQI (B).

subjects included consumed one or two alcoholic beverages per day detected only mild elevations of liver enzymes within the normal range following the intake of up to 4 g/day paracetamol [10]. In line with the latter study, Temple et al. [11] demonstrated that patients with impaired liver function neither had higher NAPQI levels nor liver enzyme elevations following repeated doses of 4 g/day paracetamol. Other studies support the view that short-term use of paracetamol at 4 g/day in alcoholics, particularly when abstinent, and subjects with hepatitis C virus (HCV) infection is safe [12,13].

From these data it can be concluded – leaving a margin of safety – that paracetamol dosed at or below 2 g/day can be given to patients with pre-existing liver diseases, whereas doses up to 4 g/day should not be given long term, particularly when regular alcohol consumption is an issue.

Nonsteroidal anti-inflammatory drugs

Nonsteroidal anti-inflammatory drugs (NSAIDs) are potent agents used for the treatment of chronic mild to moderate pain. NSAIDs are among the most widely used drugs worldwide, either via prescription or as over-the-counter preparations. However, non-selective NSAIDs, also known as cyclooxygenase (COX) inhibitors, carry an increased risk of serious upper gastrointestinal complications, including gastroduodenal ulcers, perforation and bleeding, and liver injury. Regarding the latter, along with anti-infectious agents, they top the list for causes of DILI [14]. The incidence of liver disease induced by NSAIDs reported in clinical studies is fairly uniform, ranging 0.3–9 per 100 000 depending on the drug under scrutiny, but considerable under-reporting of asymptomatic, mild cases prevent a precise assessment of the actual risk of DILI along with NSAIDs [15]. Following numerous cases of severe liver injury including fulminant hepatic failure, several NSAIDs, such as bromfenac, ibufenac, and benoxaprofen, have either been withdrawn from the market, or, as for nimesulide, are licensed with tight restrictions [16].

Although liver-related hepatotoxicity induced by NSAIDs generally reveals a low incidence in the general population, several agents appear to carry a higher risk such as sulindac, diclofenac, and nimesulide. While the incidence of NSAID-associated DILI in patients with preexsting liver disease has not been systematically investigated, several agents should not be used under certain circumstances:

1 Physicians are advised to avoid any type of NSAID in patients with end-stage liver disease because of the risk of gastrointestinal bleeding and kidney failure aggravating latent hepatorenal syndrome [17,18];
2 Aspirin is considered more hepatotoxic in patients with cirrhosis, possibly due to hypoalbuminemia [19], and may cause Reye's syndrome, a sequel of metabolic acidosis, hepatic encephalopathy, hypoglycemia, coagulopathy, and azotemia following mitochondrial dysfunction for as yet unclear reasons [20];
3 Ibuprofen, which is frequently used to the treat flu-like syndrome along with interferon-based treatment of HCV infection, has been associated with acute hepatitis in this context [21,22], but appears to be safe when used in small doses on an "on demand" basis.

Antirheumatic agents

Methotrexate is an efficacious and cost-effective treatment for rheumatoid arthritis and psoriasis, but associated with significant safety issues, particularly regarding hepatotoxicity. Among the risk factors predisposing to methotrexate-related liver injury are female gender, steatosis, regular alcohol consumption, a higher duration and cumulative methotrexatedose, and possibly, cotherapy with acitretin, a synthetic retinoid [23]. However, weighing the risks against the possible benefits of methotrexate, a clear contraindication for its use in patients with liver diseases appears inappropriate, also because noninvasive biomarkers and novel follow-up tools such as transient elastography (Fibroscan^{TM}) are available [24]. Bearing this in mind, regular liver biopsies after each 1.5 g of cumulative methotrexatedose – as recommended by several guidelines – seems inordinate, even in those with coexisting liver pathologies.

Mok et al. [25] retrospectively investigated the safety of the use of disease modifying antirheumatic drugs (sulfasalazine, chloroquine, gold, methotrexate) in patients with rheumatoid arthritis, either with chronic HBVand HCV infection (n = 30) or without (n = 62), and found that all of the disease-modifier drugs were associated with significantly higher rates of liver enzyme elevations, with a single case HBV reactivation in a patient on azathioprine. In clinical practice, liver enzymes should be monitored during the start of therapy, and HBV carriers be treated with an antiviral drug to prevent reactivation.

Particular prudence must be applied when treating patients with novel "biologicals" such as infliximab, etanercept, adalimumab, or certolizumab who are infected with HBV, because reactivation of viral replication and subsequent severe courses of acute hepatitis are well described. In a recent systematic review of published cases, HBV reactivation was reported in 39% of HBsAg+ carriers, and overall more likely to occur in patients previously treated with immunosuppressive agents, and lower in those who received antiviral prophylaxis (23% vs. 62%; $P = 0.003$). Notably, acute liver failure was reported in five patients, four of whom died [26].

This remarkable risk of biologicals in causing potentially fatal sequelae of acute hepatitis in HBV carriers does not apply to patients with chronic HCV in whom the safety profile of anti-TNF-α agents seems to be acceptable with only minor and rare incidents of liver enzyme elevations [27].

Opiate replacement therapy

Buprenorphine, a synthetic molecule derived from thebaine, has been marketed in numerous countries as an opiate replacement therapy in drug addicts, a subpopulation of patients often afflicted with chronic infection with HCV and human immunodeficiency viruses (HIV). At recommended sublingual doses, buprenorphine is well tolerated, although a mild increase in serum ALT activity can occasionally occur in some patients. Some heroin addicts inject buprenorphine intravenously and may develop plasma peak concentrations severalfold higher than with sublingual administration. Several case series have reported on acute cytolytic hepatitis with marked jaundice following both intravenous [28] and sublingual administration of buprenorphine [29,30]. Of note, most patients in these series were anti-HCV positive. An interesting report described two HCV-positive individuals who developed acute hepatitis following intravenous buprenorphine, and cleared HCV-RNA after hepatitis subsided [31].

However, more recent and larger series of intravenous drug users receiving opiate replacement therapy with buprenorphine, either infected with HCV or HIV, documented no evidence of hepatotoxicity when buprenorphine was taken in recommended doses [32,33]. Thus, for clinical guidance, patients taking buprenorphine should be advised to take it only via the recommended route, and at doses considered safe. Specific follow-up guidelines are not warranted, but clinicians should take buprenorphine hepatotoxicity into account once liver enzyme elevations occur in a patient.

Naltrexone, a long-acting opioid antagonist that possesses no opioid agonist activity, was approved by the US Food and Drug Administration (FDA) for the treatment of opiate dependence in 1984 and alcoholism in 1994. A black box warning by the FDA indicates that naltrexone can cause liver damage and demands that users should be informed about this prior to prescription. However, this view has been challenged by many, and observational studies have not confirmed the hepatotoxicity risk ascribed to naltrexone neither when used in alcoholics nor in patients with HCV coinfection [34,35].

As opposed to naltrexone and buprenorphine, no reports on hepatotoxicity from methadone have been published so far.

Antituberculosis agents

Derelict alcoholics with advanced alcoholic liver injury or HIV-positive individuals with coexistent HBV or HCV infection may be afflicted by tuberculosis in a substantial proportion, and must be treated with antituberculosis agents. It is important to note that up to 20% of patients receiving isoniazide develop asymptomatic elevation of liver enzymes, often without a tendency to further deteriorate clinically. However, an increased risk for isoniazide hepatotoxicity exists for elderly patients, those who regularly drink alcohol, in malnourished individuals, and in combinations of isoniazide with other antituberculosis drugs [36]. In addition, as described in a previous study by Ungo et al. [37], HIV positive individuals revealed a fourfold higher risk of DILI from antituberculosis drugs, a fivefold higher risk among subjects with chronic HCV, and a remarkable 14.4-fold risk in those coinfected with HIV and HCV. Another study showed similar hazard ratios for patients with chronic HBV infection receiving antituberculosis agents [38].

Apart from isoniazide, rifampicin can also affect hepatic function as it competes with bilirubin for binding to the bile salt export pump, and can lead to otherwise harmless hyperbilirubinemia [39]. However, in rare instances, rifampicin may also elicit acute hepatocellular injury, likely via a hypersensitivity reaction [40]. Similarly, pyrazinamide can also produce dose-dependent hepatotoxicity and should be used with extreme caution in combination with other antituberculosis drugs [41]. Guidelines issued by the American Thoracic Society for patients with tuberculosis and coexisting chronic liver diseases call for liver enzyme surveillance and recommend treatment discontinuation if levels increase fivefold, or threefold if accompanied by hyperbilirubinemia [37]. In those with isoniazidecontraindications such as cirrhotic patients with or without decompensation, alternative regimens consisting of rifampicin, with/without ethambutol and fluoroquinolones (moxifloxacin, levofloxacin), are recommended.

Antibiotics

Results of a recent US multicenter prospective study on DILI-induced fulminant hepatic failure identified antimicrobials as the leading group of causative agents with 46% of all cases associated with their intake [42]. The most frequent single agents were sulfur-containing antibiotics and nitrofurantoin. Genome-wide association studies identified HLA genotypes as host genetic susceptibility factors associated with flucloxacillin [43] and amoxicillin–clavulanic acid [44] hepatotoxicity. Whether there exists an increased risk of DILI due to antibiotics among patients with concomitant acute or chronic liver diseases is not known, and evidence-based guidelines are not available.

Drugs to treat HIV infection

The mainstays of highly active antiretroviral therapy (HAART) in HIV-infected patients comprise nucleoside reverse transcriptase inhibitors (NRTI), non-nucleosidic reverse transcriptase inhibitors (NNRTI), and protease inhibitors. All of these drug classes have been associated with DILI, particularly in patients coinfected with HBV and HCV [45,46]. Among the clinical consequences derived from HAART-related liver toxicity are events with the potential to be fatal and, for this reason, many anti-HIV agents are labelled with a liver-related FDA black box warning (Table 23.2).

Without exception, all HAART agents can lead to a phenomenon termed "immune reconstitution" in the

Table 23.2 HAART agents with increased hepatotoxicity in patients with coexisting chronic viral hepatitis B/C.

Drug	Hepatotoxicity rate (%)	Other risk factors	Hepatic failure in literature	Proposed mechanism
NRTIs				
Abacavir	6	HLA-B*5701 polymorphism	+	Mitochondrial toxicity
Didanosine	6	Co-therapy with ribavirin	+	Immune reconstitution
Stavudine	13	Co-therapy with didanosine/ hydroxyurea	+	
NNRTIs				
Efavirenz	20	High CD4 counts (>250)	+	Hypersensitivity reaction
Etravirine	3		+	Idiosyncratic reaction
Nevirapine	19		+	
Protease inhibitors				
Atazanavir/ritonavir	15	High dose ritonavir	–	Harmless
Darunavir	7		+	hyperbilirubinemia
Ritonavir	26		+	Idiosyncratic reaction
Tipranavir/ritonavir	20		+	
Saquinavir	17		–	
CCR5 blockers (maraviroc)	Unclear data		+	Unclear
Integrase inhibitor (raltegravir)	27		–	Unclear

setting of viral hepatitis, which clinically presents with aminotransferase elevation and is considered a result of an increased immunocompetence subsequent to effective HAART [47]. For example, among the NRTIs, zidovudine, stavudine, and didanosine are associated with symptomatic lactic acidosis and steatohepatitis due to mitochondrial dysfunction with an incidence of approximately 1–4 per 1000 patient-years which often progresses to multi-organ failure with a high mortality, even if the medication is stopped [48]. Another NRTI, abacavir, has been linked to drug-induced hypersensitivity reactions with clinical signs of skin rash, fever, and pronounced fatigue, and cytolytic hepatitis which can be fatal, particularly in an event of re-exposure to abacavir [49]. Interestingly, abacavir-associated drug hypersensitivity shows an association with a HLA-B*5701 polymorphism [50].

Didanosine is more likely to cause DILI in HIV–HCV coinfected patients treated with ribavirin as part of an interferon-based combination to eradicate HCV. The mechanism behind this interaction is an increased intracellular phosphorylation of didanosine due to ribavirin, leading to an increased risk of mitochondrial toxicity [51].

For many NNRTIs, a higher rate of DILI among HIV-infected individuals with chronic viral hepatitis can be observed, and in this regard, nevirapine seems to be a particularly frequent cause in up to 20% of HIV–HCV coinfected subjects. Sulkowski et al. [52] found the highest rate of liver enzyme elevations among patients with HCV coinfection receiving nevirapine compared to those without. A typical pattern is drug-induced hypersensitivity which typically occurs early within 3 months of therapy, but idiosyncratic reactions without signs of autoimmunity are also possible. Additional risk factors for DILI due to NNRTIs are concomitant therapy with protease inhibitors, CD4 cell numbers of >250 in women and >400 in men, low body mass index, and certain host genetic factors, which, however, are not part of the regular decision-making algorithm when selecting the type of HAART [53]. As for nevirapine in patients with HCV coinfection, CD4 cell levels above 200 in females and 250 in males should make prescribers refrain from its use [54].

Protease inhibitors may cause harmless hyperbilirubinemia not indicative of hepatotoxicity; however, significant liver injury has been observed with ritonavir, nelfinavir, saquinavir, and indinavir. Among these, ritonavir in full dose is the most likely agent to induce DILI, especially in patients coinfected with HBV and HCV. Thus, in such patients, ritonavir should be given in a reduced dosage [55].

With novel directly acting antivirals (e.g., boceprevir, telaprevir) for the treatment of HCV infection now available, and many more under scrutiny in phase II and III trials, their use in HIV-infected subjects in the future increases the risk of interactions with HAART components, and close pharmacovigilance will lead to the identification of new risk constellations, and likely, contraindications.

Drugs acting on the central nervous system

Antidepressants

Patients with advanced liver damage including cirrhosis reveal a high prevalence of depressive symptoms either as a result of liver disease, its treatment, or as a separate entity. Pharmacotherapy may be indicated in some, and the selection of antidepressant with a low hepatotoxic risk is warranted. However, antidepressant drugs are not devoid of adverse effects, including hepatotoxicity with all classes currently used. Liver impairment shows clinicopathologic features that range from transient liver enzyme elevations to even fulminant hepatic failure. Traditional antidepressants such as monoamine oxidase inhibitors or tricyclic antidepressants appear to have the highest risk to induce liver damage compared with the novel selective serotonin reuptake inhibitors (SSRIs) [56,57]. In some databases of drug-induced liver diseases, antidepressants account for up to 5% of reported cases, while SSRIs have a low incidence of hepatotoxicity from 1.28 to 3.62 cases per patient-year and, among them, the incidence with sertraline is the lowest of its group with 1.28 (0.42–3) cases per patient-year [58]. Among the SSRIs, the highest number of reports is available for paroxetine, possibly due to its frequent use, whereas nefazodone, a serotonin–norepinephrine reuptake inhibitor, can cause liver failure due to mitochondrial injury and is the only antidepressant agent that carries a FDA black box warning regarding hepatotoxicity [59].

Whether any of the antidepressants are more likely to cause DILI in patients with pre-existing liver disease is not known, but it appears prudent to extrapolate the evidence above to this group of patients to avoid superimposed DILI in such patients, and to opt for agents with the best safety record such as sertraline, when indicated from the psychiatric point of view.

Antipsychotics

Antipsychotic neuroleptics including phenothiazines, butyrophenones, and clozapine have been recognized as causes of DILI in a variable but small proportion of users and therefore can be considered unpredictable or idiosyncratic. Presentation enzyme patterns can be hepatocellular, mixed, or cholestatic.

Phenothiazines such as chlorpromazine were among the first neuroleptics recognized as causes of DILI, mostly with a cholestatic presentation due to ductopenia, but are less frequently used nowadays [59]. Butyrophenones, such as haloperidol and bromperidol, are rare cases of DILI which resembles that of phenothiazines [60]. Atypical neuroleptics such as clozapine or olanzapine are increasingly used, and thus reports on their hepatotoxicity have emerged [61,62]. Increased liver enzymes are reported to affect 30–50% of patients treated with clozapine [62,63]. As with antidepressants, no data exist as to whether patients with pre-existing liver diseases, and particularly those with cirrhosis, have an increased risk of neuroleptic-associated DILI than those with apparently healthy liver status, and physicians should not be deterred from using them with appropriate laboratory follow-up when indicated.

Anticonvulsants

Some liver diseases are associated with generalized convulsions, such as alcoholic liver diseases, which require appropriate pharmacotherapy. Several anticonvulsants have been associated with DILI.

Phenytoin has long been used to treat epilepsy, and in some countries, monitoring of liver enzymes monthly during the first quarter of the year, and then 6-monthly, is recommended. The risk of both acute and chronic liver injury associated with the use of phenytoin, although generally low, has been well described and is presumed idiosyncratic in nature, as no studies have shown a correlation between serum phenytoin concentrations and hepatotoxicity [64]. Phenytoin can elicit a hepatocellular pattern of injury, although a cholestatic or mixed pattern is more common and, in the majority of cases, associated with hypersensitivity features early during treatment [65]. In addition to acute liver injury, chronic liver damage has also been reported as associated with phenytoin [66]. Data on the incidence of phenytoin-associated DILI in patients with liver diseases have not been published as yet, and thus pre-existing liver disease poses no contraindication for phenytoin.

Valproic acid is an antiepileptic used in the treatment of bipolar disorder, and its toxicity profile is characterized by a rare but well-documented hepatotoxicity. Fatal hepatic failure associated with valproic acid occurs in 1 in 5000–10 000 of exposed patients who are predominantly male, of young age (<10 years), and often mentally retarded [67]. Liver injury associated with valproic acid is of four main subtypes: transient and reversible elevation in liver tests (in up to 50% of patients), toxic hepatitis, hyperammonemia, and Reye-like syndrome. Valproic acid carries a boxed warning from the FDA and should only be used with frequent liver enzyme monitoring, and even more carefully used, if at all, in patients with cirrhosis as elimination of valproic acid is reduced up to 50% [68].

Similar to phenytoin, carbamazepine can cause acute liver injury with hypersensitivity features, albeit at lower frequency [64]. Persistently high levels of gamma-glutamyltranspeptidase and alkaline phosphatase should raise the suspicion of ductopenia. Again, the risk of carbamazepine-associated DILI is particularly high in children and after longer therapy. If indicated, carbamazepine can be used in patients with pre-existing liver diseases but requires regular monitoring of liver enzymes.

Most other anticonvulsants, including lamotrigine, phenobarbital, and topiramate can be used safely in patients with liver diseases as reports on hepatotoxicity are rare exceptions.

Miscellaneous agents

Antihyperglycemic drugs

At the time of its introduction onto the market, troglitazone was an effective antidiabetic drug with a fundamentally new mechanism of action, until individual cases of liver injury and failure were reported subsequent to its use [69]. Concerns about a possible class effect of the glitazones could be ruled out and post-marketing pharmcovigilance has neither found significant hepatotoxicity in diabetics nor in patients with liver diseases with the use of rosiglitazone and pioglitazone. To the contrary, data from several clinical trials indicate a potential benefit on liver enzyme levels and histology of these agents in the treatment of nonalcoholic fatty liver disease [70,71].

While package inserts and prescription information state that metformin should not be used in patients with liver dysfunction because of the risk of lactic acidosis, only few cases have been reported, and toxicity often occurred in patients with alcoholic cirrhosis [72,73]. Considering the potential benefits from metformin in patients with nonalcoholic fatty liver disease, its use in patients with liver disease cannot be discouraged.

Hormonal drugs

Tamoxifen, an antiestrogen used as an adjuvant therapy of breast cancer, has been recognized as a potential cause of DILI, and cases of toxic hepatitis, massive hepatic steatosis, multifocal hepatic fatty infiltration, hepatic necrosis, and cirrhosis have been described [74]. Among these lesions, steatosis is particularly frequent in more than 30% of breast cancer patients treated with adjuvant tamoxifen. A risk factor for DILI following tamoxifen is insulin resistance as in patients with nonalcoholic fatty liver disease which is associated with steatosis. However, no clear contraindication for its use in patients with liver diseases is defined.

In contrast, antiandrogens such as flutamide and cyproterone acetate have been associated with fulminant hepatic failure [75], and appear to carry a higher risk in patients with chronic viral hepatitis [76].

Statins

Much concern has been raised over the safety of cholesterol-decreasing statins (atorvastatin, simvastatin, rosuvastatin), but which appears inappropriate considering the low frequency of adverse hepatic reactions following their use [77]. Clinical trials aiming at assessing the frequency of liver-related adverse reactions in patients with nonalcoholic fatty liver disease [78] and chronic hepatitis C [79] could not detect higher risk of DILI in comparison to patients without liver abnormalities, and one study even demonstrated improved transaminase levels [80]. The latter effect was ascribed to the metabolic improvements achieved with statin treatment.

Although idiosyncratic liver injury along with statins can be severe, it is very rare and thus they can be safely used in patients with pre-existing liver diseases.

Complementary herbal medicines and dietary supplements

Systematic investigations on the safety of complementary herbal medicines and dietary supplements are scarce, and not available in the subgroup of liver-diseased patients. However, their use in this patient group is widespread [81,82]. While a number of herbal medicines show promising activity including silymarin and glycyrrhizin to inhibit HCV RNA replication, *Phyllantus amarus* in chronic HBV infection, and several herbal combinations from China and Japan that deserve testing in appropriate studies [83], reports about severe liver injury after the intake of herbals and dietary supplements are accumulating [84,85]. However, the evidence supporting the use of such products in healthy subjects is poor and the same applies to individuals with liver diseases. Bearing in mind the possible adverse hepatic reactions resulting from their intake, the use of complementary herbal medicines and dietary supplements cannot be recommended.

Assessment of DILI in patients with cirrhosis

Recognition of adverse hepatic drug reactions in patients with cirrhosis is sometimes particularly difficult as elevations of indicative serum liver enzyme tests are either due to the underlying or worsening liver disease or due to the intake of a certain drug. However, if the enzyme levels are well-documented, a significant rise above those levels or a changing pattern of laboratory abnormalities should raise the suspicion of superimposed DILI. For DILI in general, and for cirrhotics in particular, early recognition of a precipitating drug as the cause of liver injury is crucial as it appears to reduce the risk of progression to acute liver failure or chronic liver damage [86]. Since DILI can resemble other acute and chronic liver injuries, and because specific tests are needed to ascertain whether drugs are the cause of the liver injury, diagnosis depends largely on the exclusion of other etiologic causes and a high degree of clinical judgment and suspicion from the physician in charge.

For DILI causality assessment, several standardized scores have been proposed which rely on numeric scales, probability, and expert opinion. While some of these assessment systems are widely in use, all are compromised by the fact that they are not validated, because there is no gold standard method in establishing the diagnosis of DILI. This particularly accounts for patients with confirmed cirrhosis. Nevertheless, diagnostic scales

Table 23.3 Causality score proposed by the Council for the International Organization of Medical Sciences (CIOMS).

Axis	Points
Chronologic criteria:	
From drug intake until onset	+1 to +2
From drug withdrawal until onset	0 to +1
Course of reaction	−2 to +3
Risk factors	0 to +2
Concomitant medication	−3 to 0
Exclusion of other causes	−3 to +2
Published evidence of hepatotoxicity of suspected drug	0 to +2
Rechallenge	−2 to +3
Causality level:	
>8 points – defintive	
6–8 points – probable	
3–5 points – possible	
1–2 points – unlikely	
≤0 points – excluded	

Source: Danan et al., 1993 [87]. Reproduced with permission of Elsevier.

and algorithms provide a helpful management checklist for guiding the collection of clinical data required for diagnosis. Among the many assessment tools, a scale introduced by the Council for International Organizations of Medical Sciences (CIOMS) is currently the preferred method when suspecting DILI, in combination with clinical judgment [87]. The scale was published as the Roussel Uclaf Causality Assessment Method (RUCAM) in 1993 and includes seven domains of which each is given a numerical weight (Table 23.3). When first validated, the CIOMS score has shown 86% sensitivity, 89% specificity, and a positive and negative predictive value of 93% and 78%, respectively. Other scores, such as the Maria and Victorino scale or the Digestive Disease Week-Japan (DDW-J) scale consider similar aspects in the setting of a suspected adverse hepatic drug reaction (e.g., exclusion of other causes, chronology, rechallenge) and perform similarly well in the assessment of DILI. Another approach to assign or reject causality is distinct from using numerical scores and based on expert judgment. As relying on the opinion of a single expert would be too subjective, all crucial data available are considered by three experts to reach a consensus. This concept is used as a standardized method by the DILI network study group [88], and outscored other numerical scores in some studies [89]. However, a clear limitation of this strategy is the absence of expert panels who can be contacted in daily routine.

In summary, assessing causality between certain drugs and liver injury in a patient with cirrhosis does not differ from the assessment in noncirrhotic individuals. However, due to the limited hepatic reserve of cirrhotic patients to withstand additional liver insults, immediate recognition and subsequent cessation of suspected medication is particularly important. An algorithm of how to proceed is proposed in Figure 23.2.

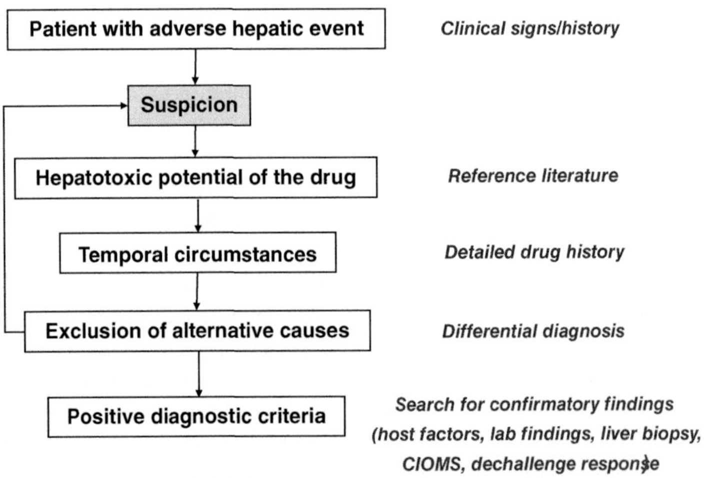

Figure 23.2 Diagnostic algorithm in the management of adverse hepatic drug reactions. CIOMS, Council for International Organizations of Medical Sciences.

References

1 Verbeeck RK. Pharmacokinetics and dose adjustment in patients with hepatic dysfunction. Eur J Clin Pharmacol 2008;64:1147–61.

2 Mohutsky MA, Romeike A, Meador V, et al. Hepatic drug-metabolizing enzyme induction and implications for pre-clinical and clinical risk assessment. Toxicol Pathol 2010;38:799–809.

3 Ilan Y. Review article: the assessment of liver function using breath tests. Aliment Pharmacol Ther 2007;26:1293–302.

4 Lucena MI, García-Cortés M, Cueto R, et al. Assessment of drug-induced liver injury in clinical practice. Fundam Clin Pharmacol 2008;22:141–58.

5 Ostapowicz G, Fontana RJ, Schiødt FV, et al. Results of a prospective study of acute liver failure at 17 tertiary care centers in the United States. Ann Intern Med 2002;137: 947–54.

6 Mitchell JR, Jollow DJ, Potter WZ, et al. Acetaminophen-induced hepatic necrosis. 1. Role of drug-metabolism. J Pharmacol Exp Ther 1973;187:185–94.

7 Thummel KE, Slattery JT, Ro H, et al. Ethanol and production of the hepatotoxic metabolite of acetaminophen in healthy adults. Clin Pharmacol Ther 2000;67:591–9.

8 Watkins PB, Kaplowitz N, Slattery JT, et al. Aminotransferase elevations in healthy adults receiving 4 grams of acetaminophen daily: a randomized controlled trial. JAMA 2006;296:87–93.

9 Zimmerman HJ, Maddrey WC. Acetaminophen (paracetamol) hepatotoxicity with regular intake of alcohol: analysis of instances of therapeutic misadventure. Hepatology 1995;22: 767–73.

10 Heard K, Green JL, Kuffner EK, et al. A randomized trial to determine the change in alanine aminotransferase during 10 days of paracetamol (acetaminophen) administration in subjects who consume moderate amounts of alcohol. Aliment Pharmacol Ther 2007;26:283–90.

11 Temple AR, Lynch JM, Vena J, et al. Aminotransferase activities in healthy subjects receiving three-day dosing of 4, 6, or 8 grams per day of acetaminophen. Clin Toxicol (Phila) 2007;45:36–44.

12 Dart RC, Green JL, Kuffner EK, et al. The effects of paracetamol (acetaminophen) on hepatic tests in patients who chronically abuse alcohol: a randomized study. Aliment Pharmacol Ther 2010;32:478–86.

13 Kuffner EK, Green JL, Bogdan GM, et al. The effect of acetaminophen (four grams a day for three consecutive days) on hepatic tests in alcoholic patients – a multicenter randomized study. BMC Med 2007;5:13

14 Andrade RJ, Lucena MI, Fernández MC, et al. Drug-induced liver injury: an analysis of 461 incidences submitted to the Spanish registry over a 10-year period. Gastroenterology 2005;129:512–21.

15 Bessone F. Non-steroidal anti-inflammatory drugs: what is the actual risk of liver damage? World J Gastroenterol 2010;16:5651–61.

16 Aithal GP, Day CP. Nonsteroidal anti-inflammatory drug-induced hepatotoxicity. Clin Liver Dis 2007;11:563–75.

17 Laffi G, Lavilla G, Pinzani M, et al. Arachidonic acid derivatives and renal function in liver cirrhosis. Semin Nephrol 1997;17:530–48.

18 Deledinghen V, Heresbach D, Fourdan O, et al. Anti-inflammatory drugs and variceal bleeding: a case–control study. Gut 1999;44:270–3.

19 Russell AS, Sturge RA, Smith MA. Serum transaminases during salicylate therapy. Br Med J 1971;2:428–9.

20 Soller RW, Stander H. Association between salicylates and Reye's syndrome. JAMA 1983;249:883

21 Andrade RJ, Lucena MI, García-Cortés M, et al. Chronic hepatitis C, ibuprofen, and liver damage. Am J Gastroenterol 2002;97:1854–5.

22 Riley TR, Smith JP. Ibuprofen-induced hepatotoxicity in patients with chronic hepatitis C: a case series. Am J Gastroenterol 1998;93:1563–5.

23 Ahern MJ, Smith MD, Roberts-Thomson PJ. Methotrexate hepatotoxicity: what is the evidence? Inflamm Res 1998;47: 148–51.

24 Barker J, Horn EJ, Lebwohl M, et al. Assessment and management of methotrexate hepatotoxicity in psoriasis patients: report from a consensus conference to evaluate current practice and identify key questions toward optimizing methotrexate use in the clinic. J Eur Acad Dermatol Venereol 2011;25:758–64.

25 Mok MY, Ng WL, Yuen MF, et al. Safety of disease modifying anti-rheumatic agents in rheumatoid arthritis patients with chronic viral hepatitis. Clin Exp Rheumatol 2000;18:363–8.

26 Pérez-Alvarez R, Díaz-Lagares C, García-Hernández F, et al. Hepatitis B virus (HBV) reactivation in patients receiving tumor necrosis factor (TNF)-targeted therapy: analysis of 257 cases. Medicine (Baltimore) 2011;90:359–71.

27 Brunasso AM, Puntoni M, Gulia A, Massone C. Safety of anti-tumour necrosis factor agents in patients with chronic hepatitis C infection: a systematic review. Rheumatology (Oxford) 2011;50:1700–11.

28 Berson A, Gervais A, Cazals D, et al. Hepatitis after intravenous buprenorphine misuse in heroin addicts. J Hepatol 2001;34:346–50.

29 Hervé S, Riachi G, Noblet C, et al. Acute hepatitis due to buprenorphine administration. Eur J Gastroenterol Hepatol 2004;16:1033–7.

30 Zuin M, Giorgini A, Selmi C, et al. Acute liver and renal failure during treatment with buprenorphine at therapeutic dose. Dig Liver Dis 2009;41:e8–10.

31 Peyrière H, Tatem L, Bories C, et al. Hepatitis after intravenous injection of sublingual buprenorphine in acute hepatitis C carriers: report of two cases of disappearance of viral

replication after acute hepatitis. Ann Pharmacother 2009;43: 973–7.

32 Bogenschutz MP, Abbott PJ, Kushner R, et al. Effects of buprenorphine and hepatitis C on liver enzymes in adolescents and young adults. J Addict Med 2010;4:211–6.

33 Vergara-Rodriguez P, Tozzi MJ, Botsko M, et al. Hepatic safety and lack of antiretroviral interactions with buprenorphine/naloxone in HIV-infected opioid-dependent patients. J Acquir Immune Defic Syndr 2011;56(Suppl 1):S62–7.

34 Yen MH, Ko HC, Tang FI, et al. Study of hepatotoxicity of naltrexone in the treatment of alcoholism. Alcohol 2006;38:117–20.

35 Brewer C, Wong VS. Naltrexone: report of lack of hepatotoxicity in acute viral hepatitis, with a review of the literature. Addict Biol 2004;9:81–7.

36 Saukkonen JJ, Cohn DL, Jasmer RM, et al. Antituberculosis Therapy Subcommittee. An official ATS Statement: hepatotoxicity of antitiberculosis therapy. Am J Respir Crit Care Med 2006;174:935–52.

37 Ungo JR, Hones D, Ashkin D, et al. Antituberculosis drug-induced hepatotoxicity. The role of hepatitis C virus and the human immunodeficiency virus. Am J Respir Crit Care Med 1998;157:1871–6.

38 Wong WM, Wu PC, Yuen MF, et al. Antituberculosis drug-related liver dysfunctionin chronic hepatitis B infection. Hepatology 2000;31:201–6.

39 Byrne JA, Strautnieks SS, Mieli-Vergani G, et al. The human bile salt export pump: characterization of substrate specificity and identification of inhibitors. Gastroenterology 2002;123: 1649–58.

40 Fountain FF, Tolley EA, Jacobs AR, Self TH. Rifampin hepatotoxicity associated with treatment of latent tuberculosis infection. Am J Med Sci 2009;337:317–20.

41 Centers for Disease Control Prevention. Update: fatal and severe liver injuries associated with rifampin and pyrazinamide treatment for latent tuberculosis infection. MMWR Morb Mortal Wkly Rep 2002;51:998–9.

42 Reuben A, Koch DG, Lee WM. Drug-induced acute liver failure: results of a U.S. multicenter, prospective study. Hepatology 2010;52:2065–76.

43 Daly AK, Donaldson PT, Bhatnagar P, et al. HLA-B*5701 genotype is a major determinant of drug-induced liver injury due to flucloxacillin. Nat Genet 2009;41:816–9.

44 Lucena MI, Molokhia M, Shen Y, et al. Susceptibility to amoxicillin-clavulanate-induced liver injury is influenced by multiple HLA class I and II alleles. Gastroenterology 2011;141:338–47.

45 Sulkowski MS. Viral hepatitis and HIV coinfection. J Hepatol 2008;48:353–67.

46 Lacombe K, Rockstroh J. HIV and viral hepatitis coinfections: advances and challenges. Gut 2012;61 Suppl 1:i47–58.

47 Martin-Blondel G, Mars LT, Liblau RS. Pathogenesis of the immune reconstitution inflammatory syndrome in HIV-infected patients. Curr Opin Infect Dis 2012;25:312–20.

48 Ogedegbe AE, Thomas DL, Diehl AM. Hyperlactataemia syndromes associated with HIV therapy. Lancet Infect Dis 2003;3:329–37.

49 Bannister WP, Friis-Moller N, Mocroft A, et al. Incidence of abacavir hypersensitivity reactions in euro-SIDA. Antivir Ther 2008;13:687–696.

50 Mallal S, Phillips E, Carosi G, et al. HLA-B*5701 screening for hypersensitivity to abacavir. N Engl J Med 2008;358:568–579.

51 Balzarini J, Lee C, Herdewijn P, et al. Mechanism of the potentiating effect of ribavirin on the activity of 2′,3′-dideoxyinosine against human immunodeficiency virus. J Biol Chem 1991;266:21509–14.

52 Sulkowski MS, Thomas DL, Mehta SH, et al. Hepatotoxicty associated with nevirapine or efavirenz-containing antiretroviral therapy: a role of hepatitis C and B infections. Hepatology 2002;35:182–9.

53 Núñez M. Clinical syndromes and consequences of antiretroviral-related hepatotoxicity. Hepatology 2010;52:1143–55.

54 Torti C, Costarelli S, De Silvestri A, et al. Analysis of severe hepatic events associated with nevirapine-containing regimens: CD4+ T-cell count and gender in hepatitis C seropositive and seronegative patients. Drug Saf 2007;30:1161–9.

55 Sulkowski MS, Thomas DL, Mehta SH, et al. Hepatotoxicity associated with antiretroviral therapy in adults infected with human immunodeficiency virus and the role of hepatitis C or B virus infection. JAMA 2000;283:74–80.

56 Sedky K, Nazir R, Joshi A, et al. Which psychotropic medications induce hepatotoxicity? Gen Hosp Psychiatry 2012;34:53–61.

57 Lucena MI, Carvajal A, Andrade RJ, Velasco A. Antidepressant induced hepatotoxicity. Expert Opin Drug Saf 2003;2: 249–62.

58 Carvajal GPA, del Garcia PJ, Sanchez AS, Velasco MA, de Rueda CAM, Lucena MI. Hepatotoxicity associated with the new antidepressants. J Clin Psychiatry 2002;63:135–7.

59 Dykens JA, Jamieson JD, Marroquin LD, et al. In vitro assessment of mitochondrial dysfunction and cytotoxicity of nefazodone, trazodone, and buspirone. Toxicol Sci 2008; 103:335–45.

60 Dincsoy H, Saelinger D. Haloperidol-induced chronic cholestatic liver disease. Gastroenterology 1982;83:694–700.

61 Manceaux P, Constant E, Zdanowicz N, et al. Management of marked liver enzyme increase during olanzapine treatment: a case report and review of the literature. Psychiatr Danub 2011;23(Suppl 1):S15–7.

62 Keane S, Lane A, Larkin T, Clarke M. Management of clozapine-related hepatotoxicity. J Clin Psychopharmacol 2009;29:606–7.

63 Macfarlane B, Davies S, Mannan K, et al. Fatal acute fulminant liver failure due to clozapine: a case report and review of clozapine-induced hepatotoxicity. Gastroenterology 1997; 112:1707–9.

64 Björnsson E. Hepatotoxicity associated with antiepileptic drugs. Acta Neurol Scand 2008;118:281–90.

65 Vittorio C, Muglia J. Anticonvulsant hypersensitivity syndrome. Arch Intern Med 1995;155:2285–90.

66 Andrade RJ, Lucena MI, Kaplowitz N, et al. Outcome ofacute idiosyncratic drug-induced liver injury: long-term follow-up in a hepatotoxicity registry. Hepatology 2006;44:1581–8.

67 Koenig SA, Buesing D, Longin E, et al. Valproic acid-induced hepatopathy: nine new fatalities in Germany from 1994 to 2003. Epilepsia 2006;47:2027–31.

68 Klotz U, Rapp T, Müller WA. Disposition of valproic acid in patients with liver disease. Eur J Clin Pharmacol 1978;13: 55–60.

69 Kohlroser J, Mathai J, Reichheld J, et al. Hepatotoxicity due to troglitazone: report of two cases and review of adverse events reported to the United States Food and Drug Administration. Am J Gastroenterol 2000;95:272–6.

70 Boettcher E, Csako G, Pucino F, et al. Meta-analysis: pioglitazone improves liver histology and fibrosis in patients with non-alcoholic steatohepatitis. Aliment Pharmacol Ther 2012;35:66–75.

71 Ratziu V, Giral P, Jacqueminet S, et al. Rosiglitazone for nonalcoholic steatohepatitis: one-year results of the randomized placebo-controlled Fatty Liver Improvement with Rosiglitazone Therapy (FLIRT) Trial. Gastroenterology 2008;135: 100–10.

72 Cone CJ, Bachyrycz AM, Murata GH. Hepatotoxicity associated with metformin therapy in treatment of type 2 diabetes mellitus with nonalcoholic fatty liver disease. Ann Pharmacother 2010;44:1655–1659.

73 Brackett CC. Clarifying metformin's role and risks in liver dysfunction. J Am Pharm Assoc 2010;50:407–410.

74 Elefsiniotis IS, Pantazis KD, Ilias A, et al. Tamoxifen induced hepatotoxicity in breast cancer patients with pre-existing liver steatosis: the role of glucose intolerance. Eur J Gastroenterol Hepatol 2004;16:593–8.

75 Miquel M, Soler A, Vaqué A, et al. Suspected cross-hepatotoxicity of flutamide and cyproterone acetate. Liver Int 2007;27:1144–7.

76 Pu YS, Liu CM, Kao JH, et al. Antiandrogen hepatotoxicity in patients with chronic viral hepatitis. Eur Urol 1999;36:293–7.

77 Björnsson E, Jacobsen EI, Kalaitzakis E. Hepatotoxicity associated with statins: reports of idiosyncratic liver injury postmarketing. J Hepatol 2012;56:374–80.

78 Chalasani N, Aljadhey H, Kesterson J, et al. Patients with elevated liver enzymes are not at higher risk for statin hepatotoxicity. Gastroenterology 2004;126:1287–92.

79 Khorashadi S, Hasson NK, Cheung RC. Incidence of statin hepatotoxicity in patients with hepatitis C. Clin Gastroenterol Hepatol 2006;4:902–7.

80 Lewis JH, Mortensen ME, Zweig S, et al. Efficacy and safety of high-dose pravastatin in hypercholesterolemic patients with well-compensated chronic liver disease: results of a prospective, randomized, double-blind, placebo-controlled, multicenter trial. Hepatology 2007;46:1453–63.

81 Flora KD, Rosen HR, Brenner KG. The use of neuropathic remedies for chronic liver disease. Am J Gastro 1996;91: 2654–5.

82 Strader DB, Bacon BR, Lindsay KL, et al. Use of complementary and alternative medicine in patients with liver disease. Am J Gastro 2002;97:2391–7.

83 Stickel F, Schuppan D. Herbal medicine in the treatment of liver diseases. Dig Liver Dis 2007;39:293–304.

84 Navarro VJ. Herbal and dietary supplement hepatotoxicity. Semin Liver Dis 2009;29:373–82.

85 Stickel F, Kessebohm K, Weimann R, Seitz HK. Review of liver injury associated with dietary supplements. Liver Int 2011;31:595–605.

86 Andrade RJ, Lucena MI, Kaplowitz N, García-Munoz B, Borraz Y, Pachkoria K, et al. Outcome of acute idiosyncratic drug-induced liver injury: long-term follow-up in a hepatotoxicity registry. Hepatology 2006;44:1581–8.

87 Danan G, Benichou C. Causality assessment of adverse reactions to drugs-I. A novel method based on the conclusions of international consensus meetings: application to drug-induced liver injuries. J Clin Epidemiol 1993;46: 1323–30.

88 Rockey DC, Seeff LB, Rochon J, Freston J, Chalasani N, Bonacini M, et al. Causality assessment in drug-induced liver injury using a structured expert opinion process: comparison to the Roussel-Uclaf causality assessment method. Hepatology 2010;51:2117–26.

89 Macedo AF, Marques FB, Ribeiro CF. Can decisional algorithms replace globalintrospection in the individual causality assessment of spontaneously reported ADRs? Drug Saf 2006;29:697–702.

CHAPTER 24

Changing outcomes with antiviral or antifibrotic therapies

Gamal Esmat and Maissa El Raziky
Faculty of Medicine, Cairo University, Cairo, Egypt

Introduction

When the term cirrhosis was coined two centuries ago by Laennec, it meant – by definition – an end-stage irreversible liver disease. Nowadays this word encompasses a whole range of disorders including some degree of reversibility [1]. The issue of regression or reversal of cirrhosis was first noticed in animal models upon the discontinuation of injurious agents to the liver or initiating treatment with antifibrotic agents [2], but this regression was not fully demonstrated in humans. Evidence of fibrotic and/or cirrhotic regression were reported in chronic viral hepatitis [3–5], alcoholic and nonalcoholic steatohepatitis [6,7], and autoimmune hepatitis [8]. However, these studies concluded that, in spite of a variable degree of fibrosis regression there was no complete reversal of cirrhosis [3–8].

In hepatitis B virus (HBV) related cirrhosis, the use of nucleot(s)ide analogs showed advantages for Child–Turcotte–Pugh (CTP) score improvement and transplant-free survival, and the incidence of hepatocellular carcinoma (HCC) was reduced [9]. Interferon treatment for patients with hepatitis C virus (HCV) related cirrhosis inhibits the development of HCC [10] and improves survival [11]. In situations where treating the underlying process is not possible, specific antifibrotic therapy is highly recommended [12].

HBV-Related Cirrhosis

Treatment is mandatory in patients with compensated or decompensated cirrhosis and detectable HBV DNA, independently of alanine aminotransferase (ALT) levels. Patients with no HBV DNA detectable by current sensitive tests should be monitored. Before treatment, the following factors should be considered: age, HBV DNA levels, hepatic performance, whether the cirrhosis is compensated or decompensated, presence of esophagogastric varices, comorbidities and cofactors potentially worsening liver disease, and the prospect of liver transplantation (LT) [13].

Nucleot(s)ide analog therapy can achieve sustained suppression of HBV replication, remission of liver disease, and has been shown to halt disease progression and prevent long-term complications, such as decompensation and HCC [9].

Nucleos(t)ide analogs in compensated cirrhosis

Since its introduction in the 1990s, lamivudine has been considered as a safe and effective drug in suppression of HBV replication [14]. It was reported that in patients with compensated cirrhosis, prolonged therapy with lamivudine was well tolerated and resulted in improved serum biochemical values and loss of HBV DNA together with clinical improvements in the form of decrease in CTP scores, an improvement in albumin, and a reduced incidence of ascites [15]. However, reports of long-term antiviral treatment resistance and selection of antiviral-resistant mutations with subsequent reduction of clinical benefit may be associated with flares of the disease; even frank hepatic decompensation was frequently described with lamivudine [16]. Thus, other treatment strategies, such as add-on therapies with another agent that lacks cross-resistance, are most often necessary for suppression of viral replication and prevention of further worsening of disease [17].

Cirrhosis: A practical guide to management, First Edition. Edited by Samuel S. Lee and Richard Moreau.

Adefovir was the first nucleotide analog to be used in cases of lamivudine resistance [18]. A number of studies have clearly demonstrated that adding adefovir to ongoing lamivudine was associated with a lower risk of adefovir-resistance than switching to adefovir in both hepatitis Be antigen (HBeAg)-positive and HbeAg-negative patients with lamivudine-resistant HBV [19,20]. Current guidelines recommend that when adefovir is used as an add-on therapy in patients with lamivudine-resistant HBV infection, lamivudine should be continued indefinitely to decrease the risk of hepatitis flares during the transition period and to reduce the risk of subsequent adefovir resistance [21]. Randomized, placebo-controlled studies demonstrated that this add-on therapy was safe and associated with substantial virologic and biochemical improvement after 1–2 months of treatment [17]. The European Association for the Study of the Liver (EASL) guidelines recommend that in lamivudine-resistant YMDD mutations, tenofovir monotherapy should be started [22].

Among entecavir-treated patients with advanced liver fibrosis, improvement in fibrosis was observed in almost 60% of nucleos(t)ide-naive HBeAg-positive or HBeAg-negative patients. The treatment was well tolerated. The performance of entecavir relative to that of lamivudine in patients with advanced liver fibrosis and/or cirrhosis was comparable with the relationship observed in noncirrhotic patients. Virologic response to entecavir is associated with a lower probability of disease progression in patients with cirrhosis, even after correction for possible baseline confounders. When using a threshold of 2000 IU/mL, the association between viral replication and disease progression was reduced, suggesting that complete viral suppression is essential for nucleos(t)ide analog treatment, especially in patients with cirrhosis, whether compensated or decompensated [23,24].

For chronic hepatitis B (CHB) patients with cirrhosis, telbivudine can improve CTP score at 48 weeks of treatment. One of the major drawbacks with long-term telbivudine treatment is the development of drug resistance [25].

Tenofovir is considered one of the first line drugs for treatment-naïve patients. Having a potent antiviral activity, low resistance rate and toxicity, it can be used in the long term for effective HBV DNA suppression. Tenofovir is useful in patients with lamivudine, telbivudine, and entecavir resistance; it is cost-effective for patients with cirrhotic CHB [26].

CHB patients with advanced fibrosis are often not considered for treatment with pegylated interferon (PEG-IFN) because IFN therapy may precipitate immunologic flares, potentially inducing hepatic decompensation. Treating HBeAg-positive CHB patients with advanced fibrosis and/or cirrhosis with compensated liver disease, with 52 weeks of PEG-IFN-α-2b (100 μg/week) alone or in combination with lamivudine (100 mg/day), resulted in virologic response in about 25% of patients. Improvement in liver fibrosis occurred in two-thirds of patients. The authors concluded that PEG-IFN is effective and safe for HBeAg-positive patients with advanced fibrosis. Patients with advanced fibrosis or cirrhosis but compensated liver disease should not be excluded from PEG-IFN treatment [27].

Nucleos(t)ide analogs in decompensated cirrhosis

Patients with decompensated HBV cirrhosis at initial presentation have a poor short-term prognosis, with an estimated 5-year survival of only 10–15% [4]. Although LT is an effective treatment option for decompensated HBV cirrhosis, shortage of donor organs and limited availability of resources worldwide precludes the majority of HBV patients in endemic areas from undergoing transplantation, raising the issue of considering antiviral therapy as an alternative option [28].

Pooled 1-year data of treating patients with decompensated cirrhosis showed benefit favoring lamivudine vs. untreated controls for CTP score improvement by at least 2 points and transplant-free survival [14]. Adefovir monotherapy was less successful in achieving undetectable HBV DNA at 1-year in 41% than with lamivudine and entecavir. Overall, 1-year transplant-free survival rates varied from 78% with lamivudine to 95% and 94% with tenofovir and telbivudine, respectively [9].

The 1-year incidence of drug-resistant HBV was almost null with adefovir, entecavir, and tenofovir and around 10% with lamivudine although telbivudine was associated with almost 30% incidence at 2 years. Drug-related adverse events were infrequently reported. All the oral antiviral agents were associated with improved virologic, biochemical, and clinical parameters at 1 year. However, the efficacy of lamivudine is limited by drug resistance, and adefovir is limited by its slower onset of action [29].

Other beneficial effects with the oral nucleo(t)side agents included removal from the LT waiting list in 6% of patients receiving adefovir, 21% receiving lamivudine, and 11% treated with entecavir. Development of HCC at 1 year was reported to be lower in treated patients. However, lamivudine was not more effective in reducing the incidence of HCC at 1 year compared to untreated patients [9].

The largest amount of data involved lamivudine monotherapy in decompensated HBV cirrhosis, presumably due to the fact that this agent has been available for over 15 years in many countries. Resistance to lamivudine, which occurred in 10% of patients at 1 year, has emerged as a major limitation especially in patients with advanced disease who cannot tolerate biochemical flares with emergence of drug-resistant HBV. HBV cirrhosis patients had a higher rate of clinical outcomes when they developed drug resistance during follow-up and a higher mortality rate [14].

The data of entecavir monotherapy in patients with decompensated HBV cirrhosis showed no evidence of entecavir-resistant HBV at 1 year despite the presence of lamivudine-resistant HBV in some of these patients [24,30,31].

Data on the use of tenofovir and telbivudine in decompensated HBV cirrhosis are restricted by the small numbers of studies for each drug. Tenofovir was as effective and potent as entecavir with a similar side-effect profile and no evidence of drug-resistance. Tenofovir-treated patients were able to achieve HBeAg seroconversion [32,33].

Drug safety is an important consideration when treating patients with decompensated cirrhosis who have impaired drug metabolism, protein binding, and renal functions. Lamivudine had the fewest number of serious adverse effects. Renal insufficiency with associated renal tubular dysfunction was reported in adefovir, tenofovir, or entecavir-treated decompensated patients, especially in those with low baseline glomerular filtration rate (GFR) [9]. Recent studies have demonstrated an increasing frequency of serum creatine phosphokinase (CPK) elevations with prolonged tenofovir use. Thus, telbivudine may be a second line agent for patients with decompensated HBV cirrhosis due to safety concerns. There are also some concerns regarding the long-term safety of tenofovir in patients with malnutrition and low vitamin D levels.

Another concern with the prolonged use of nucleos(t)ide analogs is the potential for mitochondrial toxicity and lactic acidosis, which may present with myopathy, neuropathy, and rhabdomyolysis [34].

Hepatitis B virus-related acute-on-chronic liver failure

HBV-related acute-on-chronic liver failure (ACLF) has an extremely poor prognosis. The 3-month survival rate was higher with those treated with entecavir or lamivudine than in nontreated patients. Short-term antiviral treatment with entecavir or lamivudine rapidly suppressed HBV replication, increased the short-term survival rate, and reduced recurrence. Early administration of long-term nucleoside analog treatment is recommended for the prevention of recurrence of HBV-related ACLF [35].

Hepatitis B virus-related liver transplantation

In patients eligible for LT, treatment with nucleoside analogs should be started in collaboration with a reference transplant center. This should aim to control the risk of clinical deterioration, reduce viremia to as low as possible before transplantation to reduce the risk of HBV reactivation, and prevent the emergence of HBV-resistant mutants (Figure 24.1). After transplantation, the standard of prophylaxis is a combination of nucleoside analogs and anti-HBV immunoglobulins (HBIG). Post-LT experience has been mostly reported with lamivudine and/or adefovir. Data on entecavir, tenofovir, and telbivudine are rare [36].

HCV-related cirrhosis

The clinical significance of treating patients with established cirrhosis has been a matter of debate. Earlier studies on the treatment of HCV-related cirrhosis failed to demonstrate the benefit of viral eradication in subjects with advanced liver disease [37,38]. However, retrospective, longitudinal study of cirrhotic patients treated with IFN, and who were followed-up for 5 years, showed that the annual incidence of HCC was 2.3% for untreated and 1.0% for treated patients, whereas the incidence of hepatic decompensation was 1.5% and 5.7%, respectively, which supports the claim that eradication of HCV infection prevents progression to potentially fatal complications by fibrosis regression and lowering portal hypertension, thus effectively confronting the debate of reversibility of cirrhosis [39,40].

The analysis of four randomized trials, pooling data of 3010 treatment-naive patients treated with different

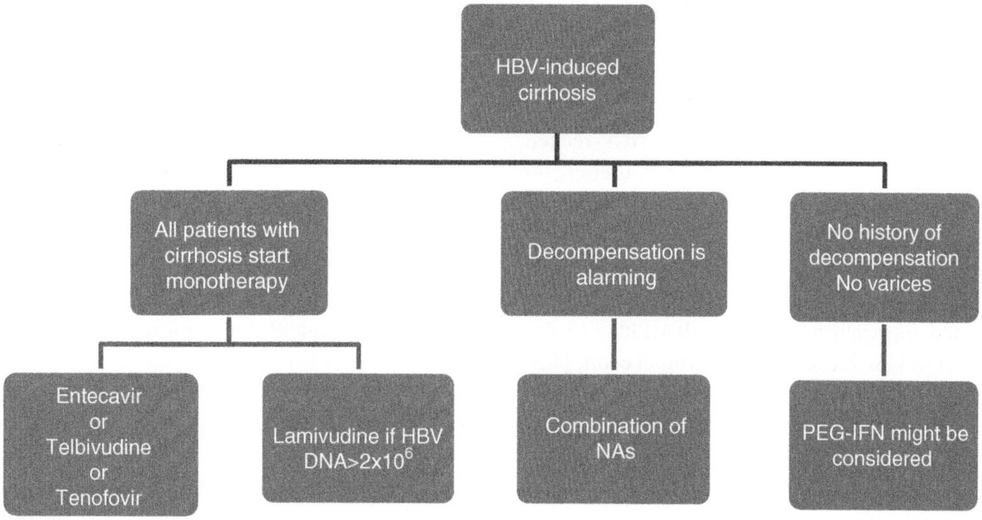

Figure 24.1 Algorithm for the treatment of hepatitis B virus (HBV) induced cirrhosis. NA, nucleot(s)ide analog.

regimens of standard IFN-α or PEG-IFN-α, with or without ribavirin, demonstrated the reversal of cirrhosis in half of patients with baseline cirrhosis. Cirrhotic patients who have cleared HCV infection showed lower rates of liver decompensation, HCC development, and liver-related death [11]. Another international, multicenter, long-term follow-up study from five large hospitals in Canada and Europe of 530 patients with chronic HCV infection who received an IFN-based treatment concluded that sustained virologic response (SVR) was associated with lower all-cause mortality [41].

Anti-HCV treatment in compensated cirrhosis

Anti-HCV treatment in cirrhotic patients is less effective than in noncirrhotics. Based on effectiveness and tolerability reports, therapy has a significant effect in patients with compensated cirrhosis, while decompensated patients need to re-evaluate the risks versus benefits of treatment [42].

The Markov model for cost-effectiveness of HCV therapy demonstrated that the treatment of patients with compensated cirrhosis was found to be the most cost-effective strategy and resulted in improved survival and decreased cost in comparison with all other strategies [43].

The rates of SVR to PEG-IFN in combination with ribavirin ranged 10–44% for HCV genotypes 1/4 to 33–72% for genotypes 2/3 in compensated cirrhosis, compared with 29–55% for genotypes 1/4 and 70–80% for genotypes 2/3 in noncirrhotic patients. HCV clearance was associated with a reduced risk of liver decompensation, HCC development, liver-related mortality, and hepatitis recurrence after LT during a mean follow-up of 7.7 years [11].

Triple therapy using telepravir or boceprevir had good results for the treatment of treatment-naïve patients affected by genotype 1 HCV with advanced fibrosis and cirrhosis: F3–F4 as compared to SOC therapy [44]. IFN treatment without achieving SVR does not seem to protect against HCC [40]. In genotype I HCV compensated cirrhosis triple therapy with boceprevir, IFN, and ribavirin improved SVR rates in patients with F3/4, with good safety profile [45,46]; however, triple therapy with telaprevir or boceprevir showed poor outcome and high rates of serious adverse events in patients with advanced liver disease with low platelet count and serum albumin [47].

Discontinuation rates in compensated cirrhosis ranges from 5% to 53%. Dose modification, mainly to hematologic toxicity of antiviral therapy, is more frequent in patients with compensated cirrhosis (13–68%) than in patients with less severe liver disease [11].

Anti-HCV treatment in decompensated cirrhosis

A few uncontrolled, single-center studies have investigated the role of standard IFN mono- or combined therapy with ribavirin in decompensated HCV-related cirrhosis. Reports concluded that antiviral therapy in patients with decompensated cirrhosis is possible and may prevent HCV recurrence after transplantation in a proportion of cases. However, potentially fatal side effects of infections and of death related to infections were reported, especially in patients with MELD >18 and those with a low baseline absolute neutrophil count [42].

SVR rates ranged 0–16% and 44–57% in genotypes 1/4 and 2/3, respectively, in the decompensated stage regardless of the type of PEG-IFN used or absence or presence of esophageal varices [48,49]. Decompensation during 30-month follow-up occurred in 23% of responders compared with 69% of nonresponders or untreated patients [11]. Viral eradication was also associated with reduced mortality. The use of colony-stimulating factors and erythropoietin allowed better treatment tolerance [50].

Escalating the dosage of PEG-IFN2α starting at 90 μg/week and escalating to 180 μg/week if tolerated was tried in a small group of patients on low dose ribavirin was associated with a significant reduction in all-cause mortality and nononcologic liver-related morbidity in this trial [51].

Hepatitis C virus-related liver transplantation

The aim of establishing a pre-transplantation antiviral therapy is either to attain an SVR at transplantation, or an on-treatment HCV RNA clearance at transplantation. The mere reduction of viral load should not be an aim because, unlike in HBV cirrhotic patients, this has not been proven to decrease the rate and/or severity of recurrence in HCV cases. In post-LT cases, minimizing allograft failure due to recurrence of HCV infection has also been reported in the literature (Figure 24.2) [52].

Antifibrotic therapy

The concept of reversibility of liver fibrosis and cirrhosis is not a recent one [53]; updates in our understanding of the cellular and molecular bases of fibrogenesis over the last two decades have led to the development of novel therapeutic targets, and provided a framework for therapeutic approaches to prevent, slow down, or even reverse fibrosis and cirrhosis [12,54]. Antifibrotic therapies may be directed against different areas in the fibrogenic process, including inhibition of matrix deposition, collagen synthesis, inhibiting stellate cell activation, enhancing matrix degradation, or activation of stellate cell death or apoptosis [54,55]. Many drugs with specific "antifibrotic activity" were studied in human trials but

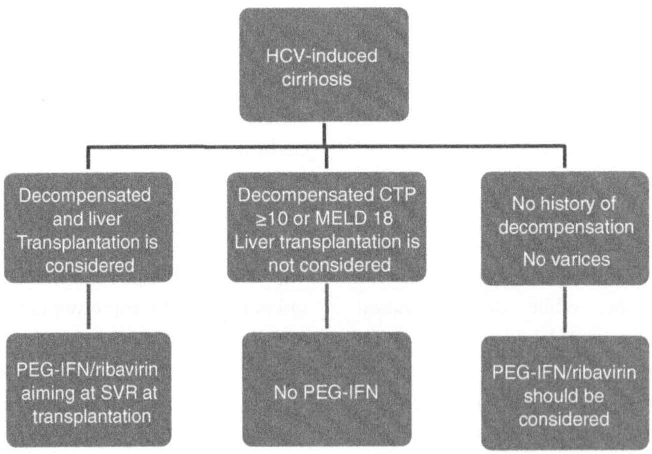

Figure 24.2 Algorithm for the treatment of hepatitis C virus (HCV) induced cirrhosis. CTP, Child–Turcotte–Pugh score; MELD, model for end-stage liver disease; PEG-IFN, pegylated interferon; SVR, sustained virologic response.

the results of these studies have been conflicting [12]. Although some of the drugs and agents detailed below have demonstrated promising initial results as antifibrotic agents in clinical trials, they have yet to become part of routine care for a variety of reasons. For some drugs, the only results available are small uncontrolled pilot studies, for others, the literature shows conflicting results.

Specific antifibrotic therapies studied in human subjects

Colchicine

Colchicine is a plant alkaloid that inhibits collagen secretion through inhibiting polymerization of microtubules. The antifibrotic effect of this compound is thought to be by preventing collagen secretion and deposition. Colchicine inhibited collagen formation effectively in experimental animal models [56], but human studies led to conflicting results. Some authors concluded that colchicine does not appear to reduce hepatic fibrosis, and it cannot therefore be recommended as a primary antifibrotic treatment [57], while others reported colchicine to be an effective antifibrotic drug for long-term treatment of chronic liver disease in which fibrosis progresses towards cirrhosis after 5 years [58,59]. Colchicine is generally safe (although one report concluded that it may suppress the response to IFN-α based anti-HCV therapy [60]. In alcoholic cirrhosis treated with colchicine for up to 6 years, overall liver-specific mortality was not reduced, but fewer patients developed hepatorenal syndrome [61].

In primary biliary cirrhosis, the addition of colchicine to ursodeoxycholic acid has resulted in a significant reduction in disease progression [62]. Colchicine may lower the incidence of the development of HCC in virally related cirrhosis possibly through its anti-inflammatory effect [12].

Angiotensin II antagonists

The angiotensin II system is a promising antifibrotic target, as it is overproduced in the injured liver; it has a role in stimulating stellate cell activation and fibrogenesis. Studies in humans to test the effects of angiotensin receptor blockers in patients with advanced liver disease in an attempt to reduce portal pressure or to potentiate fibrosis regression reported that both losartan and candesartan were effective in decreasing the hepatic venous pressure gradient but fibrosis regression was not evident [63,64].

γ-Interferon

IFN-γ has been shown to specifically inhibit extracellular matrix formation by fibroblasts. This cytokine inhibited stellate cell activation. Nine-month IFN-γ treatment significantly reduced the fibrosis score in patients with chronic HBV infection [65]. In one study, the authors did not find a long-term benefit according to histologic criteria. IFN-γ1b was safe and well tolerated in humans with HCV infection and advanced fibrosis in a dose of 100 or 200 μg [66].

Peroxisomal proliferator activated receptor gamma ligands

The peroxisomal proliferator activated receptor (PPAR) is a family of nuclear hormone receptors and hepatic stellate cell activation during liver injury is associated with reduced PPAR-γ expression. Treatment of underlying nonalcoholic steatohepatitis using thiazolidinediones may be associated with an improvement in fibrosis [67].

Pirfenidone

Pirfenidone is a small, orally bioavailable molecule that appears to downregulate collagen synthesis, but its molecular mechanism of action is not clearly understood. Pirfenidone has been shown to have antifibrotic effects in a variety of fibrogenic animal models and a few human studies, including the lung, kidney, and liver [68].

Compounds with a potential antifibrotic activity secondary to upstream effects

Many compounds seem to be capable of affecting fibrogenesis by having an effect on important biologic events such as lipid peroxidation, immune system modulation, or others.

Silymarin

Silymarin reduces lipid peroxidation. It has been reported to have variable effects. One study revealing lowered mortality in patients with alcohol-induced liver disease was debated [69]. As silymarin is considered to be safe and is commonly used as a complementary medicine, studies in patients with nonalcoholic steatohepatitis or in those who have failed standard of care antiviral therapy for HCV infection were initiated [70].

Ursodeoxycholic acid

Being a non-toxic bile acid, ursodeoxycholic acid is considered cytoprotective by means of binding to hepatocyte membranes thus reducing inflammation and downstreams fibrogenesis. It is important to stress that no studies indicate a primary antifibrotic effect of ursodeoxycholic acid in the liver. However, a variety of reports suggest that ursodeoxycholic acid may delay progression of fibrosis in primary biliary cirrhosis through its effects on biliary ductal inflammation, particularly if initiated early in the course of the disease [71].

Polyenylphosphatidy icholine

Polyenylphosphatidy icholine is derived from purified soybean extract. Having both antioxidant and antifibrotic properties, it gained considerable interest in the treatment of patients with liver injury, especially alcohol-induced [72].

Interleukin-10

As a potent immune-modulator, interleukin-10 can downregulate production of pro-inflammatory T-cell cytokines. Endogenous interleukin-10 appears to slow down the intrahepatic inflammatory response and reduce fibrosis in several models of liver injury. Direct antifibrotic effect for interleukin-10 has not been established [73].

Miscellaneous antioxidants and anti-inflammatory compounds

Methotrexate

Methotrexate has an anti-inflammatory activity and has also been shown to have profibrogenic activity, although the risk of fibrosis progression when used in patients with skin or rheumatologic disease may be less than commonly thought [74]. In patients with primary biliary cirrhosis, improvement in disease and fibrosis have been reported, but data on methotrexate show either no or minimal effects, with or without colchicine [75].

Corticosteroids

Corticosteroids have been used to treat a variety of liver diseases, especially autoimmune hepatitis [8].

One of the major challenges in the field of fibrosis therapy currently is how to monitor fibrosis. No antifibrotics are currently licensed for use in humans. The ideal antifibrotic agent that is safe when used over a long period of time, potent, orally administrated, specific to the liver and nontoxic to hepatocytes, but inexpensive has not yet been developed.

Conclusions

- The antifibrotic effect of colchicine is thought to be by preventing collagen secretion and deposition.
- The angiotensin II system is a promising antifibrotic target.
- IFN-γ specifically inhibits extracellular matrix formation by fibroblasts.
- Compounds with potential antifibrotic activity secondary to upstream effects include silymarin, ursodeoxycholic acid, and interleukin-10.

References

1 Balabaud C, Bioulac-Sage P. Cirrhosis: what else? Gastroenterol Clin Biol 2010;34:252–4.

2 Kershenobich D, Vargas F, Garcia-Tsao G, et al. Colchicine in the treatment of cirrhosis of the liver. N Engl J Med 1988;318:1709

3 Serpaggi J, Carnot F, Nalpas B, et al. Direct and indirect evidence for the reversibility of cirrhosis. Hum Pathol 2006;37:1519–26.

4 Poynard T, McHutchison J, Manns M, et al. Impact of pegylated interferon alfa-2b and ribavirin on liver fibrosis in patients with chronic hepatitis C. Gastroenterology 2002;122:1303–13.

5 Dienstag JL, Goldin RD, Heathcote EJ, et al. Histological outcome during long-term lamivudine therapy. Gastroenterology 2003;124:105–17.

6 Wakim-Fleming J, Mullen KD. Long-term management of alcoholic liver disease. Clin Liver Dis 2005;9:135–49.

7 Dixon JB, Bhathal PS, Hughes NR, O'Brien PE. Nonalcoholic fatty liver disease: improvement in liver histological analysis with weight loss. Hepatology 2004;39:1647–54.

8 Dufour JF, DeLellis R, Kaplan MM. Reversibility of hepatic fibrosis in autoimmune hepatitis. Ann Intern Med 1997;127:981–5.

9 Singal AK, Fontana RJ. Meta-analysis: oral anti-viral agents in adults with decompensated hepatitis B virus cirrhosis. Aliment Pharmacol Ther 2012;35:674–89.

10 Cheinquer N, Cheinquer H, Wolff F, et al. Effect of sustained virologic response on the incidence of hepatocellular carcinoma in patients with HCV cirrhosis. Braz J Infect Dis 2010;14:457–61.

11 Vezali E, Aghemo A, Colombo M. A review of the treatment of chronic hepatitis C virus infection in cirrhosis. Clin Ther 2010;32:2117–38.

12 Rockey DC. Current and future anti-fibrotic therapies for chronic liver disease. Clin Liver Dis 2008;12:939–64.

13 Carosia G, Rizzettob M, Albertic A. Treatment of chronic hepatitis B: update of the recommendations from the 2007 Italian Workshop. Dig Liver Dis 2011;43:259–65.

14 Liaw YF, Sung JJ, Chow WC, et al. Lamivudine for patients with chronic hepatitis B and advanced liver disease. N Engl J Med 2004;351:1521–31.
15 Liaw YF, Lee CM, Chien RN, et al. Switching to adefovir monotherapy after emergence of lamivudine-resistant mutations in patients with liver cirrhosis. J Viral Hepat 2006;13: 250–5.
16 Shaw T, Bartholomeusz A, Locarnini S. HBV drug resistance: mechanism, detection and interpretation. J Hepatol 2006;44:593–606.
17 Perrillo RP, Hann HW, Schiff E, et al. Extended treatment with lamivudine and adefovir dipivoxil in chronic hepatitis B patients with lamivudine resistance. Hepatol Int 2011;5: 654–63.
18 Perrillo R, Schiff E, Yoshida E, et al. Adefovir dipivoxil for the treatment of lamivudine-resistant hepatitis B mutants. Hepatology 2000;32:129–34.
19 Lampertico P, Vigano M, Manenti E, et al. Adefovir rapidly suppresses hepatitis B in HBeAg negative patients developing genotypic resistance to lamivudine. Hepatology 2005;42: 1414–9.
20 Fabien Z, Perrillo R. Hepatitis B: reflections on the current approach to antiviral therapy. J Hepatol 2008;48:S2–19.
21 Lok ASF, McMahon BJ. AASLD practice guidelines, chronic hepatitis B. Hepatology 2007;47:507–39.
22 EASL Clinical Practice Guidelines. Management of chronic hepatitis B virus infection. J Hepatol 2012;57:167–85.
23 Schiff E, Simsek H, Lee WM, et al. Efficacy and safety of entecavir in patients with chronic hepatitis B and advanced hepatic fibrosis or cirrhosis. Am J Gastroenterol 2008;103: 2776–83.
24 Sadler M, Coffin C, Lee S. Entecavir for the treatment of patients with hepatitis B virus-related decompensated cirrhosis. Expert Opin Pharmacother 2013;14:1363–9.
25 Zoulim F. Hepatitis B virus resistance to antiviral drugs: where are we going? Liver Int 2011;31 (Suppl 1): 111–6.
26 Van Bommel F, de Man RA, Wedemeyer H, et al. Long-term efficacy of tenofovir monotherapy for hepatitis B virus monoinfected patients after failure of nucleoside/nucleotide analogues. Hepatology 2010;51:73–80.
27 Buster EH, Hansen BE, Buti M, et al. Peginterferon alpha-2b is safe and effective in HBeAg-positive chronic hepatitis B patients with advanced fibrosis. Hepatology 2007;46:388–94.
28 Hui AY, Chan HL, Leung NW, et al. Survival and prognostic indicators in patients with hepatitis B virus-related cirrhosis after onset of hepatic decompensation. J Clin Gastroenterol 2002;34:569–72.
29 Fontana RJ. Side effects of long-term oral antiviral therapy for hepatitis B. Hepatology 2009;49:S185–95.
30 Shim JH, Lee HC, Kim KM, et al. Efficacy of entecavir in treatment-naivepatients with hepatitis B virus-related decompensated cirrhosis. J Hepatol 2010;52:176–82.
31 Pellicelli AM, Barbarini G, Romano M, et al. Entecavir therapy for lamivudine resistant HBV cirrhotic patients waiting for OLT: viral and biochemical outcomes at one year. Hepatology 2009;50:514A.
32 Woo G, Tomlinson G, Nishikawa Y, et al. Tenofovir and entecavir are the most effective antiviral agents for chronic hepatitis B: a systematic review and Bayesian meta-analyses. Gastroenterology 2010;139:1218–29.
33 Gane EC, Chan HL, Choudhuri G, et al. Treatment of decompensated HBV-cirrhosis: results from 2-years randomized trial with telbivudine or lamivudine. J Hepatol 2010;52:S1–21.
34 Fleischer RD, Lok AS. Myopathy and neuropathy associated with nucleos(t)ide analog therapy for hepatitis B. J Hepatol 2009;51:787–91.
35 Chen T, He Y, Liu X, Yan Z. Nucleoside analogues improve the short-term and long-term prognosis of patients with hepatitis B virus-related acute-on-chronic liver failure. Clin Exp Med 2012;12:159–64.
36 Ahn J, Cohen SM. Prevention of hepatitis B recurrence in liver transplant patients using oral antiviral therapy without long-term hepatitis B immunoglobulin. Hepat Mon 2011; 11:638–45.
37 Zeuzem S. Treatment of chronic hepatitis C virus infection in patients with cirrhosis. J Viral Hepat 2000;7:327–34.
38 Testino G, Ansaldi F, Andorno E, et al. Interferon therapy does not prevent hepatocellular carcinoma in HCV compensated cirrhosis. Hepatogastroenterology 2002;49:1636–8.
39 Braks RE, Ganne-Carrie N, Fontaine H, et al. Effect of sustained virological response on long-term clinical outcome in 113 patients with compensated hepatitis C-related cirrhosis treated by interferon alpha and ribavirin. World J Gastroenterol 2007;13:5648–53.
40 Puig Del Castillo I, Miquel Planas M, Vergara Gómez M, et al. Five-year follow-up of patients with chronic C hepatitis and sustained virological response. Rev Esp Enferm Dig 2011;103:56–61.
41 Van der Meer A, Veldt B, Feld J, et al. Association between sustained virological response and all-cause mortality among patients with chronic hepatitis C and advanced hepatic fibrosis. JAMA 2012;308:2584–93.
42 Iacobellis A, Siciliano M, Perri F, et al. Peginterferon alfa-2b and ribavirin in patients with hepatitis C virus and decompensated cirrhosis: a controlled study. J Hepatol 2007;46: 206–12.
43 Saab S, Hunt DR, Stone MA, et al. Timing of hepatitis C antiviral therapy in patients with advanced liver disease: a decision analysis model. Liver Transpl 2010;16:748–59.
44 Shiffman ML, Esteban R. Triple therapy for HCV genotype 1 infection: telaprevir or boceprevir? Liver Int 2012;32 (Suppl 1): 54–60.
45 Bruno Vierling J, Esteban R, et al. Efficacy and safety of boceprevir plus peginterferon-ribavirin in patients with HCV G1 infection and advanced fibrosis/cirrhosis. J Hepatol 2013; 58:479–87.
46 Vierling J, Zeuzem S, Poordad F, et al. Safety and efficacy of boceprevir/Peg interferon/ribavirin combination therapy for

chronic HCv G1 patients with compensated cirrhosis: a meta-analysis of five phase 3 clinical trials. J Hepatol 2013;58:576–7.
47 Rutter K, Ferlitsch A, Maieron A, et al. Safety with triple therapy with telaprevir or boceprevir in hepatitis C patients with advanced liver disease-predictive factors for sepsis. J Hepatol 2013;58:30
48 Crippin JS, McCashland T, Terrault N, et al. A pilot study of the tolerability and efficacy of antiviral therapy in hepatitis C virus-infected patients awaiting liver transplantation. Liver Transpl 2002;8:350–5.
49 Everson GT. Treatment of chronic hepatitis C in patients with decompensated cirrhosis. Rev Gastroenterol Disord 2004;4: 31–8.
50 Lebray P, Nalpas B, Vallet-Pichard A, et al. The impact of haematopoietic growth factors on the management and efficacy of antiviral treatment in patients with hepatitis C virus. Antivir Ther 2005;10:769–76.
51 Tanwar S, Wright M, Foster GR, et al. Randomized clinical trial: a pilot study investigating the safety and effectiveness of an escalating dose of peginterferon α-2a monotherapy for 48 weeks compared with standard clinical care in patients with hepatitis C cirrhosis. Eur J Gastroenterol Hepatol 2012;24: 543–50.
52 Selzner N, Renner EL, Selzner M, et al. Antiviral treatment of recurrent hepatitis C after liver transplantation: predictors of response and long-term outcome. Transplantation 2009; 88:1214–21.
53 Perez-Tamayo R. Cirrhosis of the liver: a reversible disease? Pathol Ann 1979;14:183–213.
54 Gutiérrez-Ruiz M, Gómez-Quiroz L. Liver fibrosis: searching for cell model answers. Liver Int 2007;27:434–9.
55 Jonathan A. Fallowfield therapeutic targets in liver fibrosis. Am J Physiol Gastrointest Liver Physiol 2011;300:G709–15.
56 Rodriguez L, Cerbon-Ambriz J, Munoz ML. Effects of colchicine and colchiceine in a biochemical model of liver injury and fibrosis. Arch Med Res 1998;29:109
57 Rambaldi A, Gluud C. Colchicine for alcoholic and non-alcoholic liver fibrosis or cirrhosis. Liver 2001;21:129
58 Kershenobich D, Vargas F, Garcia-Tsao G, et al. Colchicine in the treatment of cirrhosis of the liver. N Engl J Med 1988; 318:1709
59 Muntoni S, Rojkind M, Muntoni S. Colchicine reduces procollagen III and increases pseudocholinesterase in chronic liver disease. World J Gastroenterol 2010;16:2889–94.
60 Angelico M, Cepparulo M, Barlattani A, et al. Unfavourable effects of colchicine in combination with interferon-alpha in the treatment of chronic hepatitis C. Aliment Pharmacol Ther 2000;14:1459
61 Morgan TR, Nemchausky B, Schiff ER, et al. Colchicine does not prolong life in patients with advanced alcoholic cirrhosis: results of a prospective, randomized, placebo-controlled trial. Gastroenterology 2002; 641A.
62 Miller LC, Sharma A, McKusick AF, et al. Synthesis of interleukin-1 beta in primary biliary cirrhosis: relationship to treatment with methotrexate or colchicine and disease progression. Hepatology 1995;22:518
63 De BK, Bandyopadhyay K, Das TK, et al. Portal pressure response to losartan compared with propranolol in patients with cirrhosis. Am J Gastroenterol 2003;98:1371
64 Debernardi-Venon W, Martini S, Biasi F, et al. AT1 receptor antagonist candesartan in selectedcirrhotic patients: effect on portal pressure and liver fibrosis markers. J Hepatol 2007;46:1026
65 Yi-Jun Wu, Wei-Min Cai, Qi Li. Long-term antifibrotic action of interferon-γ treatment in patients with chronic hepatitis B virus infection. Hepatobiliary Pancreat Dis Int 2011;10:51–7.
66 Pockros PJ, Jeffers L, Afdhal N, et al. Final results of a double-blind, placebo-controlledtrial of the antifibrotic efficacy of interferon-gamma1bin chronic hepatitis C patients with advanced fibrosis or cirrhosis. Hepatology 2007;45: 569–78.
67 Lutchman G, Modi A, Kleiner DE, et al. The effects of discontinuing pioglitazone in patients with nonalcoholic steatohepatitis. Hepatology 2007;46:424
68 Schaefer CJ, Ruhrmund DW, Pan L, et al. Antifibrotic activities of pirfenidone in animal models. Eur Respir Rev 2011;20: 85–97.
69 Féher J, Lengyel G. Silymarin in the prevention and treatment of liver diseases and primary liver cancer. Curr Pharm Biotechnol 2012;13:210–7.
70 Fried MW, Navarro VJ, Afdhal N, et al. Silymarin in NASH and C Hepatitis (SyNCH) Study Group. Effect of silymarin (milk thistle) on liver disease in patients with chronic hepatitis C unsuccessfully treated with interferon therapy: a randomized controlled trial. JAMA 2012;308: 274–82.
71 Poupon R. Treatment of primary biliary cirrhosis with ursodeoxycholic acid, budesonide and fibrates. Dig Dis 2011; 29:85–8.
72 Gundermann KJ, Kuenker A, Kuntz E, et al. Activity of essential phospholipids (EPL) from soybean in liver diseases. Pharmacol Rep 2011;63:643–59.
73 Thompson K, Maltby J, Fallowfield J, et al. Interleukin-10 expression and function in experimental murine liver inflammation and fibrosis. Hepatology 1998;28:1597
74 Aithal GP, Haugk B, Das S, et al. Monitoring methotrexate-induced hepatic fibrosis in patients withpsoriasis: are serial liver biopsies justified? Aliment Pharmacol Ther 2004; 19:391
75 Kaplan MM, Cheng S, Price LL, et al. A randomized controlled trial of colchicine plus ursodiol versusmethotrexate plus ursodiol in primary biliary cirrhosis: ten-year results. Hepatology 2004;39:915

CHAPTER 25
Bone disorders

Jane Collier
John Radcliffe Hospital, Oxford, UK

Introduction

Osteomalacia, osteoporosis, and osteonecrosis are bone diseases seen in patients with liver disease. Osteomalacia is surprisingly uncommon in adults with cirrhosis, despite the high prevalence of vitamin D deficiency in this population. Osteonecrosis, usually of the femoral neck, is a rare condition seen predominately post-liver transplantation, partly related to immunosuppressive therapy [1]. This leaves osteoporosis as the most common bone disease affecting patients with cirrhosis.

Osteonecrosis

In a study of 360 patients with primary sclerosing cholangitis (PSC) and primary biliary cirrhosis (PBC) requiring liver transplantation, only 1.4% had a history of osteonecrosis [1]. This was often bilateral and usually at the femoral neck. Not all patients were on steroids which is the major risk factor. Although rare, the condition should be considered in patients on steroids who develop hip, shoulder, or knee pain, particularly on movement, as it is easy to miss.

Osteomalacia

The classic description of osteomalacia is of hypocalcemia, hypophosphotemia, increased alkaline phosphatase and parathyroid hormone, although serum calcium and phosphate levels are often normal. Hepatic osteomalacia as defined histologically by bone biopsy is now rare in adults with cirrhosis and cholestatic liver disease. In a study from the Mayo Clinic of 33 patients with end-stage PBC and PSC undergoing liver transplantation, no cases of osteomalacia were identified on bone biopsy and none were seen in 60 patients undergoing liver transplantation at another center in the UK [2,3]. Case reports of osteomalacia complicating cirrhosis in the literature are confined to patients with malabsorption such as in celiac disease and cystic fibrosis. It may also occur in untreated chronic cholestatic disease of childhood. In contrast to osteomalacia, vitamin D deficiency is common in cirrhotic patients [4].

Vitamin D deficiency

Vitamin D deficiency has been defined as 25-hydroxyvitamin D levels <20 ng/mL (50 nmol/L) with sufficient levels as >30 ng/mL (72 nmol/L) [5]. Of patients awaiting liver transplantation, 90–96% have low vitamin D levels [1,4]. In a study of 43 hepatitis C cirrhotic patients, 78% were vitamin deficient [6]. The severity of vitamin D deficiency has been associated with liver dysfunction rather than etiology [7].

Vitamin D is obtained from endogenous skin synthesis following exposure to sunlight leading to production of cholecalciferol (D3), both ergocalciferol (D2) and vitamin D3 are also acquired through food (reviewed in [5]). The liver is involved in bile salt production, absorption of vitamin D, and subsequent 25-hydroxylation of vitamin D. Intestinal absorption of cholecalciferol and 25-hydroxycholecalciferol is only affected in the presence of severe cholestasis where patients are jaundiced. Subsequent hepatic 25-hydroxylation of vitamin D3 has not been studied in humans but in cirrhotic rats this process is not impaired.

Although low vitamin D does not lead to osteomalacia it is a associated with reduced bone mineral density (BMD), high bone turnover, and increased risk of hip fracture in the elderly. The precise contribution of low vitamin D levels to osteoporosis in patients with cirrhosis is unclear [8].

Cirrhosis: A practical guide to management, First Edition. Edited by Samuel S. Lee and Richard Moreau.

Osteoporosis

Background

Osteoporosis is a major risk factor for fragility fractures, which impact on morbidity including quality of life. Osteoporotic fractures of the vertebral spine tend to occur about a decade before those in the femoral neck. Corticosteroids tend to cause vertebral rather than hip fractures. The former are often initially asymptomatic and are often detected incidentally in cirrhotic patients on cross-sectional imaging (e.g., CT scans looking for hepatocellular carcinoma) (Figure 25.1).

BMD also falls in the first 3 months following liver transplantation leading to an increase in fractures in the first 2 years post-transplant. Although the rates of post-transplant fracture have fallen with the reduction in post-transplant steroid dosage, it is important to detect in the small proportion of cirrhotic patients suitable for liver transplantation.

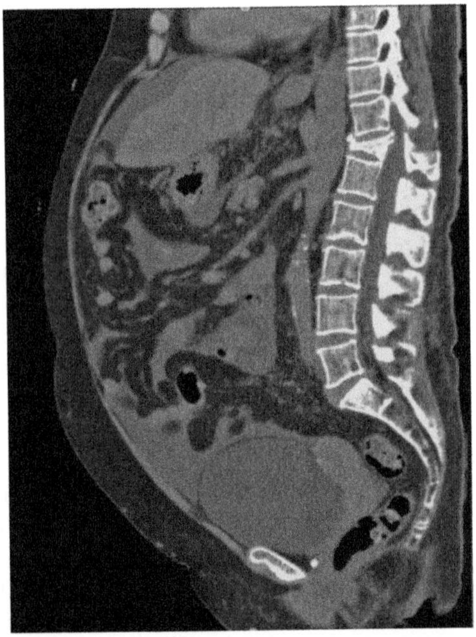

Figure 25.1 Thoracic spine osteoporotic fracture seen on a computed tomography (CT) scan in a 64-year-old woman with diuretic-resistant ascites due to alcoholic cirrhosis. She presented with a myopathy leading to the diagnosis of cirrhosis. The fracture was identified on a CT scan showing ascites and a small liver prior to a transjugular intrahepatic portosystemic shunt (TIPS). She was treated with alendronate once-weekly based on the presence of an osteoporotic fracture without bone mineral density (BMD) assessment. She had normal vitamin D levels of 52.9 nmol/L and no other risk factors of osteoporosis apart from cirrhosis and alcohol excess. BMD is not needed to start treatment but may be useful as a baseline to assess if therapy needs to be continued after 5 years, ideally with ascites drained.

Osteoporosis is characterized by loss of bone mass and strength. Peak bone mass is reached in the third decade and then declines in both sexes but more rapidly in women. The risk of fracture depends on bone density but also on trabecular architecture and bone turnover as well as the tendency to fall. The latter often occurs in cirrhotic patients, because of low body mass index (BMI) and loss of muscle mass, as well as in alcoholics.

Bone density is measured by dual-energy X-ray absorptiometry (DEXA) scan but is only part of the assessment of fracture risk (Figure 25.2).

Risk factors

Risk factors for osteoporosis are frequently found in patients with cirrhosis: poor nutrition, excess alcohol, corticosteroid use, and hypogonadism (Table 25.1). Patients with end-stage PBC are also usually post-menopausal women. Corticosteroid use, the equivalent of 5 mg prednisolone taken for more than 3 months, is a particularly important independent risk factor for fractures (reviewed in [9]). Previous fracture is a further major clinical risk factor for further fractures independently of BMD. Once a vertebral fracture has occurred, the risk of a further vertebral fracture increases 10-fold and that of a hip fracture two- to threefold. The 5–10 year risk of fracture in an individual with low BMD can be calculated using several algorithms such as the World Health Organization's fracture risk assessment tool (FRAX index) [10,11]. Although cirrhosis has been incorporated into the FRAX index (as secondary osteoporosis), the relative increased contribution of cirrhosis to fracture risk in an individual is not clear because of the relatively small numbers of liver disease patients in prospective studies. However, FRAX is useful tool in showing how age, BMI, and so on contribute to fracture risk. It is less reliable in patients on corticosteroids as it uses femoral neck BMD rather than that of the lumbar spine.

Prevalence

Various studies over the last two decades have shown that the prevalence of osteoporosis in patients with cirrhosis is between 12% and 55% (Table 25.2) [12–14]. The difference between studies is probably a reflection of

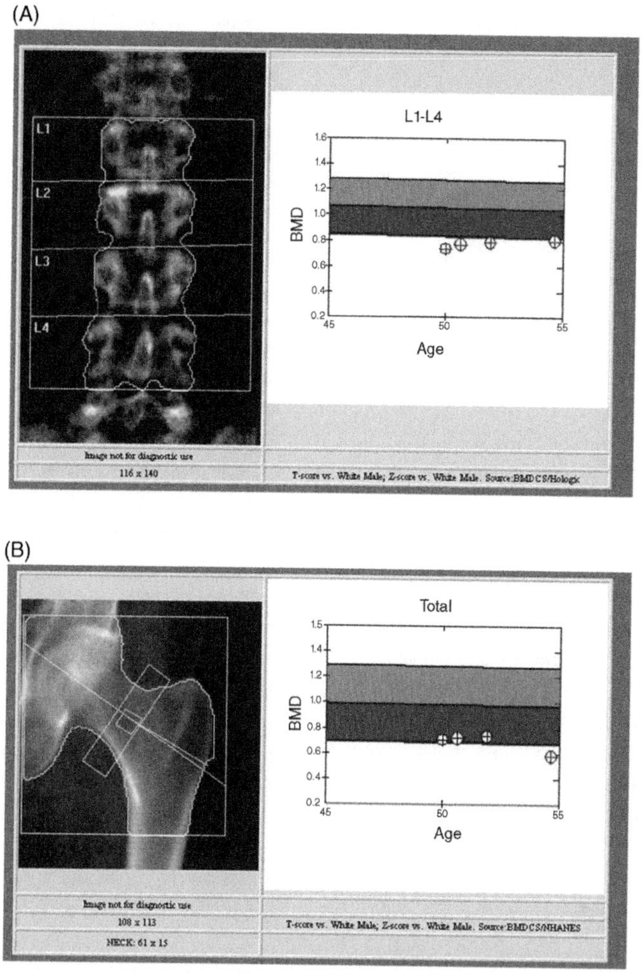

Figure 25.2 Bone mineral density in a patient with cirrhosis: (A) lumbar spine; (B) femoral neck. This 57-year-old man with a biliary cirrhosis due to combined variable immunodeficiency has a T score of –2.7 at vertebral spine and –3.0 at the femoral neck. His other risk factors for fracture include malabsorbtion due to chronic cryptosporidia and a budesonide-treated enteropathy. He has a low vitamin D level of 42 nmol/L. According to the FRAX index his fracture risk is 15% at 10 years and that of a femoral neck fracture 8.4%. The FRAX index underestimates the risk on steroids and its reliability in the presence of cirrhosis is unknown. He was treated with a single dose of zoledronic acid intravenously because of malabsorption – ibandronic acid would have been an alternative – and his vitamin D levels corrected. (See colour plate section.)

Table 25.1 Risk factors for osteoporosis independent of cirrhosis.

Age
Previous fragility fracture
Oral glucocorticoid therapy (>5 mg for 3 months)
Body mass index <19 kg/m^2
Alcohol intake >3–4 units/day
Maternal/paternal history of hip fracture
Premature menopause <45 years

differences in age, etiology of liver disease, nutritional state, hypogonadism, and severity of liver disease. In a study of 58 patients with viral cirrhosis, the risk of osteoporosis was shown to be associated with the severity of cirrhosis, with Child–Pugh A patients having a higher BMD than those with Child–Pugh C disease [15]. In a study of 243 patients with mixed end-stage liver disease requiring transplantation, the only independent risk factors for osteoporosis were lower BMI in women and

Table 25.2 Prevalence of osteoporosis and fractures in cirrhosis and chronic biliary disease [12].

n	Type of cirrhosis	Osteoporosis (%)	Referred OLT	Fractures (%)	Reference
60	Mixed	47			12
74	Viral	20	No	6.7	12
58	Mixed	43	Yes		12
32	Viral	55	No		12
81	PSC	16	No	3	12
243	Mixed	37	Yes		12
207	HCV + alcohol	20	Yes		12
104	Mixed	12	Yes		12
156	PBC	43.7	Yes	22	12
204	PSC	32.5	Yes	16	12
84	Viral[a]	43	No		13
185	PBC	31		20	14

HCV, hepatitis C virus; OLT, orthotopic liver transplantation; PBC, primary biliary cirrhosis; PSC, primary sclerosing cholangitis.
[a] Postmenopausal women in clinic setting and no difference in prevalence of osteoporosis between healthy controls.

increasing age [16]. Osteoporosis in hemochromatosis has been associated with the degree of iron overload [17].

There are fewer data on fracture prevalence in patients with cirrhosis. The limited data available suggest that cirrhosis alone increases the risk of fracture by about twofold. The severity of cholestasis is also related to the risk of fractures, and in patients with cholestatic disease undergoing transplant assessment fractures were identified in 20% [1,12].

Diagnosis

Measurement of BMD should be considered in all patients with cirrhosis (Figure 25.3). Those patients who should certainly be targeted for investigation include older female patients, alcoholics, those with low BMI and those with cholestatic liver disease. The consensus on indications for bone density in cirrhosis is summarized in Table 25.3 [18–20]. All patients receiving corticosteroids equivalent to >5 mg prednisolone for

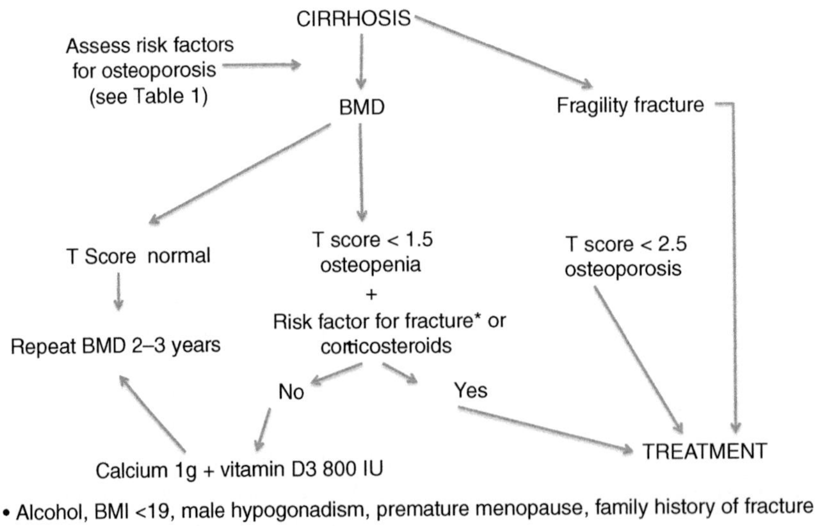

Figure 25.3 Algorithm for investigation of bone disease. BMD, bone mineral density; BMI, body mass index.

Table 25.3 Indications for bone mineral density in chronic liver disease.

Indication	AGA	EASL
Cirrhosis	+	+
Liver transplant assessment	+	+
Corticosteroids	+	+
Previous fracture		+
PBC at diagnosis	+	+
Postmenopausal and other risk factors for osteoporosis[a]	+	+
Male hypogonadism		+
Alcohol misuse		+
Cholestatic chronic liver disease	++	+
Hemochromatosis		+

Data from AGA Clinical Practice Committee [18] and European Association for the Study of the Liver [20].
PBC, primary biliary cirrhosis.
[a] Premature menopause; low body mass index, maternal history of hip fracture.

longer than 3 months should have their BMD measured. Bone density should also be part of the liver transplant assessment because of the fall in BMD seen following transplantation.

Care needs to be taken in interpreting results in the presence of ascites as a volume of over 4 L has been shown to reduce BMD measurements at the lumbar spine [21].

The benefits of measuring vitamin D levels in cirrhotic patients without osteoporosis remains unclear as there are currently no studies assessing whether this reduces fracture rates in patients with osteopenia or normal BMD or has any other beneficial effects. Adequate vitamin D intake through diet and/or supplementation with vitamin D3 is usually recommended in the presence of osteoporosis in postmenopausal women and so measurement of vitamin D levels in this group is not unreasonable.

In patients identified as having osteoporosis, other factors contributing to low bone mass should be checked, such as celiac serology. Hypogonadism, which is a cause of male osteoporosis, is common in male cirrhotic patients and testosterone levels should be measured together with steroid binding hormone levels to correct for low serum albumin levels.

Treatment

The evidence for treatment of osteoporosis in patients with liver disease is based on trials in patients with postmenopausal osteoporosis. There are only a few small studies in patients with cirrhosis, the majority in PBC, and improvement in BMD rather than more clinically important fracture rates have been used as outcome measurements (reviewed in [12,18,19]). An algorithm is shown in Figure 25.4.

Vitamin D

Calcium and vitamin D supplementation has been shown to reduce fractures in elderly patients living in sheltered accommodation and consequently most patients in trials of other treatment modalities for osteoporosis are routinely given vitamin D and calcium, usually 800 IU/day

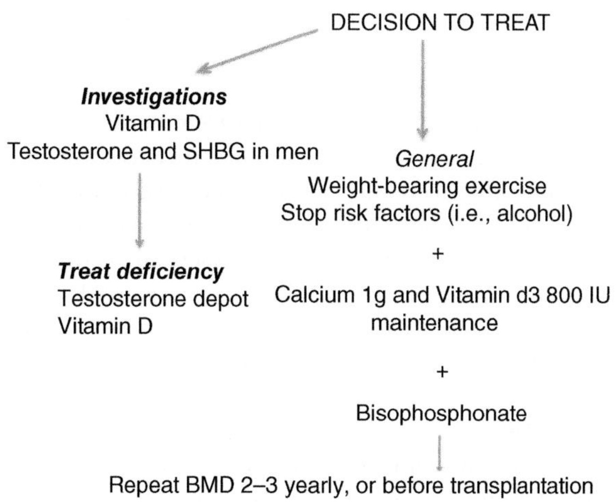

Figure 25.4 Algorithm for treatment of osteoporosis. SHBG, steroid hormone binding globulin.

vitamin D3 and 1 g/day calcium supplementation, as it is difficult to obtain adequate vitamin D intake by diet alone.

Recommended doses of vitamin D replacement in deficiency states vary from 50 000 IU/day orally for 6 days of 25-hydroxyvitamin vitamin D (D2) followed by 50 000 IU/month for patients with levels of <25 nmol/L (local guidelines) to 50 000 IU/week for 16 weeks and then 50 000 IU maintenance dose [5]. It is unclear whether higher doses are needed in the presence of cirrhosis. In one study, patients with alcoholic cirrhosis had a better response to a single oral high dose (300 00 IU) of cholecalciferol (D3) than to a similar dose of ergocaliciferol (D2) [22]. In a second study, 65 patients with cirrhosis, one-third with a vitamin D level <25 mnol/L, were given low dose vitamin D replacement with only 1000 IU/day ergocalciferol orally (D2), cholecalciferol D3 (50 µg), with only 25% replete after 4 months, indicating the need for high doses in cirrhotic patients [23].

The effect of treating vitamin D deficiency on BMD in cirrhosis is less clear but in a nonrandomized study of 25 patients with alcoholic cirrhosis and low serum vitamin D levels, hydroxyvitamin D3 supplementation did increase BMD over baseline values [24]. In a further study of 76 patients with cirrhosis, 1-alpha, 25-hydroxyvitamin D3 resulted in a small increase in BMD at the lumbar spine but no data were given on the effect on fractures [25].

Bisphosphonates

Alendronate, etidronate, ibandronate, and risedronate, which prevent bone resorption, are used for treating postmenopausal osteoporosis. These drugs are usually given with calcium and vitamin D. They have been only studied in a small number of patients with chronic liver disease and so data on their efficacy in this setting are lacking [12]. Most studies have been conducted in patients with PBC [26]. In PBC, alendronate increases bone mass. In a study comparing weekly alendronate with monthly ibandronate given over a 2-year period, the improvement in lumbar BMD was similar but compliance was better in the ibandronate group [27]. Markers of bone turnover also fell with alendronate although no lumbar spine fractures were seen in either group [12,18,19]. There were no esophageal complications from daily alendronate although another study in PBC has suggested that once-weekly alendronate is better tolerated than once-daily. There are no studies of safety or efficacy of bisphosphonates in cirrhosis but anecdotally once-weekly bisphosphonates appear to be well tolerated although it would be reasonable to exert caution in using the drug in patients with recent esophageal banding. If safety or compliance is an issue then bisphosphanates can be given parenterally either monthly (ibandrabonate) or yearly by intravenous infusion with zoledronic acid.

Hormone replacement therapy

This has become less widely used in those with postmenopausal osteoporosis because of the concern about the risks of thromboembolic disease and gynecologic malignancy. It can be used safely in patients with chronic liver disease and is ideally given transdermally. There are no studies of efficacy in patients with cirrhosis and only one small randomized controlled trial in patients with PBC and noncirrhotic patients. In PBC, transdermal hormone replacement therapy (HRT) was shown to improve BMD after 2 years but the study was not powered to show any effect on fractures [28]. In a further open-labeled study of 18 patients with PBC, only one patient had to stop the transdermal HRT because of rising transaminase levels [29].

Testosterone

Hypogonadal patients with chronic liver disease should be treated with transdermal testosterone as it leads to stable hormone levels avoiding the exposure of the liver to surges in levels seen with oral or depot preparations. A concern about restoring testosterone levels to normal in cirrhotic patients has been the theoretical risk of increasing the risk of hepatocellular carcinoma, though this has never been demonstrated.

Other treatments

Strontium reduces vertebral and nonvertebral fractures in postmenopausal osteoporosis with the main side effect of diarrhea. Its mechanism of action remains unclear and to date there are no studies of its efficacy in chronic liver disease. Its use may be considered in patients intolerant of bisphosphonates.

Recombinant parathyroid hormone has been used for secondary prevention of fragility fractures in postmenopausal women intolerant of bisphosphonates. It acts by stimulating new bone formation.

Denosumab is a monoclonal antibody to nuclear factor κβ ligand (RANKL) that mediates osteoclast activity and survival. It has been shown to reduce vertebral fractures in postmenopausal women after 3 years from 7.2% to 2.3% but there are no studies in patients with cirrhosis. RANKL is also expressed on immune cells and so could potentially increase infection rates in cirrhotic patients [30].

Monitoring therapy

Serum markers

The effects of therapy can be monitored with repeat BMD and/or by biochemical monitoring of serum markers of bone turnover. Biochemical markers allow detection of bone turnover within 3 months whereas radiographic methods take 12–24 months to detect changes in BMD. The two problems with using serum markers in cirrhosis are that it is still unclear whether short-term measures of bone turnover can predict long-term fracture risk and serum markers are also not specific to bone. Biochemical markers of bone formation include procollagen peptides of type 1 collagen, amino-terminal and carboxylterminal (PICP) and osteocalcin. Markers of bone resorption include urinary excretion of deoxypyridinoline, pyridinoline, and serum type 1 collagen cross-linked N telopeptide (P1NP). In several small studies of patients with cirrhosis, both markers of bone resorption and bone formation have been found to be independently affected by the degree of liver fibrosis, severity of liver disease, and coexistent renal function [31,32]. This means that repeat BMD is currently the only way of assessing the efficacy of treatment for osteoporosis in patients with cirrhosis.

Length of therapy

In postmenopausal osteoporosis, concern has been raised about the potential affects of long-term bisphosphonates on bone structure after 5 years and the theoretical risk of microfractures. Bisphosphonates such as alendronate and zolendronate are retained in bone and suppress bone turnover for up to 18 months after drug withdrawal. BMD should be repeated at 3 years to ensure no progressive fall in bone mass on treatment. The need for continuing bisphosphonates should be reassessed at 5 years and it may be possible to stop in young patients with improved BMD who have not had a fracture and where some of the initial risk factors have gone (e.g., abstinence from alcohol or cessation of steroids) [33].

Conclusions

- Osteoporosis is common in cirrhosis.
- Vertebral fractures occur about a decade before hip fractures.
- Prevalence is related to severity of liver disease.
- Risk of fractures remains highest in those with previous fracture and on steroids.
- Vitamin D deficiency affects >50% of cirrhotic patients.
- Hypogonadism should be excluded in men with osteoporosis.
- Bisphosphonates are well tolerated and form the treatment of choice.

References

1 Guichelaar M, Schmoll J, Malinchoc M, Hay EJ. Fractures and avasular necrosis before and after OLT: long-term follow-up and predictive factors. Hepatology 2007;46:1198–207.

2 Guichelaar MMJ, Kendall R, Schmoll J, et al. Bone mineral density before and after OLT; longterm follow-up and predictive factors. Liver Transpl 2006;12:1390–402.

3 Vedi S, Ninkovic M, Garrahan, NJ, et al. Effects of a single infusion of pamidronate prior to liver transplantation: a bone histomorphometric study. Transpl Int 2002;15:290–5.

4 Crawford BA, Labio ED, Strasser SI, et al. Vitamin D replacement for cirrhosis-related bone disease. Nat Clin Pract Gastroenterol Hepatol 2006;3:689–99.

5 Holick MF. Vitamin D deficiency. N Engl J Med 2007;357:266–81.

6 Arteh J, Narra S, Nair S. Prevalence of vitamin D deficiency in chronic liver disease. Dis Dis Sci 2010;55:2624–8.

7 Malham M, Peter Jorgensen S, Ott P, et al. Vitamin D deficiency in cirrhosis related to liver dysfunction rather than aetiology. World J Gastrenteol 2011;17:922–5.

8 Kitson MT, Roberts SK. D-livering the message: the importance of vitamin D status in chronic liver disease. J Hepatol 2012;57:897–907.

9 Weinstein RS. Glucocorticosteroid-induced bone disease. N Engl J Med 2011;365:62–70.

10 World Health Organization. FRAX: WHO fracture risk assessment tool. www.shef.ac.uk/FRAX/tool.jsp (accessed September 5, 2014).

11 Papaioannou A, Morin S, Cheung AM, et al. 2010 clinical practice guidelines for the diagnosis and management of osteoporosis in Canada: summary. CMAJ 2010;182:1864–73.

12 Collier J. Bone disorders and chronic liver disease. Hepatology 2007;46:1271–8.

13 Gonzalex-Calvin JL, Mundi JL, Casado-Calbaellero FJ, et al. Bone mineral density and serum levels of soluble tumour necrosis factors, estradiol and osteoprotegerin in post-menopausal wpmen with cirrhosis after viral hepatitis. J Clin Endocrinol Metab 2009;94:4844–50.
14 Guanabens N, Cerda D, Monegal A, et al. Low bone mass and severity of cholestasis affect fracture risk in patients with primary biliary cirrhosis. Gastroenterology 2010;138: 2348–56.
15 Monegal A, Navasa M, Guanabens N, et al. Osteoporosis and bone mineral metabolism disorders in cirrhotic patients referred for orthotopic liver transplantation. Calcif Tissue Int 1997;60:148–54.
16 Ninkovic M, Love SA, Yom B, et al. High prevalence of osteoporosis in patients with chronic liver disease prior to liver transplantation. Calcif Tissue Int 2001;69:321–8.
17 Valenti L, Varenna M, Fracanzani AL. Association between iron overload and osteoporosis in patients with hereditary hemochromatosis. Ostetoporos Int 2009;20:549–55.
18 AGA, Clinical Practice Committee. AGA technical review on osteoporosis in hepatic disorders. Gastroenterology 2003: 125;941–66.
19 Guanabens N, Pares A. Management of osteoporosis in liver disease. Clin Res Hepatol 2011;35:438–45.
20 European Association for the Study of the Liver (EASL). EASL clinical practice guidelines. Management of cholestatic liver disease. J Hepatol 2009;51:237–67.
21 Guanabens N, Monegal A, Muxi A, et al. Patients with cirrhosis and ascites have false values of bone density: implications for the diagnosis of osteoporosis. Osteoporos Int 2012;23:1481–7.
22 Malham M, Peter Jørgensen S, Lauridsen A, et al. The effect of a single megadose of vitamin D provided as either ergocalciferol (D2) or cholecalciferol (D3) in alcoholic liver cirrhosis. Eur J Gastroenterol Hepatol 2012;24:172–8.
23 Rode A, Fourlanos S, Nicoll A. Oral vitamin D replacement is effective in chronic liver disease. Gastroenterol Clin Biol 2010;34:618–20.
24 Crawford BA, Labio ED, Strasser SI, et al. Vitamin D replacement for cirrhosis-related bone disease. Nat Clin Pract Gastroenterol Hepatol 2006;3:689–99.
25 Shiomi S, Masaki K, Habu D, et al. Calcitriol for bone disease in patients with cirrhosis of the liver. J Gastroenterol Hepatol 1999;14:547–52.
26 Angulo P. Strengthening the bones in primary biliary cirrhosis. Hepatology 2013;58:1871–3.
27 Guanabens N, Monegal A, Cerda D. Randomised trial comparing monthly ibandronate and weekly alendronate for osteoporoais in patients with primary biliary cirrhosis. Hepatology 2013;58:2070–8.
28 Pereira SP, O'Donohue J, Moniz C, et al. Transdermal hormone replacement therapy improves vertebral lobe density in primary biliary cirrhosis: results of a 1 year controlled trial. Aliment Pharmocol Ther 2004;19:563–70.
29 Rudic JS, Poropat G, Krstic MN, Bjelakovoc G, Gluud C. Hormone replacement for osteoporosis in women with primary biliary cirrhosis. Cochrane Database Syst Rev 2011;12: CD009146.
30 Prockop DJ. New targets for osteoporosis. N Engl J Med 2012;367:2353–4.
31 Moller S, Hansen M, Hillingso J, et al. Elevated carboxy terminal cross linked telopeptide of type 1 collagen in alcoholic cirrhosis: relation to liver and kidney function and bone metabolism. Gut 1999;44:417–23.
32 Crosbie OM, Freaney R, McKenna MJ, et al. Bone density, vitamin D status and disordered bone remodelling in end-stage chronic liver disease. Calcif Tissue Int 1999;64:295–300.
33 Whittaker M, Kehoe T, Benson G. Bisphosphonates for osteoporosis: where do we go from here? N Engl J Med 2012; 366:2048–51.

CHAPTER 26
Pruritus

Nora V. Bergasa
Metropolitan Hospital Center, New York; New York Medical College, Valhalla, New York, USA

Pruritus, or itch, is an unpleasant sensation that triggers the need to scratch. The pruritus of cholestasis can be severe, associated with sleep deprivation, and it may lead to suicidal ideations. It can be generalized, localized to some areas, constant or intermittent, and in some patients it can increase in the premenstrual period [1]. Violent scratching can lead to excoriations, which may become secondarily infected, and prurigo nodularis; however, it is difficult for patients not to scratch because pain from heavy scratching can be associated with the relief of itch [2]. Pruritus, the most troubling symptom in women with cholestasis of pregnancy, resolves after delivery; if it does not, liver disease has to be excluded.

A retrospective study from the United States found that 5% of patients with chronic hepatitis C presented with pruritus, which correlated with advanced disease [3], and from a retrospective review from a center in Europe, it was reported that 40% of patients with chronic pruritus from liver disease had chronic viral hepatitis B or C [4].

In patients with primary biliary cirrhosis (PBC), the presence of intrahepatic florid bile duct lesions and granulomata were significantly related to the severity of pruritus (and fatigue), as assessed on the day of the biopsy [5]. The prutitus has not been consistently reported to correlate with biologic markers of disease [6]. An increased likelihood of reporting symptoms (and not responding to ursodeoxycholic acid, the drug approved for the treatment of this disease) was reported to correlate with presentation of PBC at less than 50 years of age in a study from the United Kingdom [7].

An internet survey conducted in members of the PBCers, an organization that supports education in PBC, revealed that 69% of patients experienced pruritus [1], consistent with the prevalence reported in other studies [8]. The itch preceded the diagnosis of liver disease by some years in a substantial number of patients [1]. In most patients (65%), the itch was worse at night, and sleep was affected in 74%. Only a minority of the patients who participated in the survey had the pruritus addressed by their physician [1], underscoring the need to educate the medical establishment and patients regarding the association between pruritus and liver disease.

It has been inferred that the pruritogens that mediate pruritus are made in the liver and excreted in bile, and, as a result of cholestasis, accumulate in body tissues. In support of a hepatic origin of the pruritogen(s) or its cofactors are the following observations.

1 In patients with cholestasis, the cessation of itch portends liver failure [9], as if some degree of liver function were necessary for the pruritogen(s) to be made, or for the sensation to be perceived.
2 Patients with pruritus report the disappearance of their symptom after liver transplantation [10].
3 Complete relief of cholestasis from mechanical obstruction (e.g., common duct stones) is associated with disappearance of pruritus [8].

If the liver is the source of the pruritogen(s) and the pruritogen(s) is excreted in bile, genetic polymorphisms in the genes that code for biliary transporters may be relevant in the biliary excretion of pruritogenic substances. In the hepatocyte, MRP2 (ABCC2) mediates the transport of several organic anions [11] and, interestingly, in the context of the pruritus of cholestasis, opioid ligands are substrates of MRP2 [11]. A single nucleotide polymorphism (SNP) characterized by the substitution of valine for glutamate (V1188E) in exon 25 of the MRP2 gene was found in heterozygosity in a group of patients with PBC [11], and significantly associated with the presence of pruritus. Thus, V1188E in MRP2 may change the way the pruritogen(s) or its

Cirrhosis: A practical guide to management, First Edition. Edited by Samuel S. Lee and Richard Moreau.

cofactors are transported from the hepatocyte into the bile canalicula or into the central nervous system (CNS). SNP in relevant genes may explain, in part, why not all patients with cholestasis experience pruritus [8].

Pathogenesis of the pruritus of cholestasis

Clinical research in the pruritus of cholestasis was stimulated by the landmark publication by Thornton and Losowsky [12] in which it was reported that patients with PBC and pruritus experienced an opiate withdrawal-like reaction and a marked decrease in the pruritus after the intake of an opiate antagonist (i.e., nalmefene) [12]. The reaction, which included high blood pressure, insomnia, and abdominal pain, was in sharp contrast to the absence of any reaction in normal volunteers who, in other studies, had taken 60 times the dose of the drug administered to the patients with cholestasis [12]. The relief of the pruritus by nalmefene was proposed to be from the inhibition of release of pruritogens by the opiate antagonist [12]. The results of this study stimulated a reassessment of the mechanism by which nalmefene had relieved pruritus in the patients reported [12]. An alternative interpretation was submitted as a hypothesis: "increased availability of endogenous opiate [opioid] agonist ligands at central opiate [opioid] receptors may contribute to the pruritus of cholestasis" [13]. The basis for this hypothesis was: (i) the opiate withdrawal-like reaction precipitated by the opiate antagonist nalmefene in patients with cholestasis [12], hence suggesting that central opioid neurotransmission was increased, and (ii) the pruritus associated with the pharmacologic increase in opioidergic neurotransmission (tone) by the central administration of drugs (i.e., morphine) with agonist activity at the opioid receptors (i.e., mu opioid receptor according to current knowledge) that can be prevented and ameliorated by opiate antagonists [14].

If cholestasis is associated with increased opioidergic tone [13], and the pruritus of cholestasis is mediated, at least in part, by this type of neurotransmission, opiate antagonists should decrease the sensation and its behavioral manifestation, scratching activity. Indeed, evidence in support of this hypothesis has been provided by controlled clinical trials that have documented a significant relief in the perception of pruritus [15–21] and a significant decrease in hourly scratching activity, measured by a scratching activity monitoring system that records scratching activity independent from gross body movements [15,16,19,20]. The results of a meta-analysis that included five trials of opiate antagonists, three that tested the effect of opiate antagonists administered orally (i.e., naltrexone and nalmefene) and two that tested the effect of intravenous naloxone, with a total of 84 participants, also support an ameliorating effect of this type of drug on the pruritus of cholestasis [22]. Accordingly, the use of opiate antagonists to treat patients with this type of pruritus is specific, and supported by scientific evidence from controlled clinical trials, based on a clear rationale [15–21]. Studies exploring the role of single types of opioid receptors have identified an antiscratching effect of kappa agonists [8]. In this regard, nalfurafine, an agonist at the kappa opioid receptor, has been reported to decrease the sensation of pruritus in patients with uremia in controlled studies [23]. Thus, there is a rationale to study this type of drug in patients with the pruritus of cholestasis.

One question that arises is whether an increase in serum concentration of some endogenous opioids in patients with cholestasis, and the potential liver origin of these peptides, as suggested by the enhanced hepatic expression of Met-enkephalin immunoreactivity in liver disease [24,25], are related to the high central opioidergic tone of cholestasis. In this context, however, some transporters that can transport opiates *in vitro* are common to the basolateral domain of the hepatocyte, to the choroid plexus, and to the blood–brain barrier [11]. Accordingly, it is plausible that they can also transport periphery-derived opioids into the CNS, which would increase central opioidergic tone. In this regard, the results of brain scans by single photon emission computed tomography and functional magnetic resonance methodology in patients with cholestasis during periods of itch and no itch have suggested that the limbic system is the primary CNS pathway involved in the perception of itch, and that the findings support a central origin for this type of pruritus [26]. In addition, a central component of the pruritus may also arise from central sensitization for itch, which has been suggested to result from the constant stimuli of C-pruriceptors in conditions associated with chronic itch, which allow for nociceptive stimuli to facilitate itch instead of inhibiting it, leading to nonpruritogenic stimuli to be perceived as pruritus.

In regards to opioid receptors, the SNP A118G in the gene that codes for the mu opioid receptor 1 (OPRM1), to which morphine and opiate drugs bind, was found in heterozygosity 1.5 times more frequently in DNA samples from a group of patients from the United States with PBC who had not experienced pruritus than in the rest of the samples, which were from patients from Italy [27]. These results may suggest that patients with the A118G SNP in the OPRM1 may be protected from the itch in cholestasis [27]. Indeed, the presence of the G or A allele in A118G SNP has been associated with a difference in the degree of pruritus secondary to epidural morphine [28]. In addition, ethnicity may inform the experience of side effects, including pruritus, from the administration of intravenous morphine in children [29]. Thus, SNP in the gene that codes OPRM1 may also explain, in part, why not all patients with cholestasis report pruritus (see above) [8,11]. Accordingly, genetic analyses that apply techniques including genome-wide association studies may be useful in identifying specific features in the group of genes that code for transport proteins in the hepatobiliary system, in the CNS, and those involved in the activation of sensory neurons including the phospholipase C B3 pathway [30].

Bile acids accumulate in the tissues of patients with cholestasis [9]. They were reported to trigger local "itch" when injected intracutaneously in normal volunteers [31]; however, this is not a model of the pruritus of cholestasis. Intake of synthetic bile acids, including cholylsarcosine and ursodeoxycholic acid, has been associated with pruritus in patients with liver disease (i.e., PBC). These reports alone cannot be interpreted as evidence to support a role of bile acids as the pruritogens in liver disease, as pruritus is intermittent and triggered by a variety of factors including foodstuffs [32]. Furthermore, (i) in liver failure, when bile acids are maximally elevated, pruritus tends to cease [9], (ii) some patients with cholestasis and marked elevations of serum bile acids do not experience pruritus throughout the course of their disease, and (iii) pruritus can fluctuate and even remit spontaneously without concomitant changes in serum bile acid concentrations. A certain profile of serum bile acids may contribute to the pruritus but, based on current data, a role of bile acids in the mediation of the pruritus of cholestasis has not been demonstrated. In this context, a study published in abstract form revealed that the administration of obeticholic acid to patients with PBC was associated with itch, severe enough to require discontinuation of the drug, in contrast to the placebo intervention [33]. Obeticholic acid is a synthetic derivative of chenodeoxycholic acid, which is an agonist at the farsenoid nuclear receptor (FXR), and which has choleretic properties [33]. FXR is a bile acid sensor associated with a decrease in bile acid production [8]. The relevance of this observation to the pruritus from liver disease is unknown.

Substance P is an excitatory neurotransmitter that acts through the NK-1 receptor synthesized by primary afferent nociceptors and released into the spinal cord after noxious stimuli. In animal studies, increased opioidergic tone activates mechanisms that promote pain (e.g., nociception) in association with stimulation of the NK-1 receptor and substance P expression in the dorsal root ganglia [34]. Increased opioidergic tone in cholestasis may also contribute to a state of enhanced nociception and perceived as pruritus mediated, in part, by substance P. In this regard, the mean serum concentration of substance P in patients with liver disease and pruritus was significantly higher than in patients with liver disease without pruritus, and that of a control group of subjects [34]. These data suggest that substance P may mediate some of the manifestations of liver disease, including pruritus. In this context, the substance P antagonist aprepitant was reported to relieve pruritus in an uncontrolled study that used subjective methodology and that was comprised of a heterogeneous group of patients [35]. These findings seem to support a rationale to study aprepitant to treat pruritus in patients with liver disease in controlled clinical trials.

Serum histamine concentrations were reported to be increased in patients with liver disease and pruritus [36]. However, antihistamines do not ameliorate the pruritus of cholestasis, suggesting that histamine does not have a major role in the pathogenesis of this type of pruritus. However, this type of medication is associated with drowsiness, which may facilitate sleep in some patients, a definite aim in the management of patients with pruritus.

In animal studies, it has been reported that lipophosphatidic acid (LPA) induces nociception through substance P release from peripheral nerve endings [37], and it has been implicated as a mediator in animal and in *in vitro* neural models that explore signals associated with pain [38–40]. A role of LPA and the enzyme that generates its production, autotaxin, has been recently proposed to participate in the mediation of the pruritus of cholestasis [41,42]. It was reported that the concentration of several LPA species was significantly higher in the sera from patients with pruritus from cholestasis of pregnancy than in the sera from pregnant women matched for gestation term [41]. The activity of autotaxin was reported to: (i) be higher in the serum from women with cholestasis of pregnancy, and that from patients with cholestasis and pruritus from other liver diseases, and not in the serum of patients with pruritus from uremia, and from "Hodgkin's disease" [42]; (ii) have decreased in the serum from patients with liver disease and pruritus who had responded to the antibiotic rifampicin; (iii) have not decreased in the serum from patients with cholestasis and pruritus who had participated in a controlled trial of colesevalan, in which the resin was reported not to relief pruritus [43]; (iv) correlate with a decrease in the severe pruritus of patients who had been treated with the Molecular Adsorbent Recirculating System (MARS™) or with nasobiliary drainage; and (v) not be found in the bile of patients treated with nasobiliary drainage and who had responded to the treatment with a decrease in pruritus, although it was reported to have returned to pretreatment levels when the pruritus recurred [42]. The antibiotic rifampicin induces drug-metabolizing enzymes and transporters, through activation of the pregnane X receptor (PXR) [44]. The idea that the reported antipruritic effect of this drug results from either the enhanced metabolism of the *pruritogens* or its transport has been suggested [32]. The inhibition of the expression of autotaxin by rifampicin *in vitro* in HepG2 hepatoma cells and in hepatoma cells overexpressing PXR, and not on cells in which PXR had been knocked out, was interpreted to suggest that a decrease in autotaxin by rifampicin may be the mechanism by which this drug decreases pruritus in some patients with cholestasis [42]. How this relates to patients with liver disease who do not respond to rifampicin with relief of their pruritus was not addressed [45]. It was concluded that autotaxin may be a therapeutic target for the treatment of the pruritus of liver disease [42]. Potential or factual mechanisms by which autotaxin or LPA may mediate the pruritus of liver disease were not provided in this report [42]. It should be noted that the effect of rifampicin on hepatoma cells, not a model of pruritus, and the presence or changes in the serum activity or concentration of autotaxin and LPA, respectively, in patients with pruritus are not evidence to support a role of these substances in the pathogenesis of the pruritus of cholestasis. Accordingly, whether autotaxin or LPA contribute in any way to the pruritus of cholestasis is unknown.

A role of gastrin-releasing peptide receptor (GRPR) in the mediation of scratching behavior from pruritogenic stimuli in genetically engineered mice has been identified [46]. It is uncertain whether this receptor is relevant in the mediation of pruritus from liver disease; interesting, however, is the connection reported between GRPR and an isoform of the mu opioid receptor 1, in the mediation of morphine-induced scratching behavior in mice [47].

The approach to the patient with the pruritus of cholestasis

Primary skin diseases must be excluded in patients with liver disease and pruritus. As recommended for dry skin, low temperature in the home environment and the use of mild laundry detergent may be helpful. Gentle soaps including Dove® and Eucerin® may be preferable. After bathing, the application of moisturizers such as Aquaphor® and Caress® to damp skin also helps to keep it moist. Patients suffering from intractable pruritus may require admission to hospital for intravenous therapy with naloxone [16] (Figure 26.1) or anesthetics [48]; intravenous antihistamines lead to sedation, which can be helpful. Psychiatric support may be necessary in patients with depression from this chronic maddening complication of liver disease. Referral for liver transplant evaluation is indicated in patients with intractable pruritus.

Selected therapies for the pruritus of cholestasis are provided in Table 26.1, guidelines for treatment in Figure 26.1, and some relevant information regarding some therapeutic regimens in this section, where other treatments are also described and classified according to the aim that they seem to pursue; however, a rationale for the use of certain interventions is not always apparent.

Nonabsorbable resins

The most commonly used drug to treat this form of pruritus is cholestyramine [49], which seems to be associated with relief in some patients by an unknown mechanism. The side effects of this resin tend to be minor in most patients (e.g., bloating).

Several interventions aimed at the removal of pruritogens from the circulation include anion adsorption and plasma separation [8], and Prometheus ™ and MARS™ [50], which combine albumin adsorption with hemodialysis [8], and have been associated with relief of intractable pruritus. Analysis of plasma contents removed from patients with severe pruritus via MARS™ was reported to reveal 60 proteins, one of which, SLURP1, was three times higher in the samples from patients with cholestasis than in those from the control group [50]; the relevance of any of these proteins in the

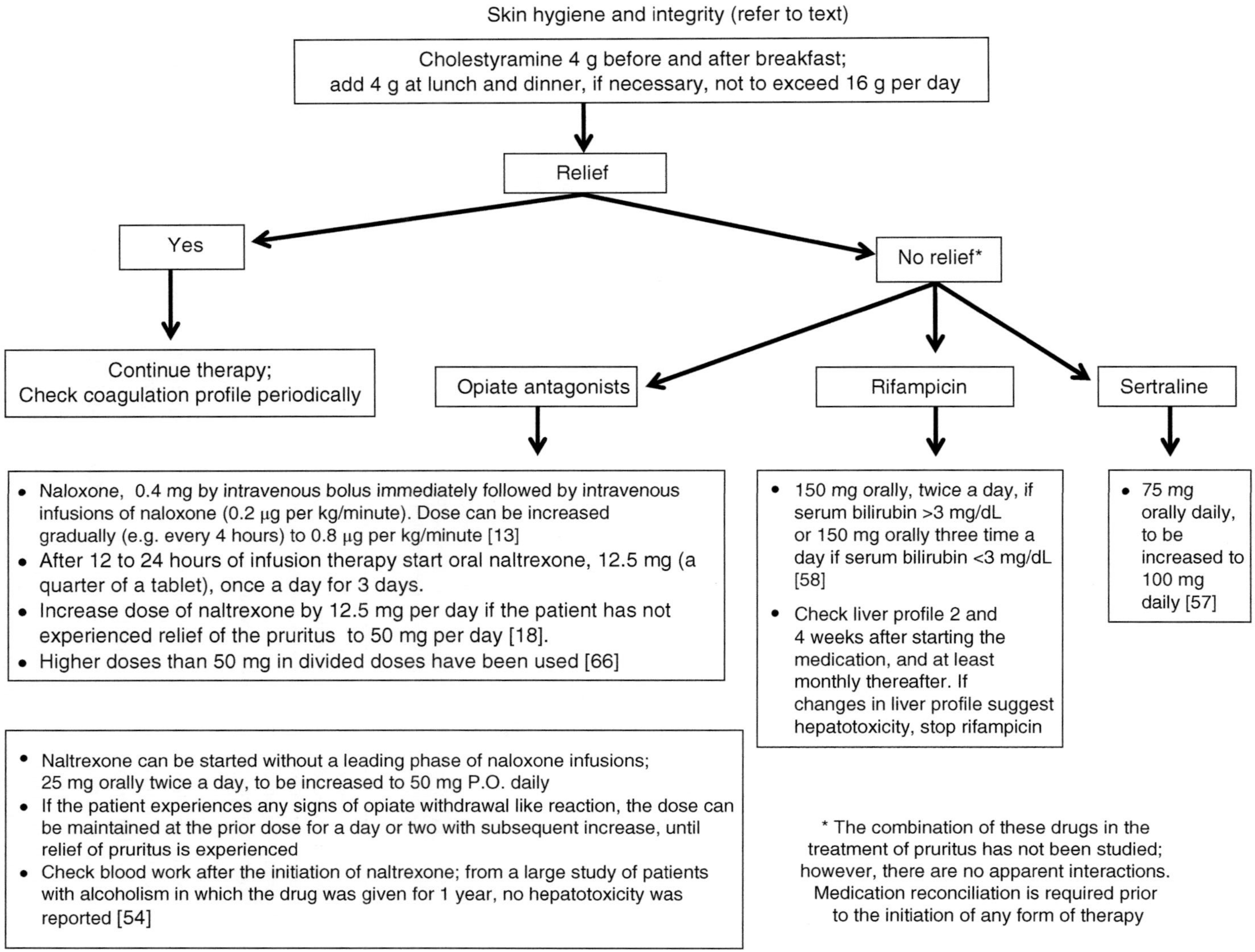

Figure 26.1 Treatment of the pruritus of cholestasis.

Table 26.1 Selected publications on the treatment of itch from liver disease.

Medication	Aim	Dose/mode of administration/ frequency	Type of study/ duration	n	End points on pruritus and/or scratching	Results	Reference
Cholestyramine	Removal of pruritogen(s)	3.3–12 g/PO/ daily	Single blind, open label/placebo controlled crossover[a]/6–32 months	27	Not reported	23 patients experienced relief of pruritus[1]	[49]
Rifampicin	Unknown	150 mg/PO/BID if serum bilirubin >3 mg/dL; 150 mg/PO/TID if serum bilirubin <3	Double blind, randomized placebo controlled crossover/4 weeks[b]	9	Change in VAS[a]	Highly significant decrease in the 7-day summed VAS[b]	[58]
Naloxone	To decrease opioidergic tone	0.2 μg/kg/min/IV continuous infusions preceded by 0.4 mg IV bolus	Double blind, placebo controlled, randomized cross-over/4 consecutive days	29	Change in HSA	Geometric mean HSA 34% lower on naloxone than on placebo	[16]
Naltrexone	To decrease opioidergic tone	25 mg/PO/BID on day 1 followed by 50 mg/PO/daily	Randomized placebo controlled/ 4 weeks[c]	16	Change in VAS	Daytime VAS down by 54% and night-time VAS down by 44%	[18]
Sertraline	To change serotoninergic tone	75–100 mg/PO/ daily	First phase, dose finding study/4 weeks Second phase, randomized, double placebo controlled, cross-over design/6 weeks	21 12	Change in VAS, decrease in skin excorations	Decrease in mean VAS by 53% in first phase and decrease in mean VAS by 33% from baseline on sertraline	[57]

BID, two times daily; HAS, hourly scratching activity; n, total number of patients; PO, per os, orally; VAS, visual analog score.
[a] Compared with an observational control group that did not receive cholestyramine but that received norethandrolone or no treatment.
[b] The use of cholestyramine was allowed to continue; the number of cholestyramine packs per day that the patients used was counted. Mean change in VAS not reported; VAS graphed per patient.
[c] Concomitant use of antipruritic medications were allowed.

pathogenesis of the pruritus is unknown. Although the placebo effect of these interventions may be substantial, and the relief provided temporary, the tremendous need to provide relief from pruritus supports the use of this type of intervention in controlled environments.

Nasobiliary drainage in patients with PBC [51], and in patients with familial intrahepatic cholestasis syndromes, partial external diversion of bile, and ileal diversion [8], are also aimed at the removal of pruritogens. A decrease in the degree of cholestasis may contribute to the relief associated with these interventions.

Changes in neurotransmission

Opiate antagonists

Naloxone and naltrexone are opiate antagonists that have been tested for the treatment of the pruritus of cholestasis in adults [15–18,21,52] and in children [53]. If at any point of the dose increase the patient reports signs of withdrawal, the dose can be maintained at the prior dosage for a day or two with subsequent increases until relief of the pruritus is experienced. The opiate withdrawal-like reaction runs its course on the dose that triggered it; thus, it is not necessary to stop the medication if such a reaction occurs. Patients should be evaluated with a liver profile after the initiation of naltrexone although, from a large study of patients with alcoholism in which the drug was given for 1 year, no hepatotoxicity was reported [54]. The metabolism of naltrexone is slow in patients with compensated and decompensated cirrhosis, leading to drug accumulation [55]. However, pruritus tends to cease in patients with hepatic synthetic dysfunction; thus, naltrexone is not commonly needed for patients with decompensated liver disease [9].

Pain, probably as a result of blocking endogenous analgesia mediated by opioids, was reported to occur in three patients with inflammatory conditions and with liver disease who had responded to naltrexone with relief of pruritus [8]. If pain occurs, the dosage of the opiate antagonist can be decreased or the drug stopped, if necessary.

Butorphanol, an antagonist at the mu opioid receptor and an agonist at the kappa receptor, has been reported to ameliorate the pruritus of cholestasis [8]. The addiction potential of butorphanol, initially considered to be low, is important [8]. Thus, the use of this drug, for example, in short courses, for the treatment of the pruritus of cholestasis must be considered in light of this possible complication. The effect of butorphanol on this type of pruritus has to be reconciled with preliminary reports of codeine, an agonist at the mu opioid receptor, and also of buprenorphine, an agonist at the mu and an antagonist at the kappa receptor, which have been reported to relieve the pruritus of cholestasis [8].

Serotonin antagonists

Ondansetron was reported to have a marginal ameliorating effect on the pruritus of cholestasis in a controlled study that applied behavioral methodology [56].

Serotonin reuptake inhibitors and other centrally acting drugs

Sertraline was reported to relieve pruritus of cholestasis in a controlled study [57]. Other centrally acting medications including the noradrenergic and serotoninergic antidepressant mertazapine, have been reported to relieve this type of pruritus in a small heterogeneous group of patients with malignancy and uremia [8] and in patients with nocturnal itch from skin diseases [8]. Thus, in concert, these reports may suggest that in addition to the serotonin neurotransmitter system, noradrenaline may participate in the mediation of pruritus not limited to that from liver disease.

Antiobiotics

Rifampicin is a ligand of the PXR, whose stimulation induces drug-metabolizing enzymes and transporters [44]. It has been concluded from several clinical studies that rifampicin is associated with a decrease in the pruritus of cholestasis [58,59]; however, some patients do not report relief on this drug [45]. It was reported from a meta-analysis that rifampicin was safe, and not associated with hepatotoxicity in the short term [60]. Rifampicin, however, can be hepatotoxic, and associated with liver dysfunction [61]; accordingly, close follow-up of patients on this drug is necessary, and the drug should be stopped if changes suggestive of hepatotoxicity are detected.

Miscellaneous interventions

Antioxidants, phenobarbital, grapefruit juice, *S*-adenosylmethionine, and dronabinol have been reported to decrease the pruritus of cholestasis [8]. Gabapentin may only be useful in a selective group of patients with high expectations for relief from the drug [62].

Steroids and tracolimus have been reported in association with relief of this type of pruritus [8]. Controlled studies on the use of immunosuppressants for this indication, however, have not been published.

The rationale for the use of phototherapy to the skin, which has been associated with relief of pruritus in patients with liver disease, is not readily apparent [63]. Bright light phototherapy (10 000 lux), based on the potential light regulation of pruritus and scratching suggested by the 24-hour rhythm in hourly scratching activity in some patients with cholestasis [16], was associated with a decrease in the bouts of scratching over the 24–48 hour periods recorded in patients with liver disease [64].

The administration of anesthetics including propofol [8] and lidocaine [48] has been associated with relief from the pruritus of cholestasis. The response to lidocaine may support the involvement of the transient receptor potential vanilloid receptor-1, which has been identified as relevant in the mediation of scratching behavior in mice [65].

Conclusions

The pathogenesis of the pruritus of cholestasis, is most likely, multifactorial, and its perception may be modified by the genetic composition of the patient. The pruritus may have central and peripheral components. The design of studies of pruritus is challenging because pruritus is a perception, and, as a perception, is individual-specific and cannot be directly quantitated. In contrast, scratching activity, the behavioral manifestation of pruritus, can be quantitated [15,16,19,20]. The inclusion of behavioral methodology in clinical trials allows for the measurement of clear end-points (i.e., change in scratching activity) to be assessed, rather than changes in arbitrary measures. Oral reports on the effect of drugs on the intensity of pruritus are also extremely relevant, and should be included in clinical trials of pruritus: patients can respond yes or no to the question of relief. Development of improved portable instruments for the specific continuous recording of scratching activity is feasible in the current technological environment. Clinicians attending patients with liver disease can contribute to the elucidation of the pathogenesis of the pruritus by referring patients to studies of pruritogenic neurotransmission and to clinical trials of antipruritic medications.

References

1 Rishe E, Azarm A, Bergasa NV. Itch in primary biliary cirrhosis: a patients' perspective. Acta Derm Venereol 2008;88:34–7.
2 Aoki T. Pleasure of "scratch" is a complex sensation of itch an pain. In: Second International Workshop for the Study of Itch. Toyama; 2003. p. 11.
3 Chia SC, Bergasa NV, Kleiner DE, Goodman Z, Hoofnagle JH, Di Bisceglie AM. Pruritus as a presenting symptom of chronic hepatitis C. Dig Dis Sci 1998;43:2177–83.
4 Huesmann M, Huesmann T, Osada N, Phan NQ, Kremer AE, Stander S. Cholestatic pruritus: a retrospective analysis on clinical characteristics and treatment response. J Dtsch Dermatol Ges 2013;11:158–68.
5 Poupon R, Chazouilleres O, Balkau B, Poupon RE. Clinical and biochemical expression of the histopathological lesions of primary biliary cirrhosis. UDCA-PBC Group. J Hepatol 1999;30:408–12.
6 Newton JL, Bhala N, Burt J, Jones DE. Characterisation of the associations and impact of symptoms in primary biliary cirrhosis using a disease specific quality of life measure. J Hepatol 2006;44:776–83.
7 Carbone M, Mells G, Pells G, et al. Sex and age are determinants of the clinical phenotype of primary biliary cirrhosis and response to ursodeoxycholic acid. Gastroenterology 2013;144:560–9.
8 Bergasa NV. Pruritus in primary biliary cirrhosis: pathogenesis and therapy. Clin Liver Dis 2008;12:385–406.
9 Lloyd-Thomas HG, Sherlock S. Testosterone therapy for the pruritus of obstructive jaundice. Br Med J 1952;2:1289–91.
10 Mezey E, Burns C, Burdick JF, Braine HG. A case of severe benign intrahepatic cholestasis treated with liver transplantation. Am J Gastroenterol 2002;97:475–7.
11 Floreani A, Carderi I, Variola A, Rizzotto ER, Nicol J, Bergasa NV. A novel multidrug-resistance protein 2 gene mutation identifies a subgroup of patients with primary biliary cirrhosis and pruritus. Hepatology 2006;43:1152–4.
12 Thornton JR, Losowsky MS. Opioid peptides and primary biliary cirrhosis. BMJ 1988;297:1501–4.
13 Jones EA, Bergasa NV. The pruritus of cholestasis: from bile acids to opiate agonists. Hepatology 1990;11:884–7.
14 Ballantyne JC, Loach AB, Carr DB. The incidence of pruritus after epidural morphine. Anaesthesia 1989;44:863
15 Bergasa NV, Talbot TL, Alling DW, et al. A controlled trial of naloxone infusions for the pruritus of chronic cholestasis. Gastroenterology 1992;102:544–9.
16 Bergasa NV, Alling DW, Talbot TL, et al. Effects of naloxone infusions in patients with the pruritus of cholestasis. A double-blind, randomized, controlled trial. Ann Intern Med 1995;123:161–7.
17 Carson KL, Tran TT, Cotton P, Sharara AI, Hunt CM. Pilot study of the use of naltrexone to treat the severe pruritus of cholestatic liver disease. Am J Gastroenterol 1996;91: 1022–3.
18 Wolfhagen FHJ, Sternieri E, Hop WCJ, Vitale G, Bertolotti M, van Buuren HR. Oral naltrexone treatment for cholestatic pruritus: a double-blind, placebo-controlled study. Gastroenterology 1997;113:1264–9.
19 Bergasa NV, Schmitt JM, Talbot TL, et al. Open-label trial of oral nalmefene therapy for the pruritus of cholestasis. Hepatology 1998;27 (3): 679–84.
20 Bergasa NV, Alling DW, Talbot TL, Wells MC, Jones EA. Oral nalmefene therapy reduces scratching activity due to the pruritus of cholestasis: a controlled study. J Am Acad Dermatol 1999;41:431–4.
21 Terg R, Coronel E, Sorda J, Munoz AE, Findor J. Efficacy and safety of oral naltrexone treatment for pruritus of cholestasis, a crossover, double blind, placebo-controlled study. J Hepatol 2002;37:717–22.
22 Tandon P, Rowe BH, Vandermeer B, Bain VG. The efficacy and safety of bile acid binding agents, opioid antagonists, or rifampin in the treatment of cholestasis-associated pruritus. Am J Gastroenterol 2007;102:1528–36.
23 Kumagai H, Ebata T, Takamori K, Muramatsu T, Nakamoto H, Suzuki H. Effect of a novel kappa-receptor agonist, nalfurafine hydrochloride, on severe itch in 337 haemodialysis

patients: a Phase III, randomized, double-blind, placebo-controlled study. Nephrol Dial Transplant 2010;25:1251–7.
24 Bergasa NV, Liau S, Homel P, Ghali V. Hepatic Met-enkephalin immunoreactivity is enhanced in primary biliary cirrhosis. Liver 2002;22:107–13.
25 Boyella VD, Nicastri AD, Bergasa NV. Human hepatic met-enkephalin and delta opioid receptor-1 immunoreactivities in viral and autoimmune hepatitis. Ann Hepatol 2008;7: 221–6.
26 Barnes LB, Devous MD, Harris TS, Mayo MJ. The central nervous system activity profile of cholestatic pruritus. Hepatolgy 2009;50:375, Abstract 153.
27 Wei LX, Floreani A, Variola A, El Younis C, Bergasa NV. A study of the mu opioid receptor gene polymorphism A118G in patients with primary biliary cirrhosis with and without pruritus. Acta Derm Venereol 2008;88:323–6.
28 Tsai FF, Fan SZ, Yang YM, Chien KL, Su YN, Chen LK. Human opioid mu-receptor A118G polymorphism may protect against central pruritus by epidural morphine for post-cesarean analgesia. Acta Anaesthesiol Scand 2010;54: 1265–9.
29 Jimenez N, Anderson GD, Shen DD, et al. Is ethnicity associated with morphine's side effects in children? Morphine pharmacokinetics, analgesic response, and side effects in children having tonsillectomy. Paediatr Anaesth 2012;22: 669–75.
30 Xie W, Samoriski GM, McLaughlin JP, et al. Genetic alteration of phospholipase C beta3 expression modulates behavioral and cellular responses to mu opioids. Proc Natl Acad Sci U S A 1999;96:10385–90.
31 Varadi DP. Pruritus induced by crude bile and purified bile acids: experimental production of pruritus in human skin. Arch Dermatol 1974;109:678–81.
32 Bergasa NV. The pruritus of cholestasis. J Hepatol 2005; 43:1078–88.
33 Mason A, Luketic V, Lindor K, et al. Farsenoid-X-receptor agonist: a new class of drug for the treatment of PBC? An international study evaluating the addition of obeticholic acid (INT-747) to ursodeoxycholic acid. Hepatology 2010;52:80A.
34 Trivedi M, Bergasa NV. Serum concentrations of substance P in cholestasis. Ann Hepatol 2010;9:177–80.
35 Stander S, Siepmann D, Herrgott I, Sunderkotter C, Luger TA. Targeting the neurokinin receptor 1 with aprepitant: a novel antipruritic strategy. PLoS One 2010;5:e10968.
36 Gittlen SD, Schulman ES, Maddrey WC. Raised histamine concentrations in chronic cholestatic liver disease. Gut 1990;31:96–9.
37 Renback K, Inoue M, Ueda H. Lysophosphatidic acid-induced, pertussis toxin-sensitive nociception through a substance P release from peripheral nerve endings in mice. Neurosci Lett 1999;270:59–61.
38 Renback K, Inoue M, Yoshida A, Nyberg F, Ueda H. Vzg-1/lysophosphatidic acid-receptor involved in peripheral pain transmission. Brain Res Mol Brain Res 2000;75:350–4.
39 Cohen A, Sagron R, Somech E, Segal-Hayoun Y, Zilberberg N. Pain-associated signals, acidosis and lysophosphatidic acid, modulate the neuronal K(2P)2.1 channel. Mol Cell Neurosci 2009;40:382–9.
40 Ahn DK, Lee SY, Han SR, et al. Intratrigeminal ganglionic injection of LPA causes neuropathic pain-like behavior and demyelination in rats. Pain 2009;146:114–20.
41 Kremer AE, Martens JJ, Kulik W, et al. Lysophosphatidic acid is a potential mediator of cholestatic pruritus. Gastroenterology 2012;139:1008–18.
42 Kremer AE, van Dijk R, Leckie P, et al. Serum autotaxin is increased in pruritus of cholestasis, but not of other origin, and responds to therapeutic interventions. Hepatology 2012;56:1391–400.
43 Kuiper EM, van Erpecum KJ, Beuers U, et al. The potent bile acid sequestrant colesevelam is not effective in cholestatic pruritus: results of a double-blind, randomized, placebo-controlled trial. Hepatology 2010;52:1334–40.
44 Tirona RG, Kim RB. Nuclear receptors and drug disposition gene regulation. J Pharm Sci 2005;94:1169–86.
45 Woolf GM, Reynolds TB. Failure of rifampin to relieve pruritus in chronic liver disease. J Clin Gastroenterol 1990;12:174–7.
46 Sun YG, Chen ZF. A gastrin-releasing peptide receptor mediates the itch sensation in the spinal cord. Nature 2007;448:700–3.
47 Jordan BA, Cvejic S, Devi LA. Opioids and their complicated receptor complexes. Neuropsychopharmacology 2000;23: S5–18.
48 Villamil AG, Bandi JC, Galdame OA, Gerona S, Gadano AC. Efficacy of lidocaine in the treatment of pruritus in patients with chronic cholestatic liver diseases. Am J Med 2005;118: 1160–3.
49 Datta DV, Sherlock S. Cholestyramine for long term relief of the pruritus complicating intrahepatic cholestasis. Gastroenterology 1966;50:323–32.
50 Gay M, Pares A, Carrascal M, et al. Proteomic analysis of polypeptides captured from blood during extracorporeal albumin dialysis in patients with cholestasis and resistant pruritus. PLoS One 2011;6:e21850.
51 Beuers U, Gerken G, Pusl T. Biliary drainage transiently relieves intractable pruritus in primary biliary cirrhosis. Hepatology 2006;44:280–1.
52 Mansour-Ghanaei F, Taheri A, Froutan H, et al. Effect of oral naltrexone on pruritus in cholestatic patients. World J Gastroenterol 2006;12:1125–8.
53 Zellos A, Roy A, Schwarz KB. Use of oral naltrexone for severe pruritus due to cholestatic liver disease in children. J Pediatr Gastroenterol Nutr 2010;51:787–9.
54 Krystal JH, Cramer JA, Krol WF, Kirk GF, Rosenheck RA. Naltrexone in the treatment of alcohol dependence. N Engl J Med 2001;345:1734–9.
55 Bertolotti M, Ferrari A, Vitale G, et al. Effect of liver cirrhosis on the systemic availability of naltrexone in humans. J Hepatol 1997;27:505–11.

56 Jones EA, Molenaar HA, Oosting J. Ondansetron and pruritus in chronic liver disease: a controlled study. Hepatogastroenterology 2007;54:1196–9.
57 Mayo MJ, Handem I, Saldana S, Jacobe H, Getachew Y, Rush AJ. Sertraline as a first-line treatment for cholestatic pruritus. Hepatology 2007;45:666–74.
58 Ghent CN, Carruthers SG. Treatment of pruritus in primary biliary cirrhosis with rifampin: results of a double-blind, crossover, randomized trial. Gastroenterology 1988;94:488–93.
59 Bachs L, Parés A, Elena M, Piera C, Rodés J. Effects of long-term rifampicin administration in primary biliary cirrhosis. Gastroenterology 1992;102:2077–80.
60 Khurana S, Singh P. Rifampin is safe for treatment of pruritus due to chronic cholestasis: a meta-analysis of prospective randomized-controlled trials. Liver Int 2006;26:943–8.
61 Prince MI, Burt AD, Jones DE. Hepatitis and liver dysfunction with rifampicin therapy for pruritus in primary biliary cirrhosis. Gut 2002;50:436–9.
62 Bergasa NV, McGee M, Ginsburg IH, Engler D. Gabapentin in patients with the pruritus of cholestasis: a double-blind, randomized, placebo-controlled trial. Hepatology 2006;44: 1317–23.
63 Decock S, Roelandts R, Steenbergen WV, et al. Cholestasis-induced pruritus treated with ultraviolet B phototherapy: an observational case series study. J Hepatol 2012;57: 637–41.
64 Bergasa NV, Link MJ, Keogh M, Yaroslavsky G, Rosenthal RN, McGee M. Pilot study of bright-light therapy reflected toward the eyes for the pruritus of chronic liver disease. Am J Gastroenterol 2001;96:1563–70.
65 Kim BM, Lee SH, Shim WS, Oh U. Histamine-induced Ca(2+) influx via the PLA(2)/lipoxygenase/TRPV1 pathway in rat sensory neurons. Neurosci Lett 2004;361:159–62.
66 Jones EA, Dekker LR. Florid opioid withdrawal-like reaction precipitated by naltrexone in a patient with chronic cholestasis. Gastroenterology 2000;118:431–2.

CHAPTER 27

Quality of life and symptom management

Ayman A. Abdo[1,3] and Faisal M. Sanai[2,3]

[1]*Division of Gastroenterology, Department of Medicine, College of Medicine, King Saud University, Riyadh, Saudi Arabia*
[2]*Department of Hepatobiliary Science and Liver Transplantation, King AbdulAziz Medical City, Riyadh, Saudi Arabia*
[3]*King Saud University Liver Disease Research Center, Riyadh, Saudi Arabia*

Introduction

In a typical visit to the hepatologist or the liver transplant surgeon by a cirrhotic patient, our attention is mostly focused on what we have been well trained to do in medical schools and residency programs: reach the right diagnosis, estimate the prognosis, recommend the appropriate management, and explain these points to the patient and family.

But are these the same worries and concerns of the patient in front of us? Certainly, the patient is interested to learn about his or her diagnosis, wants to know what to expect from the disease and its associated prognosis, wishes to start treatment right away, and definitely wants to have a reasonable explanation from the doctor. However, the patient often has symptoms and complaints that are not always attended to by the doctor because they are either considered trivial or "have nothing to do with your liver disease."

Although the majority of liver diseases seen in early stages are totally asymptomatic, like inactive hepatitis B virus (HBV) infection and nonalcoholic fatty liver disease (NAFLD), it is increasingly recognized that many patients have a significant impairment in their quality of life (QoL). This reduction in their QoL, which is more pronounced in those with advanced liver disease, often becomes the first and foremost concern when they meet their doctor. Conversely, and not infrequently, the patient may actually be unaware that these systemic symptoms are either directly or indirectly related to the liver disease.

In order to address this common problem effectively, physicians need to be mindful of the systemic symptoms that are commonly faced by their patients, especially in those with end-stage liver disease (ESLD), which significantly impact their QoL. Ignoring these symptoms or simply convincing oneself that they are unrelated to the overt liver disease, or focusing on treating the liver disease and hoping that these symptoms will abate or disappear is never a successful strategy.

The ever-improving medical management of liver disease portends that the majority of patients with chronic liver disease will live with the disease rather than dying from it. The commonplace notion that chronic liver disease connotes entirely to the consequences of ESLD is fundamentally flawed. Nonetheless, there is a growing awareness that a number of systemic symptoms may occur at any point in the natural history of chronic liver disease, causing functional impairment and reduced QoL.

Health-related QoL is a concept that reflects the physical, social, and emotional attitudes and behaviors of an individual as they relate to their prior and current health state [1]. The recognition that there is an additional disease burden in patients, linked with considerable functional deprivation, the management of which is vastly unrelated to that of the specific fallout of having ESLD, represents a paradigm shift in the approach to the disease.

In this chapter, we provide a general approach to this important problem and offer a structured framework for its management. Importantly, we focus on systemic symptoms that compromise the patients' QoL rather than address specific clinical symptoms that are related to well-known sequelae of cirrhosis, like ascites and hepatic encephalopathy, because these are covered in other chapters.

Cirrhosis: A practical guide to management, First Edition. Edited by Samuel S. Lee and Richard Moreau.

Measuring functional ability and quality of life

Quality of life

The tools routinely used to assess QoL are not standardized among studies dealing with chronic liver disease [2]. In addition, most methods employed are static questionnaires that fail to adapt to the patient's responses or are not specifically designed for liver disease. This is further compounded by the fact that some of these surveys are copyrighted and do not have readily available normative data [3].

Several instruments have been validated for use in cirrhosis, specifically the Sickness Impact Profile (SIP) and the Chronic Liver Disease Questionnaire (CLDQ) [4,5]. Another commonly used questionnaire is the Short Form (36) Health Survey (SF-36). The advantage of a simple tool like the SF-36 is its brevity (36 questions) and extensive normative information, but it is disadvantaged by its static nature, being a generic instrument, and being unable to provide the depth of questioning due to its limited number of questions. Therefore, generic instruments such as the SF-36 have given mixed results when used in cirrhotic patients [6,7]. However, the SIP, which has been validated in cirrhosis [3,8], has higher coverage of social and behavioral domains, is non-disease-specific, and inquires about QoL over the last 24 hours, which may minimize its ability to capture episodic but troubling effects on QoL. Although it has good responsiveness and has been studied extensively in cirrhosis, the SIP is not routinely used because of its length (136 questions) and lack of population norms [8,9]. The CLDQ is a simple, brief (29 questions), and freely available instrument that has good responsiveness in several stages of liver disease [4,5,10]. While it has good validity in chronic liver disease and has been used in several countries, its evaluation of social and sleep disturbances is limited, and, like other paper and pencil questionnaires, remains a static instrument. As such, the search for the ideal tool that would be freely accessible, brief, and yet comprehensive, that could simplify the diagnosis of impaired QoL and increase its regular investigation, remains unfulfilled.

Functional ability

One of the most important components of a fulfilling life is functional ability. If one is unable to perform daily activities (e.g., work-related duties, family chores, and social interactions), then surely QoL will be affected. But how would one reliably measure functional ability? In the majority of cases, researchers have used patient-reported outcome measures (PROMs) to study functional ability. PROMs are self-completion tools derived using qualitative approaches which address patient experience and highlight an individual's capacity to undertake functions that they perceive as being important for daily living [11,12].

Causes for impaired quality of life

As QoL is a term that is very difficult to define and measure, factors affecting it are also hard to capture. In general, there are many factors that affect QoL in patients with liver disease, primarily the physical effects stemming from the biology of the disease. This is clearly seen in patients with advanced liver disease. Symptoms like ascites, hepatic encephalopathy, and muscle wasting would significantly impair the patients' functional ability. Fortunately, this part of the story is relatively easy to recognize and manage. In addition to the effects of symptoms and physical impairment, medical treatment also adds to the physical burden of disease: frequent physician visits, frequent testing and imaging, multiple admissions, medication side effects, and a plethora of other management-related issues, physical stress, and risk.

Second, there is the psychological component of the disease which is clearly seen across all aspects of liver disease and across all disease severity scales. These symptoms are much more difficult to recognize and manage. They include depression, anxiety, and personality disorders, among many others. In addition, the stress of obtaining, appreciating, and reacting to information related to the diagnosis and prognosis is paramount. The anxiety over the possibility of liver transplantation and the waiting list associated with it or having to identify a living related donor is also a major factor that has tremendous implications towards QoL.

Finally, there are other associated symptoms and systemic features that may be related to the biologic pathophysiology of liver disease or to its physiological consequences: fatigue, depression, sleep disturbances, cognitive impairment, and cardiac dysfunction [13]. These symptoms and systemic problems may interact with each another.

Is quality of life really impaired in patients with liver disease?

Assessing functional ability in an accurate and meaningful way is laden with difficulties in research settings, let alone the hectic schedule of an outpatient clinic. Crude measures of functional ability such as the ability to engage in hobbies or wash oneself, or employment status are indicators of function that are significantly impaired in chronic liver disease [14]. Complex processes such as being able to dress or wash oneself, let alone engage in complex social interactions are functions of daily living that are frequently taken for granted. Objective studies have confirmed that patients with chronic liver disease of many etiologies have reduced physical activity levels measured using continuous physical activity monitoring [1,15], although this approach may still underestimate the impact of disease on the complex functions required for effective daily living.

QoL and functional ability have been clearly shown to be compromised in many types of liver disease patients. In terms of functional ability, with the use of tools like PROMs, it has been established that patients with liver disease of various etiologies and at different stages of their disease have significant functional impairment [13] regardless of the etiology. For example, in a study by Elliott et al. [16], functional ability and symptom severity were compared in 103 consecutive liver transplant recipients and matched controls using the patient-reported functional outcome measure: Patient-Reported Outcomes Measurement Information System, Health Assessment Questionnaire (PROMIS HAQ). Symptoms frequently seen in chronic liver disease were quantified by: (i) Fatigue Impact Scale (FIS), (ii) Orthostatic Grading Scale (OGS: autonomic dysfunction), (iii) Cognitive Failures Questionnaire (CFQ), and (iv) Epworth Sleepiness Scale (ESS: Daytime Somnolence). There was a significant functional impairment in patients with cirrhosis which was present across all domains of functional ability and seen across different etiologies including alcoholic liver disease, NAFLD, primary biliary cirrhosis (PBC), and primary sclerosing cholangitis when compared with control subjects. This did not improve significantly after liver transplantation and liver transplant recipients exhibited a significant reduction in function across all domains of the PROMIS HAQ, suggesting that functional impairment is broad-based. Seventy-seven percent of all patients after liver transplant identified some difficulty with activities of daily living. Elevation in PROMIS HAQ score (and therefore functional impairment) was strongly associated with symptoms, particularly of fatigue, cognitive impairment, and daytime somnolence, and fatigue severity was independently associated with functional impairment.

Quality of life and patients with hepatitis C

Of all causes of liver disease, impairment in QoL has been best studied and documented in patients infected with the hepatitis C virus (HCV) [17]. Chronic HCV seems to directly alter health-related QoL. One of the largest studies, which included 642 HCV-infected patients, evaluated the impact of the virus on QoL before and after treatment with interferon-based antiviral therapy [18]. The authors clearly showed that the health-related QoL in patients with HCV was significantly reduced compared to a healthy control group, regardless of histologic severity. Ware et al. [19], as part of a study by the International Hepatitis Interventional Therapy Group, reported a significant reduction in five out of eight SF-36 concepts in patients with HCV compared with matched population norms. The reductions were seen in the physical functioning, role-physical, general health, vitality, and social functioning domains. In a British study, 72 unselected, sequential patients with chronic HCV and 30 sequential patients with chronic HBV infection were compared [20]. Patients who had any signs of cirrhosis were excluded. The SF-36 scores in all domains were greatly reduced in chronic HCV patients, implying that these patients felt that they were unwell and perceived themselves as having significantly reduced QoL. On the other hand, patients with chronic HBV infection did not report any significant reductions in their SF-36 scores except in the "mental health" and "general health perception" variables. Their SF-36 scores that assess a person's ability to conduct physical activities were only marginally affected. When the HCV and HBV patients were compared, patients with HCV infection had poorer scores in the social functioning, physical limitations, and energy and fatigue domains compared with HBV-infected patients.

However, these results were not reproduced in other populations. Sixty Japanese patients with chronic HCV were subjected to the Todai Health Index (a checklist for a self-administered scoring system of a variety of physical and psychological symptoms) and showed no characteristic subjective symptoms when compared with a healthy control group apart from a lower aggression score [21]. Another Japanese study by Fukuhara et al. [22] utilized the SF-36 questionnaire to examine a group of HCV-infected patients and found no difference between patients and control subjects. Similar results were also obtained from two studies in North America. In the first study, Davis et al. [23] used the SIP to study health-related QoL, although this instrument is insensitive in identifying changes that are clinically relevant. The second study investigated a group of American blood donors who were incidentally found to have HCV. These donors, who had a high incidence of fatigue (61%) and headache (54%) in an earlier study [24], were compared with normal healthy blood donors without HCV infection. The non-HCV group reported a fatigue rate of up to 70%, indicating no difference between the two groups. The key item of interest of this study was that it evaluated a random sample from a random population wherein HCV symptoms and status were examined in a totally independent manner, distinctly different from the majority of studies which include patients from tertiary care centers [25].

Based on the above review, it is clear that patients with HCV infection do experience multiple symptoms and disease entities that adversely affect QoL. However, it is unclear how much of the effect is really due to the infection itself and its consequent liver disease or all the other associated features and factors that are directly or indirectly related such as ethnicity, route of infection, intravenous drug use status, and social and psychologic factors. Therefore, the question remains – is it the virus or the patient [26]?

Specific symptoms or clinical syndromes affecting quality of life

Fatigue

Fatigue is probably the most studied symptom that affects QoL in patients with liver disease. It has been extensively studied in PBC and HCV. In PBC, fatigue impact qualification tools have been well developed and validated, diagnostic criteria defined, and a management approach developed [13].

There have been several uncontrolled studies that show that a significant proportion of HCV patients have fatigue. Tong et al. [27] revealed that 67% of post-transfusion HCV-infected patients complained of fatigue. In a study on Irish women with HCV due to contaminated anti-D immunoglobulin, Kenny-Walsh et al. [28] found a fatigue level of at least 81%. Of note, those who were anti-HCV-positive but not viremic also had similarly high reported levels of fatigue. Likewise, Barkhuizen et al. [29] reported that 67% of HCV-positive patients compared to 44% of HCV-negative patients from a hepatology outpatient setting experienced fatigue. In a large French study by Poynard et al. [30], 53% of 1614 patients with HCV reported fatigue at their first visit and of these 17% felt their fatigue was severe. Several factors were found to be independently associated with fatigue: age over 50 years, female gender, cirrhosis, depression, and purpura. Nonetheless, it is worthy to note that very few studies have actually investigated fatigue in HCV patients in comparison with a control group.

While fatigue is an uncommonly elicited symptom in routine physician–patient interviews in patients with NAFLD and other less common liver diseases such as primary sclerosing cholangitis and autoimmune hepatitis, many publications have confirmed a high prevalence of fatigue in these disease groups [1,31,32]. Notably, the pathogenesis of fatigue is less well understood in these patient groups. Available data suggest that the prevalence is comparable to that in PBC, indicating that common management pathways and approaches may be relevant [33]. However, fatigue in autoimmune hepatitis appears to only be a feature of acute or active disease, with only low levels being reported in patients with controlled chronic disease [34].

Sleep disturbance

Sleep disturbance is common in patients with liver disease and cirrhosis [1,35–37]. This has been well-studied in patients with PBC and has been linked to the accompanying fatigue [38]. Patients with NAFLD also experience sleep disturbances, especially obstructive sleep apnea [39]. Effective treatment in these patients has been shown to modify liver injury by improving liver steatosis [40].

Psychiatric disorders

A number of studies have reported a high incidence of depression in chronic HCV-infected patients. For instance, Dwight et al. [41] found that 28% of their HCV patients satisfied the criteria for having major depression. In an attempt to establish the incidence of psychiatric comorbidities among HCV-infected US veterans, Lehman et al. [42] used verified scoring systems to study 120 consecutive patients with chronic HCV. Almost 50% had a history of a psychiatric disorder that was unrelated to substance abuse, and about one-third of the patients were taking psychotropic medications at the time of the evaluation. Of clinical significance was that 44% had depression, 38% had anxiety, 20% had post-traumatic stress disorder, and 26% had alcohol-related problems. However, veterans typically have a high level of alcohol consumption and so the prevalence of psychiatric disorders in the HCV population may have been overestimated in this study. Fontana et al. [43] obtained similar results in a group of 220 unselected patients with compensated chronic HCV and found that 35% harbored clinically significant emotional distress. It is worth noting that most of the studies described above did not have a control group. Nevertheless, a large, controlled Italian study determined that there was a higher lifetime prevalence of major depression among HCV patients than either HBV patients or controls [44].

Cognitive impairment

Obvious symptoms of cognitive impairment can be related to a variety of disease entities. Overt hepatic encephalopathy is usually easy to distinguish and its management has been well described. Somewhat more difficult to identify and manage is minimal hepatic encephalopathy, a condition recently recognized and being intensively studied. Yet there is some evidence to suggest that there are objectively demonstrated cognitive abnormalities in patients in whom minimal hepatic encephalopathy has been excluded. This has been shown through neurophysiologic abnormalities demonstrated in patients with PBC, for instance [45]. Abnormalities have also been described on magnetic resonance imaging (MRI) [45–47]. These abnormalities are perceived to be related mainly to impaired executive function. Similar findings have been reported in patients with NAFLD [48].

Cognitive dysfunction in patients with HCV has also been well described but is very closely related to fatigue and psychiatric abnormalities [49]. In this setting, it has been shown that demonstrable abnormalities in MRI testing may be related to direct central nervous system inflammatory processes [50].

Cardiac and autonomic abnormalities

In addition to the well-established cirrhotic cardiomyopathy and hyperdynamic circulation typically seen in patients with advanced liver disease, recent evidence suggests that significant impairment of cardiac function could be demonstrated even in patients with earlier stages of liver disease [51,52]. In addition, autonomic dysfunction is frequently seen in patients with various levels of liver disease [53], including early stages [54–59], and may manifest as frequent falls, blackouts, orthostatic hypotension, and syncope. It has also been linked to sudden cardiac death and mortality [53].

General approach to evaluation and diagnosis

Assessment of functional ability and QoL concerns in any chronic illness is a challenge. Several issues need to be clearly emphasized while approaching patients with general symptoms and QoL impairment:

1 Significant attention to these symptoms must be given during history taking and physical examination. If these symptoms are not kept in mind and looked out for they might be missed. Table 27.1 contains some important symptoms that need to be asked about during the interview and some signs that need to be looked out for during the examination.
2 It is the primary responsibility of the treating physician (whether a hepatologist, gastroenterologist, transplant physician, general internist, or family physician) to identify and form a management plan for these QoL issues. It is not acceptable that the specialist is only responsible for the primary illness and not for all of its associated consequences.
3 Whenever possible, an attempt should be made to assess QoL issues objectively using standardized tests in order to assess severity, assess outcome of intervention, and provide prognostic information. Some standardized tests are suggested in Table 27.1 for each of the main clinical entities.
4 Symptom severity does not always correlate with cirrhosis or liver disease severity. Often, the symptoms of earlier disease have more profound and functionally significant effects than later stages.

Table 27.1 Common systemic symptoms in cirrhotic patients and suggested objective measurement tools.

	Symptoms	Considerations	Objective tools
Fatigue	Malaise, low power, tiredness	• Rule out other medical conditions: anemia, hypothyroidism, diabetes, cardiac problems • Consider sleep disturbances	• Fatigue impact scale (FIS) • Fatigue severity scale (FSS) (Both validated in liver disease patients)
Sleep disturbances	Daytime sleepiness, insomnia, fragmented sleep, snoring, restless leg syndrome	• Caffeine and alcohol intake • Primary sleep disorders • Medications	• Two-week sleep diary • Epworth sleepiness scale • Pittsburgh sleep index [72,73]
Cognitive disorders	Memory disturbances, difficulty in concentration, behavioral changes	• Medications • Primary neurologic disease • Rule out minimal hepatic encephalopathy	• Mini-mental state examination • Cognitive failure questionnaire
Autonomic dysfunction	Syncope, postural dizziness	• Volume depletion • Medications	• Blood pressure lying and standing • Orthostatic grading scale [74]

General management approach

- The management of general symptoms and QoL issues must be approached in a multidisciplinary fashion. A team of qualified practitioners are able to deal with these issues much more efficiently than an individual physician. This team should include a psychologist, physiotherapist or occupational therapist, social worker and nurse practitioner, among others. When functioning within clear guidelines and management plans these team members will be able to execute a comprehensive holistic approach to patients and be more likely to achieve better results.
- The use of clinical pathways for each of these symptoms and issues is highly recommended.
- For specific clinical symptoms, consider referral to a primary specialist or service that specializes in that area, such as sleep medicine, cardiology, or neurology.
- For patients with PBC, the Newcastle PBC Group developed the so-called "Treat, Ameliorate, Cope, and Empathize (TrACE)" approach (Table 27.2). This approach has been used by many other groups as a general tool to assess QoL and general symptoms in patients with liver disease and has been recommended by a recent expert review [13].

This approach could be used as a basis for having a common approach to all symptoms related to QoL in patients with liver disease. This may be summarized in the following steps:

Table 27.2 The "TrACE" approach to management [13].

Action	Components
Treat the treatable	• Associated diseases • Intercurrent diseases • Primary disease
Ameliorate that which can be ameliorated	All features known to make the symptom worse
Cope	Help patients to develop coping strategies
Empathize	Try to understand the impact of fatigue on the patient

1 Treat the underlying primary liver disease.
2 Identify and treat any other associated disease or clinical entities.
3 Identify and treat all concomitant illnesses.
4 Ameliorate all other possibly contributing factors.
5 Help patients to develop coping strategies.
6 Try to empathize with the impact of fatigue on the patient.
 - Make sure that the patient continues to be the primary person responsible for his or her own symptoms, as he or she would be the best person to assess

the impact and significance of the symptoms and evaluate treatment effects.

- It is crucial to remember that in many cases there is no direct correlation between the severity of the primary liver disease and the associated symptoms.

Treating the underlying liver disease

In general, treating the underlying liver disease does not necessarily translate into improvements in the associated symptoms and QoL [60].

The data in the case of HCV is conflicting. Multiple clinical trials have been conducted, in which measurements of health-related QoL were undertaken mainly through the SF-36 questionnaire before and after interferon therapy. Many of these studies have shown that patients experience significant improvements in multiple domains of the SF-36 questionnaire after treatment. For example, in an international study by Hassanein et al. [61], 1121 patients were treated with pegylated interferon and SF-36 scores were compared between responders and nonresponders. Responders showed significant improvement in all domains and summary scales while nonresponders showed worsening in five domains. Very similar results were found by McHutchison et al. [62] and Desmoret et al. [63]. Bernstein et al. [64] performed a pooled analysis of three randomized trials and confirmed the improvement in responders, especially in the noncirrhotic group. On the other hand, some studies did not find the same positive effect of response to therapy on health-related QoL, such as those by Mathew et al. [65] and Bini and Mehandru [66].

It is hard to assess the effect of antiviral therapy on health-related QoL for a number of reasons. First, the effect of the knowledge of response and clearing of the virus in itself probably has a significant psychological effect on the patient, thus improving many of the QoL measures. In the only study of its kind that we are aware of, patients were blinded to treatment response while the SF-36 questionnaire was undertaken. In this study on 252 patients by Bonkovsky and Woolley [18], responders showed an improvement in four scores while relapsers had a significant worsening in the physical functioning domain. Similar to the effect of knowing about treatment response and its debatable effect on health-related QoL, it is difficult to account accurately and objectively for such psychological effects in measuring QoL in liver disease patients in general. Two large studies suggest that this effect is real. In a study from Australia by Rodger et al. [67], patients who were previously admitted to hospital with acute hepatitis between 1971 and 1975 were traced and their stored serum was tested for HCV markers. Available patients (some aware and some unaware of their diagnosis) were interviewed and completed the SF-36 questionnaire. It was interesting to note that individuals who were aware of their diagnosis ($n = 15$) rated significantly worse on seven out of eight of the standard SF-36 scales than a control Australian population, while individuals unaware of their serostatus ($n = 19$) scored significantly worse on only three scales. There were no other epidemiologic, physical, or biochemical differences between the two groups. In support of these findings, when 1286 rural Egyptians who were unaware of their HCV status were prospectively interviewed by blinded investigators using the SF-12 QoL questionnaire, the 146 who turned out to be infected scored similar results to the 1140 individuals who were HCV-negative [68].

Two other interesting studies looked at patients presenting with chronic fatigue syndrome [69,70] where HCV status was assessed retrospectively to avoid the psychological effects of knowing about the HCV infection. Neither study reported an association between chronic fatigue and HCV infection. This effect of the knowledge of the diagnosis on health-related QoL has been reported in many other chronic diseases. For instance, normotensive subjects who had been misdiagnosed with hypertension were substantially more likely (30% vs. 8%) to have symptoms of depression than matched unlabelled normotensive control subjects [71].

In many of the studies mentioned above that suggest a positive effect of antiviral therapy on health-related QoL measures, mixed groups of patients were included but we are now aware that injecting drug users have additional health-related QoL issues to patients who acquired the virus through blood transfusion or via iatrogenic routes [29]. Differences between race and ethnic groups that may be related to the route of infection also have different impacts on QoL. While most studies from North America and Europe show a significant reduction in health-related QoL measures in patients infected with HCV, some studies from other parts of the world like Japan for instance do not show this [26,27]. The study from Egypt by Schwarzinger et al. [68] also did not show a significant difference, once again suggesting a strong ethnic influence.

Table 27.3 Common symptoms and suggested interventions.

Symptom	Intervention
Fatigue	No clear effective interventions for fatigue in patients with liver disease other than the ones mentioned in the general approach
Sleep abnormalities	• Treat primary sleep disorder if present • Sleeping and waking up at specific times • Avoiding coffee after 6 p.m. • Avoiding excess alcohol
Restless leg syndrome	• Check ferritin and thyroid function and treat if abnormal • Trial of pramipexole or pregabalin
Cognitive abnormalities	• Check for medication side effects • Consider neurology or psychiatry referral

Based on this literature, it is difficult to reach a definite conclusion on the effect of antiviral therapy on QoL of patients infected with HCV. Nonetheless, based on the available evidence, it is safe to infer that antiviral therapy has a positive effect on QoL. Whether this is directly related to the clearing of the virus itself or to other associated factors is unclear.

Specific interventions with possible benefits

Other than the general management approach explained here, there are some interventions that have shown some benefits in managing specific symptoms. These are summarized in Table 27.3.

Conclusions

Patients with cirrhosis develop many serious complications such as ascites, bacterial peritonitis, variceal bleeding, and hepatic encephalopathy. Although these complications significantly compromise the QoL and functional capacity of these patients, a number of other less well-recognized and harder to discover systemic symptoms and disease entities also have a significant role. These symptoms vary across a wide range of physical, psychologic, and social domains. It is therefore extremely important that physicians managing patients with liver disease and cirrhosis are able to recognize these systemic symptoms and disease entities early. It is also important to address these issues through a multidisciplinary team of healthcare providers who are able to have different professional roles in managing these symptoms in a clear, stepwise, and structured approach.

Acknowledgement

We would like to thank Ms Safiyya Ali for providing editorial assistance.

References

1 Newton JL, Jones DE, Henderson E, et al. Fatigue in non-alcoholic fatty liver disease (NAFLD) is significant and associates with inactivity and excessive daytime sleepiness but not with liver disease severity or insulin resistance. Gut 2008;57:807–13.
2 Gutteling JJ, de Man RA, Busschbach JJ, Darlington AS. Overview of research on health-related quality of life in patients with chronic liver disease. Neth J Med 2007;65:227–34.
3 Groeneweg M, Quero JC, De Bruijn I, et al. Subclinical hepatic encephalopathy impairs daily functioning. Hepatology 1998;28:45–9.
4 Younossi ZM, Guyatt G, Kiwi M, Boparai N, King D. Development of a disease specific questionnaire to measure health related quality of life in patients with chronic liver disease. Gut 1999;45:295–300.
5 Dan AA, Kallman JB, Wheeler A, et al. Health-related quality of life in patients with non-alcoholic fatty liver disease. Aliment Pharmacol Ther 2007;26:815–20.
6 Ware JE Jr. Sherbourne CD. The MOS 36-item short-form health survey (SF-36). I. Conceptual framework and item selection. Med Care 1992;30:473–83.
7 Arguedas MR, DeLawrence TG, McGuire BM. Influence of hepatic encephalopathy on health-related quality of life in patients with cirrhosis. Dig Dis Sci 2003;48:1622–6.
8 Sobhonslidsuk A, Silpakit C, Kongsakon R, Satitpornkul P, Sripetch C. Chronic liver disease questionnaire: translation and validation in Thais. World J Gastroenterol 2004;10:1954–7.
9 Prasad S, Dhiman RK, Duseja A, Chawla YK, Sharma A, Agarwal R. Lactulose improves cognitive functions and health-related quality of life in patients with cirrhosis who have minimal hepatic encephalopathy. Hepatology 2007;45:549–59.
10 Sidhu SS, Goyal O, Mishra BP, Sood A, Chhina RS, Soni RK. Rifaximin improves psychometric performance and health-related quality of life in patients with minimal hepatic encephalopathy (the RIME Trial). Am J Gastroenterol 2011;106:307–16.

11 Cella D, Yount S, Rothrock N, et al. The Patient-Reported Outcomes Measurement Information System (PROMIS): progress of an NIH Roadmap cooperative group during its first two years. Med Care 2007;45(Suppl 1):S3–S11.

12 Fries JF, Cella D, Rose M, Krishnan E, Bruce B. Progress in assessing physical function in arthritis: PROMIS short forms and computerized adaptive testing. J Rheumatol 2009;36: 2061–6.

13 Newton JL, Jones DE. Managing systemic symptoms in chronic liver disease. J Hepatol 2012;56 (Suppl 1): S46–55.

14 Scott PJ. Participation in valued roles post-liver transplant. Br J Occup Ther 2010;73:517–23.

15 Newton JL, Hudson M, Tachtatzis P, et al. Population prevalence and symptom associations of autonomic dysfunction in primary biliary cirrhosis. Hepatology 2007;45:1496–505.

16 Elliott C, Frith J, Pairman J, Jones DEJ, Newton JL. Reduction in functional ability is significant postliver transplantation compared with matched liver disease and community dwelling controls. Transpl Int 2011;24:588–95.

17 Foster GR. Hepatitis C virus infection: quality of life and side effects of treatment. J Hepatol 1999;31(Suppl 1):250–4.

18 Bonkovsky HL, Woolley JM. Reduction of health-related quality of life in chronic hepatitis C and improvement with interferon therapy. The Consensus Interferon Study Group. Hepatology 1999;29:264–70.

19 Ware JE Jr, Bayliss MS, Mannocchia M, Davis GL. Health-related quality of life in chronic hepatitis C: impact of disease and treatment response. The Interventional Therapy Group. Hepatology 1999;30:550–5.

20 Foster GR, Goldin RD, Thomas HC. Chronic hepatitis C virus infection causes a significant reduction in quality of life in the absence of cirrhosis. Hepatology 1998;27:209–12.

21 Iwasaki M, Kanda D, Toyoda M, et al. Absence of specific symptoms in chronic hepatitis C. J Gastroenterol 2002;37: 709–16.

22 Fukuhara S, Hino K, Tomita E, Yuasa S, Okushin H. Health-related QOL in patients with chronic liver disease type-C. [In Japanese with English abstract] Acta Hepatol Jpn 1997; 38:587–95.

23 Davis GL, Balart LA, Schiff ER, et al. Assessing health-related quality of life in chronic hepatitis C using the Sickness Impact Profile. Clin Ther 1994;16:334–43; discussion 271–2.

24 Shakil AO, Conry-Cantilena C, Alter HJ, et al. Volunteer blood donors with antibody to hepatitis C virus: clinical, biochemical, virologic, and histologic features. The Hepatitis C Study Group. Ann Intern Med 1995;123:330–7.

25 Wessely S, Pariante C. Fatigue, depression and chronic hepatitis C infection. Psychol Med 2002;32:1–10.

26 Abdo AA. Hepatitis C and poor quality of life: is it the virus or the patient? Saudi J Gastroenterol 2008;14:109–13.

27 Tong MJ, el-Farra NS, Reikes AR, Co RL. Clinical outcomes after transfusion-associated hepatitis C. N Engl J Med 1995;332:1463–6.

28 Kenny-Walsh E. Clinical outcomes after hepatitis C infection from contaminated anti-D immune globulin. Irish Hepatology Research Group. N Engl J Med 1999;340:1228–33.

29 Barkhuizen A, Rosen HR, Wolf S, Flora K, Benner K, Bennett RM. Musculoskeletal pain and fatigue are associated with chronic hepatitis C: a report of 239 hepatology clinic patients. Am J Gastroenterol 1999;94:1355–60.

30 Poynard T, Cacoub P, Ratziu V, et al. Fatigue in patients with chronic hepatitis C. J Viral Hepat 2002;9:295–303.

31 Al-Rifai A, Prince M, Henderson E, Jones D, Newton J, Hudson M. Fatigue in PSC patients with and without inflammatry bowel disease. Hepatology 2009;50:1004A–5A.

32 Bjornsson E, Simren M, Olsson R, Chapman RW. Fatigue in patients with primary sclerosing cholangitis. Scand J Gastroenterol 2004;39:961–8.

33 Jones DE, Gray JC, Newton J. Perceived fatigue is comparable between different disease groups. Q J Med 2009;102: 617–24.

34 Werner M, Wallerstedt S, Lindgren S, et al. Characteristics and long-term outcome of patients with autoimmune hepatitis related to the initial treatment response. Scand J Gastroenterol 2010;45:457–67.

35 Lang CA, Conrad S, Garrett L, et al. Symptom prevalence and clustering of symptoms in people living with chronic hepatitis C infection. J Pain Symptom Manage 2006;31:335–44.

36 Newton JL, Gibson GJ, Tomlinson M, Wilton K, Jones D. Fatigue in primary biliary cirrhosis is associated with excessive daytime somnolence. Hepatology 2006;44:91–8.

37 Sockalingam S, Abbey SE, Alosaimi F, Novak M. A review of sleep disturbance in hepatitis C. J Clin Gastroenterol 2010;44:38–45.

38 Hardy T, MacDonald C, Jones DE, Newton JL. A follow-up study of modafinil for the treatment of daytime somnolence and fatigue in primary biliary cirrhosis. Liver Int 2010;30: 1551–2.

39 Ahmed MH, Byrne CD. Obstructive sleep apnea syndrome and fatty liver: association or causal link? World J Gastroenterol 2010;16:4243–52.

40 Shpirer I, Copel L, Broide E, Elizur A. Continuous positive airway pressure improves sleep apnea associated fatty liver. Lung 2010;188:301–7.

41 Dwight MM, Kowdley KV, Russo JE, Ciechanowski PS, Larson AM, Katon WJ. Depression, fatigue, and functional disability in patients with chronic hepatitis C. J Psychosom Res 2000;49:311–7.

42 Lehman CL, Cheung RC. Depression, anxiety, post-traumatic stress, and alcohol-related problems among veterans with chronic hepatitis C. Am J Gastroenterol 2002;97:2640–6.

43 Fontana RJ, Hussain KB, Schwartz SM, Moyer CA, Su GL, Lok AS. Emotional distress in chronic hepatitis C patients not receiving antiviral therapy. J Hepatol 2002;36:401–7.

44 Carta MG, Hardoy MC, Garofalo A, et al. Association of chronic hepatitis C with major depressive disorders: irrespective of

interferon-alpha therapy. Clin Pract Epidemiol Ment Health 2007;3:22.

45 McDonald C, Newton J, Lai HM, Baker SN, Jones DE. Central nervous system dysfunction in primary biliary cirrhosis and its relationship to symptoms. J Hepatol 2010;53:1095–100.

46 Hollingsworth KG, Jones DE, Aribisala BS, et al. Globus pallidus magnetization transfer ratio, T(1) and T(2) in primary biliary cirrhosis: relationship with disease stage and age. J Magn Reson Imaging 2009;29:780–4.

47 Newton JL, Hollingsworth KG, Taylor R, et al. Cognitive impairment in primary biliary cirrhosis: symptom impact and potential etiology. Hepatology 2008;48:541–9.

48 Fattakhova G, Jones D, Frith F, Day C, Newton J. Cognitive symptoms are prevalent in non-alcoholic fatty liver disease (NAFLD) and unrelated to the severity of liver disease. Hepatology 2009;50:787A–8A.

49 McAndrews MP, Farcnik K, Carlen P, et al. Prevalence and significance of neurocognitive dysfunction in hepatitis C in the absence of correlated risk factors. Hepatology 2005;41: 801–8.

50 Wilkinson J, Radkowski M, Eschbacher JM, Laskus T. Activation of brain macrophages/microglia cells in hepatitis C infection. Gut 2010;59:1394–400.

51 Jones DE, Hollingsworth K, Fattakhova G, et al. Impaired cardiovascular function in primary biliary cirrhosis. Am J Physiol Gastrointest Liver Physiol. 2010 May; 298(5): G764–73.

52 Perseghin G, Lattuada G, De Cobelli F, et al. Increased mediastinal fat and impaired left ventricular energy metabolism in young men with newly found fatty liver. Hepatology 2008;47:51–8.

53 Frith J, Newton JL. Autonomic dysfunction in chronic liver disease. Liver Int 2009;29:483–9.

54 Goldblatt J, James OF, Jones DE. Grip strength and subjective fatigue in patients with primary biliary cirrhosis. JAMA 2001;285:2196–7.

55 Newton JL, Pairman J, Wilton K, Jones DE, Day C. Fatigue and autonomic dysfunction in non-alcoholic fatty liver disease. Clin Auton Res 2009;19:319–26.

56 Newton JL, Davidson A, Kerr S, et al. Autonomic dysfunction in primary biliary cirrhosis correlates with fatigue severity. Eur J Gastroenterol Hepatol 2007;19:125–32.

57 Osztovits J, Horvath T, Abonyi M, et al. Chronic hepatitis C virus infection associated with autonomic dysfunction. Liver Int 2009;29:1473–8.

58 Salerno F, Cazzaniga M. Autonomic dysfunction: often present but usually ignored in patients with liver disease. Liver Int 2009;29:1451–3.

59 Oliver MI, Miralles R, Rubies-Prat J, et al. Autonomic dysfunction in patients with non-alcoholic chronic liver disease. J Hepatol 1997;26:1242–8.

60 Patanwala I, Newton J, Elliot C, et al. P20 Functional capacity is significantly impaired in primary biliary cirrhosis and related to orthostatic symptoms. Gut 2010;59(Suppl 2): A19–A20.

61 Hassanein T, Cooksley G, Sulkowski M, et al. The impact of peginterferon alfa-2a plus ribavirin combination therapy on health-related quality of life in chronic hepatitis C. J Hepatol 2004;40:675–81.

62 McHutchison JG, Ware JE Jr, Bayliss MS, et al. The effects of interferon alpha-2b in combination with ribavirin on health related quality of life and work productivity. J Hepatol 2001;34:140–7.

63 Desmorat H, Combis JM, Pradat P. [Assessment of quality of life in chronic hepatitis C: effect of treatment]. Gastroenterol Clin Biol 2003;27:1084–90.

64 Bernstein D, Kleinman L, Barker CM, Revicki DA, Green J. Relationship of health-related quality of life to treatment adherence and sustained response in chronic hepatitis C patients. Hepatology 2002;35:704–8.

65 Mathew A, Peiffer LP, Rhoades K, McGarrity TJ. Improvement in quality of life measures in patients with refractory hepatitis C, responding to re-treatment with Pegylated interferon alpha-2b and ribavirin. Health Qual Life Outcomes 2006;4:30.

66 Bini EJ, Mehandru S. Sustained virological response rates and health-related quality of life after interferon and ribavirin therapy in patients with chronic hepatitis C virus infection and persistently normal alanine aminotransferase levels. Aliment Pharmacol Ther 2006;23:777–85.

67 Rodger AJ, Jolley D, Thompson SC, Lanigan A, Crofts N. The impact of diagnosis of hepatitis C virus on quality of life. Hepatology 1999;30:1299–301.

68 Schwarzinger M, Dewedar S, Rekacewicz C, et al. Chronic hepatitis C virus infection: does it really impact health-related quality of life? A study in rural Egypt. Hepatology 2004;40:1434–41.

69 Dale JK, Di Bisceglie AM, Hoofnagle JH, Straus SE. Chronic fatigue syndrome: lack of association with hepatitis C virus infection. J Med Virol 1991;34:119–21.

70 Mawle AC, Nisenbaum R, Dobbins JG, et al. Seroepidemiology of chronic fatigue syndrome: a case–control study. Clin Infect Dis 1995;21:1386–9.

71 Johnston ME, Gibson ES, Terry CW, et al. Effects of labelling on income, work and social function among hypertensive employees. J Chronic Dis 1984;37:417–23.

72 Johns MW. Sleepiness in different situations measured by the Epworth Sleepiness Scale. Sleep 1994;17:703–10.

73 Buysse DJ, Reynolds CF 3rd, Monk TH, Berman SR, Kupfer DJ. The Pittsburgh Sleep Quality Index: a new instrument for psychiatric practice and research. Psychiatry Res 1989;28: 193–213.

74 Schrezenmaier C, Gehrking JA, Hines SM, Low PA, Benrud-Larson LM, Sandroni P. Evaluation of orthostatic hypotension: relationship of a new self-report instrument to laboratory-based measures. Mayo Clin Proc 2005;80:330–4.

CHAPTER 28

Special considerations in children

Alejandro Costaguta[1] and Fernando Alvarez[2]
[1]Sanatorio de Niños, Santa Fe, Argentina
[2]Department of Pediatrics, CHU- Sainte Justine, University of Montreal, Quebec, Canada

Introduction

The diagnosis and management of cirrhosis in pediatric patients requires special considerations. Different etiologies, unique nutritional requirements, age-specific complications related to different stages of growth and development, as well as size constraints to adapt therapeutic procedures to small children are some of the particularities observed in children.

Cirrhosis associated with chronic cholestasis is the most prevalent category at the pediatric age group with the majority of cases resulting from biliary atresia, but cystic fibrosis and progressive familial intrahepatic cholestasis (PFIC) are also seen, among others. Cirrhosis secondary to chronic cholestasis is characterized by a variable time of development, from months to years, and frequently by relatively well-preserved liver synthetic function associated with symptoms and signs of portal hypertension [1].

Children grow and develop due to a complex interplay between hormones and nutrients in which the liver has a central role. Interference in this process often leads to permanent growth and development problems, even after removing the cause (Figure 28.1). Particular concerns have been expressed for some disorders occurring during this critical period of life, which could lead to neurodevelopmental disorders and bone disease [2–4].

Small children (weighing 10 kg or less) constitute a significant proportion of pediatric cirrhotic patients. Dealing with specific complications like variceal hemorrhage poses special challenges because of the need to adapt procedures developed for adult patients. Endoscopic variceal ligation or transjugular intrahepatic portosystemic shunt (TIPS) are common examples of therapeutic approaches that are difficult to apply at this age.

Management strategies for children with cirrhosis vary according to the natural history of the disease entity. Therefore, this chapter highlights individual disorders leading to cirrhosis in the hope of earlier diagnosis and improved management strategies.

Particular liver diseases in children (Table 28.1)

Chronic cholestasis

Biliary atresia

This necroinflammatory and obliterative process of the biliary tree, with an incidence of 1 in 10 000–15 000 newborn infants, constitutes the single most common indication for liver transplantation among children. An enigmatic characteristic of this entity is the rapid progression of fibrosis, leading to cirrhosis in the first weeks of life. A combination of genetic and environmental factors has been proposed to explain it, giving rise to a particularly intense fibrogenesis driven by an ongoing immune activation that may persist even after surgical restoration of bile flow [5,6]. After the Kasai portoenterostomy >50% of patients will clear jaundice if surgery is performed before 60 days of age but, unfortunately, almost all will already show an advanced stage of fibrosis or cirrhosis by that time (Figure 28.2) [7].

For patients who remain icteric (i.e., total serum bilirubin >2 mg% at 3 months post Kasai), liver transplantation should be offered as soon as possible, because chances of survival beyond the second year are nil [8,9]. There is no other example in hepatology in which

Cirrhosis: A practical guide to management, First Edition. Edited by Samuel S. Lee and Richard Moreau.

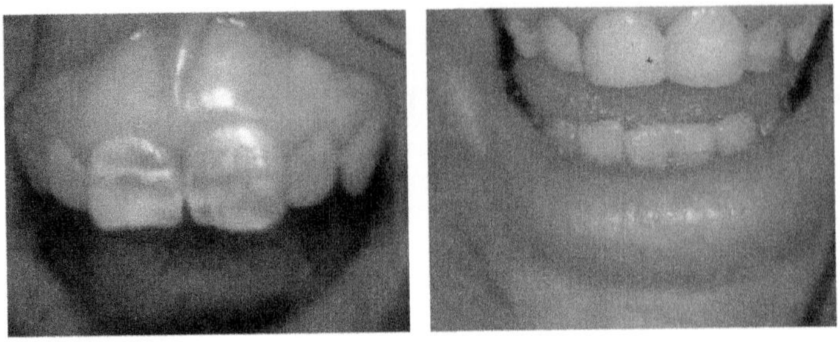

Figure 28.1 Teeth in a 12-year-old (left), and a 14-year-old (right) child with biliary atresia transplanted at the age of 6 and 8 years, respectively, because of liver failure. Permanent teeth were stained by deposition of bilirubin in dental hard tissues during their maturation. (See colour plate section.)

Table 28.1 Causes of cirrhosis in children classified according to their pathogenic mechanism.

Cholestatic causes
Biliary atresia
Cystic fibrosis
Progressive intrahepatic familial cholestasis
Histiocytosis X
Liver inflammatory diseases
Hepatitis
• Chronic hepatitis B
• Chronic hepatitis C
• Autoimmune hepatitis
Metabolic disorders
Alpha-1-antitrypsine deficiency
Wilson's disease
Glycogenosis types III and IX
Glycogenosis type IV
Tyrosinemia
Niemann–Pick type C
Toxic disorders (nutritional)
Total parenteral nutrition (TPN)

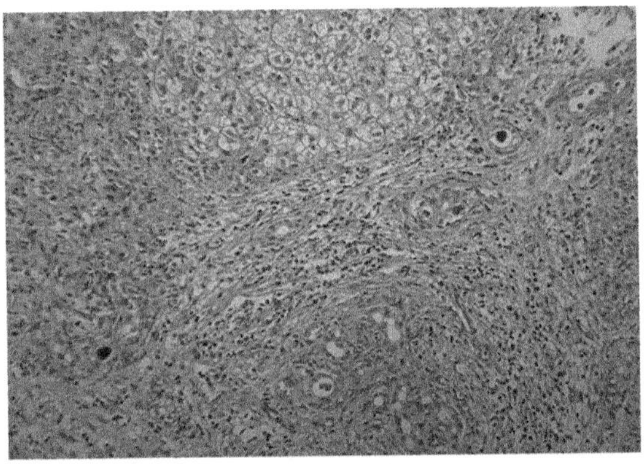

Figure 28.2 Liver biopsy (H&E staining) from a 2-month-old patient with biliary atresia, showing a rapid evolution to cirrhosis. Practically all patients with biliary atresia develop cirrhosis during the first year of life. (See colour plate section.)

the outcome can be predicted with such precision. Children who normalize serum bilirubin levels, on the other hand, face a variable clinical course mainly influenced by the presence of complications from portal hypertension, such as variceal hemorrhage, ascites, and hypersplenism. Bacterial cholangitis is a universal threat, and is associated with the worsening of fibrosis and portal hypertension, especially when recurrent episodes occur. Fifty per cent of this "initial success" group will need liver transplantation in the following years, due to complications from end-stage liver disease leaving only 20–25% of children with biliary atresia to reach adulthood with their native livers, having an almost normal life in the context of compensated cirrhosis [10–12].

Cystic fibrosis

This multiorgan disease is produced by mutations in the *CFTR* gene encoding the membrane protein, CFTR (cystic fibrosis transmembrane regulator) responsible for the efflux of chloride through the cell membrane. As a result, inspissated secretions are produced in exocrine glands with plugging and obstruction followed by activation of the inflammatory cascade, and eventually, secondary infection which stimulates the vicious circle of inflammation and destruction [13]. Liver disease occurs because the CFTR is expressed at the apical level of cholangiocytes, and the consequent biliary obstruction by the inspissated bile is followed by local deposition of collagen, giving rise to the characteristic "focal biliary cirrhosis," a hallmark of the disease [14]. This initial focal lesion eventually progresses to a multilobular cirrhosis in an estimated 5–10% of all patients with cystic fibrosis. Contributing factors involved in such progression are essentially unknown, but environmental and genetic modifiers have recently been implicated [15,16].

As survival of patients with cystic fibrosis improves due to better control of pulmonary and nutritional complications, liver disease becomes more relevant to the long-term outcome, being the third most common cause of mortality [17,18]. Cystic fibrosis liver disease is difficult to detect in its early stages because of its focal nature, hence an active work-up should be implemented involving physical findings (hepatomegaly, splenomegaly), biochemical tests, and ultrasound examination at regular intervals [19]. Liver biopsy can help in the diagnosis of liver fibrosis, although the patchy distribution of the lesions is frequently misleading and not routinely recommended by all centers caring for these patients. Cohorts followed in this way reveal that around 5% will develop clinically significant liver disease, almost all before the age of 15 which means that severe cystic fibrosis liver disease is a pediatric condition [20]. Ursodeoxycolic acid (UDCA) has been used for many years, in an attempt to halt the progression of the disease. Despite initial enthusiasm produced by some improvement in biochemical liver tests, changes in significant clinical outcomes have not been confirmed in the long term. Starting this drug in earlier stages of disease is an appealing alternative, but better tests are needed to identify patients who could benefit from it. Nevertheless, UDCA is generally used because of its safety profile and theoretical benefits in the absence of better alternatives [14].

Owing to the well-preserved synthetic liver function and multi-organ character of the disease, the best approach to manage complications from portal hypertension in patients with cystic fibrosis is controversial. Variceal hemorrhage represents a life-threatening complication usually controlled by endoscopic and pharmacologic treatments, but its recurrent tendency makes repetitive anesthetic procedures necessary in patients who are poor candidates because of suboptimal pulmonary function [21]. Moreover, hypersplenism tends to be particularly severe in patients with cystic fibrosis, who often exhibit huge and sometimes painful splenomegaly that is not resolved by endoscopic treatment. Surgical shunts or, when feasible, TIPS, offer the possibility of decompressing the portal tree and have been used for a long time in selected patients. However, concerns exist over the possible consequences in the pulmonary vascular bed and the risk of encephalopathy to which patients with cystic fibrosis are especially prone. Liver transplantation has the potential of being "curative" of cystic fibrosis liver disease, but patients should be carefully selected, and only those with a well-preserved pulmonary function should be considered. Results of single liver transplantation are very encouraging, with survival rates similar to other more common indications [17,22].

Progressive familial intrahepatic cholestasis

PFIC constitutes a heterogeneous group of diseases formerly called Byler's disease and characterized by intracellular cholestasis due to molecular defects interfering with bile formation [23]. The group exhibits signs of cholestasis from the first months of life, evolving rapidly to end-stage liver disease in a significant number of affected children. Biochemical and genetic differences allow classification into three main subtypes with different natural histories, leading to cirrhosis and liver failure mainly in the pediatric age group [24,25].

Affected patients with low gamma-glutamyl transpeptidase (GGT) levels could belong to one of two categories: FIC1 defects (*ATP8B1* mutation) or BSEP defects (*ABCB11* mutation). In the first group, the disorder is not confined to the liver given the expression of FIC1 in other cell types, particularly enterocytes and pancreatic acinar cells [26]. Phenotypic characteristics include jaundice and pruritus starting in the first months of life, typically with little impairment of liver function for many years, but with a profound impact on the quality of life, similar to recurrent benign cholestasis in the adult, which constitutes the other end of the spectrum [27,28]. Eventually, progressive fibrosis leading to complications ensues, and the decision to proceed to liver transplantation must be carefully considered given the risk of post-transplant complications in this group, like intractable diarrhea, recurrent pancreatitis, and graft steatosis. Partial external biliary diversion has been considered a better approach and should be offered early to these children [29]. Children bearing mutations in BSEP also exhibit normal GGT levels, but their clinical picture tends to be more aggressive, with progressive cholestasis and signs of liver failure during the first years. Therapy with UDCA or external diversion of bile should be offered first to these patients [30,31]. As the disease is confined to the liver, in contrast to FIC1 patients, transplantation is a *curative* option when decompensation ensues or there is suspicion of hepatocellular carcinoma, which is a worrying complication in the long term [25,32]. Milder forms have also been described [28,33], and adults with mutations in *ABCB11* and a picture of benign recurrent cholestasis have been well documented [34], highlighting the many different expressions of this entity. Recurrent cholestasis after liver transplantation has been described, secondary to an immune-related reactivity against the BSEP protein that was not expressed in the native liver [35].

Patients with high GGT levels and a normal biliary tree usually have a defect in the *MDR3* gene, giving rise to mutations in the MDR3 transporter which reduces the concentration of phospholipids in bile. Phospholipids are necessary to buffer the detergent effects of bile salts on the cholangiocyte plasma membranes. This explains a picture of generalized damage to the intrahepatic biliary tree, with a characteristic histologic picture of portal fibrosis and cholangiolar proliferation akin to obstructive bile duct diseases [36]. The clinical spectrum of the disease, again, is very broad, from neonatal cholestasis to adult cirrhosis [37]. Affected children exhibit a biochemical picture of cholestasis with variable degrees of jaundice and pruritus in the context of portal hypertension. Management is usually directed to control the complications of portal hypertension and chronic cholestasis [30]. For those who exhibit some degree of liver failure, liver transplantation is an option [38].

As a group, PFIC constitutes a growing category of diseases with a very heterogeneous picture for which a tailored approach should be taken in each case. Genotype–phenotype associations are being unraveled and as more detailed genetic testing is conducted, overlap among different categories is becoming evident, and is the focus of intense research. In addition, studies on protein sorting have led to new forms of therapy [25,39–41].

Langerhans cell histiocytosis

Progressive cholestasis has been described in children with Langerhans cell histiocytosis who go on to develop primary sclerosing cholangitis (PSC). This uncommon association should be suspected and investigated in every patient having this form of histiocytosis associated with abnormal liver tests (mainly increased GGT levels), as specific treatment protocols can result in stabilization and eventually remission of the liver disease. Progression of the disease leads to cirrhosis and development of life-threatening complications, for which liver transplantation becomes necessary. Survival rates have been comparable to other more common indications, and no relapse of the original disease has been reported so far in the transplanted liver [42]. Although this is typically a pediatric disease, rare cases among adult patients have also been reported [43].

Chronic liver inflammation

Autoimmune hepatitis

Autoimmune hepatitis (AIH) is a necroinflammatory disease of the liver of unknown etiology progressing, if untreated, to cirrhosis and liver failure in many patients. Characteristic presence of circulating autoantibodies distinguishes two types of AIH: patients with type 1 AIH have anti-smooth muscle antibodies or antinuclear factor, whereas anti-liver-kidney microsome or liver cytosol antibodies define type 2 AIH. Forty percent of type 1 AIH, and 80% of cases of type 2 AIH are diagnosed before the age of 18 years, which means that this is primarily a pediatric disease [44].

AIH is a fluctuating disease characterized by alternating periods of remission and relapses and a silent course occasionally showing a "hepatitis-like" picture with malaise, jaundice, and dark urine. Affected patients commonly develop a firm liver, with a prominent left lobe. Splenomegaly, spider nevi, palmar erythema, and occasionally ascites are signs of chronicity and should alert the physician to consider AIH among differential diagnoses. Acute liver failure, or acute decompensation of a chronic condition, can also be a form of presentation, in approximately 10% of patients [45]. Unfortunately, in a substantial number of patients, the interval from the first symptoms to the diagnosis is longer than expected, allowing the inflammatory liver injury to progress to more advanced stages of fibrosis before an effective treatment is implemented (Figure 28.3) [46].

Bile duct lesions can be seen in 20% of patients with AIH, as part of an exuberant inflammatory infiltrate of the portal tract without any abnormal changes in cholangiograms. Caution should be applied when dealing with these patients, as true bile duct lesions do not respond to immunosuppressive treatment. In addition, when stenosis and dilatation of bile ducts are observed, even in the presence of an inflammatory infiltrate similar to that found in livers from patients with AIH, the

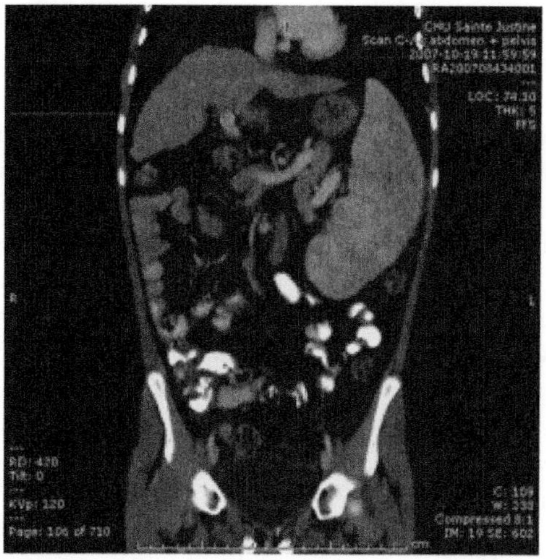

Figure 28.3 Magnetic resonance image of the abdomen of a 14-year-old girl with late diagnosis of autoimmune hepatitis showing nodular liver atrophy and large splenomegaly secondary to portal hypertension (spleen length 173 mm).

long-term outcome is that of PSC. Differential diagnosis is not always easy, considering that 30% of children with PSC show at onset characteristic features of AIH, such as the presence of autoantibodies, raised serum IgG, and interface hepatitis on histology, probably as a result of an unspecific inflammatory activation [44].

Ultimately, 40–90% of patients develop cirrhosis, with the differences probably related to the type of diagnostic procedures. When using strict histologic criteria, needle biopsy is far from ideal because the size of the sample limits the detection of large nodules so common in this post-necrotic process. Instead, laparoscopic-guided biopsy could overcome the problem, although this procedure must be reserved to special circumstances [47,48].

Immunosuppression induces remission of the disease in 80–90% of patients, for which the long-term prognosis is excellent as long as patients adhere to treatment [46,49]. There is evidence of regression of fibrosis and even cirrhosis in many of these patients, highlighting the importance of an early diagnosis in order not to delay treatment [50].

For those patients in whom there is progression of the disease despite treatment and for those not responding to therapy (approximately 10%), liver transplantation constitutes the last therapeutic alternative. A larger risk of late rejection has been described in these patients, therefore a closer follow-up and frequent adjustments of anti-rejection treatment are necessary [51]. Recent developments in the field of immunosuppressive treatment have helped to rescue formerly refractory patients, and are expected to reduce the number of liver transplantations in the near future [52,53].

Hepatitis B virus

Chronically infected children with hepatitis B virus (HBV) go through different stages in the natural history of the disease, according to the host–viral interaction. Seroconversion of e-antigen/anti-e antibody is a major event in this process and usually heralds the passage to a nonreplicative viral state. The duration of replicative state is directly related to the possibility of developing the most serious consequences of HBV liver disease (i.e., cirrhosis and hepatocellular carcinoma). The incidence of cirrhosis in HBV infected children has been estimated to be <4%, rising to 25% in those coinfected with the delta agent [54]. Well-documented cases of cirrhosis regression after long-term follow-up have been reported [55]. Children infected by vertical transmission tend to have a longer immunotolerant stage, and develop complications later than horizontally infected ones, probably as a consequence of a less vigorous immune response at the time of infection [56].

Hepatitis C virus

Hepatitis C vius (HCV) infection in children tends to run a milder course than in adults. Cohorts followed many decades after perinatal acquisition of the virus show a predominant asymptomatic state with normal or near-normal alanine aminotransferase (ALT) values [57]. Minimal histologic changes are the rule, with a prevalence of cirrhosis estimated in only 1–2% of patients. The frequency of HCV-related disease as an indication for liver transplantation among children is less than 1%, according to data from the Studies of Pediatric Liver Transplantation (SPLIT) database, in open contrast with the adult population. These data tend to confirm the idea of a relatively benign disease in the pediatric age group [58]. Differences in the rate of progression are probably related to less exposure to comorbidities, like alcohol and steatosis.

Metabolic (inherited) diseases of the liver

Alpha-1-antitrypsin deficiency

This autosomal recessive disorder is the most common genetic cause of neonatal cholestasis, with a frequency of 1 in 1500–2000 live births in Western countries. Liver disease is mainly associated with a particular structural variant of A1AT named Pi ZZ according to its characteristic migration pattern on protein electrophoresis. This mutated protein becomes misfolded, then forms aggregates that precipitate into the endoplasmic reticulum, and activate a cascade of events ending in cellular death and inflammatory response [59]. Thus, liver damage derives from the presence of the anomalous protein inside the liver cell, which has clear therapeutic implications.

Affected infants with A1AT deficiency (Pi ZZ) face different outcomes. The only population-based study showed that 17% presented with neonatal cholestasis, with nearly 20% of them developing cirrhosis some years later. The long-term outcome for the entire cohort was generally good, however, as 85% of patients showed no signs of liver disease at 18 years of age [60]. Specialized referral centers have reported an incidence of cirrhosis of 40% among A1AT PiZZ deficient patients [61]. Most children followed in those centers developed neonatal cholestasis and cleared the jaundice after a few months, but persisted with altered liver function test results. Thus, A1AT deficiency should be ruled out in any patient with cirrhosis of unknown etiology, especially in those with previous history of cholestasis in infancy. Associated pulmonary and renal disease has been described in a significant number of patients around 10 years of age [62].

Enzymatic replacement is not a therapeutic option in A1AT associated liver disease, because damage is produced by the accumulation of the intracellular misfolded protein (seen as diastase-resistant PAS-positive globules on microscopy). Currently, liver transplantation offers the only "curative" treatment, when decompensated cirrhosis ensues. Factors predicting long-term prognosis have not been fully elucidated; the disease runs a very variable course among different individuals so this has been a difficult task. Persistent jaundice and clotting deficiencies are probably the best predictors of a poor outcome [62].

Wilson's disease

This genetic disease is produced by mutations in the *ATP7B* gene resulting in an absent or dysfunctional protein, "Wilson's ATPase", which is a Golgi transmembrane transporter of Cu, expressed in liver, kidneys, CNS, and placenta. As a result of its absence or malfunction, copper excretion in bile is impaired, and its intracellular accumulation of it leads to injury owing to its intrinsic toxicity [63].

Clinical expression covers a wide range, from primary hepatic to neurologic symptoms, but hepatic forms characteristically prevail in the pediatric age group. Liver disease can be silent, as in the screening of an index case, or it can manifest itself as a most devastating acute liver failure, highlighting the need to consider Wilson's disease in every child presenting with abnormal liver tests of unknown etiology. Such a statement is of particular relevance considering that treatment is available, and effective to avoid progression of cirrhosis to liver failure when started promptly.

As copper accumulates, liver biopsy shows steatosis, necroinflammatory changes, fibrosis, and, eventually, cirrhosis. Although this usually takes years to establish, cases have been recorded as early as at the age of 3. Diagnosis is based on the demonstration of altered copper metabolism. Low serum ceruloplasmin, and high 24-hour urinary copper excretion are the most reliable screening tests, the gold standard being the quantification of copper in liver tissue (>250 μg/g dry weight). Finally, the end-point is the sequencing of the *ATP7B* gene, not possible in emergency situations before starting a specific treatment [64,65].

Treatment is aimed at copper chelation, either with penicillamine or trientine administered orally. Zinc salts can be used as well, owing to its property to induce enterocyte metallothionein, a protein with high copper affinity that acts as a natural chelator fostering its loss with the normal shedding of enterocytes in feces. Patients presenting with decompensated cirrhosis or acute liver failure most probably need liver transplantation. However, it is worthwhile to try a course of chelation in newly diagnosed patients, giving them the possibility of a favorable outcome without liver transplantation even in the acute severe forms [64].

Hereditary tyrosinemia (tyrosinemia type I; fumarylacetoacetase deficiency)

This disease is produced by the absence of the enzyme fumarylacetoacetase, and is characterized by progressive liver damage, renal tubular dysfunction, and neurologic crisis.

Affected children can present with signs of liver disease starting during the first weeks of age, ranging from an acute liver failure "sepsis-like" to a more chronic form characterized by failure to thrive, bleeding tendency, and signs of portal hypertension. Serum ALT and bilirubin tend to be minimally raised. Histologic findings evolve from micronodular to macronodular cirrhosis, and development of hepatocellular carcinoma in 10–30% of patients during the first years of life. It should also be noted, however, that these figures differ according to the time of introduction of an effective treatment, which, in turn, depends on a timely diagnosis [66].

Availability of nitisinone since 1992 has produced a dramatic change on the course of the disease, in association with the neonatal diagnosis of the deficiency. Together with dietary restriction of phenylalanine and tyrosine, nitisinone allows control of the process in more than 90% of the patients, arresting the progression to cirrhosis (and probably hepatocellular carcinoma), stabilizing the renal disease, with almost complete disappearance of neurologic crises. These remarkable results should compel the clinician to consider tyrosinemia in every child with clinical and laboratory signs of liver disease, especially in the context of renal (signs of tubular dysfunction and nephrocalcinosis) and neurologic symptoms. For those who develop carcinoma, liver transplantation is the best option [67]. In some cases, considering the potential worsening by calcineurin inhibitors of an already diminished renal function, a combined liver–kidney transplant could be indicated.

Niemann–Pick type C disease

This genetic disease is produced by an altered intracellular transport of cholesterol for which the precise mechanism is still incompletely elucidated. In the first months of life it is part of the neonatal cholestasis syndrome, being the second most common genetic cause behind A1AT deficiency, explaining 8% of cases of "neonatal cholestasis," and 25% of "neonatal hepatitis-like syndrome" [68,69]. Affected infants can exhibit signs of severe liver impairment like ascites, jaundice, and hepatomegaly. Splenomegaly is a characteristic finding, persisting even after resolution of other signs, and serves as a useful marker when neurologic deterioration is the form of presentation.

Findings on liver biopsy show different degrees of hepatocellular cholestasis, ductal proliferation, progressive fibrosis, and cirrhosis. Ductopenia has also been described, probably associated with a worse prognosis.

Currently, there is no effective treatment for this lethal condition. Liver transplantation does not avoid progression of neurologic damage, and should not be offered to these patients.

Glycogen storage disease types III and IX

Occasional patients with these two glycogen storage disease (GSD) variants show fibrosis progressing to cirrhosis in later years, usually in adolescence or young adulthood [70]. Some affected children with GSD type III can also exhibit muscular disease including cardiomyopathy, detected by raised serum values of creatine phosphokinase. These patients should not be considered for liver transplantation, and dietary therapy aimed at sustaining normal levels of serum glucose through the use of frequent feedings with complex carbohydrates is the treatment of choice. For those with only liver involvement, liver transplantation can be an option if end-stage cirrhosis develops [71]. Similar criteria apply to some GSD type IX patients, who develop cirrhosis. Clinical differentiation among these forms is very difficult, and should be based on specific tests and mutation analysis.

Glycogen storage disease type IV

Also called amylopectinosis, this disease is produced by the absence of glycogen branching enzyme, giving rise to an amylopectin-like polysaccharide instead of normal glycogen, which is insoluble and accumulates mainly in liver, striated muscle, and heart, among other tissues. In the most common hepatic form, children present with signs of progressive liver disease and early cirrhosis during the first month of life, and the only effective treatment is liver transplantation (Figure 28.4). In spite of the good results obtained initially, concern has arisen after reports of fatal outcomes with progressive myocardial involvement following liver transplantation [72]. To date there are no effective ways to predict such dismal outcomes.

Toxic (nutritional) liver disease

Total parenteral nutrition-associated liver disease

The most feared complication of total parenteral nutrition (TPN) is the development of cholestatic liver disease; this is especially true in infants with extensive resections of the small bowel and in those with inherited chronic diarrhea syndromes. Although liver complications from TPN span all ages, neonates and infants are particularly susceptible to develop the most severe forms, like cirrhosis and end-stage liver disease. Owing to the complex

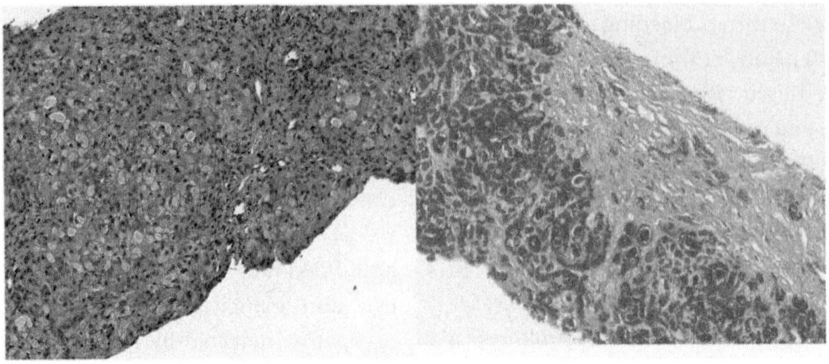

Figure 28.4 Early cirrhosis in a 6-month-old boy with glycogenosis type IV (H&E and PAS staining). (See colour plate section.)

nature of these patients, establishing a clear etiologic factor has proven elusive, and a multifactorial process is probably the best explanation. In that sense, prematurity, low birth weight, complete absence of enteral feedings, and septic complications are among the best known risk factors. Recently, some components of the administered solution have received particular attention as a significant cause of cholestasis, offering an attractive explanation for many affected patients [73].

Children who develop cholestasis during TPN are at high risk of rapid progress to portal fibrosis, cirrhosis, and decompensated liver failure. Persistent jaundice is usually the first ominous sign, with splenomegaly heralding advanced liver damage. Every effort should be made to stop progression of liver disease before cirrhosis is established, but unfortunately this is not possible in many cases because many of these patients cannot be weaned from TPN. Nevertheless, cycling perfusion, changing components of the formula, administering even minimal amounts of enteral feedings, and controlling every possible source of infection are rewarding measures that should be encouraged in every instance [74,75]. Administration of UDCA (20 mg/kg/day) is also a widely accepted therapy, unfortunately not available for intravenous administration. *N*-acetylcysteine has also been used in a similar fashion in this context. New developments in surgical techniques have allowed recovering of failing intestines through complex lengthening procedures that restore the capacity to tolerate oral feedings.

When all the above measures are insufficient, organ replacement becomes the only option. This is a complex decision, because liver disease is secondary to intestinal insufficiency, and consideration should be paid to whether liver alone, small bowel, or combined transplantation should be offered.

Conclusions

Several factors including the etiology of the liver disease in children with cirrhosis require special consideration, because of the large variety of disease entities and their variable natural history (Table 28.2). Most causes of cirrhosis considered in this chapter are exclusively detected or diagnosed in the pediatric age group. Follow-up of patients needs a detailed knowledge of the particular natural history of each of these diseases. Thanks to the improvement of care, less invasive diagnostic techniques to detect and quantify fibrosis, including the application of elastography in children, and the discovery of new treatments, most patients now reach adulthood and are currently being transferred to adult health centers. Pediatricians need to prepare their patients with chronic liver diseases for a smooth transition to adult healthcare facilities, encouraging them to be compliant for clinical visits and treatments. Unfortunately, transfer of patients has frequently been marked by nonadherence and absence of medical follow-up, resulting in adverse clinical outcomes. Hepatologists caring for these young adults

Table 28.2 Features to be considered in the management and follow-up of children with cirrhosis.

Etiology of the disease
Specific natural history
Disease stage at diagnosis
Status of growth and development
Particular nutritional deficiencies
Extrahepatic diseases
Complications of portal hypertension
Availability of therapeutic tools and local expertise
Early detection of liver failure

are thus confronted with a new challenge, and need to establish regular communication with their pediatric colleagues, as well as to update their knowledge and upgrade their experience in order to improve the quality of care given to pediatric patients transferred to them.

References

1 Leonis M, Balisteri W. Evaluation and management of end-stage liver disease in children. Gastroenterology 2008;134: 1741–51.

2 Caudle S, Katzenstein J, Karpen S, et al. Language and motor skills are impaired in infants with biliary atresia before transplantation. J Pediatr 2010;156:936–40.

3 Hogler W, Baumann U, Kelly D. Endocrine and bone metabolic complications in chronic liver disease and after liver transplantation in children. J Pediatr Gastroenterol Nutr 2012;54:313–21.

4 Alvarez F, Landrieu P, Feo C, et al. Vitamin E deficiency is responsible for neurologic abnormalities in cholestatic children. J Pediatr 1985;107:422–5.

5 Haafiz A. Liver fibrosis in biliary atresia. Expert Rev Gastroenterol Hepatol 2010;4:335–43.

6 Bezerra J. The next challenge in pediatric cholestasis: deciphering the pathogenesis of biliary atresia. J Pediatr Gastroenterol Nutr 2006;43:S23–9.

7 Weerasooriya V, White F, Sheperd R. Hepatic fibrosis and survival in biliary atresia. J Pediatr 2004;144:123–5.

8 Shneider B, Mazariegos J. Biliary atresia: a transplant perspective. Liver Transpl 2007;13:1482–95.

9 Hung P, Chen C, Chen W, et al. Long-term prognosis of patients with biliary atresia: a 25 year summary. J Pediatr Gastroenterol Nutr 2006;42:190–5.

10 Barshes N, Lee T, Balkrisham R, et al. Orthotopic liver transplantation for biliary atresia: the US experience. Liver Transpl 2005;11:1193–200.

11 Schreiber R, Barker C, Roberts E, et al. Biliary atresia: the Canadian experience. J Pediatr 2007;151:659–65.

12 Erlichman J, Hohlweg K, Haber B. Biliary atresia: how medical complications and therapies impact outcome. Expert Rev Gastroenterol Hepatol 2009;3:425–34.

13 Gaskin K. Exocrine pancreatic dysfunction: cystic fibrosis. In Walker WA, Goulet O, Kleinman RE, Sherman PM, Shneider BL, Sanderson IR (eds.) Pediatric Gastrointestinal Disease: Pathophysiology, Diagnosis, Management, 4th edn. BC Decker: Hamilton, 2004. pp. 1606–23.

14 Colombo C, Russo M, Zazzeron L, et al. Liver disease in cystic fibrosis. J Pediatr Gastroenterol Nutr 2006;43:S49–55.

15 Pereira T, Lewindon P, Greer R, et al. Transcriptional basis for hepatic fibrosis in cystic fibrosis-associated liver disease. J Pediatr Gastroenterol Nutr 2012;54:328–35.

16 Bartlett J, Friedman K, Ling S, et al. Genetic modifiers of liver disease in cystic fibrosis. JAMA 2009;302:1076–83.

17 Lamireau T, Martin S, Lallier M, et al. Liver transplantation for cirrhosis in cystic fibrosis. Can J Gastroenterol 2006; 20:475–8.

18 Colombo C, Battezzati P, Crosignani A, et al. Liver disease in cystic fibrosis: a prospective study on incidence, risk factors and outcome. Hepatology 2002;36:1374–82.

19 Patriquin H, Lenaerts C, Smith L, et al. Liver disease in children with cystic fibrosis: US-biochemical comparison in 195 patients. Radiology 1999;211; 229–32.

20 Lindblad A, Glaumann H, Strandvik B. Natural history of liver disease in cystic fibrosis. Hepatology 1999;30:1151–8.

21 Debray D, Lykavieris P, Gauthier F, et al. Outcome of cystic fibrosis-associate liver cirrhosis: management of portal hypertension. J Hepatol 1999;31:77–83.

22 Milkiewicz P, Skiba G, Kelly D, et al. Transplantation for cystic fibrosis: outcome following early liver transplantation. J Gastroenterol Hepatol 2002;17:208–13.

23 Balistreri W, Bezerra J. Whatever happened to "neonatal hepatitis"? Clin Liver Dis 2006;10:27–53.

24 Tomer G, Shneider B. Disorders of bile formation and biliary transport. Gastroenterol Clin N Am 2003;32:839–55.

25 Davit-Spraul A, Fabre M, Branchereau S, et al. ATP8B1 and ABCB11 analysis in 62 children with normal gamma-glutamyl transferase progressive familial cholestasis (PFIC): phenotypic differences between PFIC1 and PFIC2 natural history. Hepatology 2010;51:1645–55.

26 Dawson P. Liver disease without flipping: new functions of ATP8B1, the protein affected in familial intrahepatic cholestasis type 1. Hepatology 2010;51:1885–7.

27 van Mil S, Klomp L, Bull L, et al. FIC1 disease: a spectrum of intrahepatic cholestasis disorders. Sem Liver Dis 2001;21: 535–44.

28 Ooteghem N, Klomp L, van Berge-Henegouwen, et al. Benign recurrent intrahepatic cholestasis: low GGT cholestasis is a clinical continuum. J Hepatol 2002;36:439–43.

29 Shneider B. Progressive intrahepatic cholestasis: mechanisms, diagnosis and therapy. Pediatr Transplant 2004;8: 609–12.

30 Jacquemin E, Hermans D, Myara A, et al. Ursodesoxycolic acid therapy in pediatric patients with progressive intrahepatic cholestasis. Hepatology 1997;25:519–23.

31 Kurbegov A, Setchell K, Haas J, et al. Biliary diversion for progressive familial intrahepatic cholestasis: improved liver morphology and bile acid profile. Gastroenterology 2003; 125:1227–34.

32 Knisely A, Strautnieks S, Meier Y, et al. Hepatocellular carcinoma in ten children under five years of age with bile salt export pump deficiency. Hepatology 2006;44:478–86.

33 Hermeziu B, Sanlaville D, Girard M, et al. Heterozygous bile salt export pump deficiency: a possible genetic predisposition to transient neonatal cholestasis. J Pediatr Gastroenterol Nutr 2006;42:114–6.

34 Beausejour Y, Alvarez F, Beaulieu M, et al. Description of two new ABCB11 mutations responsible for type 2 benign recurrent intrahepatic cholestasis in a French-Canadian family. Can J Gastroenterol 2011;25:311–4.
35 Jara P, Hierro L, Martinez-Fernandez P, et al. Recurrence of bile salt export pump deficiency after liver transplantation. N Engl J Med 2009;361:1359–61.
36 Jacquemin E. Role of multidrug resistance 3 deficiency in pediatric and adult liver disease: one gene for three diseases. Sem Liver Dis 2001;21:551–62.
37 Jacquemin E, De Vree J, Cresteil D, et al. The wide spectrum of multidrug resistence 3 deficiency: from neonatal cholestasis to cirrhosis of adulthood. Gastroenterology 2001;120:1448–58.
38 Englert C, Grabhorn E, Richter A, et al. Liver transplantation in children with progressive familial intrahepatic cholestasis. Transplantation 2007;84:1361–3.
39 Strautnieks S, Byrne J, Pawlikowska L, et al. Severe bile salt export pump deficiency: 82 different ABCB11 mutations in 109 families. Gastroenterology 2008;134:1203–14.
40 Arnell H, Papadogiannakis N, Zemack H, et al. Follow-up in children with progressive familial intrahepatic cholestasis after partial external diversion. J Pediatr Gastroenterol Nutr 2010;51:494–9.
41 Gonzalez E, Grosse B, Cassio D, et al. Successful mutation-specific chaperone therapy with 4-phenylbutyrate in a child with progressive familial intrahepatic cholestasis type 2. J Hepatol 2012;57:695–8.
42 Braier J, Ciocca M, Latella A, et al. Cholestasis, sclerosing colangitis, and liver transplantation in Langerhans cell histiocytosis. Med Pediatr Oncol 2002;38:178–82.
43 Thompson H, Pitt H, Lewin K, et al. Sclerosing cholangitis and histiocytosis X. Gut 1984;25:526–30.
44 Alvarez F. Autoimmune hepatitis and primary sclerosing cholangitis. Clin Liver Dis 2006;10:89–107.
45 Gregorio G, Portmann B, Reid F, et al. Autoimmune hepatitis in childhood: a 20-year experience. Hepatology 1997;25:541–7.
46 Mieli-Vergani G, Heller S, Jara P, et al. Autoimmune hepatitis. J Pediatr Gastroenterol Nutr 2009;49:158–64.
47 Vajro P, Hadchouel P, hadchouel M, et al. Incidence of cirrhosis in children with chronic hepatitis. J Pediatr 1990; 117:392–6.
48 Esposito C, Garipoli V, Vecchione R, et al. Laparoscopy-guided biopsy in diagnosis of liver disorders in children. Liver 1997;17:288–92.
49 Roberts E. Autoimmune hepatitis from the pediatric perspective. Liver Int 2011;31:1424–31.
50 Bortolotti F, Guido M. Reversal of liver cirrhosis: a desirable clinical outcome and its pathogenic background. J Pediatr Gastroenterol Nutr 2007;44:401–6.
51 Cuarterolo M, Ciocca M, Lopez S, et al. Immunosuppresive therapy allows recovery from liver failure in children with autoimmune hepatitis. Clin Gastroenterol Hepatol 2011;9:145–9.
52 Cuarterolo M, Ciocca M, Cañero Velazco C, et al. Follow-up of children with autoimmune hepatitis treated with cyclosporine. J Pediatr Gatroenterol Nutr 2006;43:635–9.
53 Aw M, Dhawan A, Samyn M, et al. Mycophenolate mofetil as a rescue treatment for autoimmune liver disease in children: a 5-year follow-up. J Hepatol 2009;51:156–60.
54 Dumas L, Vergani, Mieli-Vergani G. Hepatitis B virus: something old, something new. J Pediatr Gastroenterol Nutr 2007;44:14–7.
55 Bortolotti F, Guido M, Bartolacci S, et al. Chronic hepatitis B in children after e antigen seroclearence: final report of a 29-year longitudinal study. Hepatology 2006;43:556–62.
56 Zacharakis G, Koskinas J, Kotsiou S, et al. Natural history of chronic hepatitis B virus infection in children of different ethnic origins: a cohort study with up to 12 years' follow-up in northern Greece. J Pediatr Gastroenterol Nutr 2007; 44:84–91.
57 Casiraghi M, De Paschale M, Romano L, et al. Long-term outcome (35 years) of hepatitis C after aquisition of infection through mini transfusions of blood given at birth. Hepatology 2004;39:90–6.
58 Guido M, Bortolotti F, Leandro G, et al. Fibrosis in chronic hepatitis C acquired in infancy: is it only a matter of time? Am J Gastroenterol 2003;98:660–3.
59 Greene C, McElvaney N. Z α-1 antitrypsin deficiency and the endoplasmic reticulum stress response. World J Gastrointest Pharmacol Ther 2010;1:94–101.
60 Sveger T, Eriksson S. The liver in adolescents with α-1 antitrypsin deficiency. Hepatology 1995;22:514–7.
61 Odievre M, Martin J, Hadchouel M, et al. Alpha$_1$-antitrypsin deficiency and liver disease in children: phenotypes, manifestations and prognosis. Pediatrics 1976;57:226–31.
62 Ibarguen E, Gross C, Kay Savik S, et al. liver disease in alpha-1-antitrypsin deficiency: prognostic indicators. J Pediatr 1990;117:864–70.
63 Ferenci P, Roberts E. Defining Wilson disease phenotypes: from the patient to the bench and back again. Gastroenterology 2012;142:692–6.
64 Roberts E, Schilsky M. A practical guideline on Wilson disease. Hepatology 2003;37:1475–92.
65 Nicastro E, Ranucci G, Vajro P, et al. Re-evaluation of the diagnostic criteria for Wilson disease in children with mild liver disease. Hepatology 2010;52:1948–56.
66 Mitchell G, Russo P, Dubois J, Alvarez F. Tyrosinemia. In Suchy F, Sokol R, Balistreri W (eds) Liver Disease in Children, 2nd edn. Lippincott Williams & Wilkins, Philadelphia: 2001. pp. 667–85.
67 Kvittingen E, Holme E. Disorders of tyrosine metabolism. In Fernandes J, Saudubray J, Van den Berghe G (eds.) Inborn Metabolic Diseases: Diagnosis and Treatment, 3rd edn. Springer Verlag, Berlin/Heidelberg/New York: 2000. pp. 187–94.

68 Yerushalmi B, Sokol R, Narkewicz M, et al. Niemann–Pick disease type C in neonatal cholestasis at a North American center. J Pediatr Gastroenterol Nutr 2002;35:44–50.
69 Imrie J, Dasgupta S, Besley G, et al. The natural history of Niemann–Pick disease type C in the UK. J Inherit Metab Dis 2007;30:51–9.
70 Haagsma E, Smit G, Niezen-Koning K, et al. Type IIIb glycogen storage disease associated with end-stage cirrhosis and hepatocellular carcinoma. Hepatology 1997;25:537–40.
71 Fernandes J, Smit G. The glycogen-storage diseases. In Fernandes J, Saudubray J, Van den Berghe G (eds.) Inborn Metabolic Diseases: Diagnosis and Treatment, 3rd edn. Springer Verlag, Berlin/Heidelberg/New York: 2000. pp. 87–101.
72 Willot S, Marchand V, Rasquin A, et al. Systemic progression of type IV glycogen storage disease after liver transplantation. J Pediatr Gastroenterol Nutr 2010;51:661–4.
73 Muhammed R, Bremner R, Protheroe S, et al. Resolution of parenteral nutrition-associated jaundice on changing from a soybean oil emulsion to a complex mixed-lipid emulsion. J Pediatr Gastroenterol Nutr 2012;54:797–802.
74 Fitzgibbons S, Jones B, Hull M, et al. Relationship between biopsy-proven parenteral nutrition-associated liver fibrosis and biochemical cholestasis in children with short bowel syndrome. J Pediatr Surg 2010;45:95–9.
75 Naini B, Lassman C. Total parenteral nutrition therapy, and liver injury: a histopathologic study with clinical correlation. Hum Pathol 2012;43:826–33.

Index

Page numbers in *italics* refer to illustrations; those in **bold** refer to tables

Cirrhosis: A practical guide to management, First Edition. Edited by Samuel S. Lee and Richard Moreau.

I

J

K

L

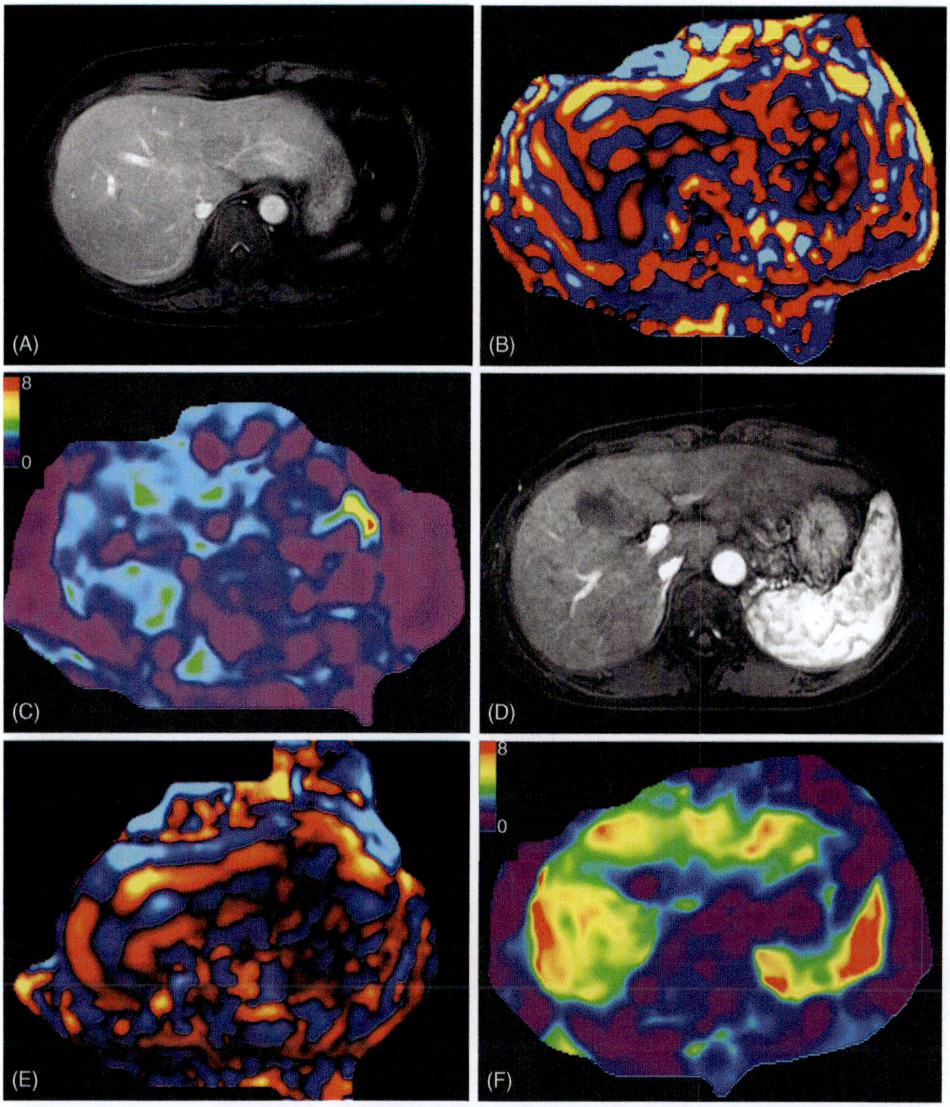

Figure 3.5 MR elastography of the normal liver (A–C) and cirrhotic liver (D–F). In the normal liver (B), shear wave passing through the liver propagates slowly compared with the cirrhotic liver (E). The elastograms show a higher mean stiffness of the cirrhotic liver (4.9 kPa; F) compared with the normal liver (1.7 kPa; C). (Courtesy of Dr. Jeong Min Lee, Department of Radiology, Seoul National University Hospital, Korea.)

Cirrhosis: A practical guide to management, First Edition. Edited by Samuel S. Lee and Richard Moreau.

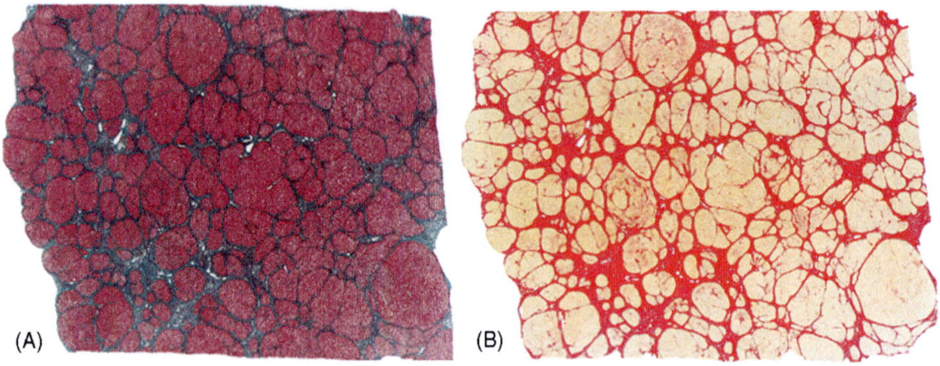

Figure 4.1 Cirrhosis at low power view. Specific stainings of fibrosis showing parenchymal nodules delineated by annular fibrous septa: (A) trichrome staining; (B) picrosirius staining.

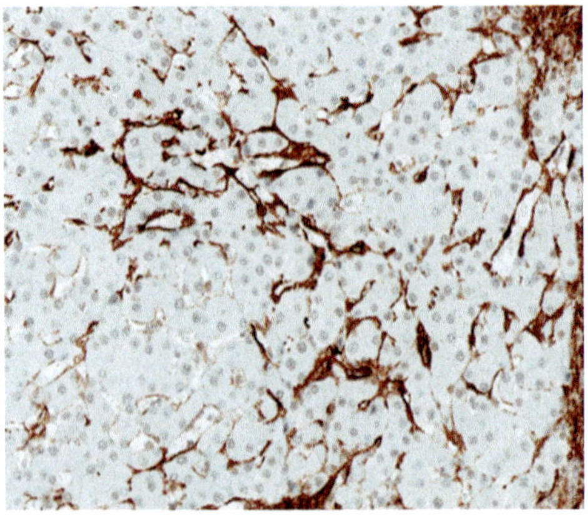

Figure 4.2 Hepatic stellate cells in cirrhosis. α-Smooth muscle actin immunostaining showing hepatic stellate cells in parenchymal nodules, located in peri-sinusoidal space (Disse space).

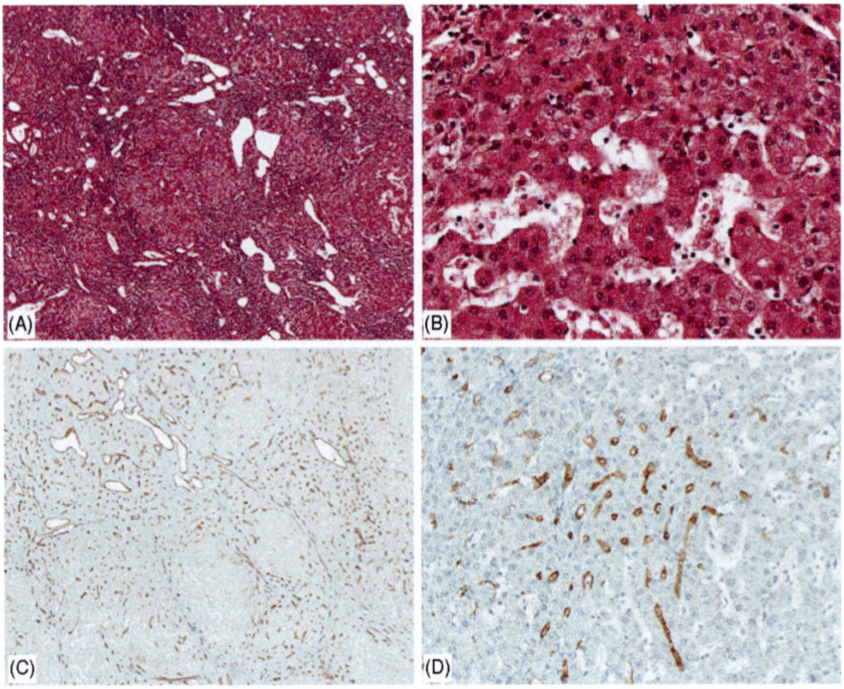

Figure 4.3 Vascular changes in cirrhosis. (A) Low magnification showing cirrhosis with vessels multiplication in fibrous septa (hematein and eosin). (B) Higher magification of cirrhotic nodule with sinusoidal dilatation. (C) CD31 immunostaining dysplaying increased vascular density. (D) Sinusoidal capillarization demonstrated by CD34 lining of endothelial cells in cirrhotic nodule.

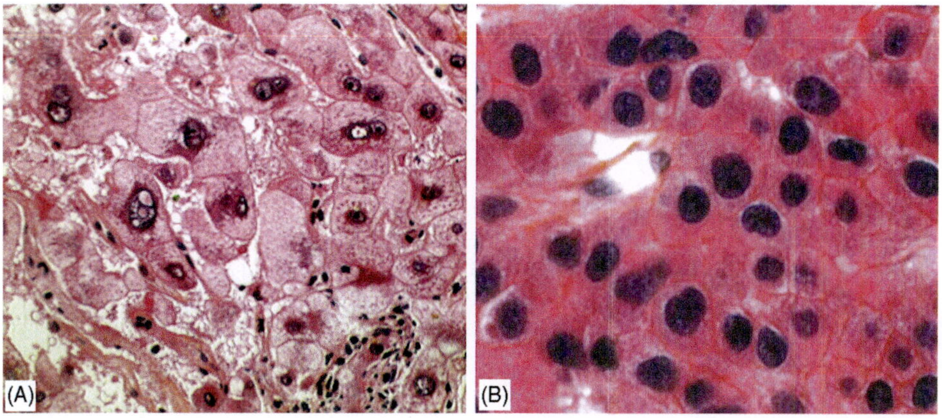

Figure 4.4 Dysplastic changes in cirrhosis. (A) Large cell change represented by large cells containing atypical nuclei of increased size. (B) Small cell change defined by foci of small hepatocytes with increased nuclear: cytoplasmic ratio (hematein and eosin).

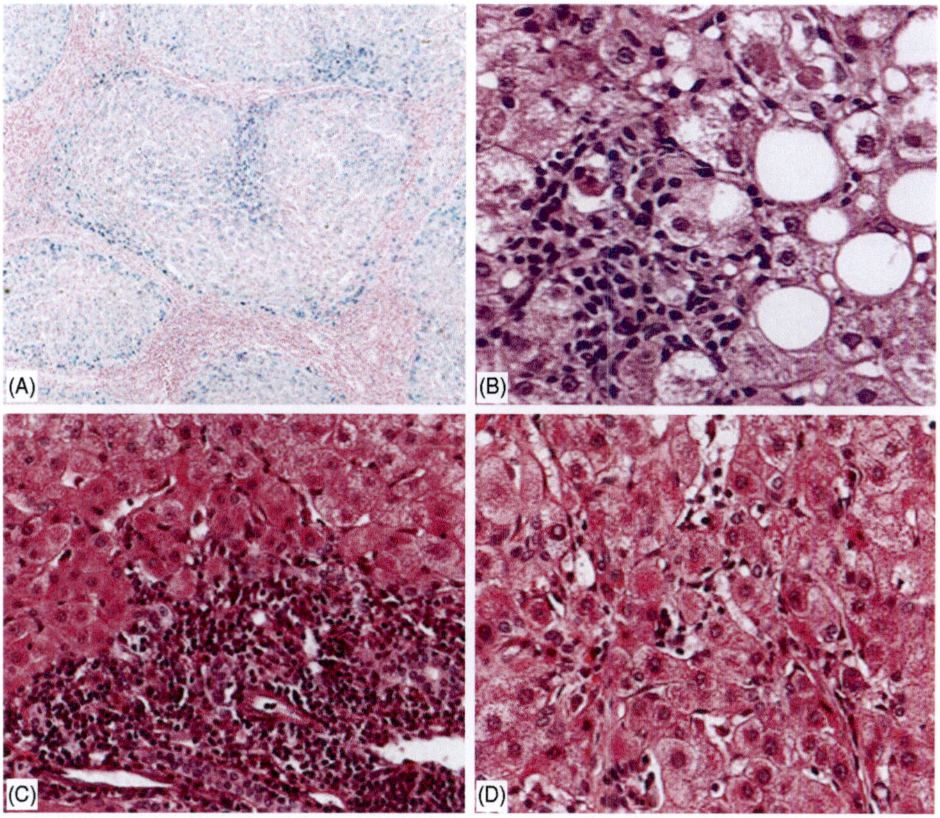

Figure 4.5 Parenchymal nodules: elementary features. (A) Iron overload in parenchymal nodules involving mainly hepatocytes with a gradient pattern (Perls' staining). (B) Steatohepatitis with ballooned hepatocytes containing Mallory–Denk bodies with inflamatory cells around (mostly lymphocytes in metabolic syndrome and neutrophil polymorphs in alcoholic diseases) (hematein and eosin). (C) Piecemeal necrosis: portal inflammation with inflammatory cells disrupting limiting plate (hematein and eosin). (D) Lobular inflammation composed of small foci of lymphocytes between hepatic cell plates (hematein and eosin).

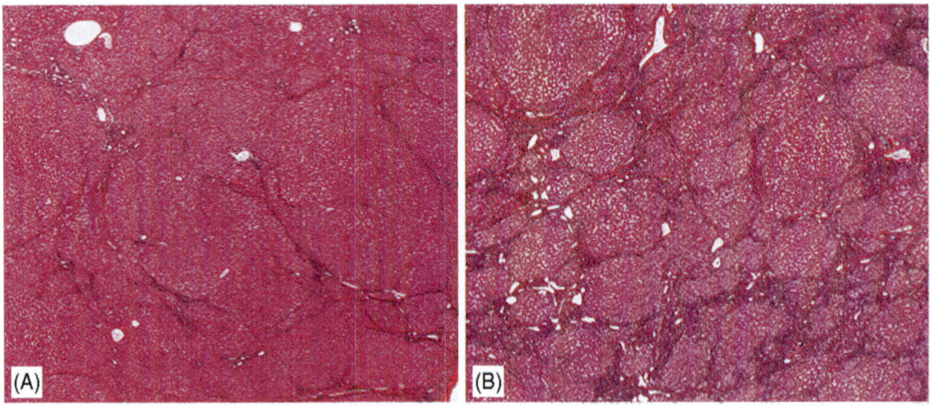

Figure 4.6 Laënnec staging. Substaging of cirrhosis is based on thickness of the fibrous septa and size of the parenchymal nodules. (A) Thin septa surrounding large sized nodules. (B) Thicker fibrous septa surrounding smaller nodules (hematein and eosin).

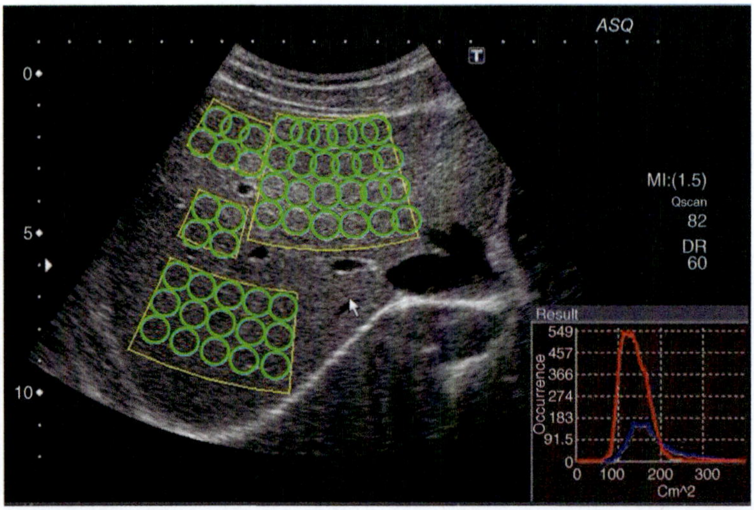

Figure 5.1 Measurement of liver stiffness using acoustic radiation force impulse. The region of interest is established by abdominal ultrasound and the stiffness of this site can be measured.

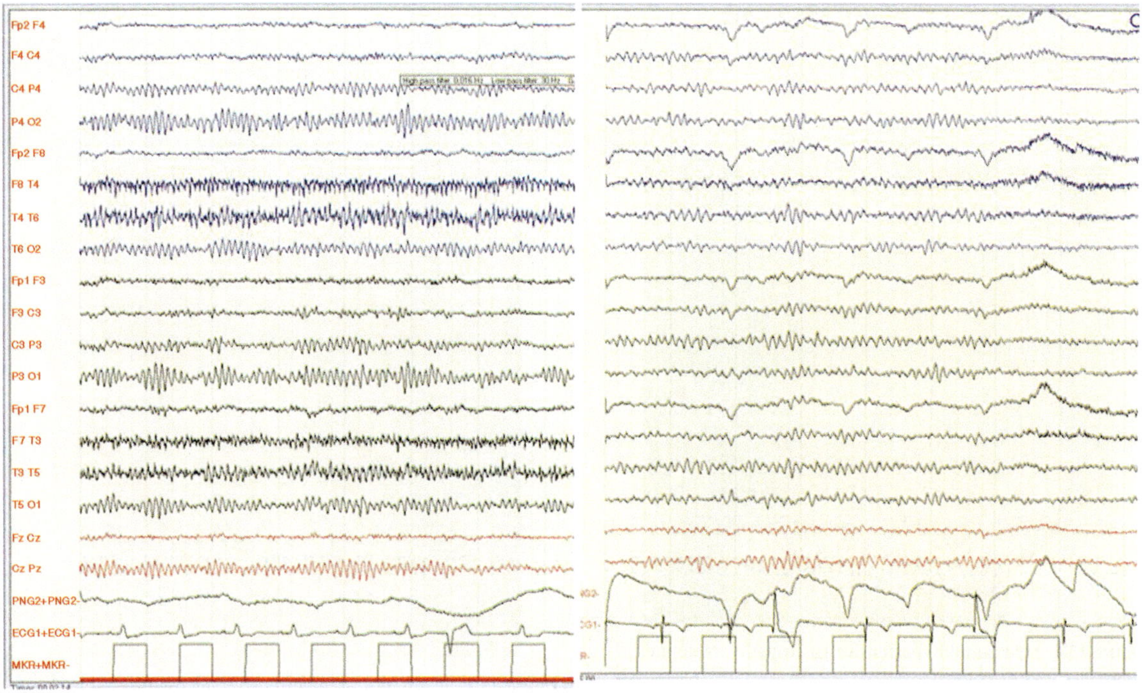

Figure 11.3 Eye closed EEG. On the left a normal tracing, on the right a tracing slowed down with interspersed theta activity (i.e., frequency <8 Hz) >35% in parietal derivation, suggesting MHE.

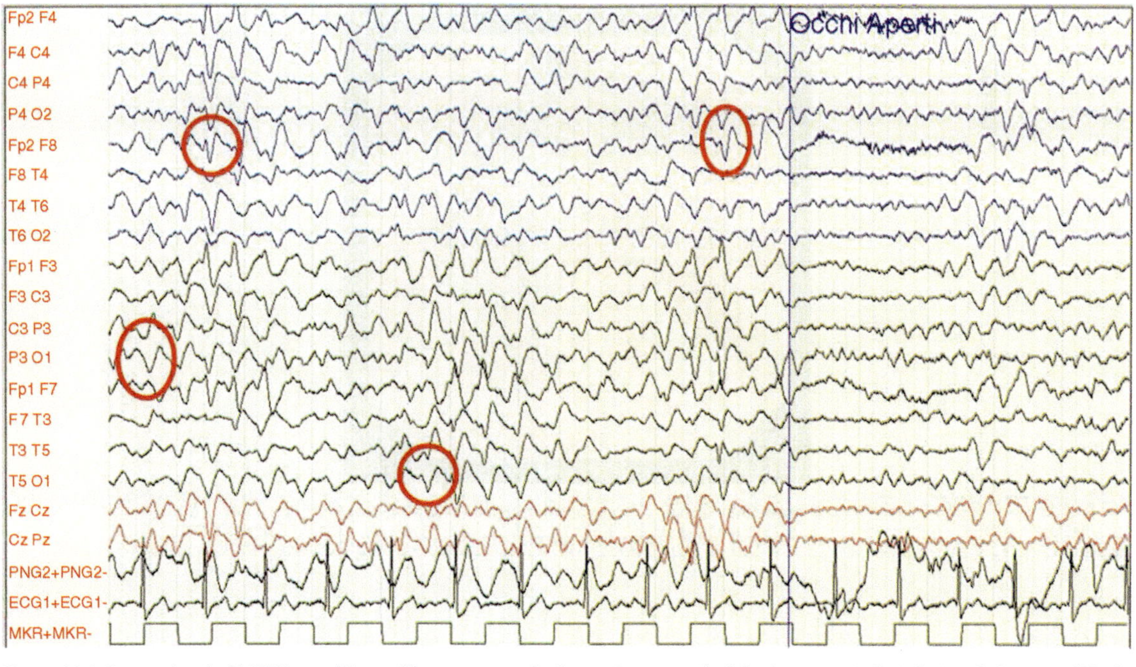

Figure 11.4 Severe (grade 3) HE in a subject with portosystemic shunt. Presence of triphasic waves (red circles) and absence of block reaction on eye opening (on the right of the vertical blue line).

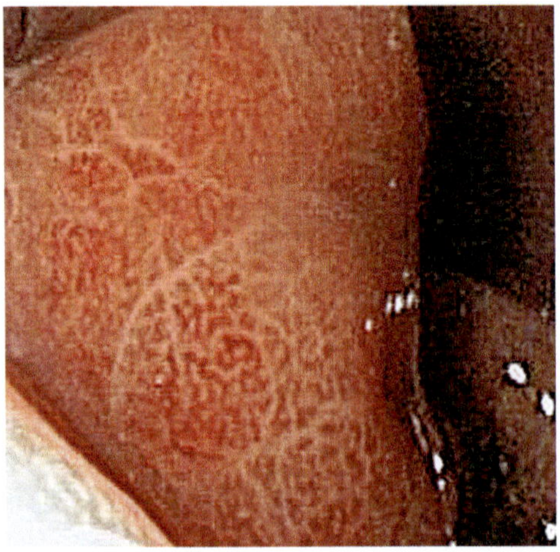

Figure 13.6 Mild portal hypertensive gastropathy. Note the snakeskin mosaic pattern.

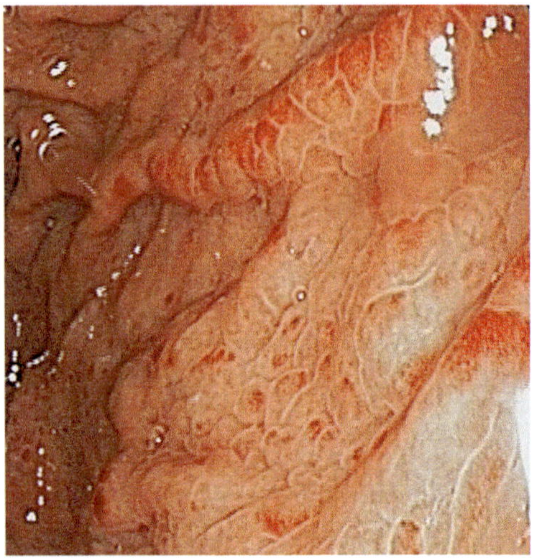

Figure 13.7 Severe portal hypertensive gastropathy. Note the snakeskin mosaic pattern with red markings.

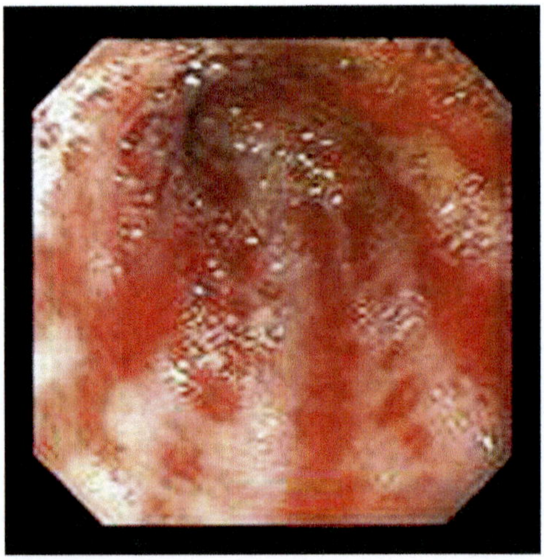

Figure 13.8 Gastric antral vascular ectasia (GAVE). Note the typical watermelon-like pattern.

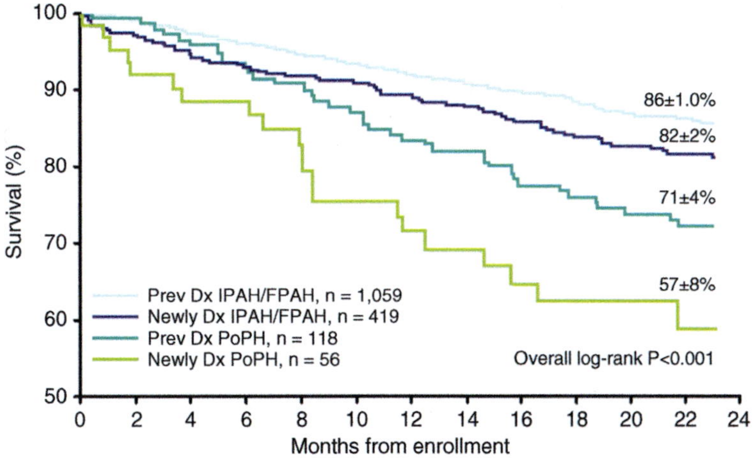

Figure 19.3 Two-year survival patterns for portopulmonary hypertension (PPH) and idiopathic pulmonary artery hypertension (IPAH) categorized by previous versus newly diagnosed at the time of entry into the registry. FPAH, familial pulmonary arterial hypertension. (Krowka et al., 2012 [22]. Reproduced with permission of Chest.)

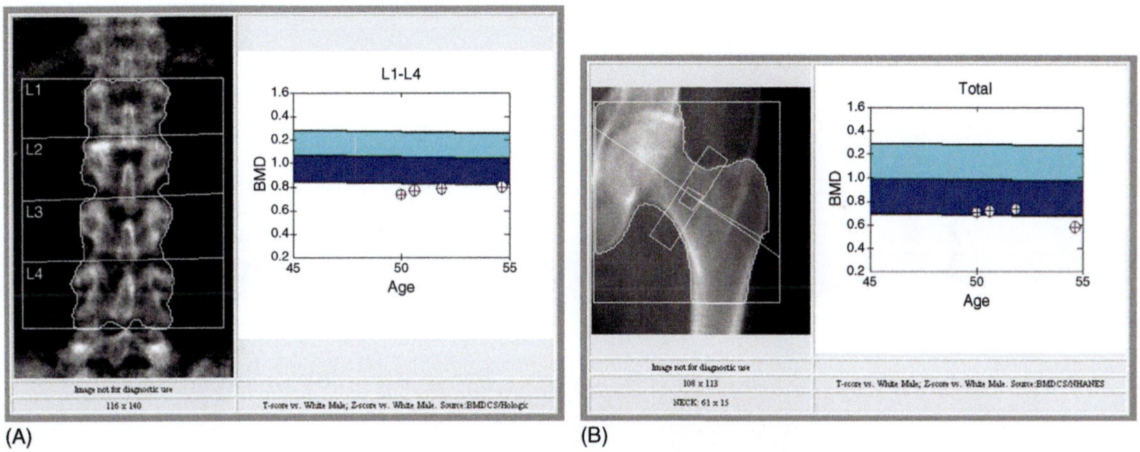

Figure 25.2 Bone mineral density in a patient with cirrhosis: (A) lumbar spine; (B) femoral neck. This 57-year-old man with a biliary cirrhosis due to combined variable immunodeficiency has a T score of –2.7 at vertebral spine and –3.0 at the femoral neck. His other risk factors for fracture include malabsorbtion due to chronic cryptosporidia and a budesonide-treated enteropathy. He has a low vitamin D level of 42 nmol/L. According to the FRAX index his fracture risk is 15% at 10 years and that of a femoral neck fracture 8.4%. The FRAX index underestimates the risk on steroids and its reliability in the presence of cirrhosis is unknown. He was treated with a single dose of zoledronic acid intravenously because of malabsorption – ibandronic acid would have been an alternative – and his vitamin D levels corrected.

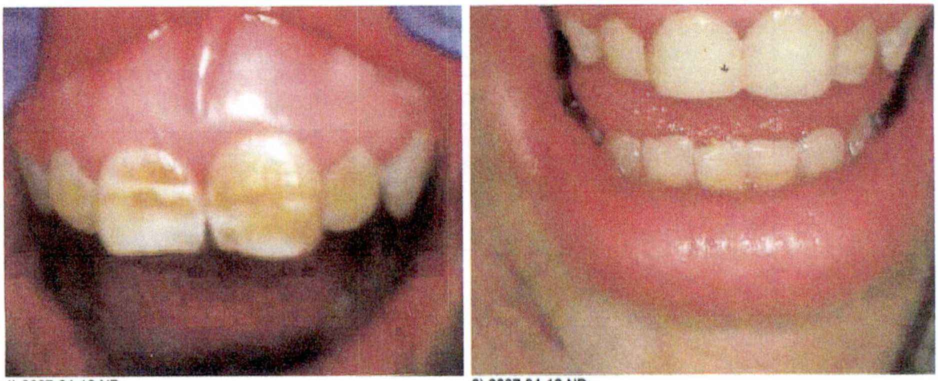

1) 2007-04-12 ND:.
.Non spécifiée

2) 2007-04-12 ND:.
.Non spécifiée

Figure 28.1 Green teeth in a 12-year-old (left), and a 14-year-old (right) child with biliary atresia transplanted at the age of 6 and 8 years, respectively, because of liver failure. Permanent teeth were stained by deposition of bilirubin in dental hard tissues during their maturation.

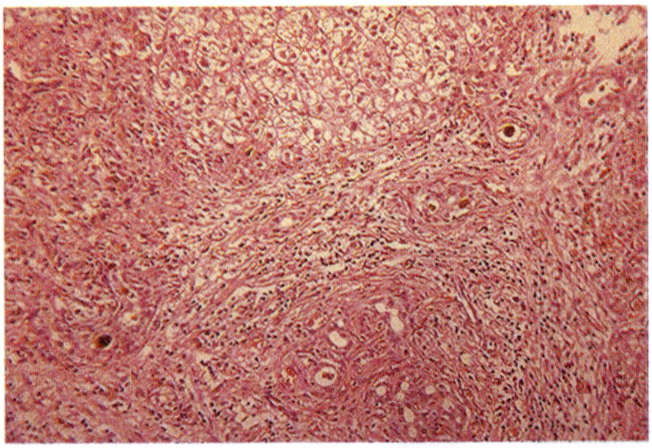

Figure 28.2 Liver biopsy (H&E staining) from a 2-month-old patient with biliary atresia, showing a rapid evolution to cirrhosis. Practically all patients with biliary atresia develop cirrhosis during the first year of life.

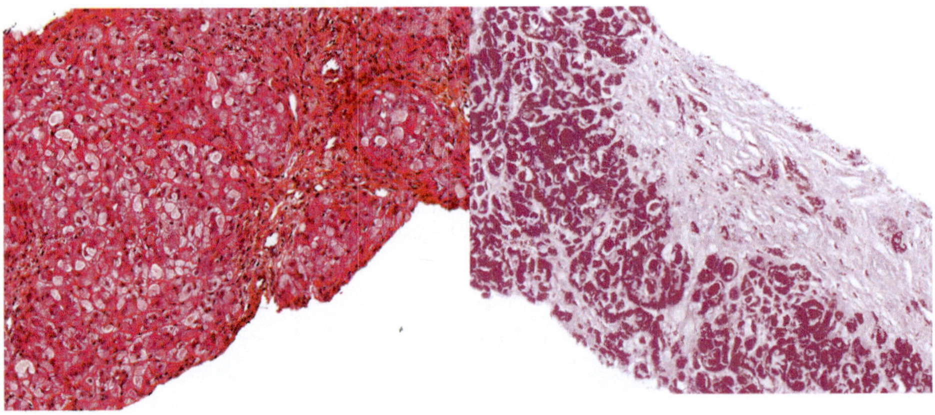

Figure 28.4 Early cirrhosis in a 6-month-old boy with glycogenosis type IV (H&E and PAS staining).

Printed and bound by CPI Group (UK) Ltd, Croydon, CR0 4YY

16/09/2026

14963474-0006